D1596469

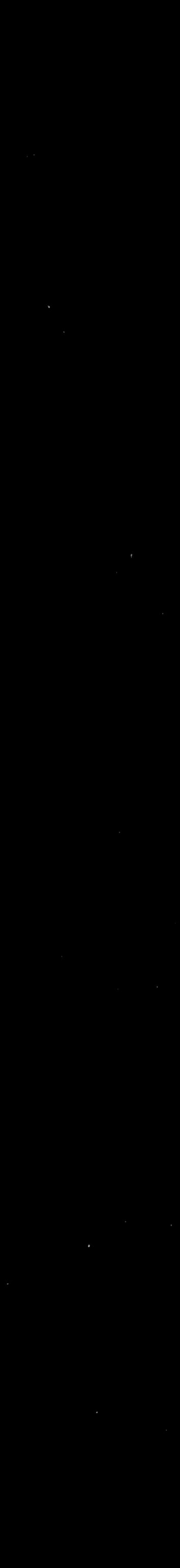

SONOGRAPHY OF THE ABDOMEN

SONOGRAPHY OF THE ABDOMEN

R. Brooke Jeffrey, Jr., M.D.

Professor of Radiology
Chief of Abdominal Imaging
Department of Diagnostic Radiology
Stanford University School of Medicine
Stanford, California

Philip W. Ralls, M.D.

Professor of Radiology
Chief of Body Imaging and Interventional Radiology
Department of Radiology
University of Southern California
School of Medicine
Los Angeles, California

Raven Press New York

Raven Press, Ltd., 1185 Avenue of the Americas, New York, New York 10036

Printed and bound in Hong Kong

Library of Congress Cataloging-in-Publication Data

Sonography of the Abdomen / editors, R. Brooke Jeffrey, Philip W. Ralls.
p. cm.
Includes bibliographical references and index.
ISBN 0-7817-0130-9
1. Abdomen—Ultrasonic imaging. I. Jeffrey, R. Brooke. II. Ralls, Philip W. (Philip Whitney), 1948-
[DNLM: 1. Abdomen—ultrasonography—atlases. WI 17 S699 1994]
RC944.S66 1994
617.5'507'542—dc20
DNLM/DLC
For Library of Congress 94-36007
CIP

The material contained in this volume was submitted as previously unpublished material, except in the instances in which credit has been given to the source from which some illustrative material was derived.

Great care has been taken to maintain the accuracy of the information contained in the volume. However, neither Raven Press nor the editors can be held responsible for errors or for any consequences arising from the use of the information contained herein.

9 8 7 6 5 4 3 2 1

To Jane, Stefanie, Catherine, and Luke Jeffrey

R.B.J.

With love to my wife Renée, whose support and patience should *be legendary, and also to my parents, Robert and Pat Ralls*

P.W.R.

Contents

Preface

This book is intended for practicing physicians, residents, and sonographers interested in abdominal sonography. The reader will note our emphasis on high-quality images and atlas format. Rather than describe and review all pathologic conditions, we have illustrated findings in those conditions encountered in the usual practice of abdominal imaging. Color flow sonography is heavily emphasized, reflecting its increasing importance as a means to enhance routine abdominal sonography. An effort has been made to correlate sonograms with other imaging modalities, especially CT and MRI, when germane.

The text is concise. It presents current clinical and imaging information. It is also a practical, realistic guide for the use of abdominal sonography. The strengths and weaknesses of sonography, along with practical suggestions, are presented in a pragmatic, straightforward way. The information and suggestions reflect the current literature and our experience using sonography in evaluating abdominal conditions. It is our view of how sonography fits in to the diagnostic and therapeutic armamentarium of medical imagers.

We hope the reader will find the images useful and beautiful, the text practical and informative. Our goal is to provide useful information to those learning abdominal sonography as well as to experienced practitioners interested in a pragmatic, practical approach to problems in imaging the abdomen.

SONOGRAPHY OF THE ABDOMEN

CHAPTER 1

Peritoneal Cavity and Gastrointestinal Tract

PERITONEAL CAVITY

Technique

The selection of ultrasound transducers and scanning techniques for evaluating peritoneal abnormalities depends on specific clinical objectives. A general abdominal survey to detect intraperitoneal fluid is best performed with a curved linear 3.5- or 5-MHz transducer. Where access is difficult, a 3.5- or 5-MHz sector transducer is often very useful. A 5-MHz linear array transducer is best for evaluation of superficial peritoneal implants and omental abnormalities. Graded compression technique with a 5-MHz linear array transducer is valuable for imaging mesenteric masses and abnormal bowel. Color Doppler sonography can clearly demonstrate important vascular landmarks such as the mesenteric artery and vein, as well as areas of increased vascularity within the bowel wall.

INTRAPERITONEAL FLUID COLLECTIONS

Many of the complex anatomic relationships of the peritoneal cavity are poorly demonstrated by sonography and are best evaluated by computed tomography (CT) (1). The main advantage of CT is its ability to directly visualize fascial planes and fat-containing structures such as the mesentery and omentum. Nevertheless, sonography excels in demonstrating intraperitoneal fluid and is often the initial imaging method of choice for detecting ascites and intraperitoneal abscesses. Sonography can detect even minute amounts of intraperitoneal fluid often in the cul-de-sac or retrovesical fossa of the pelvis. In the upper abdomen, small fluid collections are first noted in the hepatorenal fossa or paracolic gutters, especially near the caudal tip of the right lobe of the liver. Following ovulation, a small amount of fluid may normally be seen in the cul-de-sac on endovaginal scanning.

With increasing ascites, fluid is noted in the subhepatic, subphrenic, and interloop compartments. Massive ascites often results in medial displacement of bowel loops. The location and distribution of intraperitoneal fluid are influenced by patient position, the viscosity of the fluid, and the presence of peritoneal adhesions. When ascites is found unexpectedly, the abdomen must be surveyed carefully to detect evidence of underlying malignancy, lymphadenopathy, hepatic or portal vein thrombosis, cirrhosis, or portal hypertension.

Serous fluid is generally anechoic. Peritoneal fluid containing septations, low-level echoes, or debris suggests infection, hemorrhage, or carcinomatosis (Fig. 1.1). On occasion, long-standing bland ascites may contain internal septations and be loculated. Uninfected ascites usually has no mass effect and passively conforms to intraperitoneal compartments. Abscesses usually have significant mass effect and displace adjacent bowel and often indent adjacent solid organs. It may not be possible to differentiate loculated ascites from an abscess by sonographic criteria alone; diagnostic needle aspiration is often required for definitive diagnosis.

Intraperitoneal Hemorrhage

CT is the imaging method of choice to diagnose hemorrhage within the peritoneal cavity (2). Acute intraperitoneal hemorrhage is most often due to blunt trauma, ruptured ectopic pregnancy, recent surgery, or interventional procedures, such as liver biopsy (3). An important, although uncommon, cause of hemoperitoneum is spontaneous rupture of abdominal neoplasms, most often hepatic adenomas, hepatocellular carcinomas, or giant cavernous hemangiomas (4).

The sonographic appearance of intraperitoneal hemorrhage is nonspecific and varies according to its chronicity. Subacute lysed blood within the peritoneal cavity may be totally anechoic or demonstrate diffuse low-level echoes (Fig. 1.1). Acute clot formation may, however, be strikingly echogenic (5) (Fig. 1.2). A layered or lamellated appearance of clot may occur in patients with intermittent hemorrhage, which may occur with splenic

(text continues on page 3)

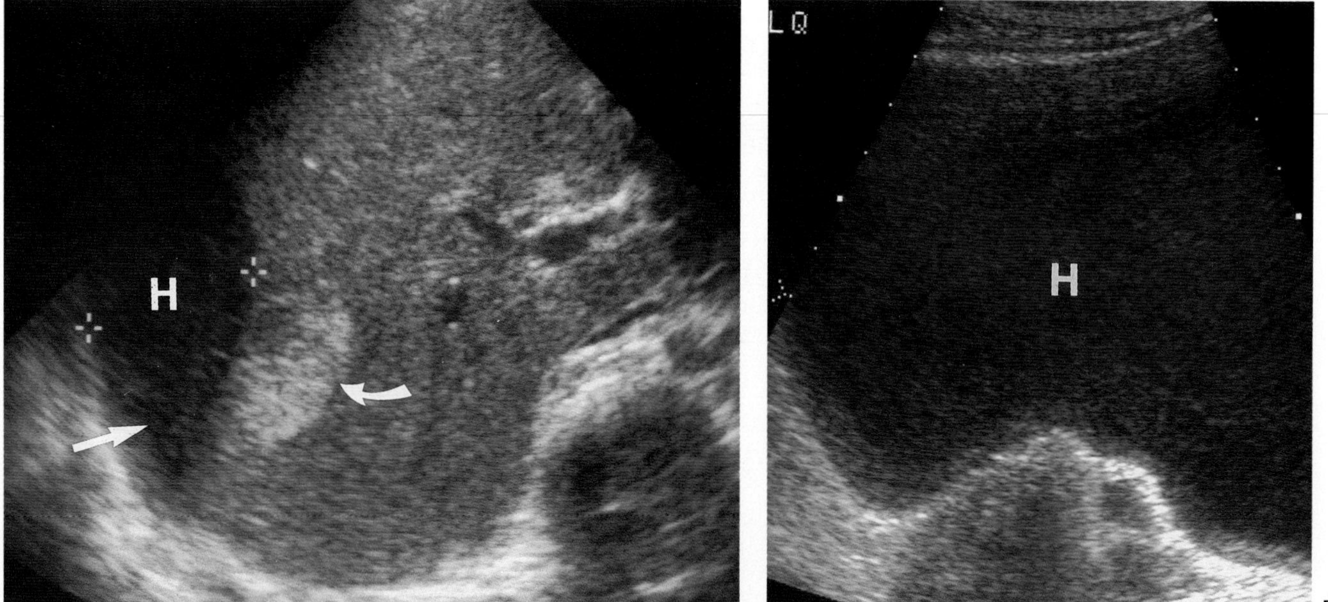

FIG. 1.1. Acute hemoperitoneum in two patients. **A:** Transverse scan of the right lobe of the liver demonstrating echogenic hepatic hematoma (*curved arrow*) and adjacent hemoperitoneum (H) due to inadvertent injury to the liver during thoracentesis. Note low-level echoes within the free lysed hemoperitoneum (*arrow*). **B:** Transverse scan of right lower quadrant in another patient demonstrating massive hemoperitoneum (H) containing diffuse low-level echoes. Patient had extensive bleeding from laparoscopic liver biopsy one day prior to sonography.

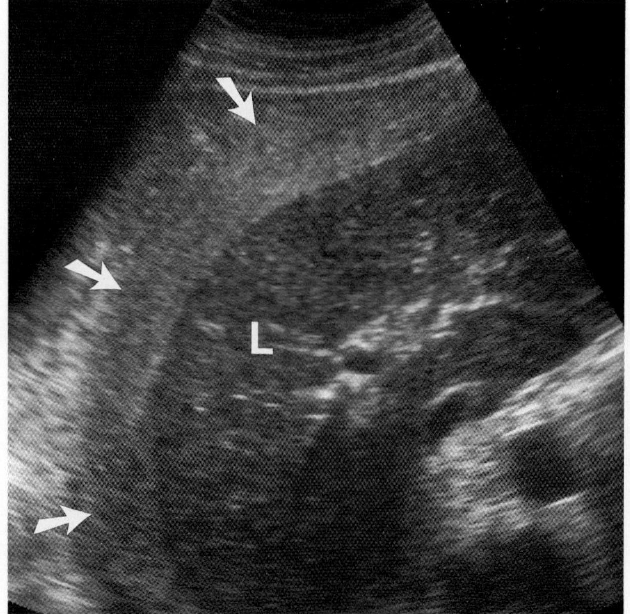

FIG. 1.2. Echogenic appearance of clotted hemoperitoneum. Clotted blood (*arrows*) adjacent to the liver (L) is strikingly echogenic. Patient had massive postoperative hemorrhage following aneurysm repair. Surgery revealed extensive perihepatic clot.

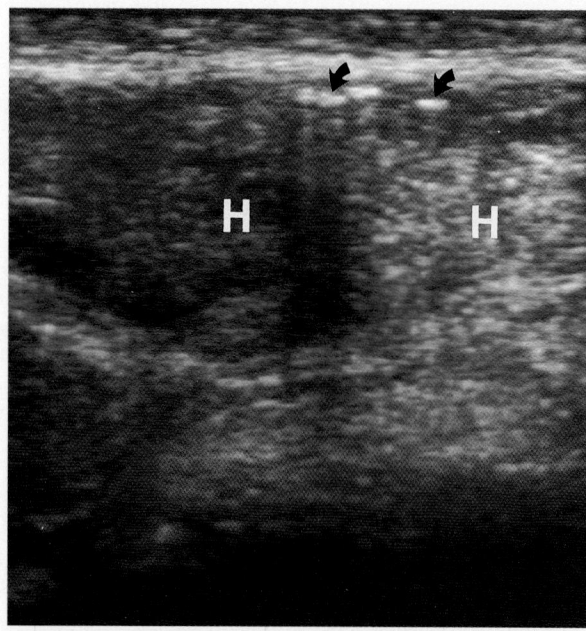

FIG. 1.3. Clotted hemoperitoneum simulating a mass. Sagittal scan of right lower quadrant in a patient operated on for ruptured spleen demonstrates large echogenic hematoma (H) and pneumoperitoneum (*arrows*) from prior laparotomy.

trauma. An acute echogenic hematoma may cause mass effect and could potentially be misconstrued as a neoplasm (Fig. 1.3). It is important to note that hematomas have no internal vascularity with color Doppler sonography. Due to the nonspecific sonographic appearance, a noncontrast CT scan is often useful to confirm the diagnosis of hemoperitoneum. In general, acute hemoperitoneum has attenuation values greater than 30 HU for free lysed blood (2). Attenuation values for clotted blood range from 45 to 60 HU (2).

Intraperitoneal Abscesses

CT and sonography are the primary imaging modalities for the diagnosis of abdominal abscesses (6–12). The predominant finding is a localized fluid collection with mass effect. Gas bubbles may or may not be present (Figs. 1.4 to 1.7). Both CT and sonography are invaluable for guiding percutaneous catheter drainage of liquefied abscesses when technically feasible and clinically appropriate. Whether CT or sonography is the initial imaging method of choice for suspected abdominal abscesses is largely determined by institutional preference, the likely location of the abscess, and the clinical status of the patient. Sonography is quite accurate for diagnosing hepatic, pericholecystic, and pelvic abscesses. However, CT is superior to sonography in demonstrating pancreatic, retroperitoneal, paraspinous, interloop, or gas-forming abscesses (12). Because open wounds and surgical drains often preclude adequate sonographic access, CT is often preferred in imaging postoperative or critically ill patients.

Compared to sonography, CT has three main advantages in evaluating patients with abdominal abscesses (12). These include (a) ability to administer intravenous contrast to distinguish a liquefied abscess from a phlegmon; (b) clear definition of thickened fascial planes, edematous fat, and small gas bubbles; and (c) superior visualization of interloop and extraperitoneal abscesses. Most liquefied abdominal abscesses have CT attenuation values ranging from 10 to 25 HU. Phlegmons, on the other hand, are not liquefied and represent indurated areas of soft tissue inflammation. Attenuation values for phlegmons range from 20 to 50 HU. The distinction between a phlegmon and a liquefied abscess is often crucial in the decision to perform percutaneous drainage (13,14). Phlegmons cannot successfully be drained percutaneously and are best treated with intravenous antibiotics.

The sonographic appearance of abdominal abscesses is variable and depends on the presence or absence of gas, septations, or solid debris. Due to attenuation of sound by proteinaceous debris, many intra-abdominal abscesses exhibit little distal enhanced through sound transmission (10). It is not uncommon for a liquefied abscess to sonographically mimic a solid hypoechoic mass (Figs. 1.5 and 1.6) (15). This potential pitfall must be kept in mind whenever an abscess is clinically suspected. Color Doppler sonography may be helpful in differentiating these two entities since liquefied abscesses lack internal vascularity.

Although most patients with abdominal abscesses demonstrate systemic signs of fever and leukocytosis, these findings are not invariably present (16,17). Fever and leukocytosis may not be present in patients with acquired immunodeficiency syndrome (AIDS) or other causes of systemic immunosuppression (16). Similarly, patients receiving steroids, antibiotics, or antipyretics may have a deceptively benign clinical presentation (17). Localized abdominal pain may be the only clinical sign of an abdominal abscess. Liberal use of diagnostic needle aspiration is advisable for all localized complex fluid collections to avoid misdiagnosis.

Gas bubbles are present in only one-third of abdominal abscesses (12). Tiny gas bubbles may be difficult to detect sonographically and are best demonstrated by CT. Abscesses containing extensive microbubbles may be quite echogenic (9). However, abscesses may be echogenic without microbubbles (Fig. 1.4B). Sonographically, gas bubbles are typically linear high-amplitude echoes with "comet tail" reverberation artifacts. There may or may not be distal acoustic shadowing (Fig. 1.3). Gas bubbles may be trapped by septations within the abscess.

Enteric abscesses secondary to gastrointestinal perforation (i.e., appendicitis, diverticulitis) have a number of relatively characteristic sonographic features. Using graded compression sonography, it is possible to make a specific diagnosis of an appendiceal abscess if a hypoechoic mass is identified adjacent to a site of necrosis of the appendiceal wall (Fig. 1.8) (15). Necrosis may be diagnosed when there is loss of visualization of the echogenic submucosal layer of the bowel wall (15). In patients with diverticulitis, gas within an infected diverticulum may appear sonographically as an intramural echogenic focus with acoustic shadowing within a thickened area of the colonic wall (18). Localized enteric abscesses are typically "walled off" by an echogenic rim of tissue representing inflamed mesenteric or omental fat.

Enteric abscesses from Crohn's disease are complex fluid collections or hypoechoic masses adjacent to a focally thickened segment of bowel (Fig. 1.5). Echogenic areas within the mesentery may be demonstrated in patients with Crohn's disease representing fibrofatty masses (i.e., "creeping fat"). On occasion, gas-containing sinus tracts may be detected sonographically as linear echogenic areas within the bowel wall and mesentery (19). In most patients with Crohn's disease, however, CT is the examination of choice if an enteric abscess is clinically suspected.

(*text continues on page 7*)

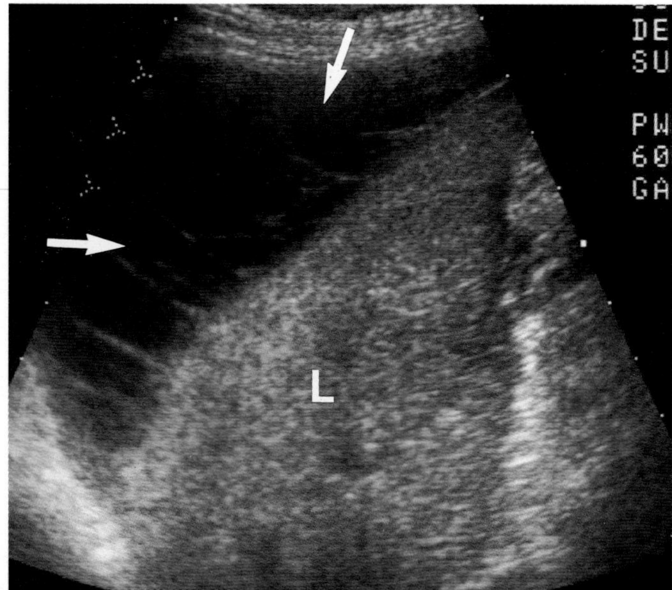

A

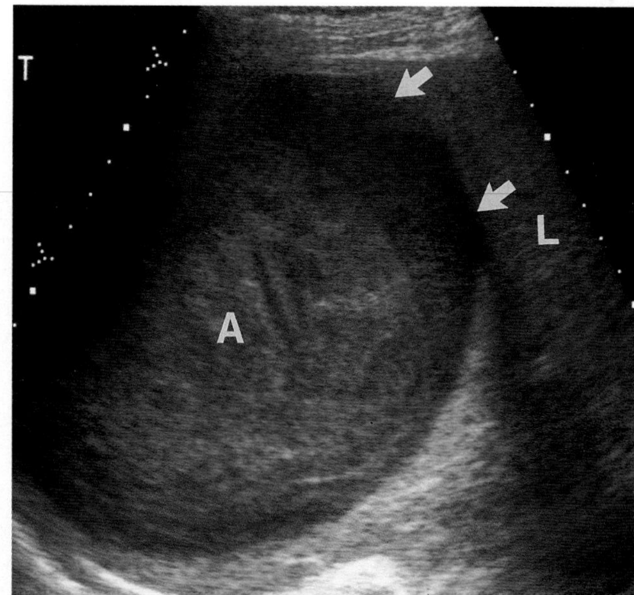

FIG. 1.4. Subphrenic abscesses following biliary surgery in two patients. Sagittal scan (**A**) demonstrates abscess (*arrows*) with numerous internal septations compressing dome of the liver (L). In another patient (**B**) transverse scan of the liver demonstrates significant mass effect (*arrows*) on liver (L) from subphrenic abscess (A). Note echogenic pus within the abscess.

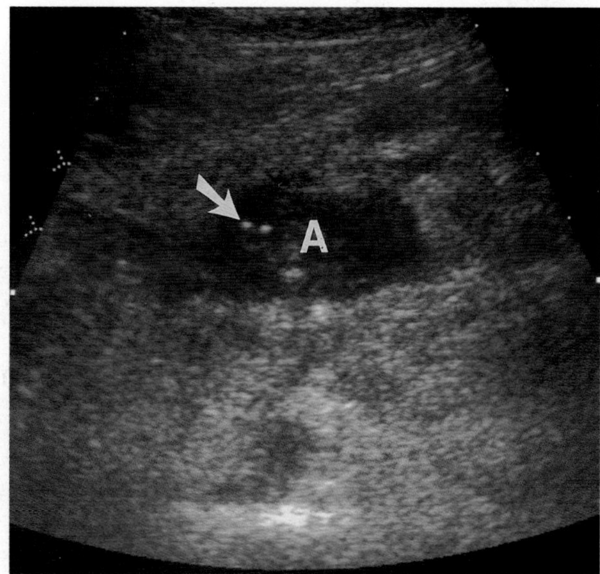

A

FIG. 1.5. Solid appearing enteric abscess. **A:** Transverse sonogram of the right lower quadrant in a patient with Crohn's disease. Note hypoechoic, rounded abscess (A) with tiny echogenic areas (*arrow*) representing gas bubbles. Abscess mimics solid lesion as there is a lack of significant distal enhanced sound transmission. **B:** Corresponding contrast CT scan demonstrating low-density abscess (A) with gas bubble (*arrow*).

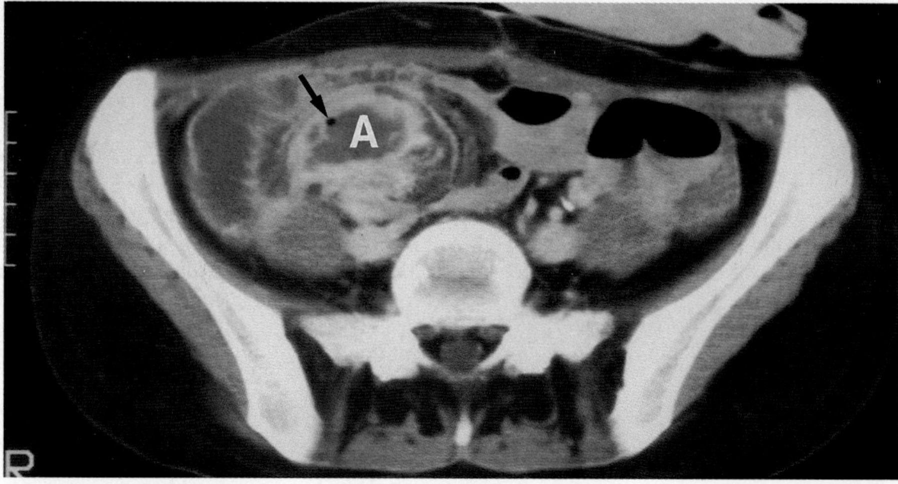

B

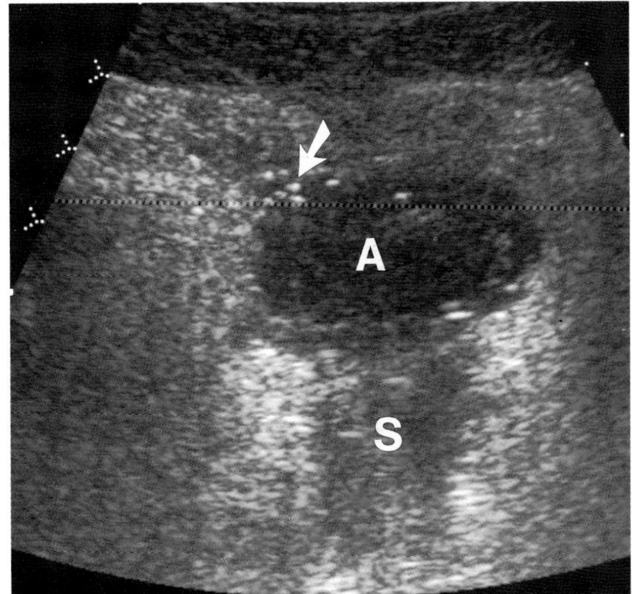

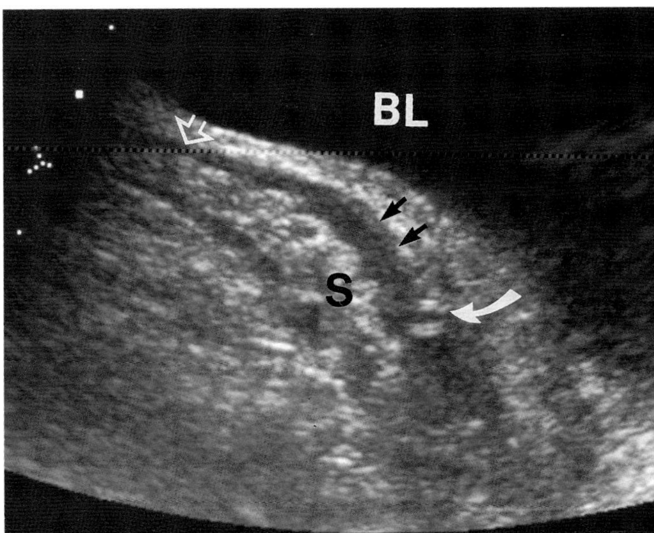

FIG. 1.6. Solid appearing diverticular abscess. **A:** Transverse sonogram of left lower quadrant demonstrating typical hypoechoic diverticular abscess (A) adjacent to sigmoid (S). Note gas bubbles (*arrow*) and lack of significant enhanced sound transmission from abscess. **B:** Sagittal sonogram following percutaneous drainage of abscess (*curved arrow*). Note residual mural thickening (*black arrows*) of sigmoid (S) adjacent to abscess catheter. Bowel wall more distally has normal mural thickness (*open arrow*). BL, bladder.

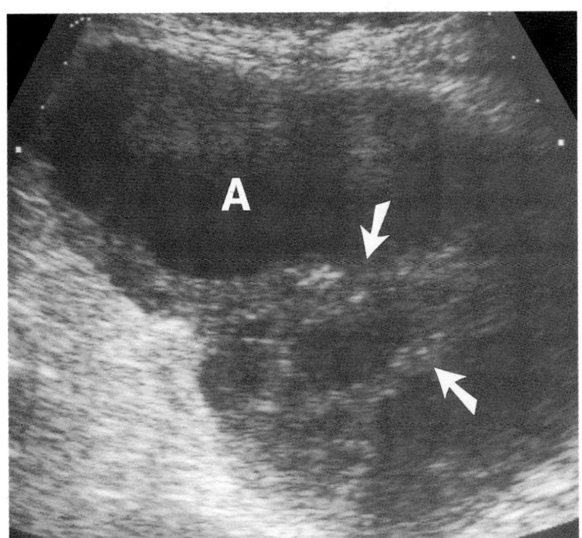

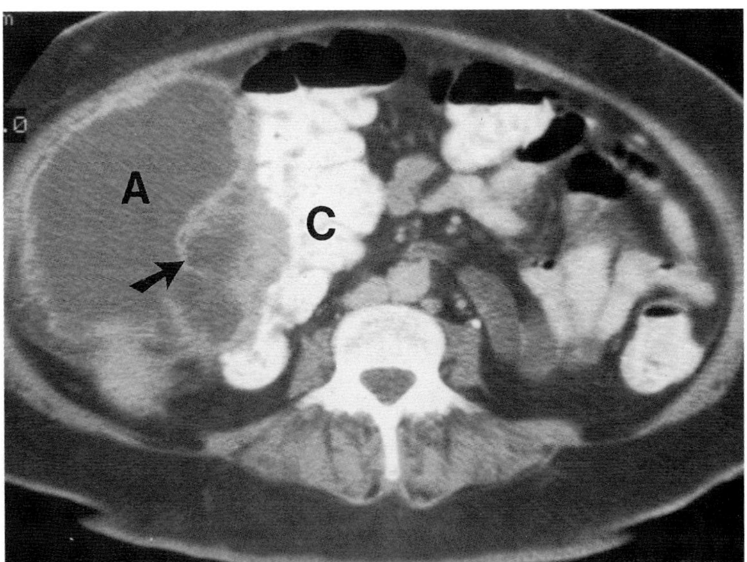

FIG. 1.7. Mass effect from intraperitoneal abscess. **A:** Transverse scan of right lower quadrant abscess (A) with thick septations (*arrows*). **B:** Corresponding CT scan demonstrates significant mass effect on right colon (C) from the abscess (A). Note septations within abscess on CT scan (*arrow*).

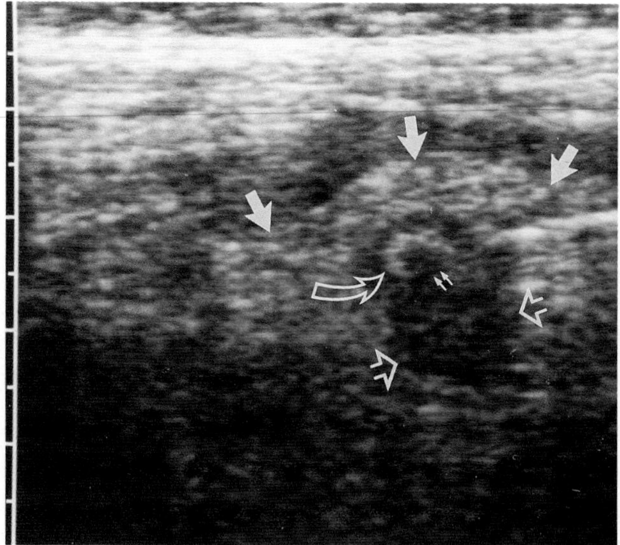

FIG. 1.8. Periappendiceal abscess with little enhanced sound transmission. Note hypoechoic abscess (*open arrows*) adjacent to appendix (*curved arrow*). Site of mural necrosis of appendix is indicated (*small arrows*) by interruption of normal submucosal layer. Note prominent periappendiceal fat (*large arrows*) (from surrounding inflammation) and relative lack of enhanced through sound transmission from the abscess.

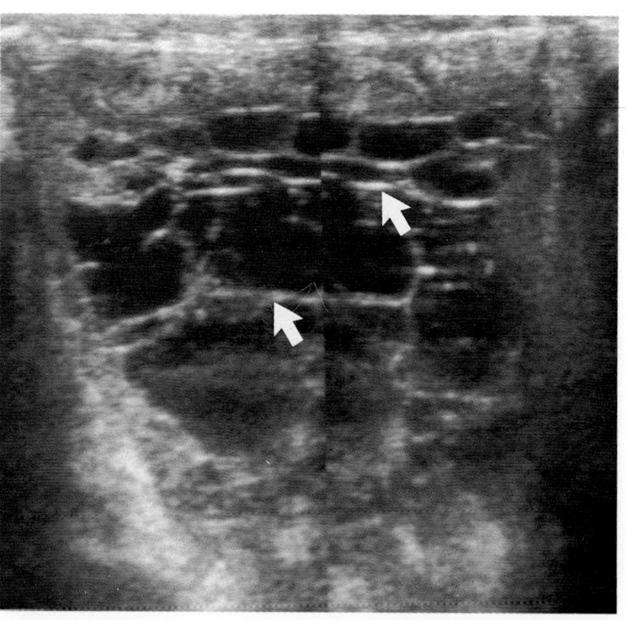

FIG. 1.9. Cytomegalovirus (CMV) peritonitis in a patient with AIDS. Transverse scan of right paracolic gutter demonstrates complex fluid collection with multiple septations (*arrows*).

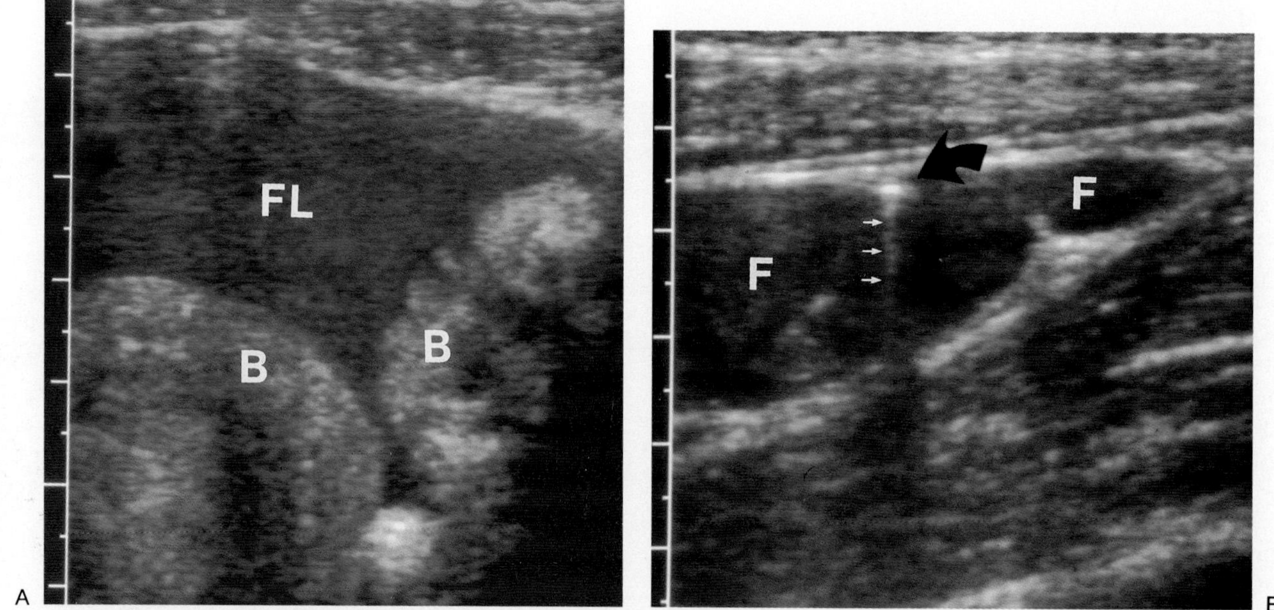

FIG. 1.10. Bacterial peritonitis in two patients. **A:** Note complex fluid (FL) with low-level echoes on sagittal scan of right lower quadrant. Note echogenic surface of small bowel (B) serosa indicative of serosal inflammation. **B:** In another patient with bacterial peritonitis, scan of right lower quadrant demonstrates free fluid (F) and pneumoperitoneum (*curved black arrow*) from perforated duodenal ulcer. Note reverberation artifact (*white arrows*) from gas bubble.

Peritonitis and Other Complex Intraperitoneal Fluid Collections

Complex intraperitoneal fluid collections, such as infected ascites, lymphoceles, bilomas, pancreatic pseudocysts, postoperative seromas, and hematomas, are all readily detected by sonography (Fig. 1.9). However, there is considerable overlap in the sonographic appearance of these fluid collections because most contain septations and low-level echoes. Because of the nonspecific sonographic features, diagnostic needle aspiration or a CT scan is almost always required for definitive diagnosis. Many patients with subacute bacterial or tuberculous peritonitis demonstrate thickened bowel loops from serosal inflammation (Fig. 1.10). Tuberculous peritonitis is a great mimic of other forms of intraperitoneal pathology. The "ascitic" form of tuberculous peritonitis may closely simulate carcinomatosis or other complex fluid collections (20,21) (Fig. 1.11). Mycobacterial cultures should therefore be obtained whenever performing sonographically guided paracentesis.

Parasitic infections such as amebiasis and echinococcal disease may occasionally involve the peritoneal cavity. Hydatid cysts may loculate intraperitoneally and produce a multicystic mass (Fig. 1.12).

Peritoneal and Mesenteric Tumors

Peritoneal metastases and mesenteric nodal masses are the most common intraperitoneal neoplasms (22). A large percentage of peritoneal implants are tiny nodular plaques on the serosal surface of the bowel or solid viscera (Fig. 1.13). Lesions less than 1 cm often cannot be visualized reliably by any imaging modality and can be detected only by surgery or laparoscopy. When visualized with sonography, peritoneal implants are hypoechoic nodules on the peritoneal surface adjacent to ascitic fluid. Malignant septations may be thickened and irregular (Fig. 1.14). CT and sonography can detect diffuse infiltration of the omentum ("omental cakes") and larger nodular implants (>1 cm) (22). CT is probably more accurate than sonography for diagnosing peritoneal or mesenteric metastases. CT scans may be performed after administration of positive intraperitoneal contrast to enhance detection of small implants.

Omental tumors are often broad, band-like masses anterior to the transverse colon. Due to its relatively superficial location, high-resolution linear array transducers (5 MHz) can routinely be used to image the omentum. Omental tumors may be either hypoechoic or echogenic (Figs. 1.15 to 1.17). Biopsy is generally required to distinguish primary peritoneal or mesenteric tumors (desmoid, carcinoid, mesothelioma, lymphoma) from metastases. Cystic or calcified peritoneal implants may occur in metastatic ovarian carcinoma.

Pseudomyxoma peritonei is a form of carcinomatosis caused by mucin-producing adenocarcinomas of the appendix, ovary, or colon (23). Peritoneal implants from pseudomyxoma peritonei are gelatinous masses that cause subtle scalloping of the liver contour (23). Spread along the falciform ligament and fissure for the ligamentum venosum is characteristic. CT is more reliable than sonography in suggesting a specific diagnosis by demonstrating low-attenuation masses. Sonographically, cystic masses from pseudomyxoma peritonei may contain echogenic areas of mucinous debris (Fig. 1.16).

Mesenteric masses are often best detected sonographically with graded compression technique using a 5-MHz linear array transducer. Visualization of the mesenteric vasculature encased by a nodal mass (the "sandwich sign") (Fig. 1.18) and displacement of adjacent bowel loops by the mass are characteristic features.

GASTROINTESTINAL TRACT

Introduction

At present, sonography of the gastrointestinal tract has a limited but growing number of clinical applications (24,25). In selected patients, sonography may provide unique diagnostic information that may aid in patient management. Barium studies, endoscopy, and CT remain the primary techniques for evaluating most gastrointestinal tract lesions. Not infrequently, however, unsuspected gastrointestinal abnormalities are identified incidentally during routine sonography performed for other indications (Fig. 1.19). The development of graded compression techniques, color Doppler sonography, and endoluminal probes have expanded the scope and applications of gastrointestinal sonography. For the most part, sonography is used as a directed examination to address specific clinical questions regarding focal inflammatory or neoplastic processes. One of the main indications for gastrointestinal sonography is evaluation of right lower quadrant pain in patients with possible appendicitis (26,27). In addition, endoluminal sonography may aid in the local staging of esophageal, gastric, and rectal carcinomas (28–30).

When compared to CT, sonography has a number of distinct advantages in imaging the gastrointestinal tract. These include rapid multiplanar imaging, real-time observation of peristalsis and response to manual compression, and color Doppler sonography of the bowel wall. The main limitation of sonography is its inability to reliably image all of the luminal gastrointestinal tract, the mesentery, and subperitoneal space due to bowel gas. Often a combination of CT and sonography yields complimentary information that cannot be obtained with either single modality.

(text continues on page 16)

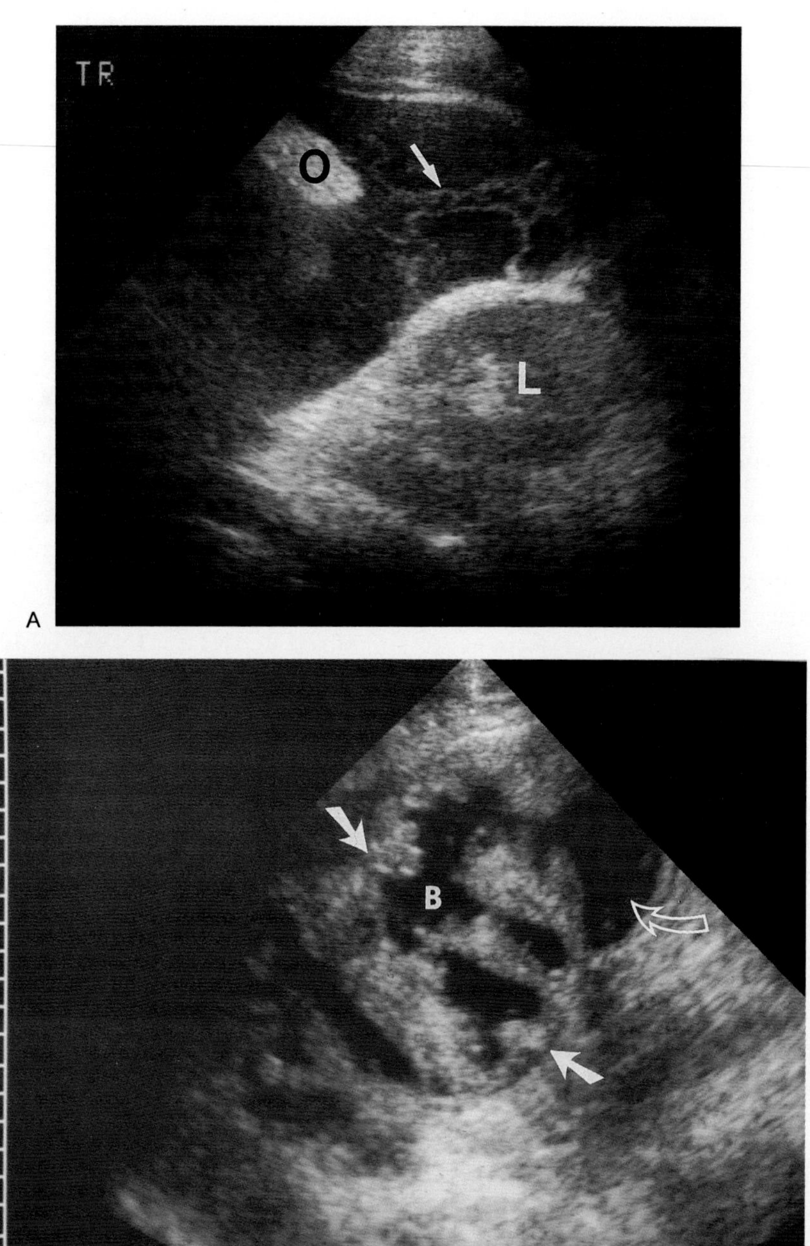

FIG. 1.11. Ascitic form of tuberculous peritonitis in two patients. **A:** Transverse scan of left upper quadrant demonstrates complex intraperitoneal fluid with numerous septations (*arrow*). Note echogenic inflamed omentum (O). L, kidney. **B:** In another patient with tuberculous peritonitis, note ascites (*curved arrow*) and mural thickening (*arrows*) of adjacent inflamed small bowel (B).

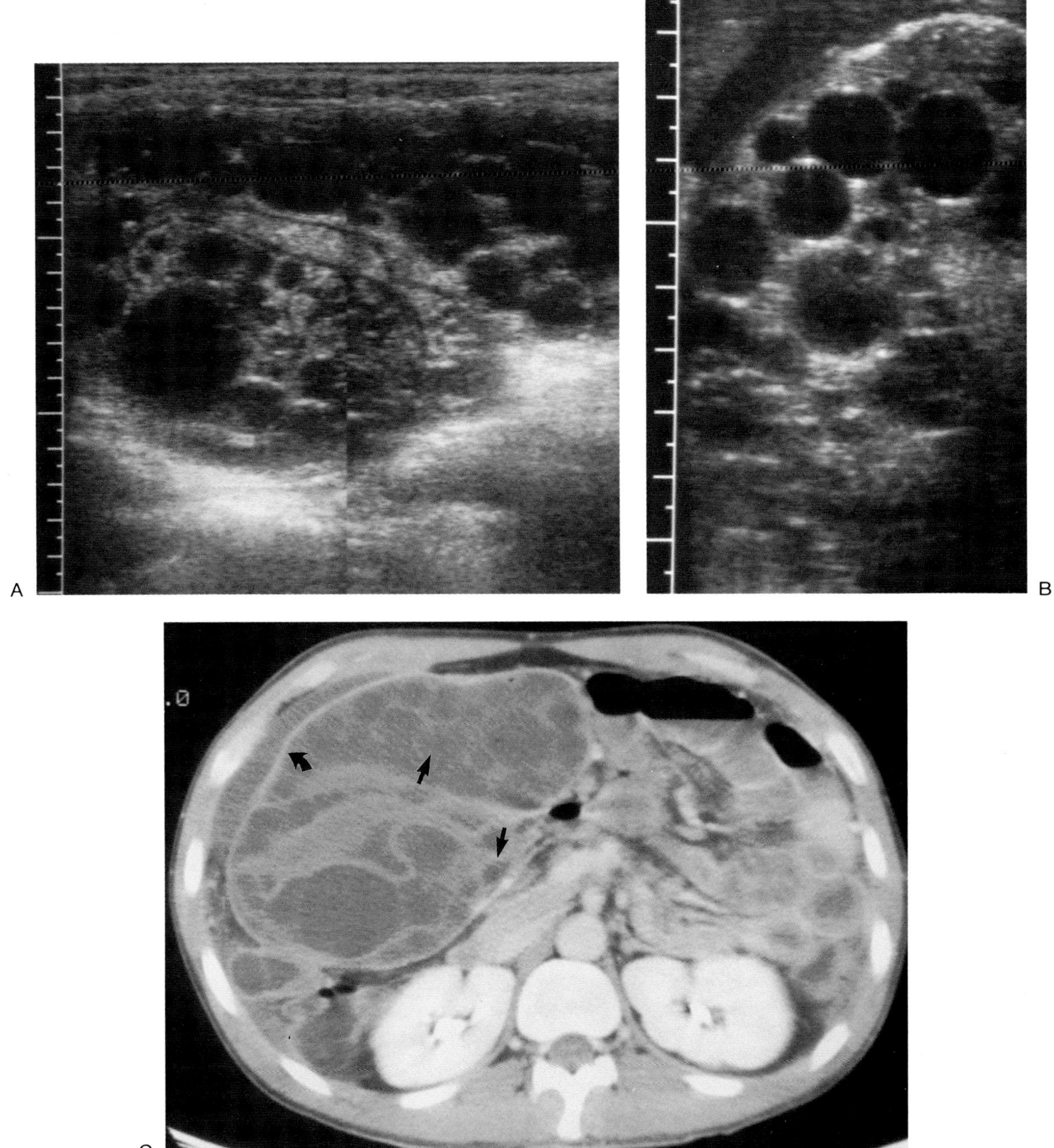

FIG. 1.12. Intraperitoneal hydatid cysts. Sagittal (**A**) and transverse (**B**) sonograms of right paracolic gutter demonstrating complex multicystic masses from intraperitoneal hydatid cysts. Corresponding CT scan (**C**) demonstrates numerous daughter cysts (*arrows*) within larger cyst membrane (*curved arrow*).

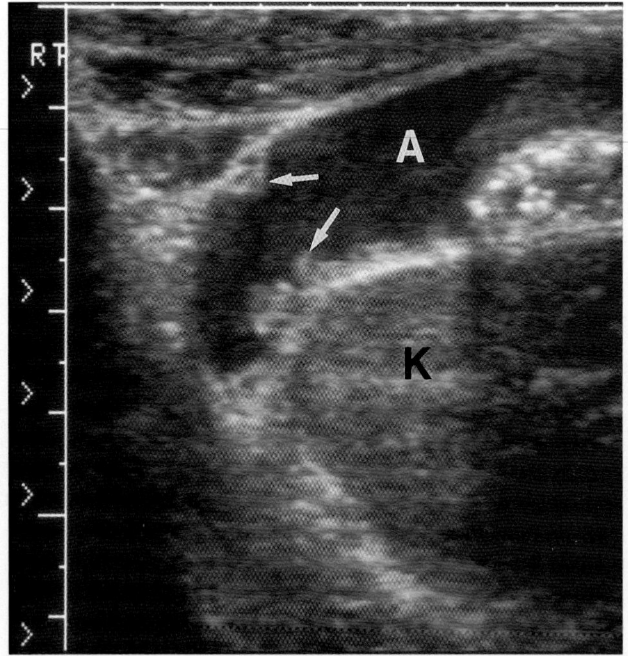

FIG. 1.13. Peritoneal implants from mesothelioma. Transverse scan of right lower quadrant demonstrates ascites (A) and plaque-like peritoneal implants (*arrows*). K, right kidney.

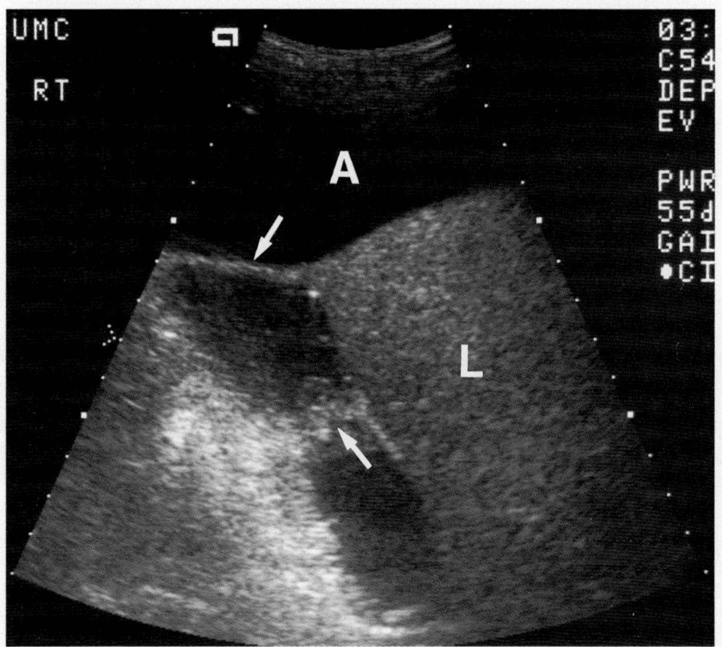

FIG. 1.14. Malignant adhesions from metastatic ovarian carcinoma. Transverse scan of liver (L) demonstrates ascites (A) and thick peritoneal adhesions (*arrows*). Laparoscopy revealed tumor cells within adhesions.

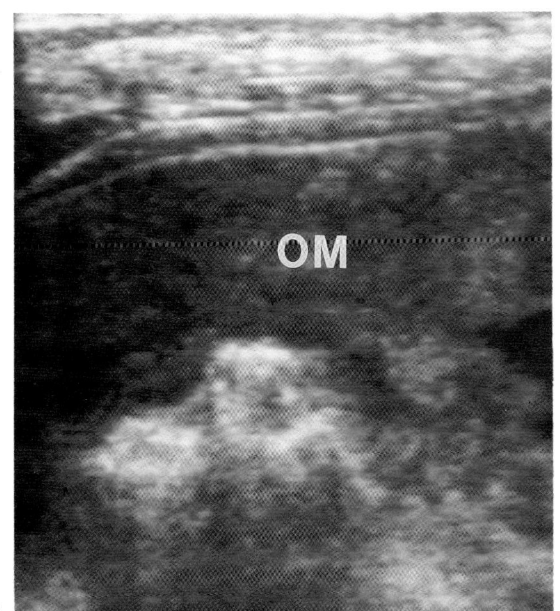

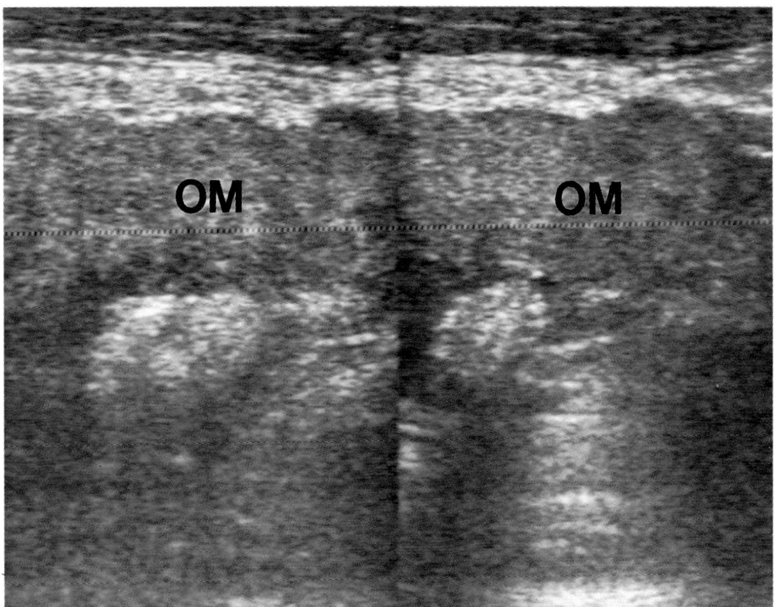

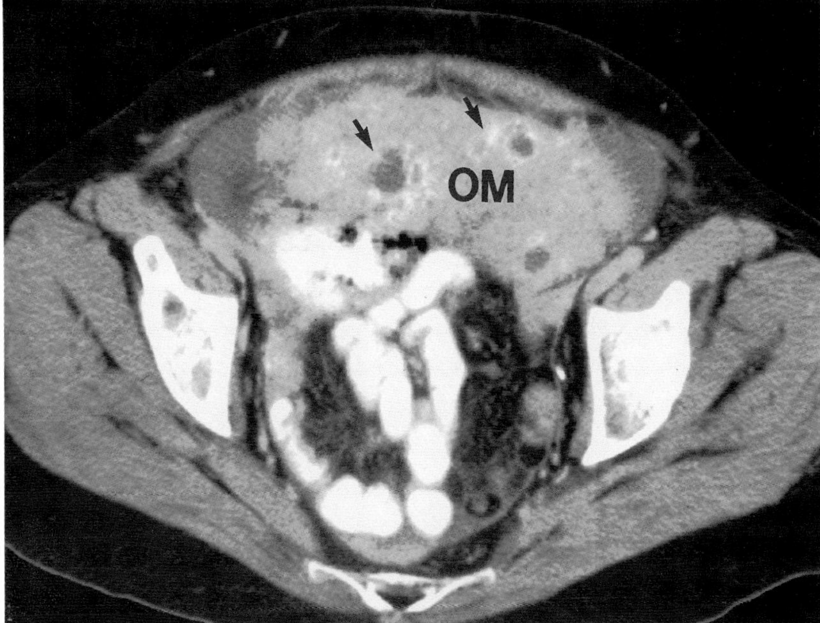

FIG. 1.15. Omental metastases in two patients. **A:** Demonstration of hypoechoic omental metastases (OM) from AIDS-related lymphoma. **B:** Demonstration of echogenic omental "cake" (OM) from metastatic ovarian carcinoma. **C:** CT scan in same patient as (B). Note areas of calcification (*arrows*) within omental "cake" (OM) not apparent on sonography.

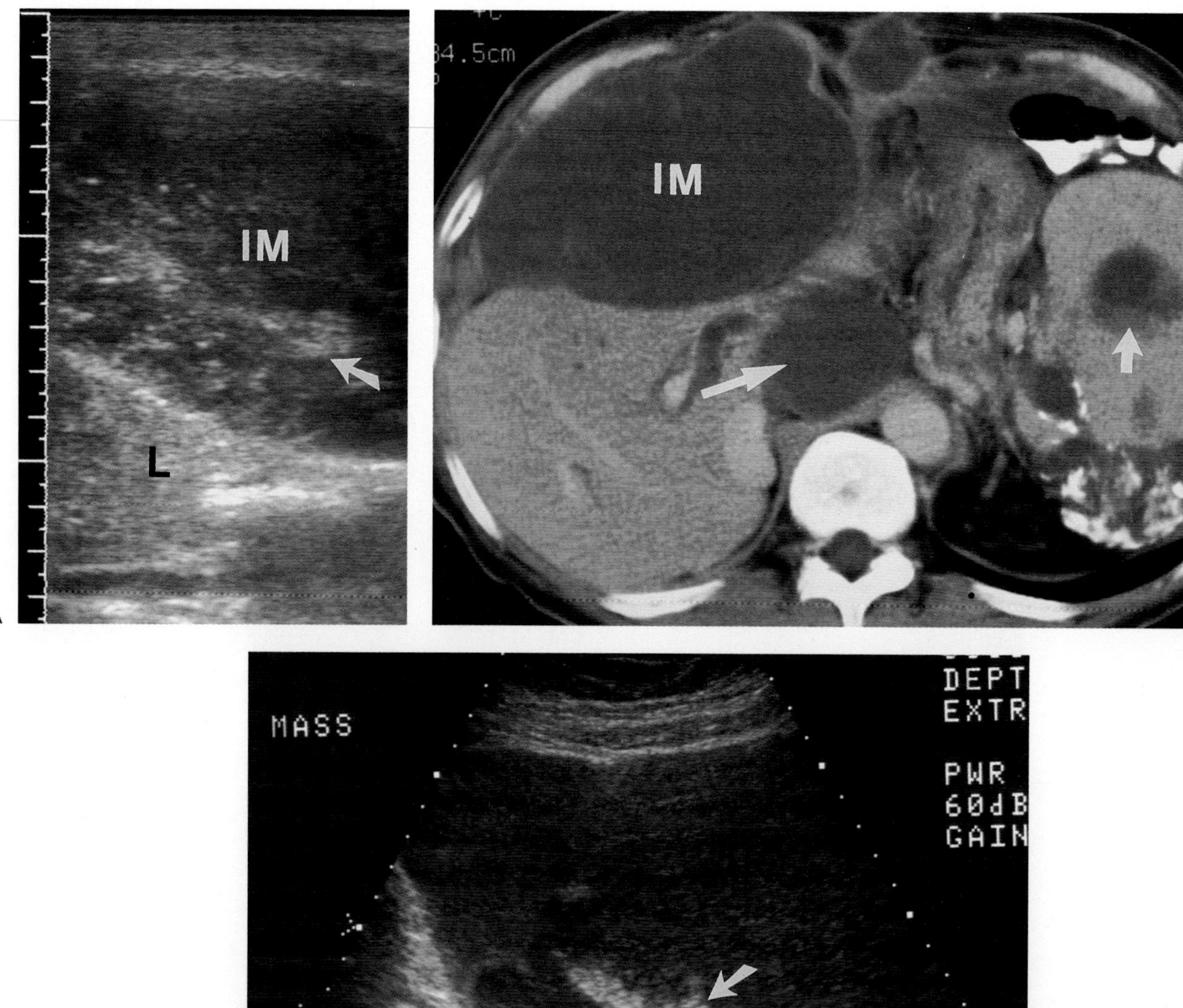

FIG. 1.16. Cystic peritoneal implants in two patients. **A:** Cystic peritoneal implant in a patient with pseudomyxoma peritonei from appendiceal carcinoma. Transverse scan of right upper quadrant demonstrates complex cystic implant (IM) adjacent to liver (L). Note echogenic mucinous debris within implant (*arrow*). **B:** Corresponding CT scan demonstrates low-density perihepatic implant (IM), cystic gastrohepatic ligament implant (*long arrow*), and splenic metastases (*short arrows*). Note calcified implants around the spleen. **C:** In another patient, a large cystic peritoneal implant from recurrent ovarian carcinoma is noted in right lower quadrant. Note solid elements within cystic mass (*arrow*).

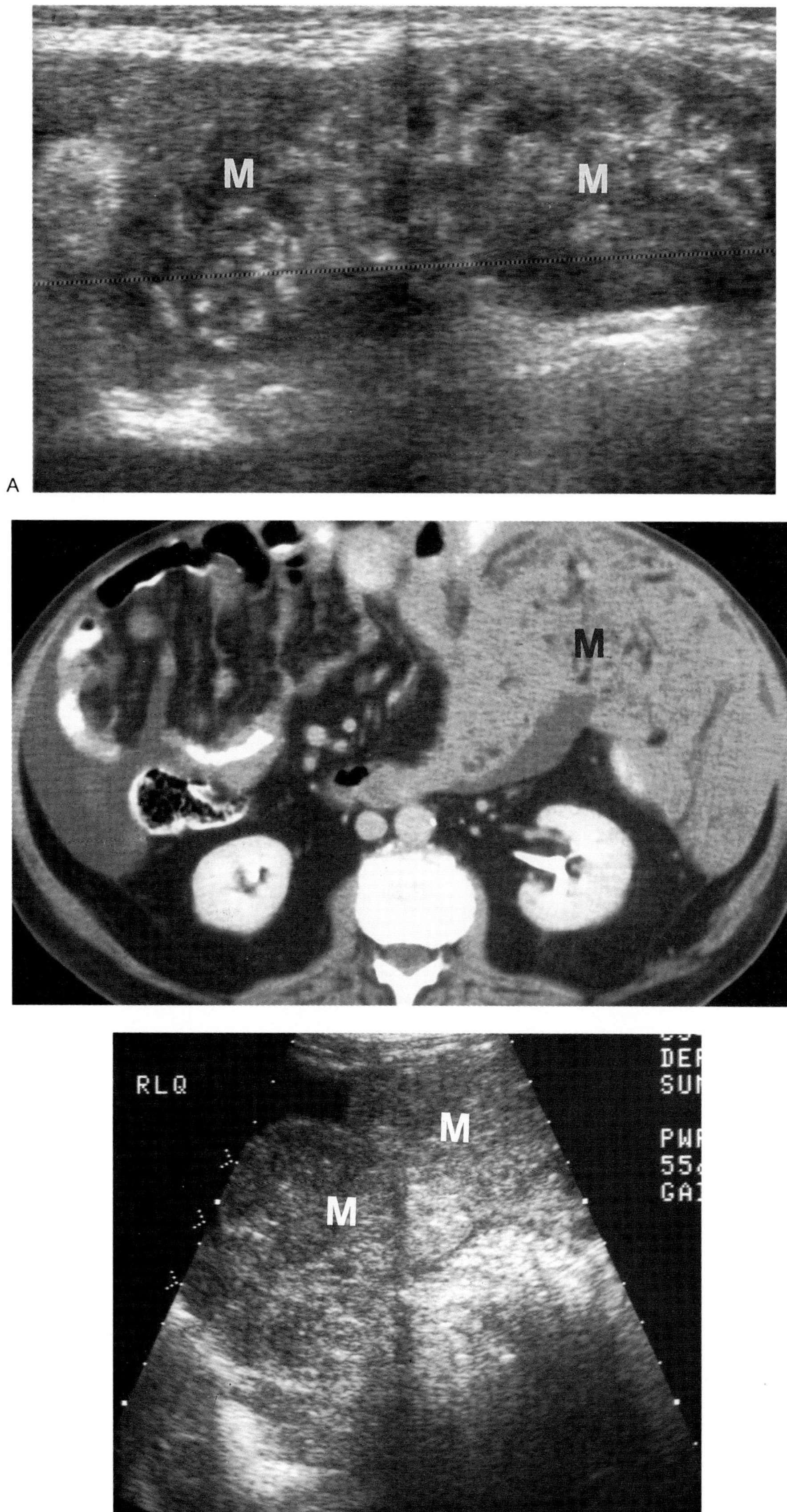

FIG. 1.17. Peritoneal mesothelioma in two patients. **A:** Sagittal scan of left flank demonstrating large heterogeneous omental mass (M) representing primary mesothelioma. **B:** Corresponding CT scan demonstrates significant contrast enhancement within the large mesothelioma (M). **C:** In another patient, transverse sonogram of right lower quadrant demonstrates mesothelioma (M) as a homogenous mass.

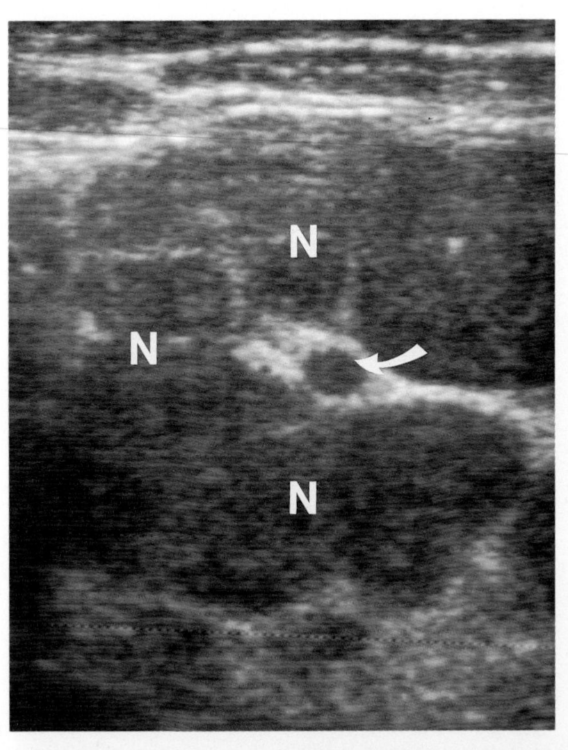

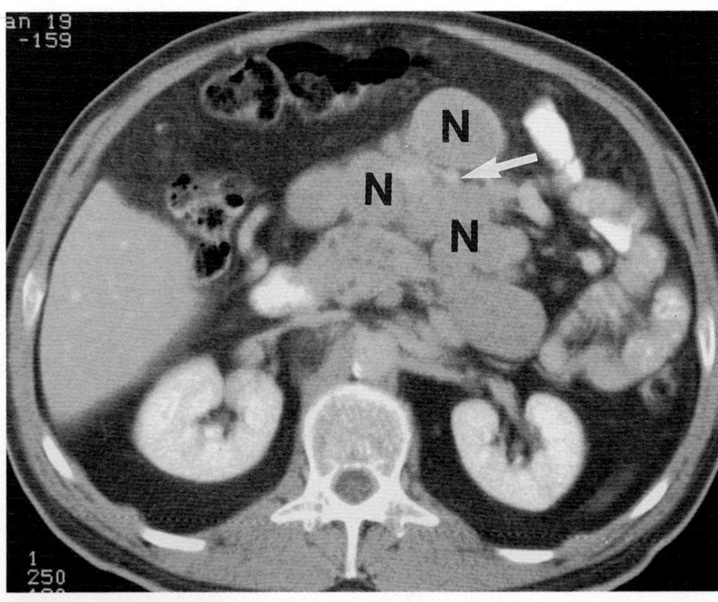

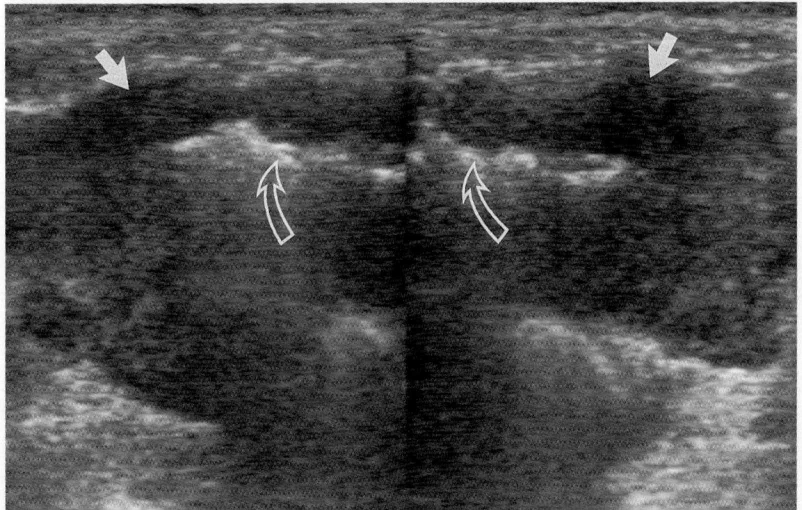

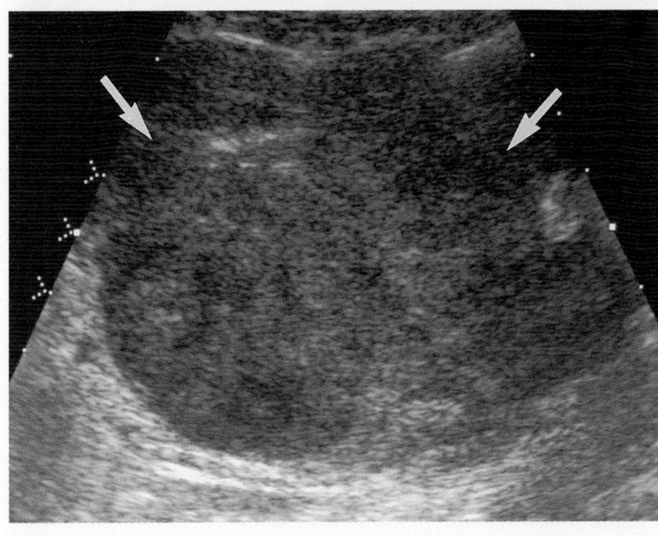

FIG. 1.18. Mesenteric masses in two patients. **A:** Graded compression sonogram of midabdomen demonstrating hypoechoic mesenteric nodes (N) encasing mesenteric vasculature (*arrows*). **B:** Corresponding CT scan demonstrates extensive mesenteric lymphadenopathy (N). Note mesenteric vasculature (*arrow*). **C:** In another patient, metastases to small bowel from melanoma result in large hypoechoic mass (*arrows*) infiltrating bowel wall. Note residual lumen of small bowel (*curved arrow*). **D:** Adjacent large mesenteric mass (*arrows*).

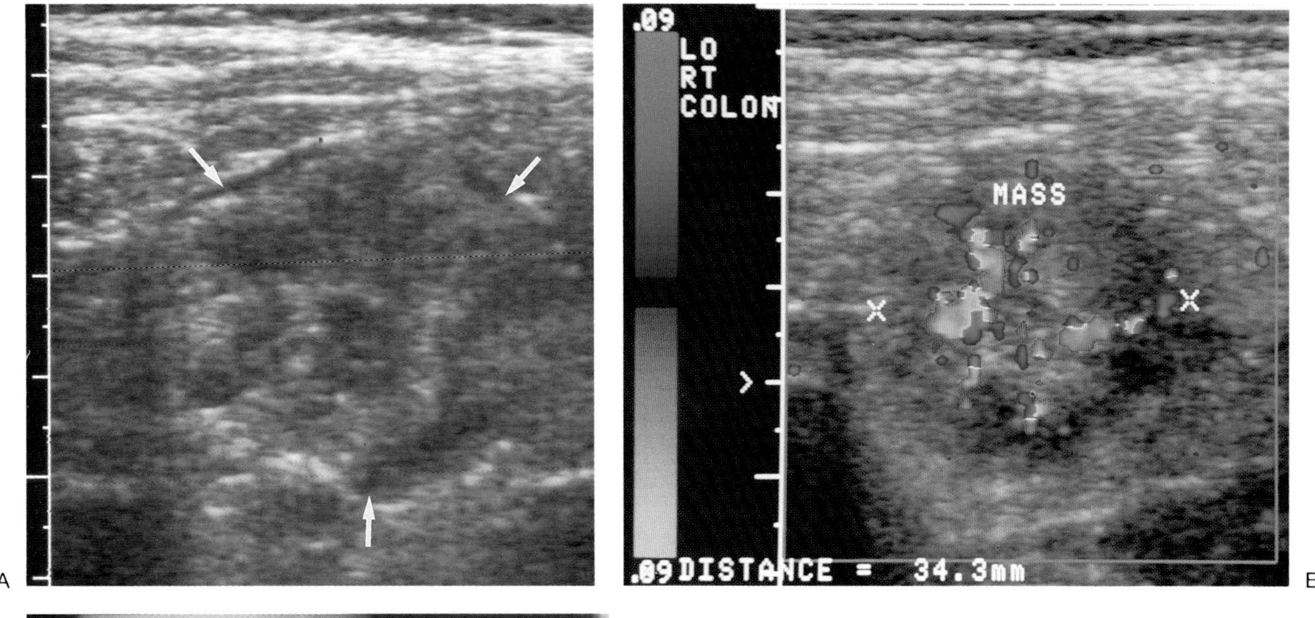

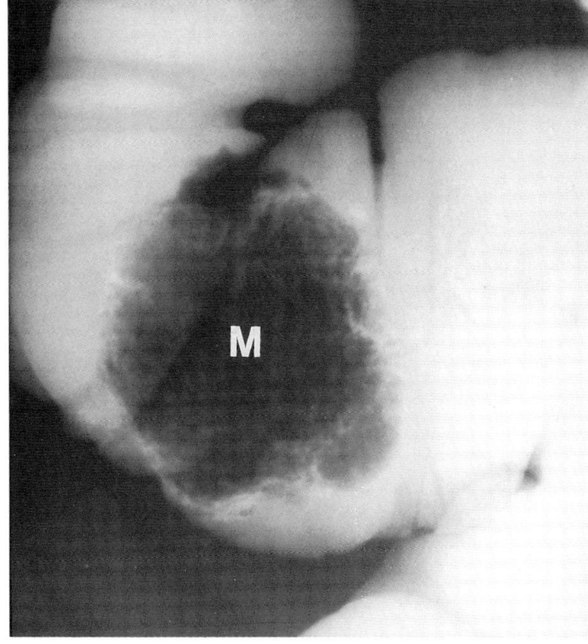

FIG. 1.19. Colonic tumor discovered incidentally during right lower quadrant sonogram for suspected appendicitis. **A:** Graded compression sonogram of right colon demonstrating vague hypoechoic mass (*arrow*). **B:** Color Doppler sonogram reveals hypervascular mass. **C:** Barium enema demonstrates large polypoid mass (M) in right colon. Surgery revealed large benign villoglandular polyp.

Technique

For most gastrointestinal studies, a combination of real-time imaging with a 5.0-MHz curved array transducer and graded compression technique with 5-MHz linear array probe yields the best results. Graded compression technique is particularly useful in evaluating patients with right lower quadrant pain and possible appendicitis (26). This technique takes advantage of the fact that the normal bowel wall is readily compressible and collapses when gentle pressure is applied with the ultrasound transducer. However, any pathologic process that infiltrates the bowel wall (tumor, inflammation, hemorrhage) alters its compliability. Normal overlying bowel loops can then be compressed away to bring pathologically thickened loops into the field of view of the high-resolution transducer. Because of superior near-field imaging capabilities, either a 5- or 7.5-MHz linear array transducer is preferred for graded compression sonography.

Color Doppler sonography may demonstrate areas of increased mural blood to the bowel in some patients with inflammatory or neoplastic lesions (Fig. 1.20). A high-resolution linear array transducer (5.0 or 7.5 MHz) must be used with graded compression technique to visualize small mural vessels. To image flow in the bowel wall, color Doppler imaging parameters must be optimized for low-flow sensitivity. Although clinical results are quite preliminary, color Doppler sonography may potentially aid in characterizing focal gut abnormalities.

Sonographic Features of the Bowel Wall

With endoluminal transducers (generally 7.5 to 12.5 MHz) it is now possible to visualize five discrete layers of the bowel wall (28–30) (Fig. 1.21). These include the echogenic mucosal interface between luminal fluid or mucus, the hypoechoic mucosa and muscularis mucosa, the echogenic submucosa, a hypoechoic muscularis propria, and an echogenic serosal or adventitial surface (28–30). With graded compression technique and abdominal transducers (5 to 7.5 MHz), it is not possible to resolve these layers of the bowel wall. However, the echogenic submucosal layer is a constant anatomic feature of the gastrointestinal tract and serves as an extremely useful landmark to identify a structure as a loop of bowel. The muscular layers of bowel wall (i.e., muscularis propria) appear as a single hypoechoic layer with 5- to 7.5-MHz transducers.

Ischemic or inflammatory processes may result in ulceration or necrosis of the submucosal layer. There is generally focal or global loss of this echogenic anatomic landmark (15). Loss of visualization of the submucosa is an important finding of transmural inflammatory disease such as gangrenous appendicitis. Neoplastic invasion of the bowel wall may cause a target or "pseudo-kidney" appearance (24). The infiltrated bowel wall appears hypoechoic (mimicking the cortex of a kidney). The echogenic mucosal surface and lumen are preserved (mimicking the renal hilar fat) (Fig. 1.22). Areas of ulceration may result in high-amplitude echoes and acoustic shadowing from gas within the submucosal layers of the bowel wall. However, it is often impossible to visualize small mucosal abnormalities without endoluminal sonography.

Gastrointestinal Inflammatory Lesions

Acute Appendicitis

In 70 percent of patients with possible acute appendicitis, classic signs and symptoms permit surgery without preliminary imaging. Graded compression sonography is a valuable technique in the remaining 30 percent of patients with uncertain clinical findings. This often includes women ages 20 to 40, children less than 5 years of age, and very elderly patients (26, 31–34). CT may also be utilized to evaluate patients with suspected appendicitis. The choice between CT or sonography depends primarily on institutional preference and the availability of expertise in each modality. Sonography's advantages include lower cost, real-time observation of bowel peristalsis, and its ability to define layers of the bowel wall. It also excels in diagnosing many of the acute gynecologic disorders that can mimic appendicitis. CT is performed in markedly obese patients or in patients likely to have an abscess.

At the outset of the sonographic examination, the patient is asked to point to the site of maximal abdominal tenderness with a single finger. This may facilitate identification of an appendix in an unusual location. Transverse scans of the right flank are obtained with gentle pressure in an attempt to identify the right colon. The right colon is the largest gastrointestinal structure in the right flank. Once identified, the right colon is scanned in a caudal direction until the tip of the cecum is identified. Although the tip of the appendix may lie in a variety of locations, the appendix always originates at the base of the cecum. Once the cecum is identified, pressure with the ultrasound transducer is gradually increased to displace normal bowel loops and to visualize the noncompressible appendix. Gentle compression is tolerated remarkably well; sedation or analgesia is rarely required. Failure to visualize the cecum or other important landmarks (the psoas muscle or iliac vessels) must be considered a nondiagnostic study. Technical failures, which occur in about 3 percent of all patients, may occur in patients with marked obesity, tense ascites, or severe pain (33). CT should be performed in patients with a technically inadequate sonogram.

(text continues on page 19)

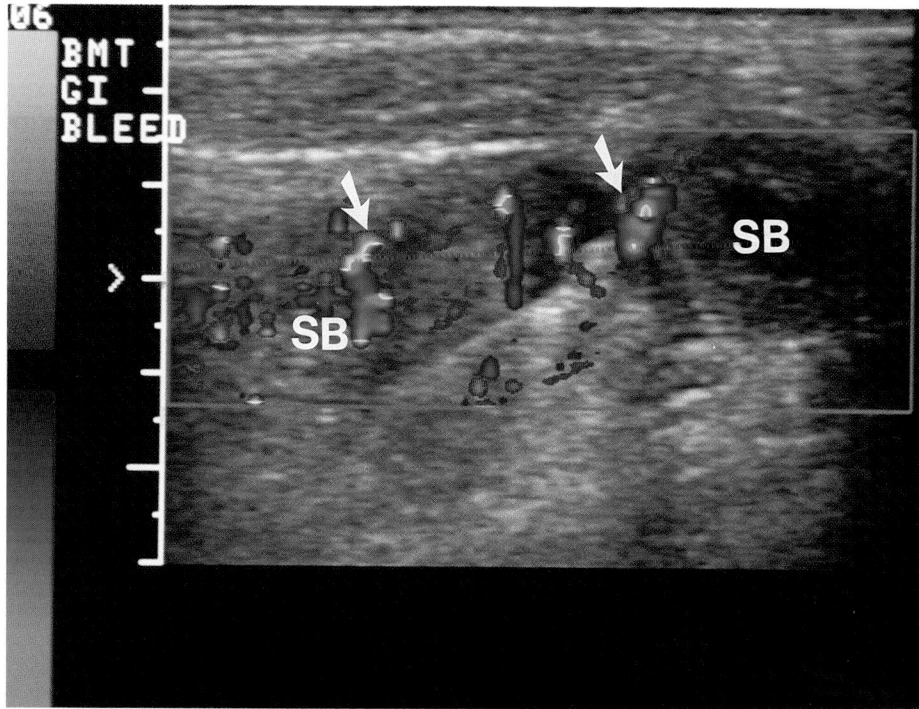

FIG. 1.20. Small bowel enteritis with increased mural vascularity demonstrated by color Doppler sonography. Patient had bone marrow transplant and developed severe small bowel enteritis with gastrointestinal bleeding. Color Doppler sonography demonstrates increased vascularity (*arrows*) of small bowel (SB).

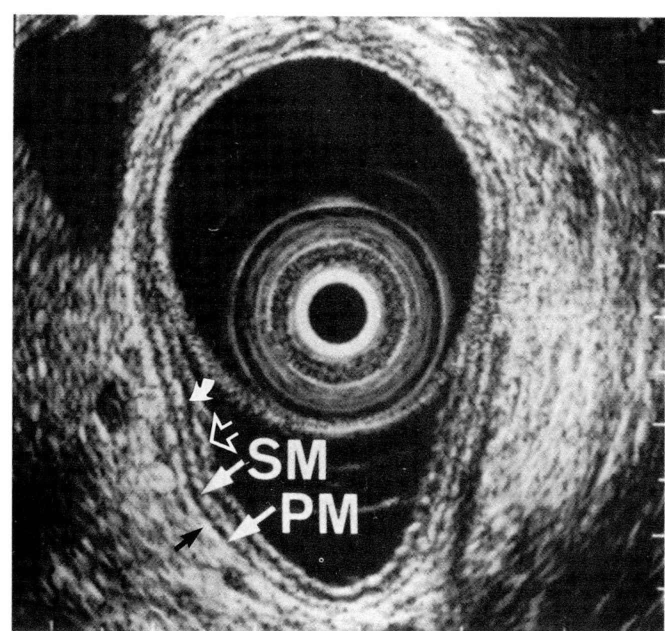

FIG. 1.21. Five normal layers of stomach demonstrated by 7.5-MHz endoluminal sonogram. First inner layer (*open arrow*) is hyperechoic mucosal interface between luminal fluid and mucus. Second layer (*curved arrow*) is hypoechoic mucosa and muscularis mucosa. Third layer (SM) is echogenic submucosa. Fourth layer (PM) is hypoechoic muscularis propria. Fifth layer (*black arrow*) is echogenic serosal surface. (Case courtesy of Jin Hong Kim, MD, Seoul, Korea.)

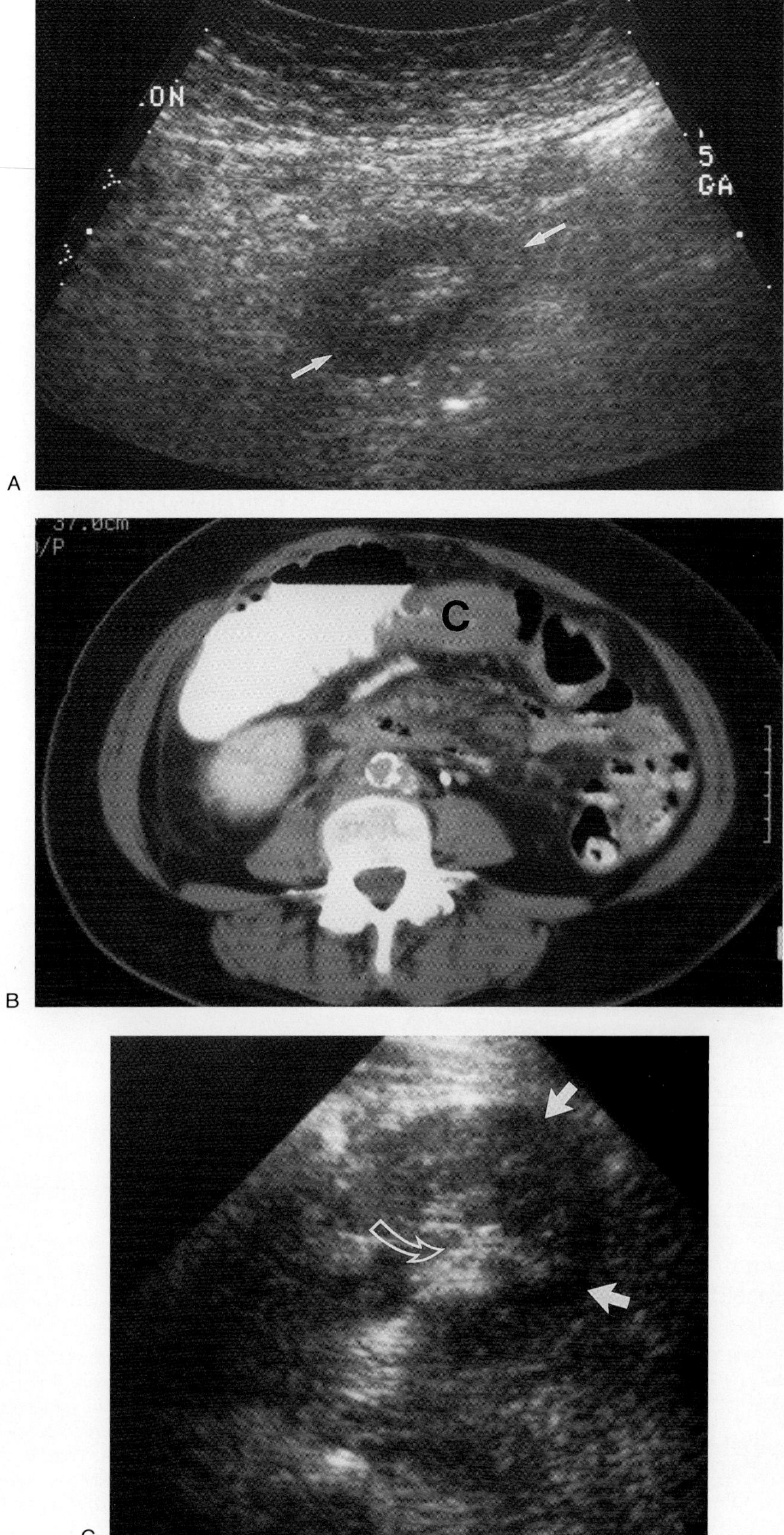

FIG. 1.22. Pseudokidney appearance of infiltrating lesions of bowel wall in two patients. **A:** Sagittal sonogram of midabdomen demonstrating mass (*arrows*) that resembles a kidney. **B:** CT scan demonstrates circumferential carcinoma (C) obstructing hepatic flexure. **C:** In another patient, pseudokidney sign (*arrows*) is noted secondary to lymphoma infiltrating bowel wall. Echogenic mesenteric fat (*curved arrow*) mimics renal sinus fat.

The normal appendix has five sonographic features: (a) origin from the base of the cecum, (b) an inner echogenic submucosal ring and an outer hypoechoic ring, (c) no peristalsis, (d) termination in a blind pouch, and (e) maximum outer diameter of 6 mm and a mural thickness of 2 mm or less (Fig. 1.23). While most authors feel that a normal appendix is infrequently visualized (32–35), Rioux (36) identified a normal appendix in 102 of 125 patients (82 percent). Sonographic criteria for acute appendicitis include (a) a noncompressible appendix measuring 7 mm or more in greatest outer anteroposterior (AP) diameter or (b) a noncompressible appendix with a mural thickness of 3 mm or greater and (c) identification of an appendicolith in an appendix of any size (Fig. 1.24) (33). Multiple clinical studies have documented a diagnostic accuracy of 90 percent or greater using these criteria (32–34).

Additional findings may be present in patients with gangrenous appendicitis: focal or global interruption of the echogenic submucosal layer from necrosis, echogenic inflamed mesenteric fat, and a localized fluid collection representing an abscess (Fig. 1.25) (15). Periappendiceal phlegmons are areas of indurated soft tissue inflammation without liquefied pus (Fig. 1.26). Phlegmons are typically poorly defined masses of mixed echogenicity (15).

The presence of an appendicolith in a noncompressible appendix indicates acute appendicitis regardless of the size measurements (33). Sonography is significantly more sensitive than plain films (82 versus 51 percent) for the detection of appendicoliths (Fig. 1.25) (37). A hypoechoic fluid collection containing an appendicolith or a fluid collection located adjacent to a gangrenous appendix is virtually diagnostic of a periappendiceal abscess (Fig. 1.26) (15). Both sonography and CT are quite valuable in guiding percutaneous drainage of larger periappendiceal abscesses (14).

When examination of the right lower quadrant is negative for acute appendicitis, the upper abdomen and pelvis should be surveyed for an alternative diagnosis. The majority of patients referred for right lower quadrant sonography, in fact, do not have appendicitis (34). Often no firm diagnosis is established and the pain resolves spontaneously. In patients with a proven cause for abdominal pain, however, sonography may detect alternative diagnoses to appendicitis in 70 percent of patients (Figs. 1.27 to 1.33) (34). These entities include salpingitis, mesenteric adenitis, cecal diverticulitis, infectious ileitis or Crohn's disease, ureteral calculi, or bowel obstruction. If multiple mesenteric nodes 5 mm or larger in size are detected, a diagnosis of mesenteric adenitis may be suggested (Figs. 1.27 and 1.28) (35). Inflammatory or neoplastic disease may cause significant mural thickening of the terminal ileum (Figs. 1.29 and 1.30). On occasion, a dilated ureter from an ureteral calculus is detected (Fig. 1.31). Endovaginal scanning in women may be useful to detect distal ureteral stones as well as to detect gynecologic abnormalities such as a pyosalpinx or a tubo-ovarian abscess. Rectus sheath hematomas may be misdiagnosed for appendicitis (Fig. 1.32). Color Doppler sonography may be useful to detect painful degenerating right-sided myomas (Fig. 1.33).

Rarely, patients with sonographic findings of acute appendicitis have spontaneous resolution of symptoms without surgery (Fig. 1.34). Some patients may have recurrent symptoms and repeat sonography demonstrating findings of acute appendicitis. Pathologically, the appendix in these patients may have evidence of acute inflammation and chronic scarring. Nevertheless, because symptoms of appendicitis may rarely spontaneously resolve, the decision for surgery must always be based on both clinical and image findings.

False-positive sonographic results may occur in patients with a dilated fallopian tube (Fig. 1.35), or secondary inflammation of the appendix due to contiguous diseases such as Crohn's disease or tubo-ovarian abscess (Fig. 1.36) (38,39).

False-negative diagnoses are uncommon in experienced hands but may occur in retrocecal appendicitis, advanced pregnancies, or perforated appendicitis (33). In patients with perforation, peritonitis may cause muscular rigidity precluding adequate compression. A gas-filled appendix may be difficult to visualize and lead to a false-negative examination (Fig. 1.37) (40). In some patients, appendicitis may be confined to the tip of the appendix. Care must be taken to image the entire length of the appendix to avoid misdiagnosis (Fig. 1.38) (41).

Diverticulitis

In most patients, CT is superior to sonography in defining inflammatory changes within the pericolonic fat and in detecting small abscesses in the sigmoid mesentery (18,42,43). CT is often the imaging method of choice in septic patients with a possible paracolonic abscess. In patients with classic clinical symptoms of left lower quadrant pain and low-grade fever, however, a contrast enema may be all that is required to establish the diagnosis. Sonography, nevertheless, may play a useful role as a screening examination in patients with confusing signs and symptoms. Percutaneous drainage of diverticular abscesses with sonography or CT may increase the number of patients eligible for a primary resection, thus obviating the need for a staged surgical procedure and a colostomy (43–48).

Sonographic findings in acute diverticulitis include mural thickening of the involved segment of bowel and echogenic adjacent mesenteric fat (Figs. 1.28 and 1.39) (49–50). The infected colonic diverticulum may be identified, particularly if it contains a gas-forming infection (Fig. 1.40). This appears as an echogenic mural focus

(*text continues on page 35*)

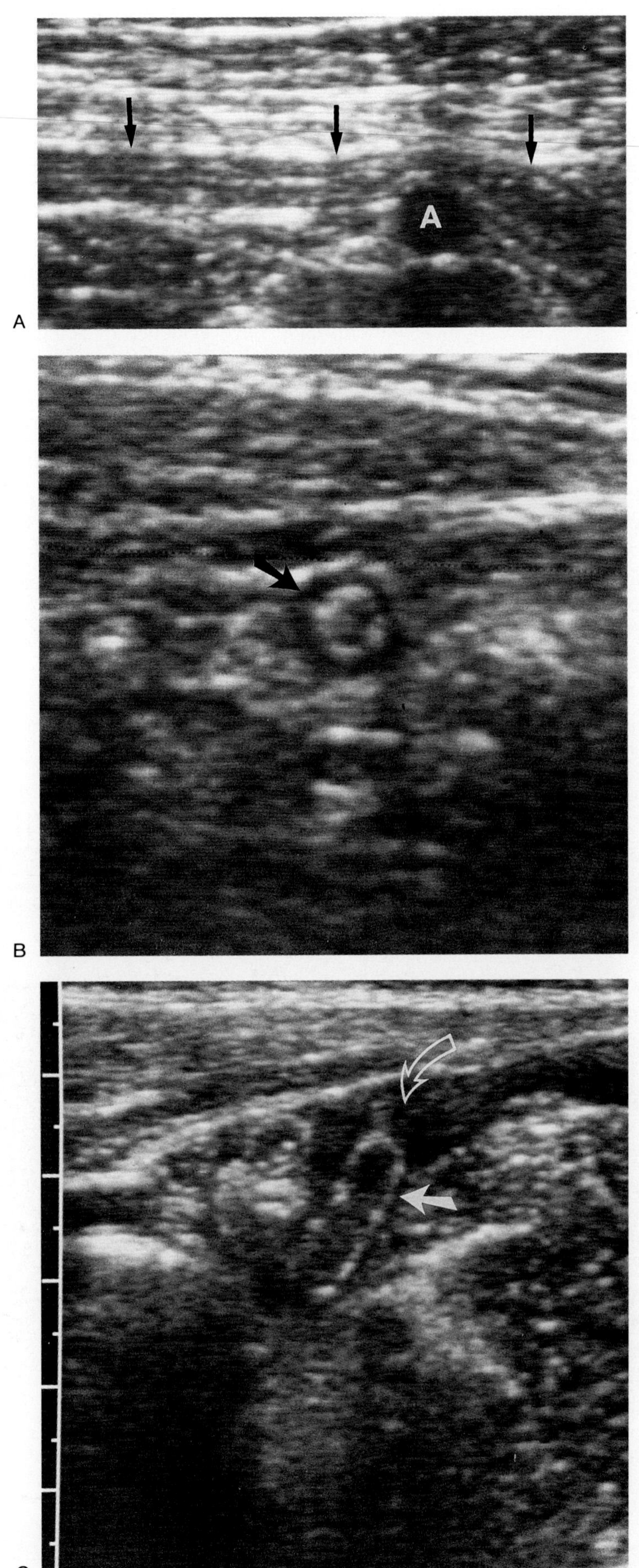

FIG. 1.23. Normal appendix visualized by sonography in three patients. **A:** Normal appendix (*arrows*) is noted anterior to external iliac artery (A). **B:** In another patient, a normal 5-mm appendix (*arrow*) is noted in cross section. **C:** In a third patient, normal appendix (*arrow*) is outlined by ascites in right flank (*curved arrow*).

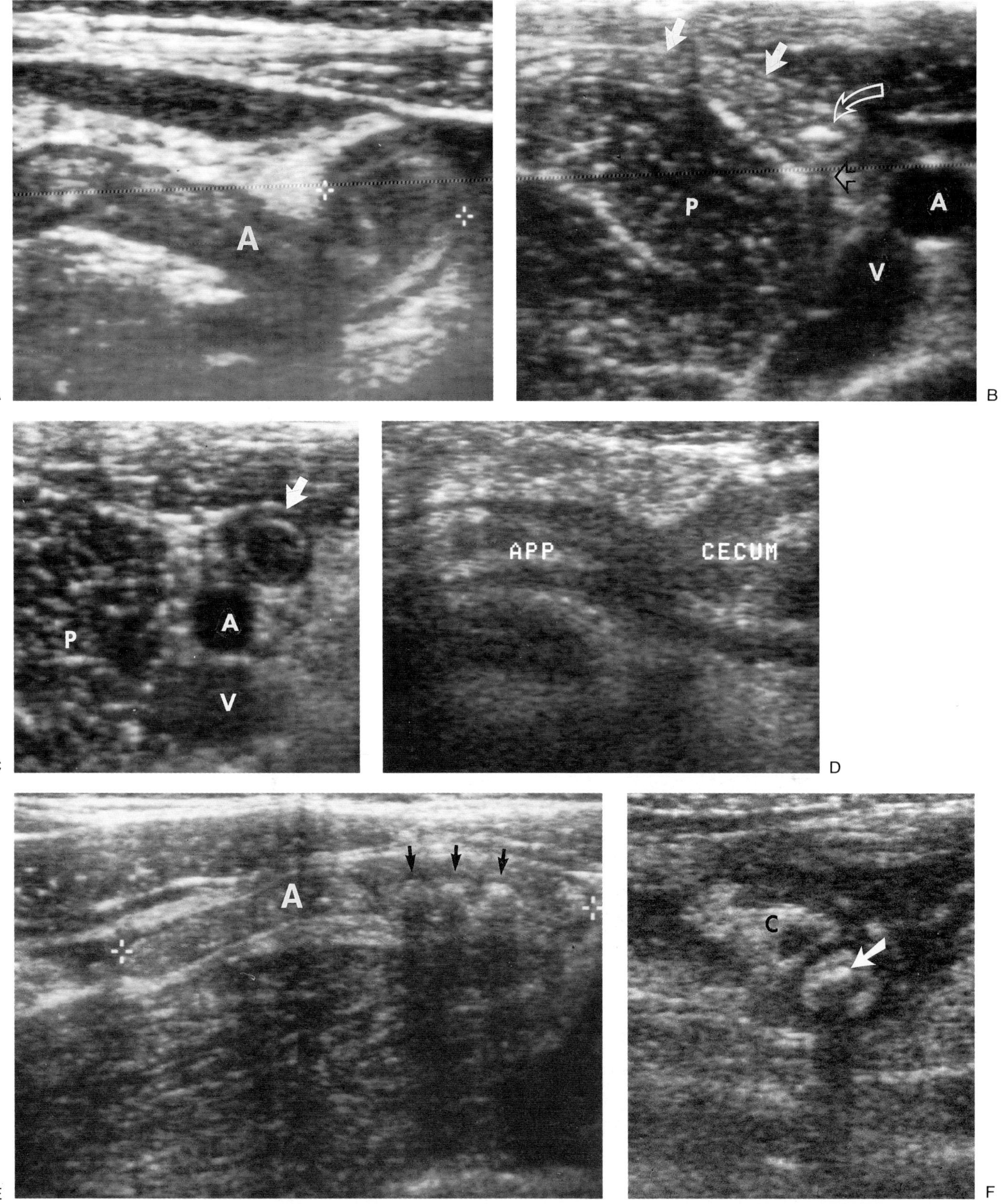

FIG. 1.24. Early acute appendicitis in six patients. **A:** Note appendix (A) with distended tip (*cursors*). **B:** A small appendicolith (*curved arrows*) is noted in the tip of the appendix (*arrows*). Note acoustic shadowing from appendicolith (*open arrow*). A, external iliac artery; V, external iliac vein. **C:** Inflamed appendix (*arrow*) is seen in cross section. P, psoas; A, external iliac artery; V, external iliac vein. **D:** Appendix (APP) originates laterally from cecum. **E:** Multiple appendicoliths (*arrows*) are noted in relatively normal size appendix (A). **F:** Retrocecal appendix with appendicolith (*arrow*) is noted. C, cecum.

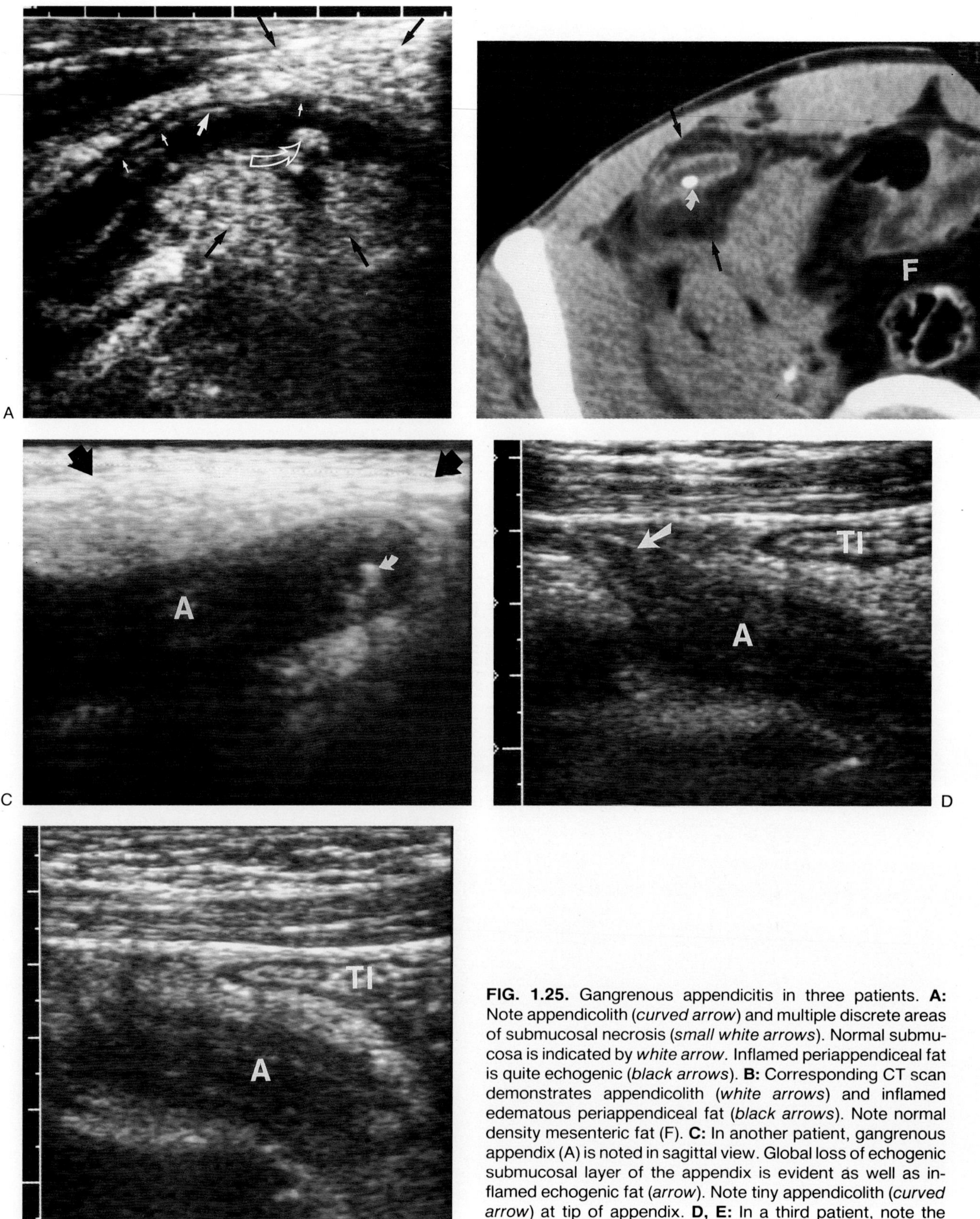

FIG. 1.25. Gangrenous appendicitis in three patients. **A:** Note appendicolith (*curved arrow*) and multiple discrete areas of submucosal necrosis (*small white arrows*). Normal submucosa is indicated by *white arrow.* Inflamed periappendiceal fat is quite echogenic (*black arrows*). **B:** Corresponding CT scan demonstrates appendicolith (*white arrows*) and inflamed edematous periappendiceal fat (*black arrows*). Note normal density mesenteric fat (F). **C:** In another patient, gangrenous appendix (A) is noted in sagittal view. Global loss of echogenic submucosal layer of the appendix is evident as well as inflamed echogenic fat (*arrow*). Note tiny appendicolith (*curved arrow*) at tip of appendix. **D, E:** In a third patient, note the relatively normal base of the appendix (*arrow* in D) with poor definition of gangrenous distal appendix (A). TI, terminal ilium.

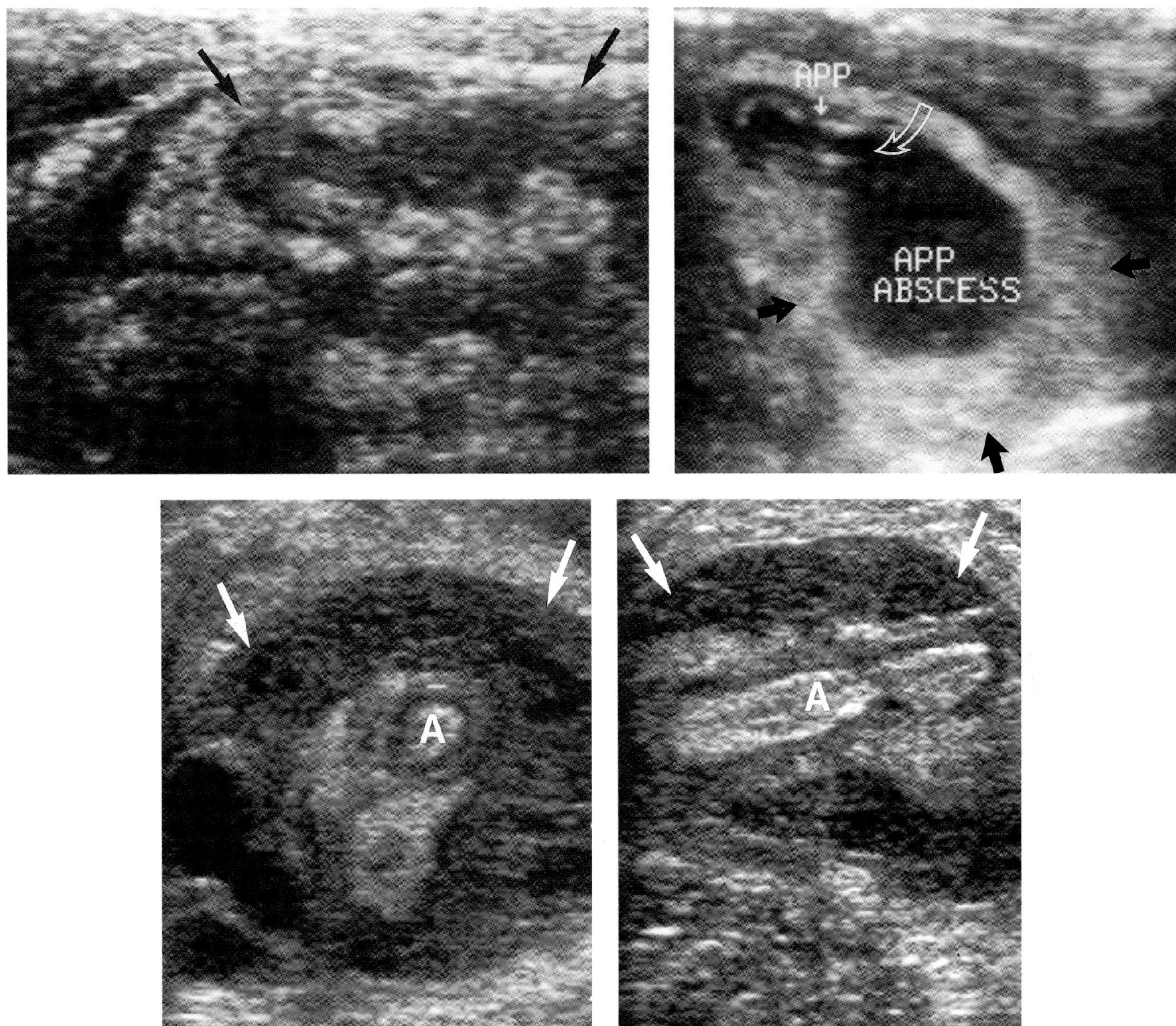

FIG. 1.26. Periappendiceal phlegmon versus abscess. **A:** A poorly defined phlegmon of mixed echogenicity is noted in the right lower quadrant (*arrows*). **B:** In another patient, a well-defined hypoechoic abscess (*black arrows*) is seen adjacent to focal area interruption of the submucosa (*curved arrows*). Note echogenic inflamed periappendiceal fat that walls off abscess. **C, D:** In another patient, large complex periappendiceal abscess (*arrows*) surrounds appendix (A).

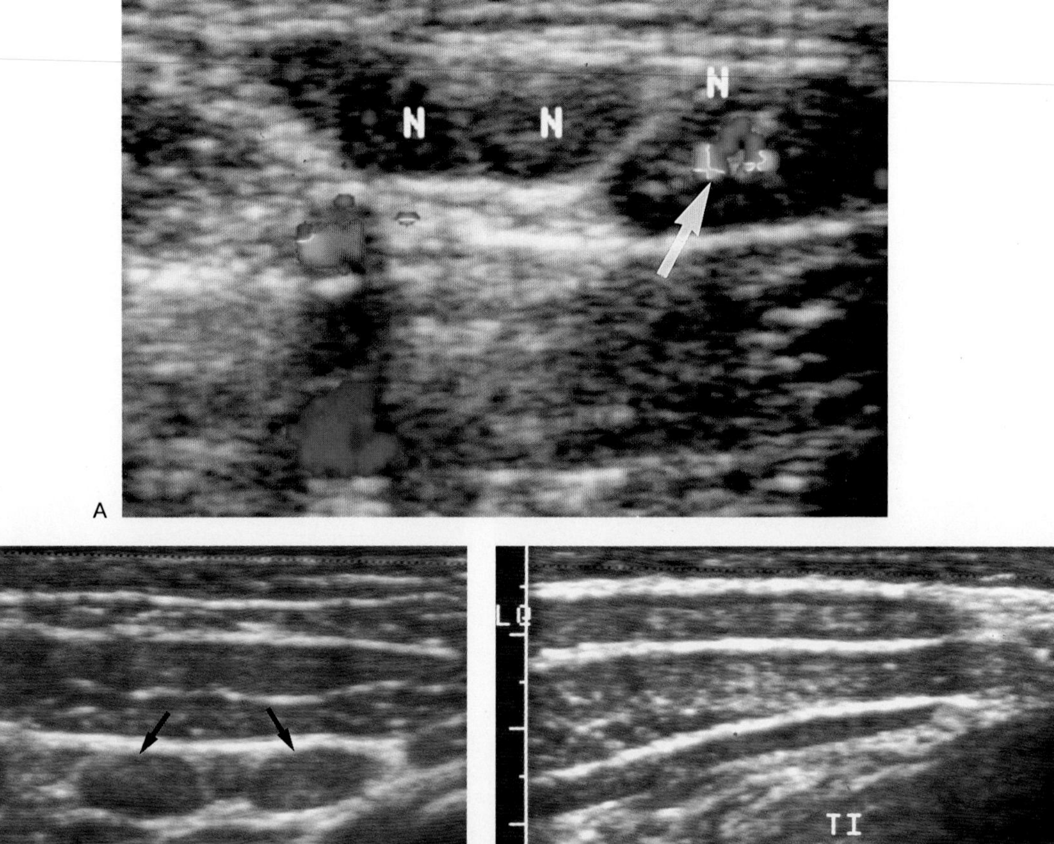

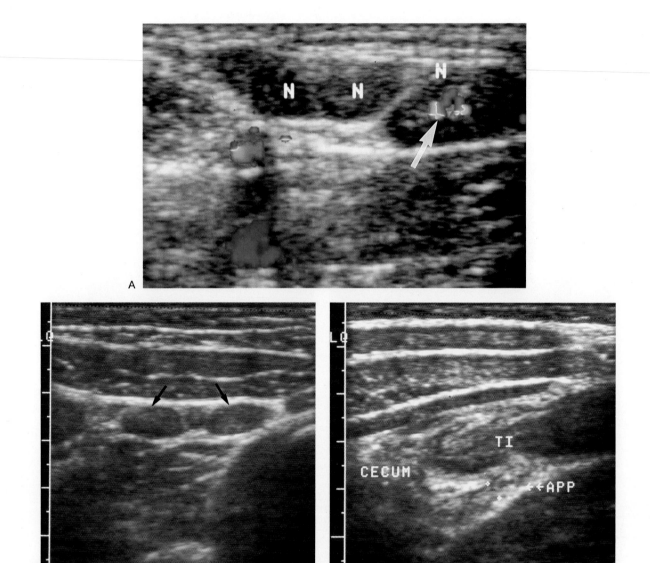

FIG. 1.27. Mesenteric adenitis in two patients. **A:** Color Doppler sonogram demonstrating multiple enlarged mesenteric nodes (N). Note central area of vascularity within (*arrow*) large reactive node. **B:** In another patient, note multiple enlarged mesenteric nodes (*arrows*). **C:** Scan of cecum, terminal ileum (TI), and normal appendix (APP).

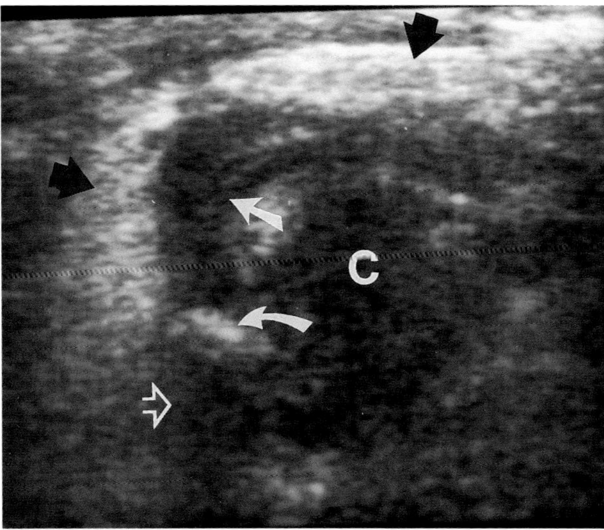

FIG. 1.28. Cecal diverticulitis mimicking appendicitis. Transverse scan of cecum (C) demonstrates mural thickening (*white arrow*) and prominent echogenic paracolonic fat (*black arrows*). Infected diverticulum is identified as echogenic intramural focus (*curved arrow*) casting an acoustic shadow (*open arrow*).

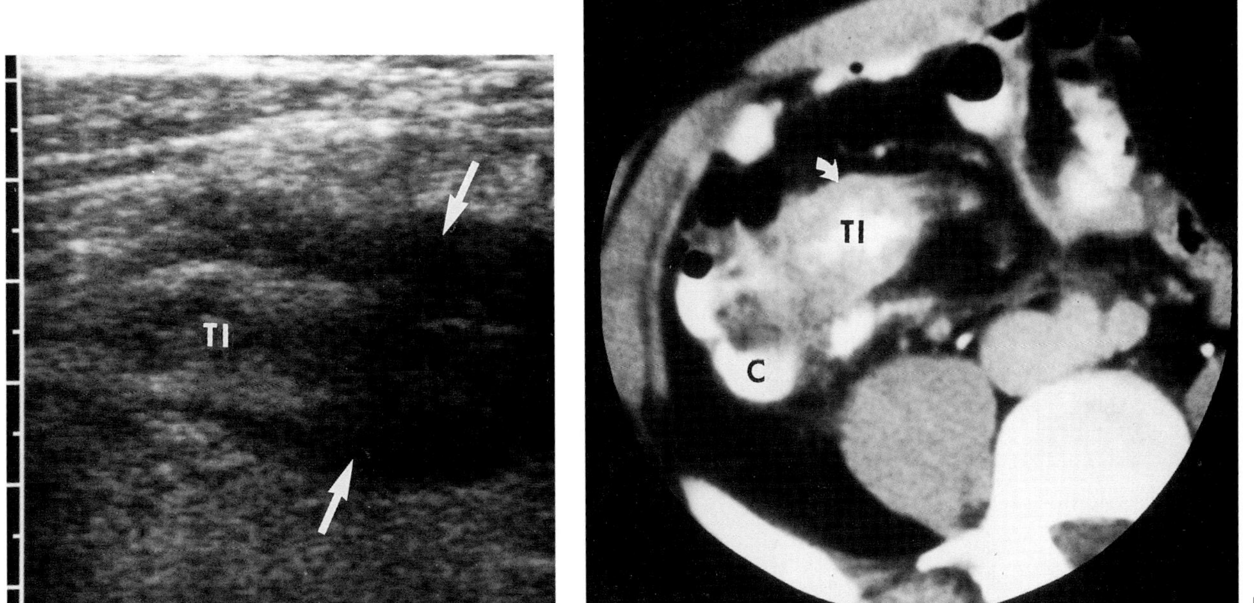

FIG. 1.29. Terminal ileitis mimicking appendicitis. Note marked thickening (*arrows*) of terminal ileum (TI) from *Campylobacter* enteritis. CT scan (**B**) confirms mural thickening (*arrow*) of terminal ileum (TI). C, cecum.

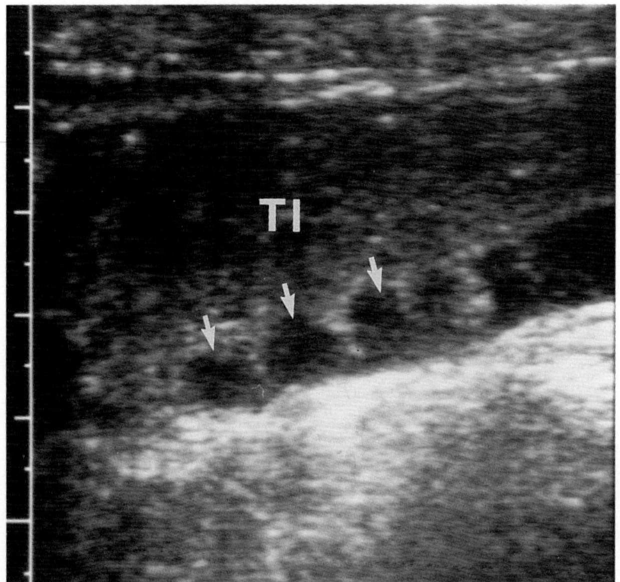

FIG. 1.30. Lymphoma of terminal ileum misdiagnosed as appendicitis. Note nodular thickening of small bowel folds (*arrows*). TI, terminal ileum.

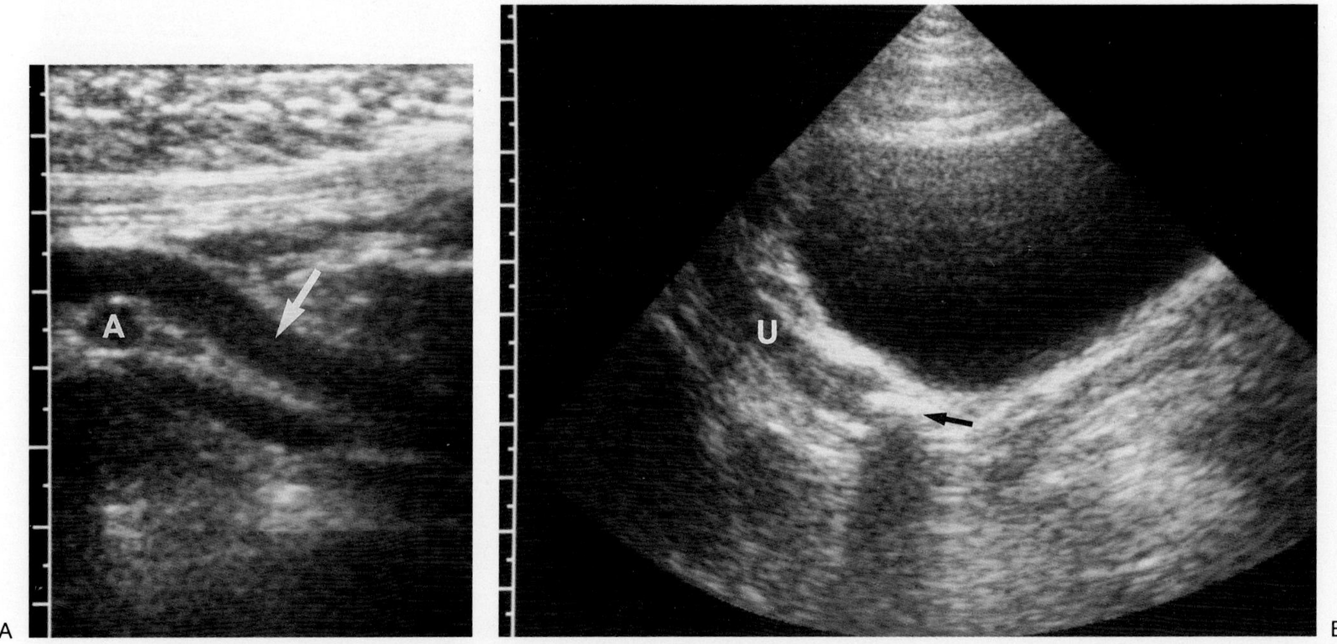

FIG. 1.31. Distal ureteral calculus mimicking acute appendicitis. **A:** Longitudinal scan of right lower quadrant demonstrates dilated ureter (*arrow*) anterior to external iliac artery (A). **B:** Sagittal scan of pelvis demonstrates distal ureteral calculus (*arrow*) and dilated ureter (U).

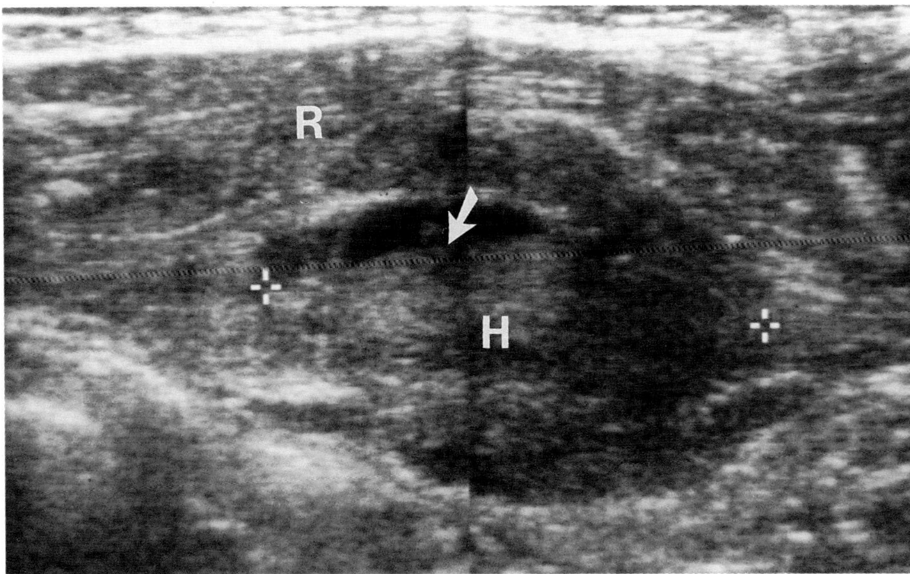

FIG. 1.32. Rectus sheath hematoma mimicking appendicitis. Note echogenic hematoma (H) with hematocrit effect (*arrow*) within rectus muscle (R).

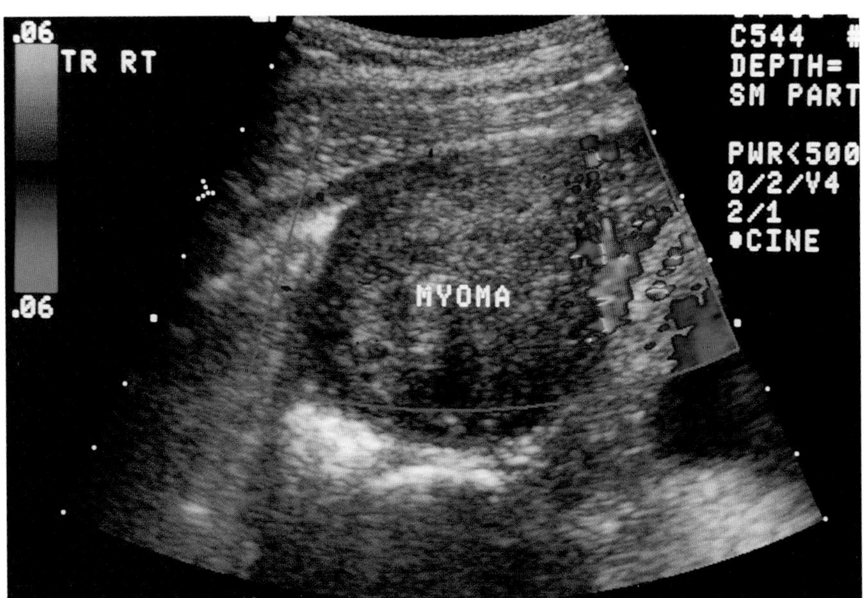

FIG. 1.33. Degenerating uterine myoma misdiagnosed clinically as appendicitis. Color Doppler sonography demonstrates large right-sided myoma with no internal vascularity. Infarcted uterine myoma found at surgery.

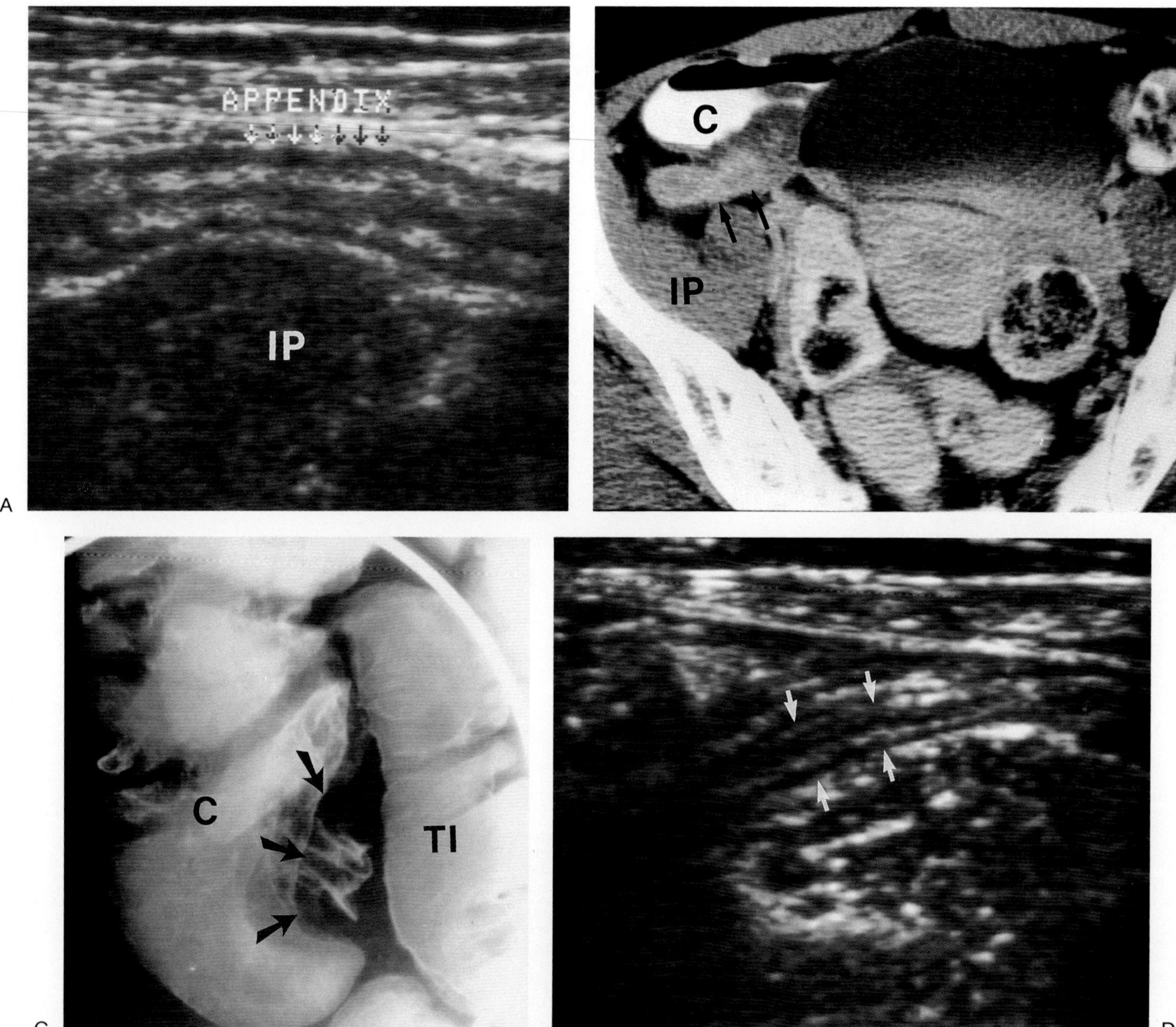

FIG. 1.34. Spontaneous resolution of acute appendicitis. **A:** Graded compression sonogram demonstrates noncompressible 9-mm appendix consistent with acute appendicitis (IP, iliopsoas muscle). **B:** Retrocecal appendicitis is confirmed by CT. Note thickened retrocecal appendix (*arrows*). C, cecum; IP, iliopsoas muscle. **C:** Barium enema performed same day reveals mass effect on cecal tip (*arrows*) and lack of filling of appendix compatible with appendicitis. Patient refused surgery. Two weeks later patient was asymptomatic. **D:** Repeat sonogram reveals normal size (6 mm) appendix (*arrows*). One year later patient had recurrent appendicitis with positive sonogram. Surgery revealed acute appendicitis with areas of chronic scarring and fibrosis.

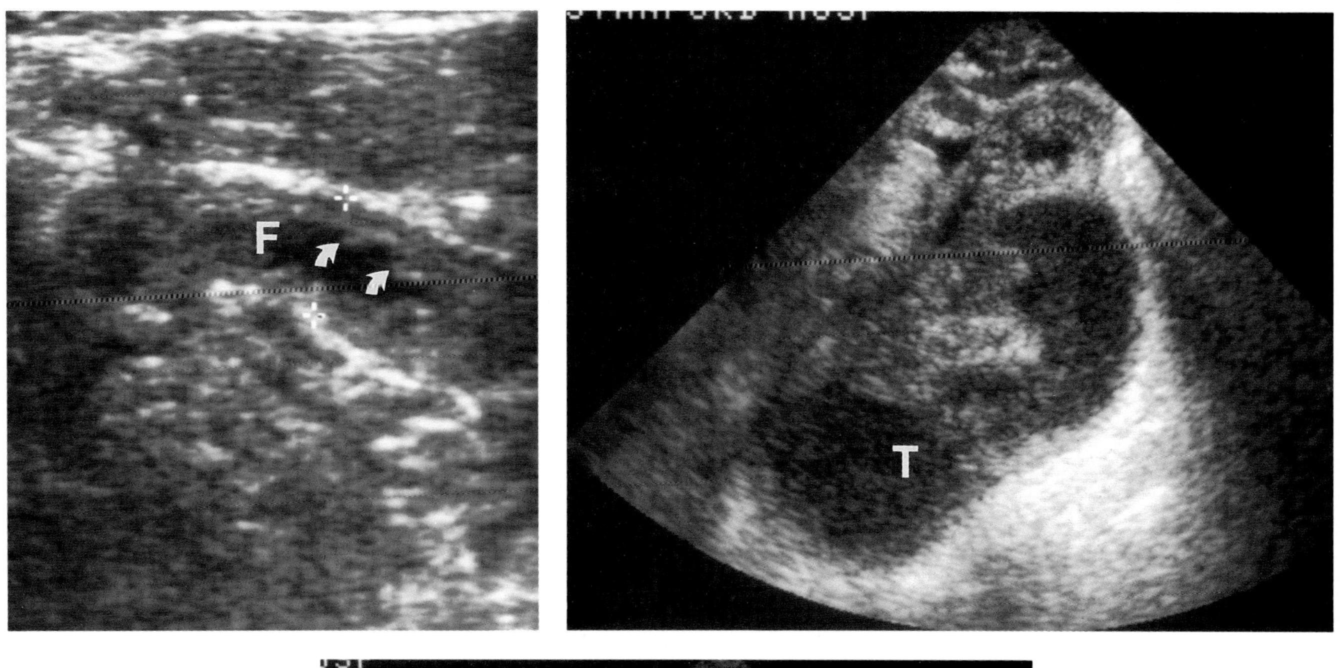

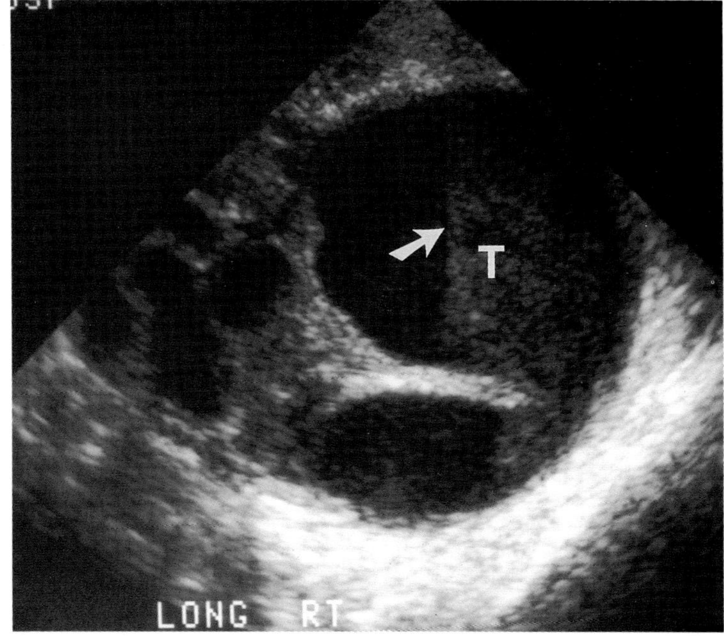

FIG. 1.35. Salpingitis mimicking appendicitis in three patients. **A:** Sonogram of right lower quadrant reveals slightly dilated fallopian tube resembling an appendix. Note undulating mucosal folds of fallopian tube (*arrows*) and lack of convincing echogenic submucosal layer. F, fallopian tube. **B, C:** In two other patients, dilated, pus-filled tubes (T) are identified with endovaginal probe. Note echogenic pus in both tubes and fluid–fluid level (*arrow* in C).

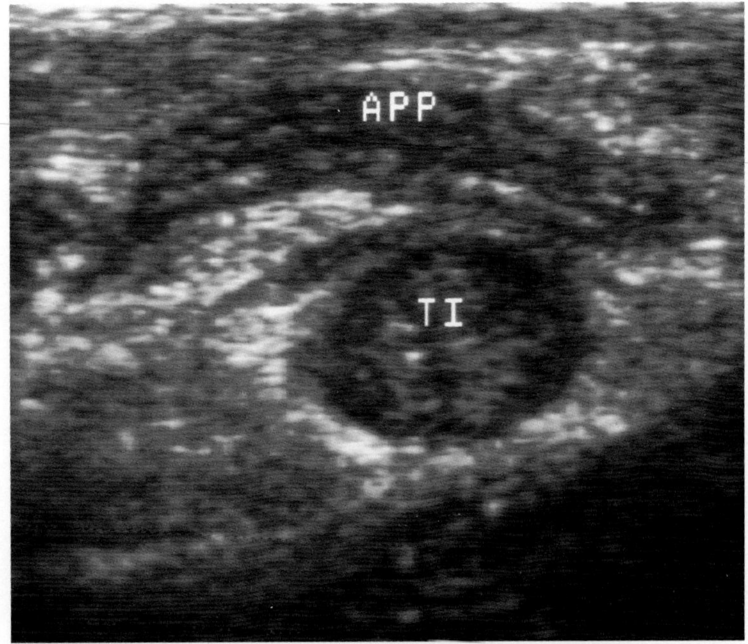

A

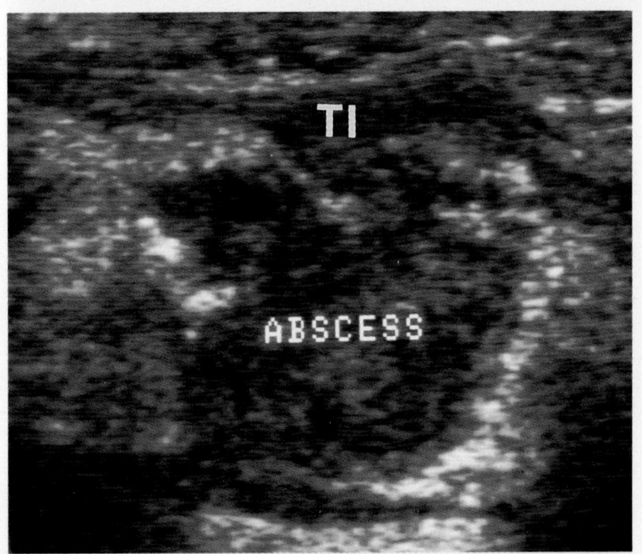

B

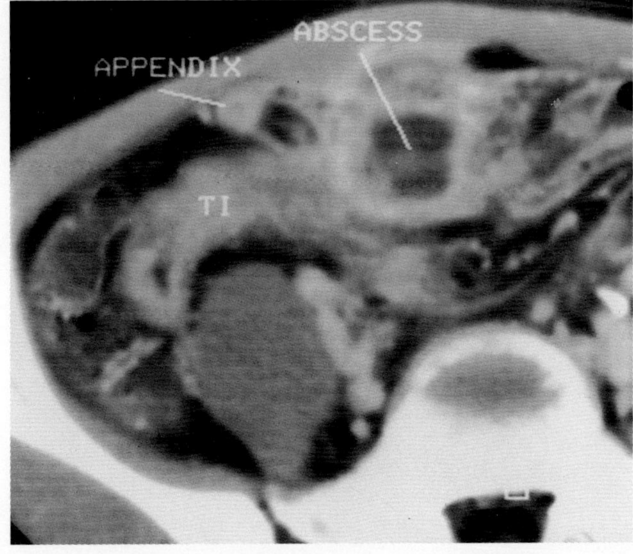

C

FIG. 1.36. Secondary inflammation of appendix (periappendicitis) caused by Crohn's disease. **A:** Enlarged noncompressible 8-mm appendix (APP) anterior to markedly inflamed terminal ileum (TI) from Crohn's disease. **B:** Abscess adjacent to terminal ileum (TI). **C:** CT scan confirms enlarged appendix anterior to thickened terminal ileum (TI). Note adjacent abscess.

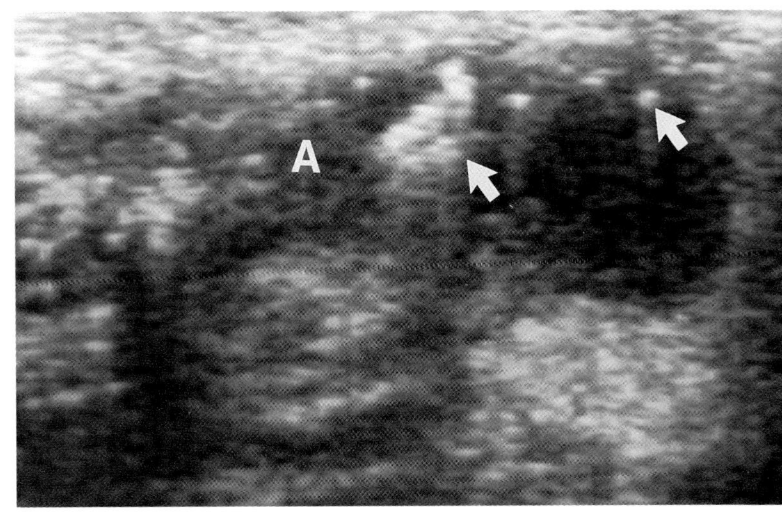

FIG. 1.37. Gas-filled inflamed appendix. Sagittal scan of appendix (A) demonstrates extensive intraluminal gas (*arrows*) almost obscuring inflamed appendix (A).

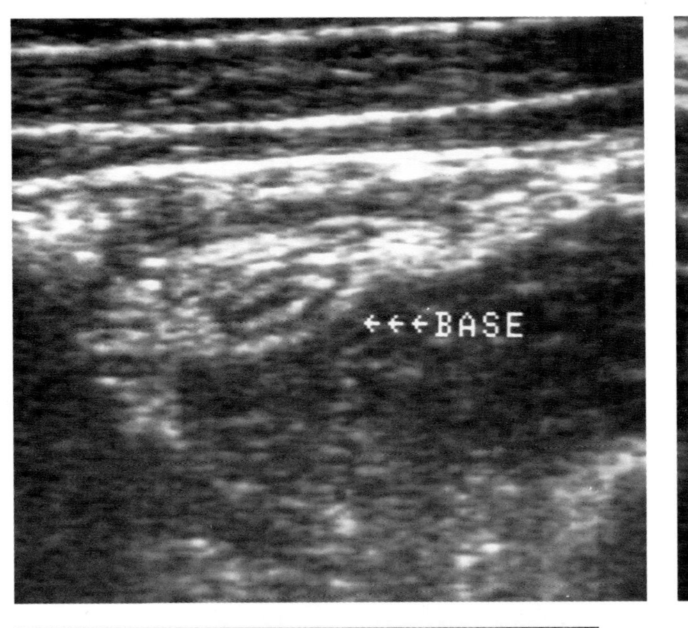

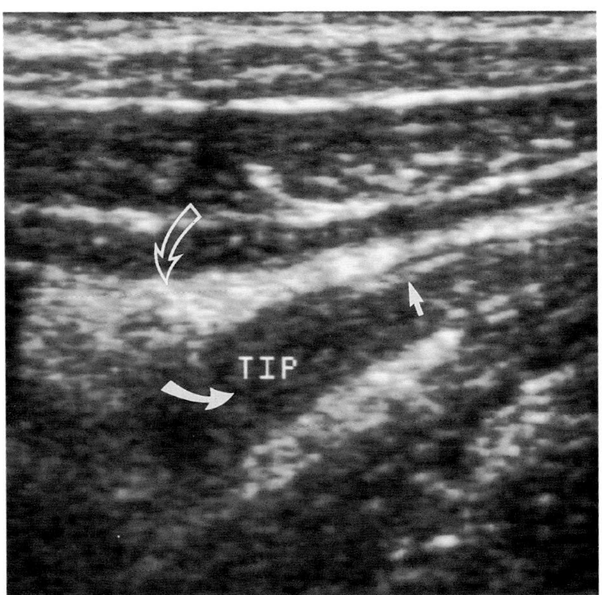

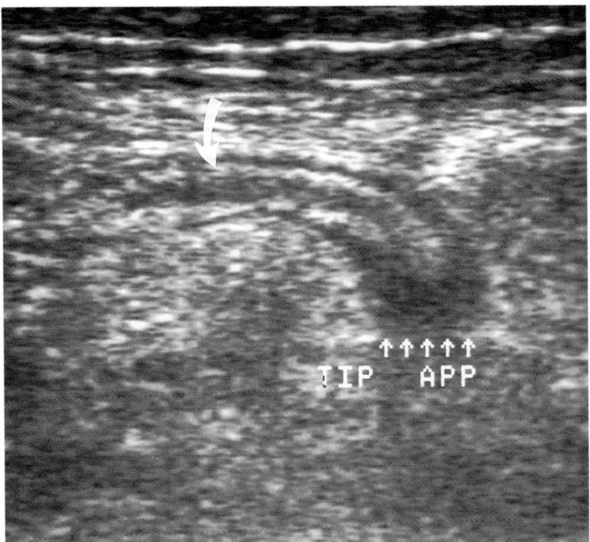

FIG. 1.38. Appendicitis confined to the tip of the appendix in two patients. **A:** Transverse scan of right lower quadrant demonstrating normal base of the appendix (*arrows*) measuring 6 mm. **B:** Tip of the appendix demonstrates significant enlargement and loss of echogenic submucosal layer (*arrow*). Note inflamed periappendiceal fat (*curved arrow*). Note intact submucosal layer in proximal appendix (*arrow*). **C:** In another patient, note enlarged hypoechoic tip (*arrows*) of appendix (APP). Note normal base of the appendix (*curved arrow*).

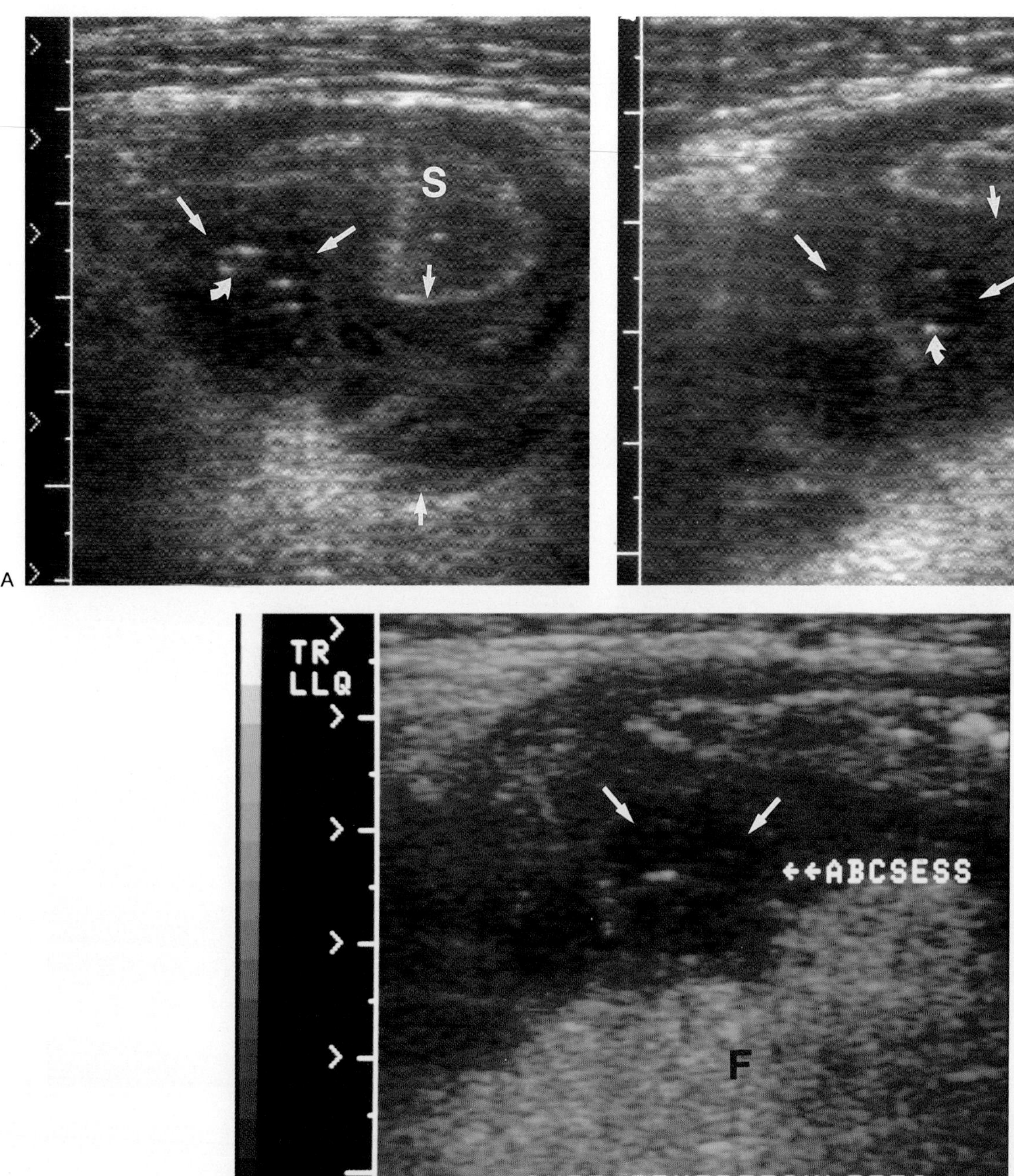

FIG. 1.39. Sigmoid diverticulitis with paracolonic abscess. Sagittal (**A**) and transverse (**B**) views of sigmoid colon (S) demonstrate marked mural thickening (*short arrows*) and hypoechoic abscess (*long arrows*). Note gas bubbles within abscess (*curved arrow*). Abscess cavity is better appreciated on B-color image (*arrows*) (**C**). Also note echogenic inflamed mesenteric fat (F). Color Doppler sonograms (**D, E**) reveal increased vascularity of sigmoid (S). Contrast CT (**F**) scan demonstrates mural thickening of sigmoid (S) and paracolonic abscess (A) with gas bubble (*curved arrow*).

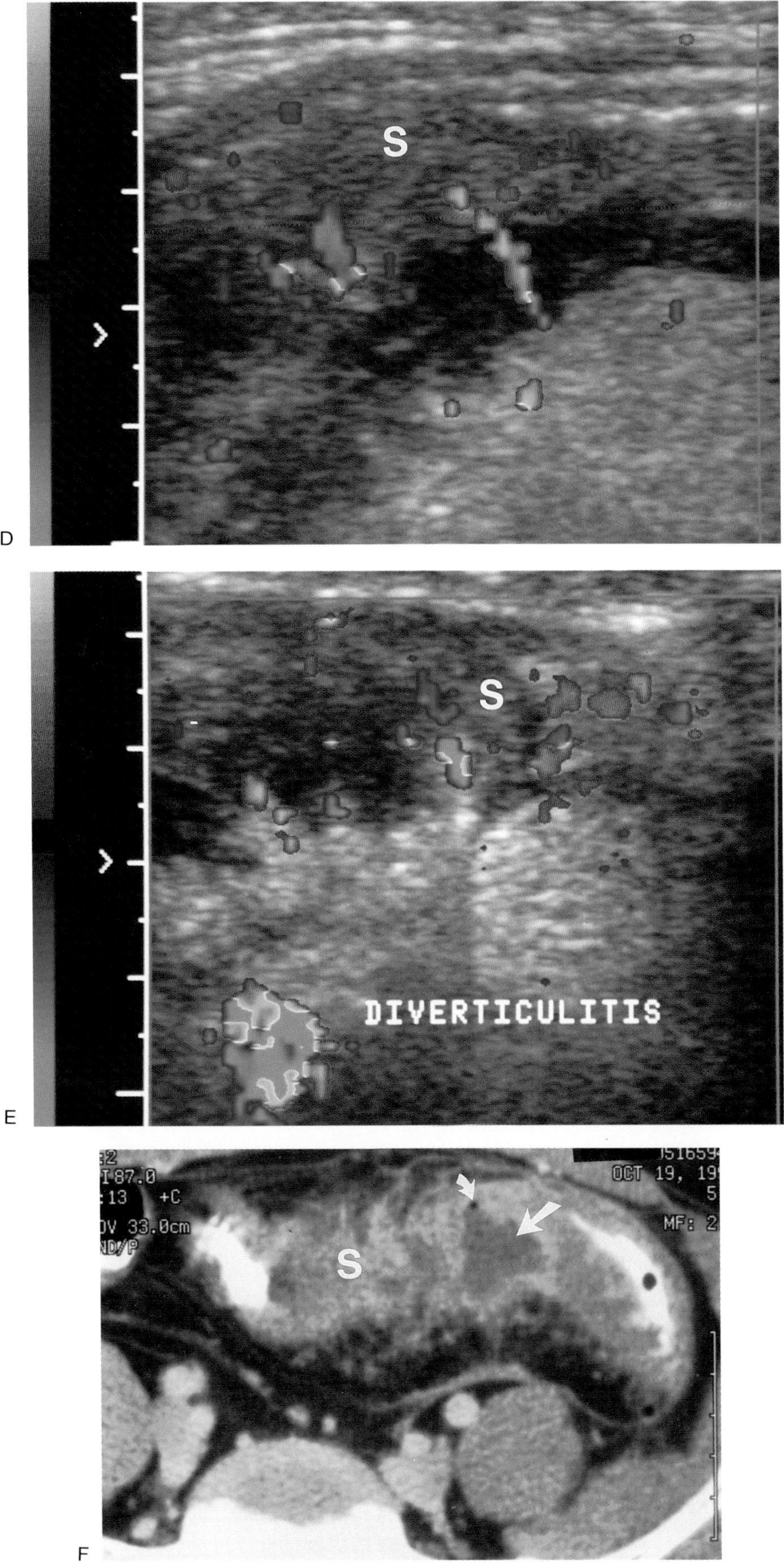

FIG. 1.39. *Continued.*

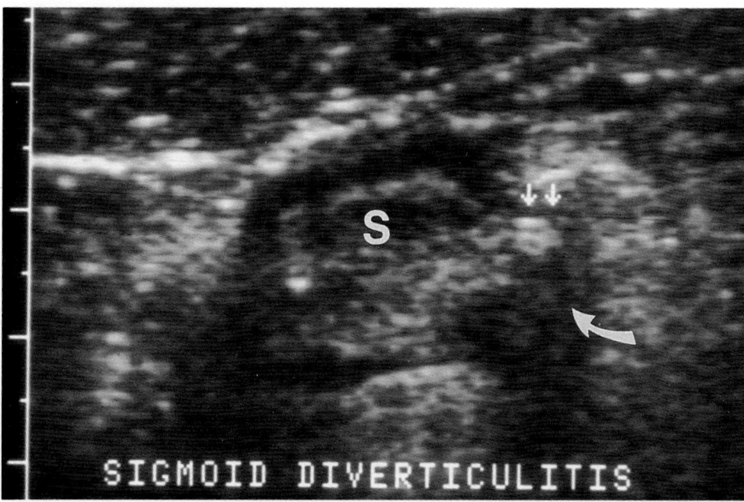

FIG. 1.40. Sigmoid diverticulitis with visualization of infected diverticulum. Note echogenic diverticulum (*arrows*) within thickened mural segment of sigmoid (S) casting an acoustic shadow (*curved arrow*).

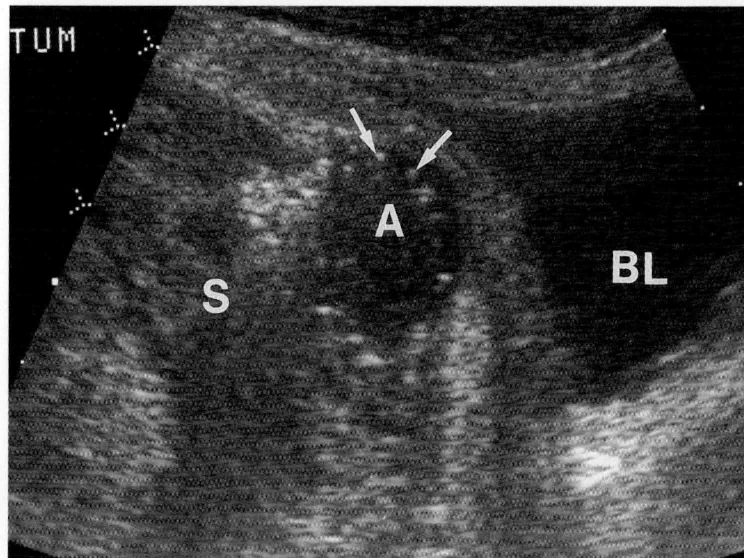

FIG. 1.41. Paracolonic abscess from diverticulitis. Sagittal scan of rectosigmoid colon (S) demonstrates well-defined intramural abscess (A) with multiple gas bubbles (*arrows*). BL, bladder.

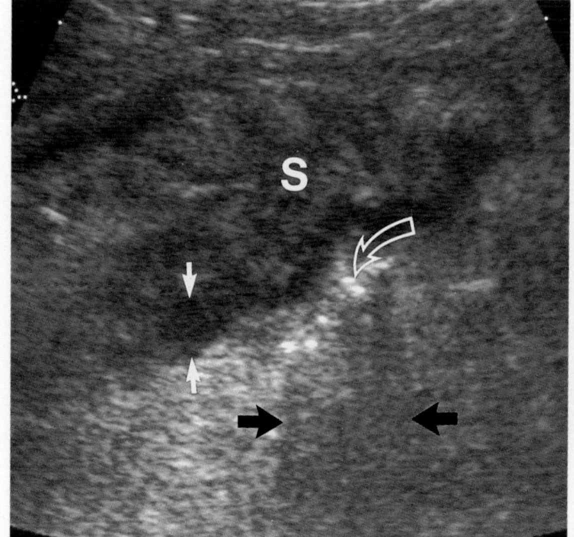

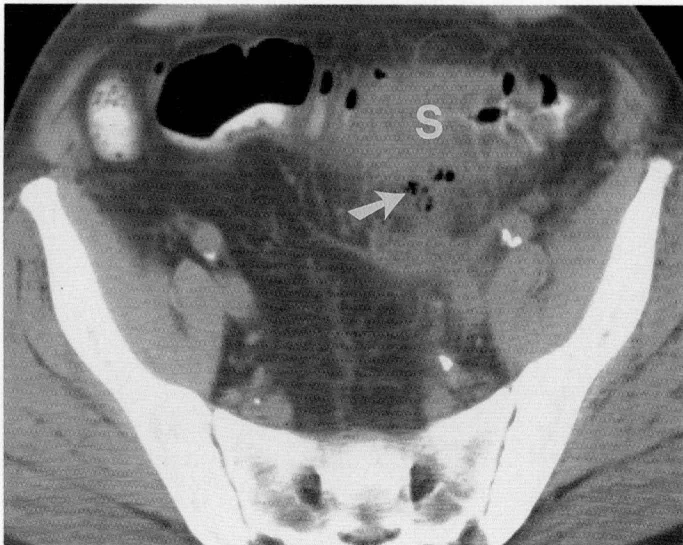

FIG. 1.42. Perforated sigmoid diverticulitis with gas bubbles in sigmoid mesentery. **A:** Sigmoid colon (S) with mural thickening (*arrows*). Note multiple gas bubbles in sigmoid mesentery (*curved arrow*). Distal acoustic shadowing is evident from gas (*black arrows*). **B:** Contrast CT scan reveals mural thickening of sigmoid (S) and multiple gas bubbles (*arrow*) in sigmoid mesentery but no discrete abscess.

with acoustic shadowing. In perforated diverticulitis, a pelvic abscess may be identified. Gas bubbles in the sigmoid mesentery appear sonographically as echogenic linear areas with or without distal shadowing (Figs. 1.41 and 1.42). Cecal diverticulitis may clinically mimic appendicitis; this entity should be considered in adult patients with mural thickening of the cecum and no evidence of an inflamed appendix (Fig. 1.28).

The CT scan or sonographic demonstration of focal mural thickening of the colon with surrounding inflammatory changes is a nonspecific finding. Although commonly due to diverticulitis, a perforated colonic neoplasm can never entirely be excluded. When acute symptoms subside, further studies such as a barium enema or endoscopy should be performed to exclude carcinoma.

Enteritis and Colitis

Stool culture, endoscopy, and barium studies remain the primary methods for diagnosis of infectious enteritis and colitis. In patients with AIDS and opportunistic infection of the gastrointestinal tract, contrast CT is the method of choice to demonstrate associated visceral microabscesses and retroperitoneal lymphadenopathy (16). Abnormalities of the gastrointestinal tract may be discovered incidentally in patients with fever and abdominal pain referred for evaluation of appendicitis or an abdominal abscess. The sonographic findings of enteritis or colitis are typically nonspecific, demonstrating focal areas of mural thickening of the bowel and echogenic inflamed mesenteric fat (51). Enteritis and colitis are common causes of an acute abdomen in patients with AIDS (Fig. 1.43) (16). Mesenteric adenopathy may be present in patients with *Campylobacter jejuni, Mycobacterium avium-intracellulare,* and *Yersinia enterocolitica* (35). It is generally not possible to distinguish infectious ileitis from Crohn's disease by sonography. Demonstration of echogenic sinus tracts within the bowel wall and mesentery favors the diagnosis of Crohn's disease.

Crohn's Disease

In patients with an acute episode or recurrence of Crohn's disease, the important clinical facts to be determined are (a) the site and extent of bowel involvement and (b) the presence of specific complications, such as stricture formation, fistulas, or abscesses. Barium studies and endoscopy are most helpful in assessing mucosal abnormalities, strictures, and fistulas. CT is of considerable value in identifying fibrofatty masses ("creeping fat"), mesenteric abscesses, and other complications, such as colovesical fistulas (52–57). Sonography plays a limited role in the patient with known Crohn's disease but may suggest the diagnosis in patients with focal mural bowel wall thickening and echogenic mesenteric fatty masses (Fig. 1.44). Color Doppler sonography of affected bowel loops may demonstrate striking increased mural vascularity (Fig. 1.44). Gas within enteric abscesses or sinus tracts may be evident sonographically but is often better demonstrated by CT (Fig. 1.45).

Pseudomembranous Colitis

It is not uncommon for postoperative patients with fever to be evaluated by sonography or CT for suspected abdominal abscesses only to discover thickening of the colon (58,59). In this clinical setting colonic thickening is often due to pseudomembranous colitis from overgrowth of *Clostridium difficile.* A history of recent antibiotic therapy is characteristic. The right colon is more commonly affected (Figs. 1.46 and 1.47) (60–63). In patients who are immunosuppressed, neutropenic colitis should also be considered in the differential diagnosis.

Mesenteric Adenitis

When there is no evidence of appendicitis or terminal ileitis, the sonographic demonstration of enlarged mesenteric lymph nodes is highly suggestive of mesenteric adenitis (Figs. 1.27 and 1.28) (51). These patients should be observed clinically without early surgical intervention as the symptoms of mesenteric adenitis will generally resolve spontaneously without specific therapy. Color Doppler sonography is particularly valuable in distinguishing mesenteric vessels from lymph nodes.

OTHER CAUSES OF ABDOMINAL PAIN

Intestinal Obstruction

In general, plain abdominal radiographs and barium studies are the primary methods to evaluate patients with suspected bowel obstruction. Sonography and CT, however, may occasionally provide important diagnostic information (64–72). Sonography is particularly valuable in patients with nondiagnostic plain radiographs due to a large amount of fluid and secretions within the lumen of the small bowel. The sonographic hallmark of small bowel obstruction is dilatation of fluid-filled loops of bowel with increased peristaltic activity on real-time examination (Fig. 1.48). A specific attempt should be made to identify a transition zone between dilated and nondilated bowel diagnostic of obstruction (Fig. 1.49). On occasion mesenteric masses, gastrointestinal tumors, and abscesses may be identified as the cause of small bowel obstruction. CT is superior to sonography in demonstrating internal hernias, closed loop, and neoplastic obstruction.

(*text continues on page 43*)

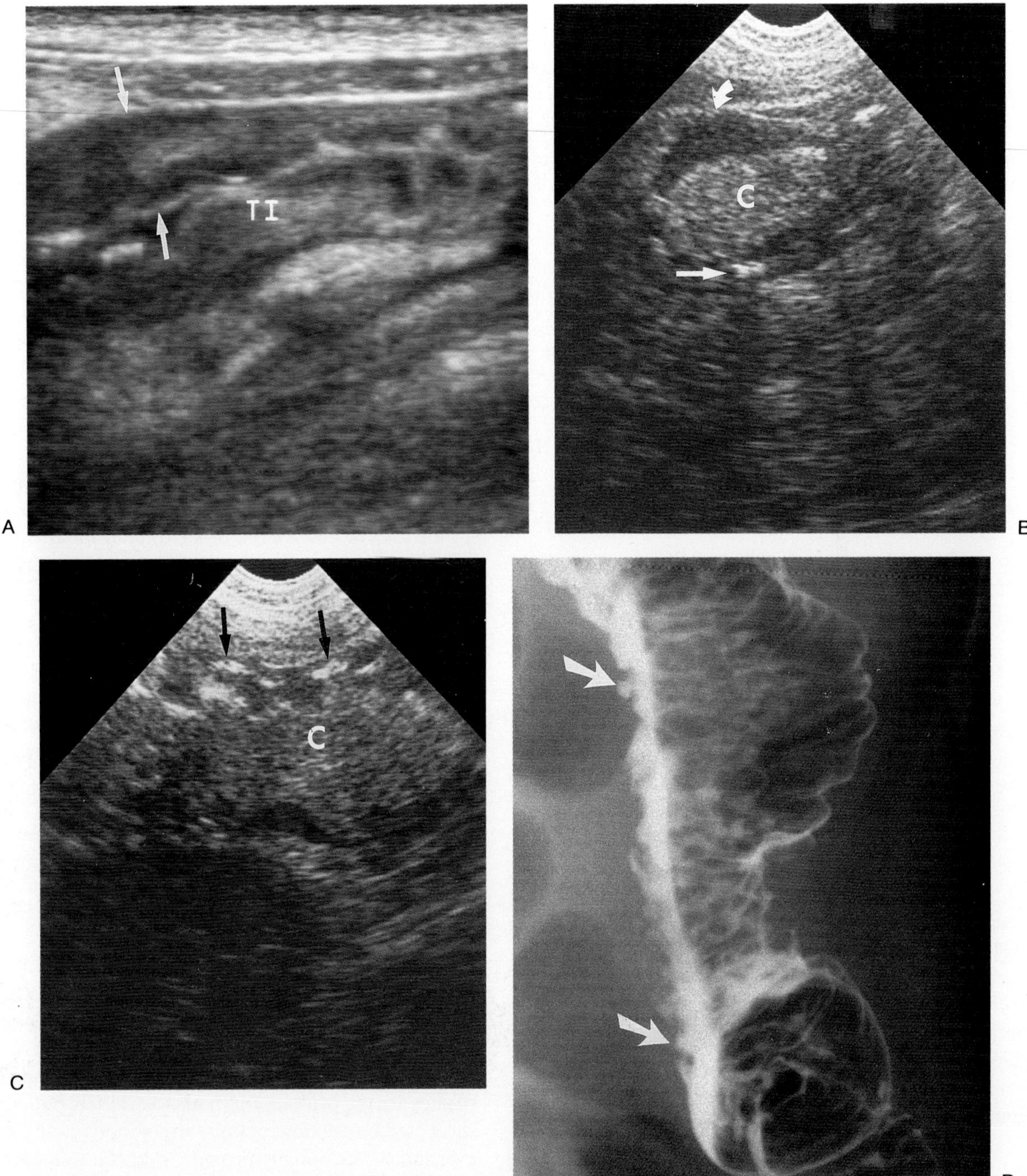

FIG. 1.43. Enteritis and colitis in two patients with AIDS. **A:** Note marked mural thickening (*arrows*) of terminal ileum (TI) due to cytomegalovirus enteritis. **B–D:** In another patient with AIDS and shigellosis of the colon, note intramural thickening (*curved arrows* in B) and pneumatosis (*arrows* in B and C) of colon (C) due to deep ulcerations seen on pneumocolon (*arrows* in D).

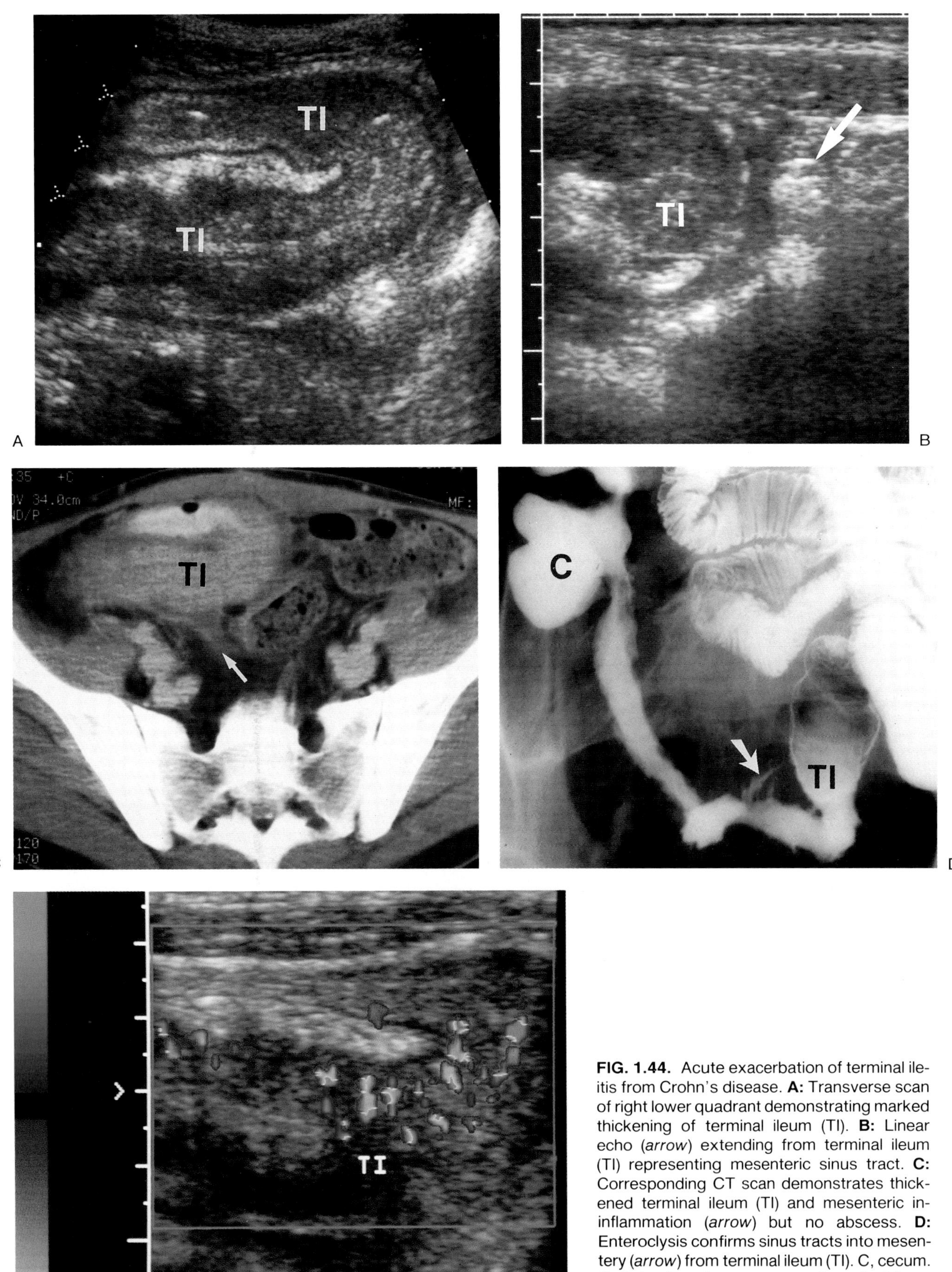

FIG. 1.44. Acute exacerbation of terminal ileitis from Crohn's disease. **A:** Transverse scan of right lower quadrant demonstrating marked thickening of terminal ileum (TI). **B:** Linear echo (*arrow*) extending from terminal ileum (TI) representing mesenteric sinus tract. **C:** Corresponding CT scan demonstrates thickened terminal ileum (TI) and mesenteric in-inflammation (*arrow*) but no abscess. **D:** Enteroclysis confirms sinus tracts into mesentery (*arrow*) from terminal ileum (TI). C, cecum. **E:** Color Doppler sonogram of terminal ileum (TI) reveals prominent mural vascularity secondary to Crohn's disease.

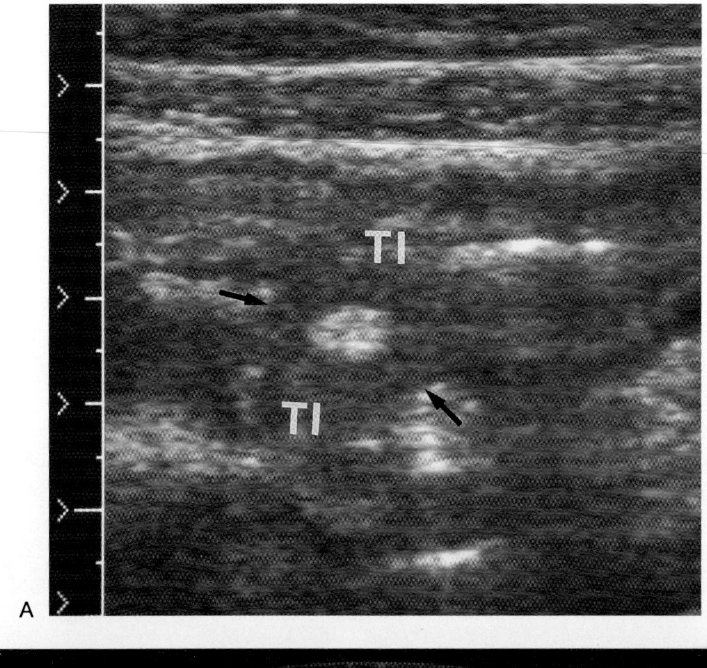

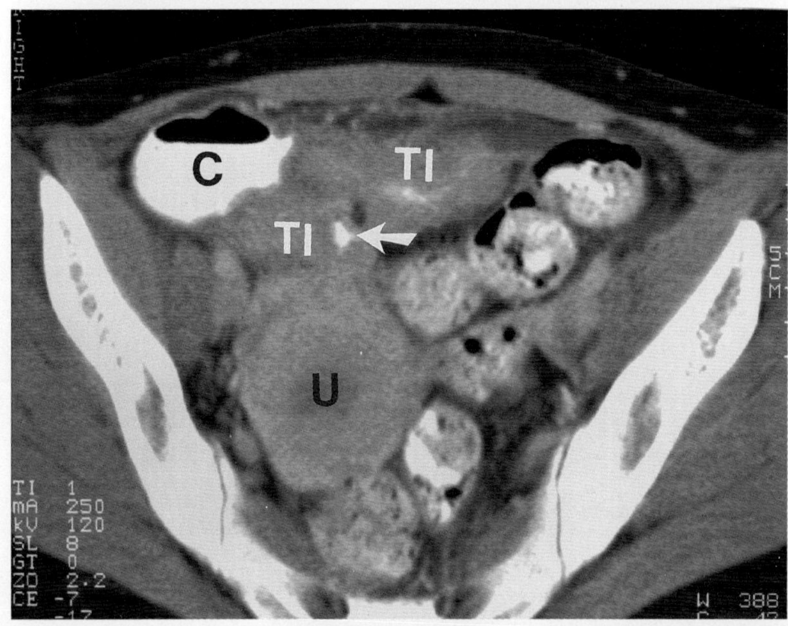

FIG. 1.45. Fistulous tracts in Crohn's disease. **A:** Transverse sonogram of terminal ileum (TI) with two discrete fistulous tracts (*arrows*). **B:** Contrast CT scan demonstrates small amount of oral contrast opacifying fistulous tract between loops of terminal ileum (TI). U, uterus; C, cecum.

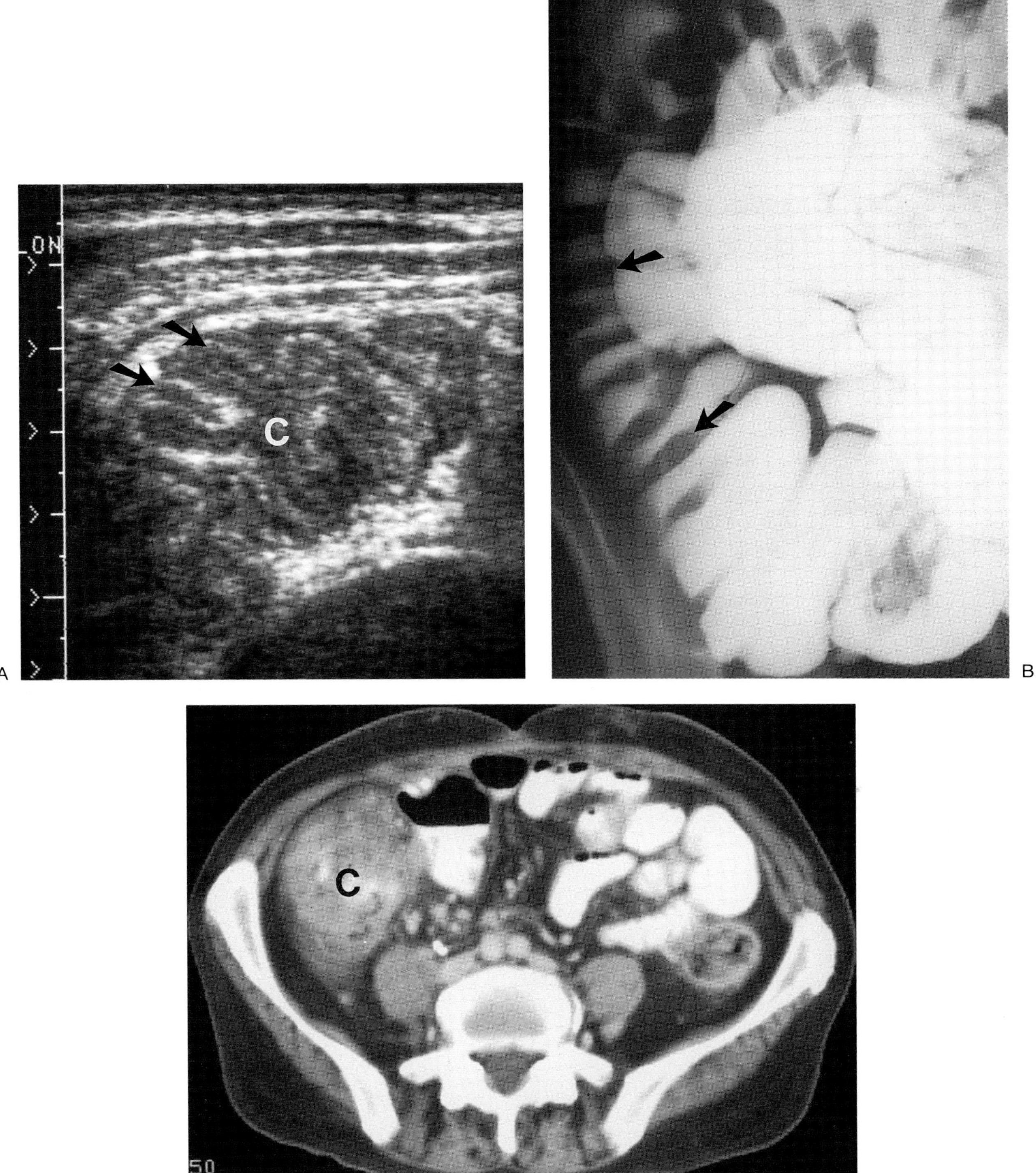

FIG. 1.46. Pseudomembranous colitis of right colon. **A:** Transverse scan of right colon (C) demonstrating mural thickening and edema of haustra (*arrows*). **B:** Barium enema confirms diffuse haustral fold thickening (*arrows*). **C:** CT scan reveals marked mural thickening of right colon (C).

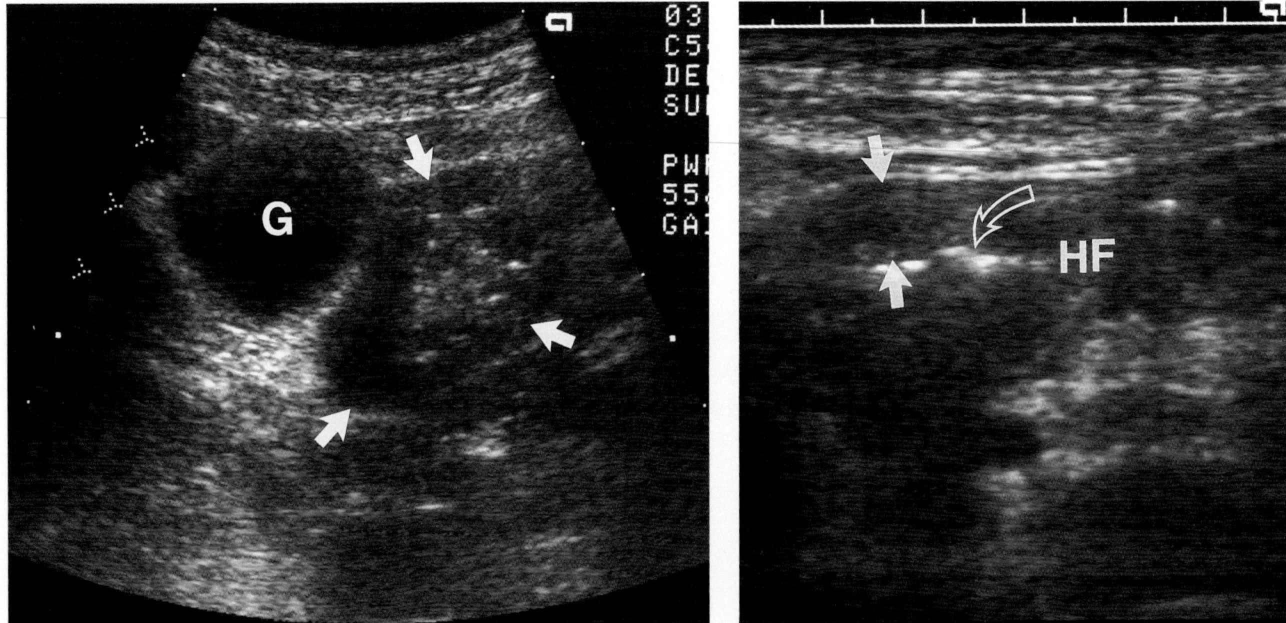

FIG. 1.47. Pseudomembranous colitis of hepatic flexure mimicking acute cholecystitis. **A:** Sagittal scan of right upper quadrant demonstrates thickened hepatic flexure of colon (*arrows*) adjacent to gallbladder (G). **B:** Transverse scan demonstrates diffuse mural thickening (*arrows*) of hepatic flexure (HF). *Curved arrow*, lumen. Patient had focal pain directly over hepatic flexure misdiagnosed as acute cholecystitis.

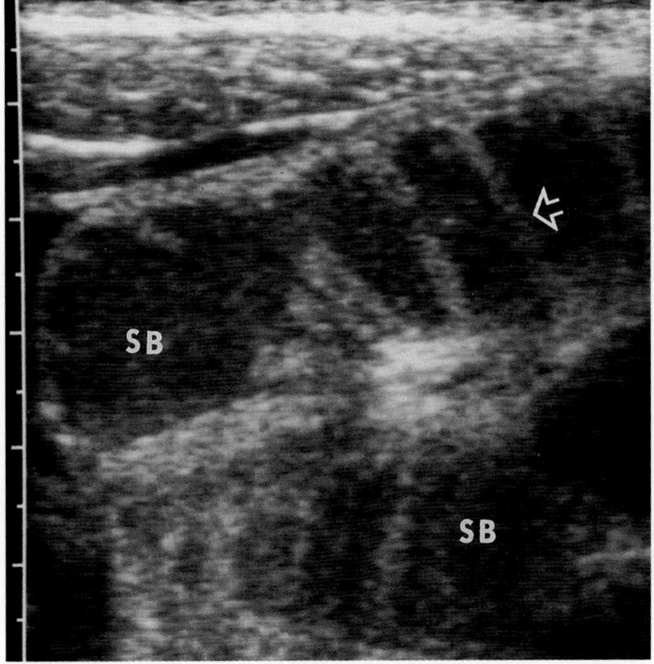

FIG. 1.48. Closed loop small bowel obstruction. Note U-shaped configuration of dilated, fluid-filled small bowel (SB). Increased peristalsis was noted on real-time examination. Closed loop obstruction from adhesions found at surgery.

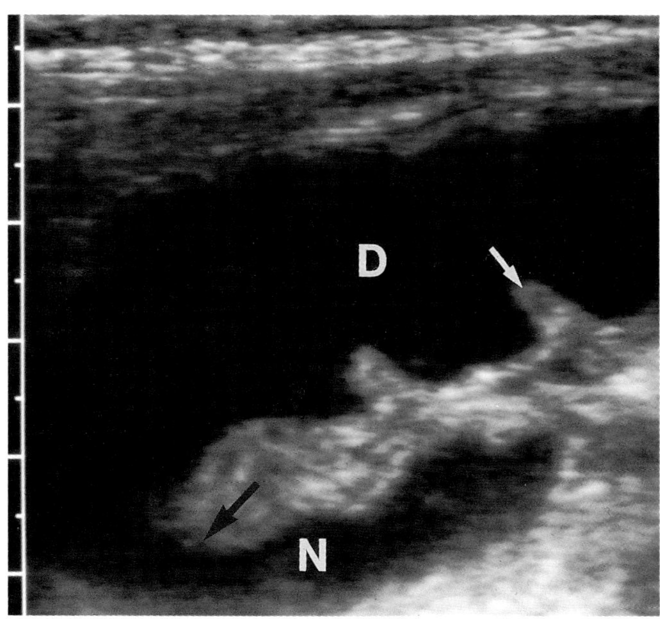

FIG. 1.49. Small bowel obstruction with transition zone identified by sonography. Transverse scan of distal small bowel demonstrates transition zone (*black arrow*) between dilated (D) and normal caliber (N) small bowel. Note thickened folds in obstructed segment (*arrow*). Adhesive band obstructing ileum found at surgery.

A

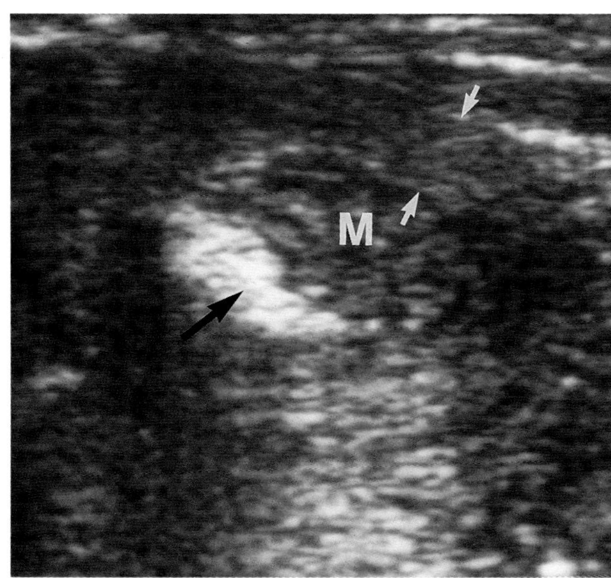

FIG. 1.50. Intussusception diagnosed by sonography and CT. **A:** Transverse scan of thickened segment of small bowel in left lower quadrant. Note crescentic area of echogenic fat (*black arrow*) from invaginated intussusceptum. Hypoechoic mass (M) is seen centrally adjacent to mesenteric fat. Note thickened wall (*white arrows*). **B:** Contrast CT scan demonstrating crescentic invaginated fat (*arrow*) diagnostic of intussusception. Lymphoma of small bowel was the lead point of the intussusception at surgery.

B

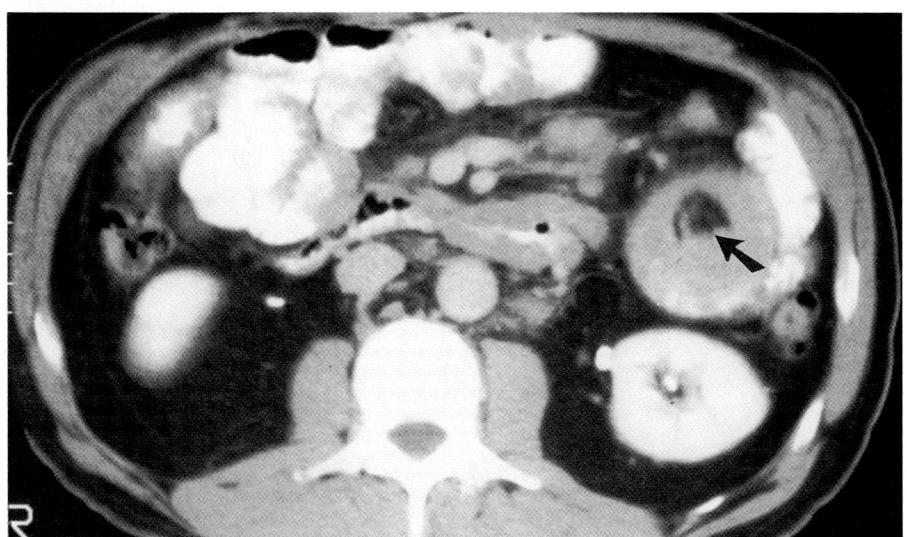

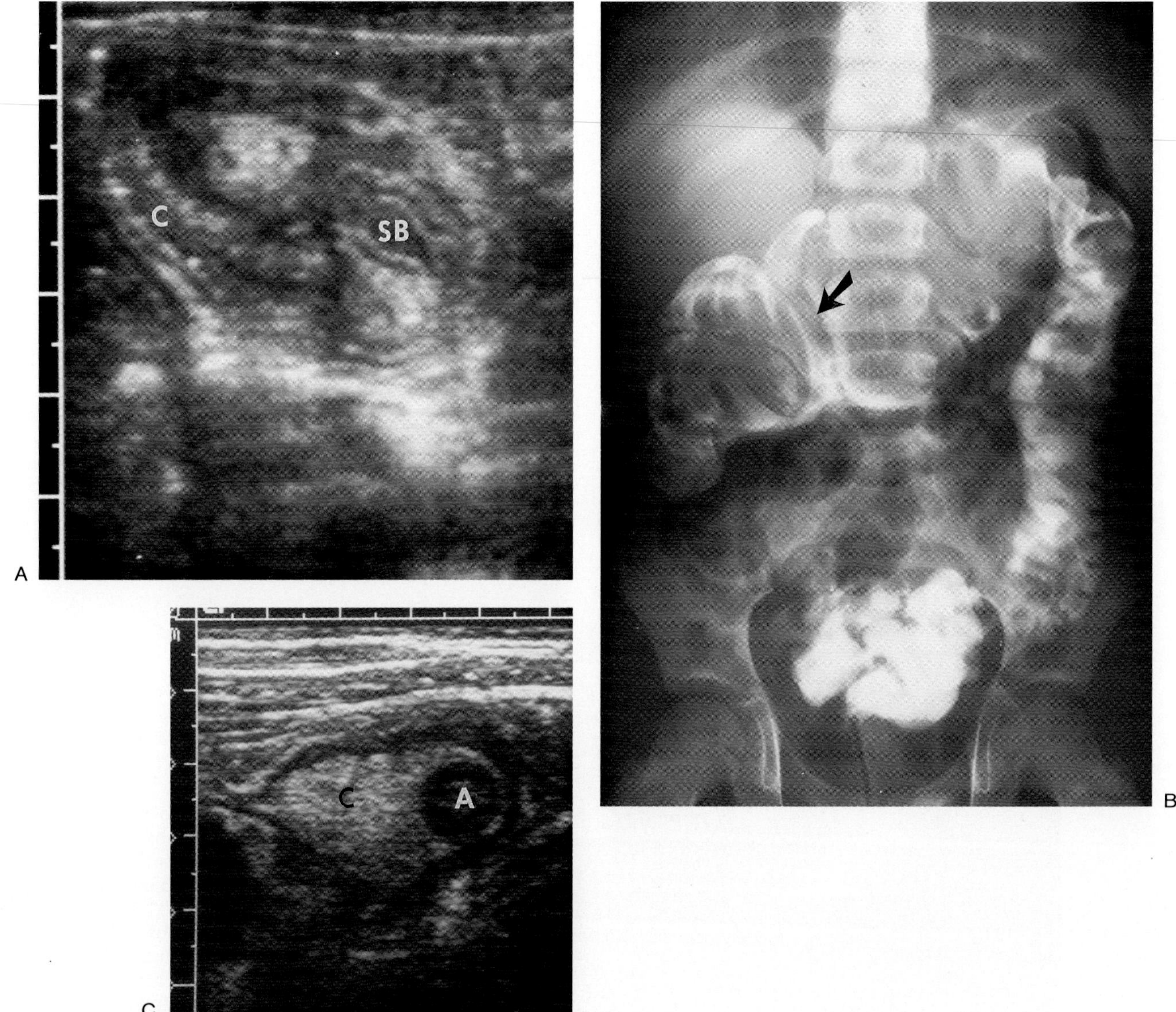

FIG. 1.51. A: Sonography of intussusception. Note intussuscepted small bowel (SB) within cecum (C). **B:** Barium enema confirms ileocolic intussusception (*arrow*). Patient had cystic fibrosis. **C:** In another patient thickened appendix (A) is seen to be invaginated within cecum (C). (A and B from ref. 68, with permission; C from ref. 69, with permission.)

Intussusception is an uncommon, but important, form of bowel obstruction. In adults, a tumor mass is typically the lead point. A key imaging observation in patients with intussusception is the invaginated mesenteric fat of the intussusceptum. Sonographically, a crescentic intraluminal area of echogenic fat is noted (Figs. 1.50 and 1.51) (68–72). In some patients intussusception may appear sonographically as a nonspecific mass (Fig. 1.52). Unless a lead point for the intussusception is a cystic mass (i.e., mucocele of the appendix), the actual cause of intussusception cannot be diagnosed with sonography. On a CT scan, a fat-containing lead mass (lipoma) can be diagnosed due to its negative attenuation values.

Gastric outlet obstruction can be suggested sonographically by observing marked retention of fluid and secretions within the stomach coupled with a collapsed duodenum. In some patients, focal thickening of the antrum from carcinoma can be identified. Similarly, in pediatric patients gastric outlet obstruction from pyloric stenosis can be diagnosed with sonography by identification of marked mural thickening of the muscular ring in the antropyloric area. In general, the mural thickness of the antrum and pylorus should be 3 mm or less. Mural thickness of 4 mm or greater is reliable evidence for the sonographic diagnosis of pyloric stenosis (Fig. 1.53) (73).

Small Bowel Infarction

Mesenteric angiography and contrast CT are the imaging methods of choice to confirm clinically suspected acute small bowel infarction (74–77). CT can reliably demonstrate focal mural thickening of the bowel wall, intramural pneumatosis, and mesenteric thrombosis. The diagnosis may be suggested sonographically when dilated atonic loops of bowel are noted with thickened small bowel folds (Fig. 1.54). Mural thickening may be due to edema or hemorrhage. An attempt should be made to evaluate the bowel wall with color Doppler sonography using graded compression technique and a 5-MHz transducer. A thickened segment of bowel with no demonstrable flow to the bowel wall should suggest the diagnosis of ischemia or infarction (Fig. 1.55). To date, the results of color Doppler sonography in small bowel infarction are quite preliminary and must be confirmed with larger clinical trials.

Intramural Hemorrhage

Intramural hemorrhage of the small bowel or colon may be due to trauma, vasculitis, coagulopathy, ischemia, or infections such as cytomegalovirus. In acute intramural hemorrhage, there is often diffuse increased echogenicity of the bowel wall (Figs. 1.56 to 1.58). In more chronic forms of hemorrhage such as ischemic colitis, the bowel wall is thickened and hypoechoic. Scalloping of the submucosal line may be present due to submucosal hemorrhage (Fig. 1.59). This corresponds to the "thumbprinting" visualized on plain films and barium studies due to subacute submucosal hemorrhage. On occasion, rectus sheath or abdominal wall hemorrhage may clinically be misdiagnosed as an intraperitoneal lesion.

Mucocele of the Appendix

Chronic obstruction of the appendix may result in a mucocele. Although typically benign, it is rarely associated with mucinous cystadenocarcinoma. Rupture of a mucocele may lead to pseudomyxoma peritonei. Mucoceles typically appear sonographically as a tubular complex cystic mass at the base of the cecum (Fig. 1.60) (78). There may be mural calcification in chronic cases. Thick mucoid elements may be echogenic on sonography.

Gastrointestinal Tract Tumors

Prior to the recent development of endoluminal sonography, the role of cross-sectional imaging in the diagnosis and staging of gastrointestinal tract neoplasms had been quite limited. On occasion, bulky gastrointestinal tract neoplasms may be discovered incidentally during routine CT or sonography (Figs. 1.61 and 1.62). Superficial mucosal lesions virtually always require bariumstudies or endoscopy for precise diagnosis. Tumors diffusely infiltrating the bowel wall cause either concentric or asymmetric mural thickening of the bowel on sonography (Figs. 1.63 to 1.65).

Precise preoperative assessment of the depth of mural invasion of gastrointestinal tract neoplasms is critical for patient management (79). This is particularly true of esophageal and rectal neoplasms. Superficial lesions may be treated with local resection with a high rate of cure. Tumors infiltrating through the muscularis propria or serosa of the bowel wall must be treated with more radical surgery. Patients with superficial rectal carcinoma may successfully undergo low anterior resection. However, lesions invading the serosa or perirectal fat virtually always require abdominal perineal resection. Infiltration of esophageal carcinoma beyond the submucosal layer precludes radical surgery and is usually treated with radiation and/or chemotherapy.

The CT and sonographic appearance of many gastrointestinal tract neoplasms is nonspecific and can be mimicked by focal inflammatory processes such as Crohn's disease, tuberculosis, pancreatitis, or even intramural hemorrhage. Exophytic gastrointestinal neoplasms, such as gastrointestinal stromal tumor (leiomyosarcoma), are bulky masses with a relatively small intramural component (Figs. 1.64 and 1.65). Gastrointestinal lymphoma has a variety of appearances and may

(text continues on page 54)

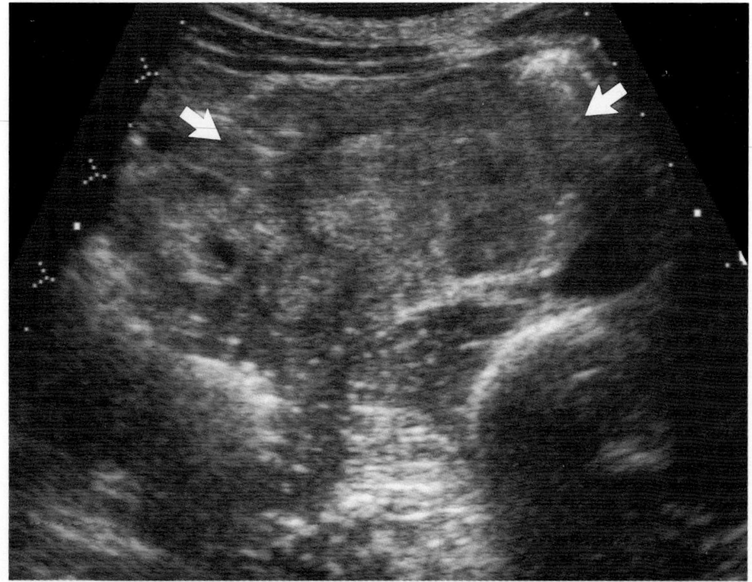

A

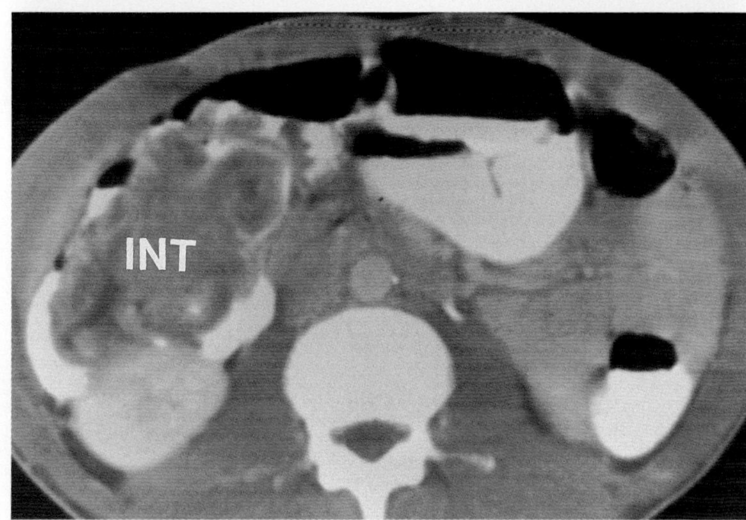

B

FIG. 1.52. Intussusception as nonspecific mass on sonography. **A:** Oblique scan of right lower quadrant demonstrating a nonspecific mass (*arrows*) of mixed echogenicity. **B:** CT scan clearly identifies intussuscepting right colonic mass. Cecal carcinoma found at surgery.

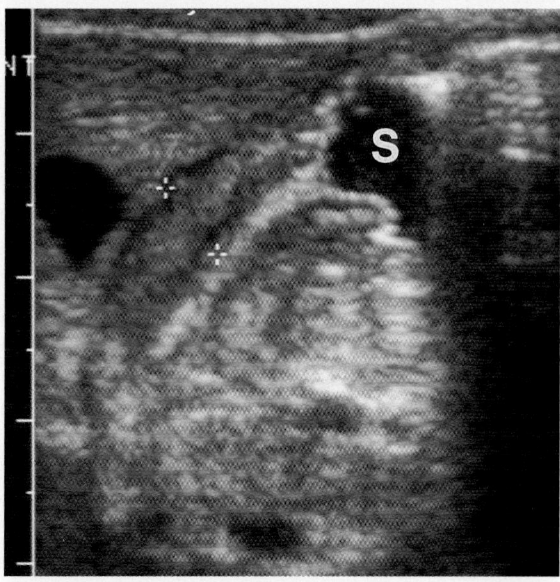

FIG. 1.53. Pyloric stenosis. Transverse scan of distal stomach (S) demonstrates marked mural thickening (6 mm) of pyloric channel (*cursors*).

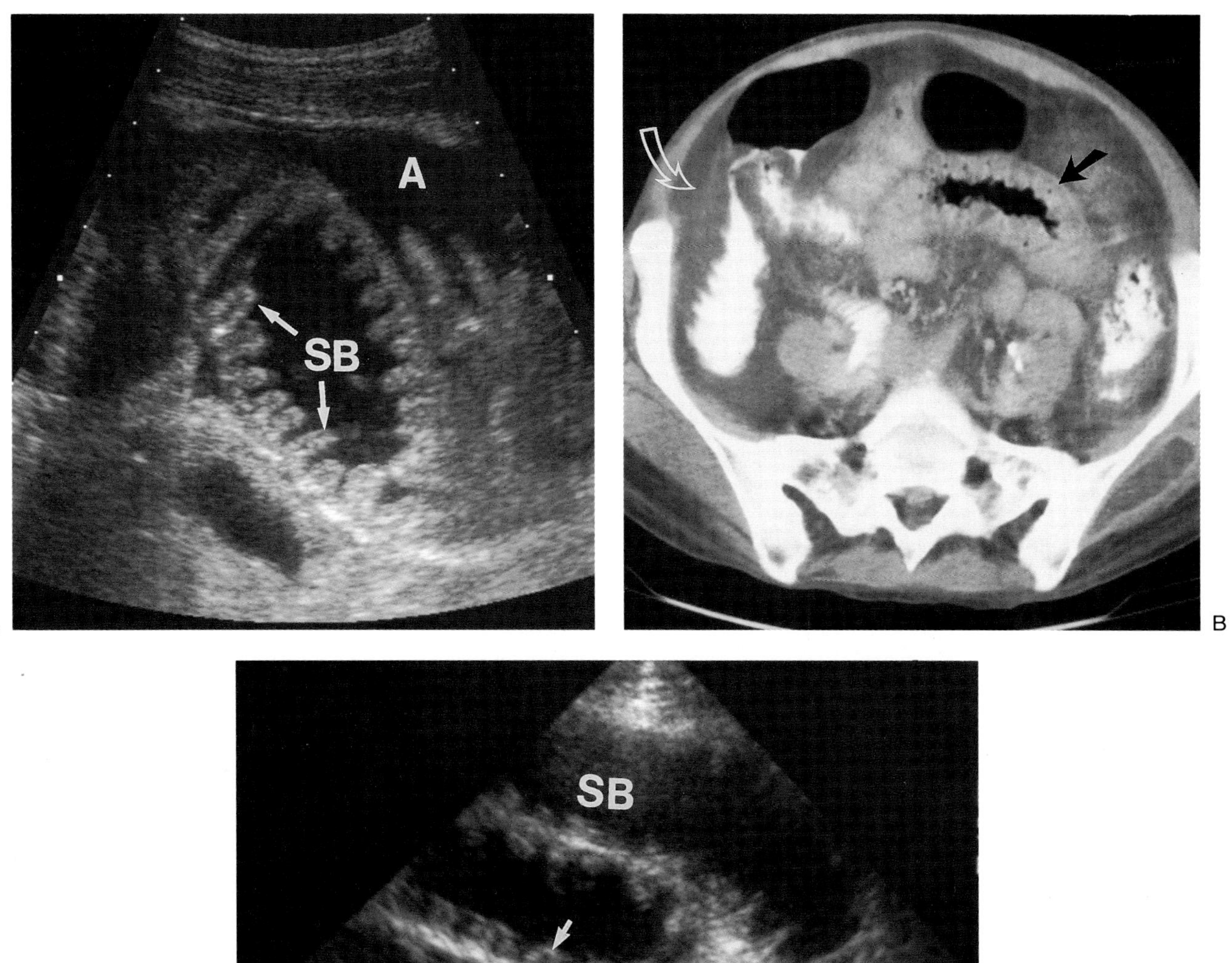

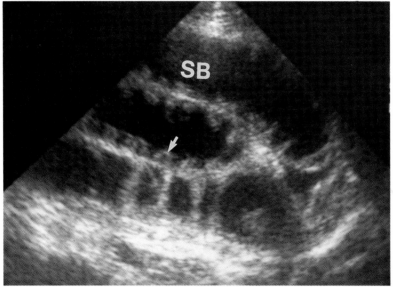

FIG. 1.54. Small bowel ischemia in two patients. **A:** Oblique sonogram of left midabdomen demonstrating dilated segment of small bowel (SB) with thickened folds (*arrows*). Note adjacent ascites (A). **B:** Corresponding CT scan demonstrates focal bowel wall thickening (*arrow*) and ascites (*curved arrow*). **C:** In another patient, dilated atonic loops of small bowel (SB) are identified in right lower quadrant. Note edema of small bowel folds (*arrow*).

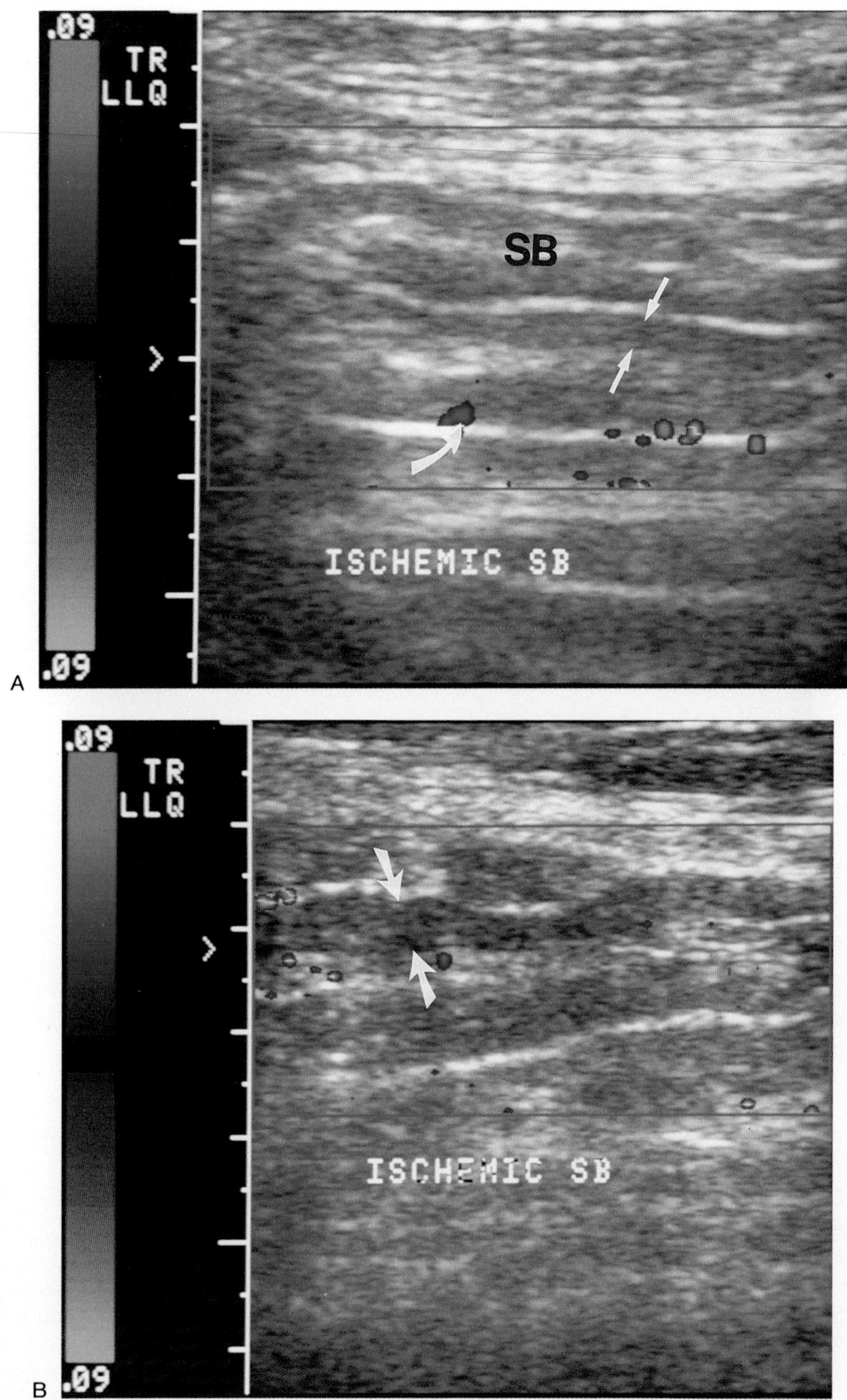

FIG. 1.55. Color Doppler sonography of small bowel infarction in two patients. **A:** Transverse scan of left lower quadrant demonstrating marked mural thickening (*arrows*) of distal small bowel (SB). No flow was noted within thickened segment despite color Doppler parameters optimized for low-flow sensitivity. Flash artifacts (*curved arrow*) are present. Infarcted small bowel found at surgery. **B:** In another patient with infarcted small bowel, note thickened wall of small bowel (*arrows*) and no discernible intramural flow on color Doppler sonogram.

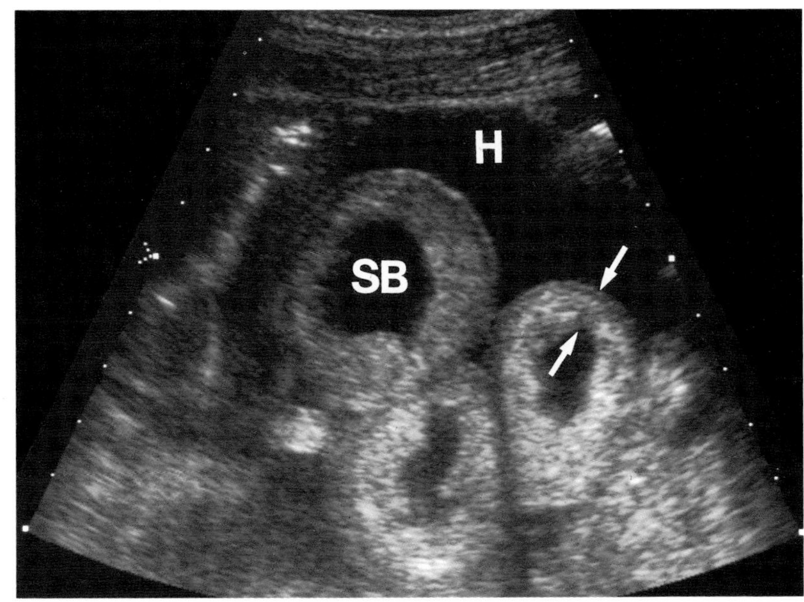

FIG. 1.56. Acute intramural hemorrhage of the small bowel secondary to excessive anticoagulation. Sagittal scan of midabdomen demonstrates small bowel (SB) with marked mural thickening (*arrows*) and diffuse increased echogenicity. Note associated hemoperitoneum (A).

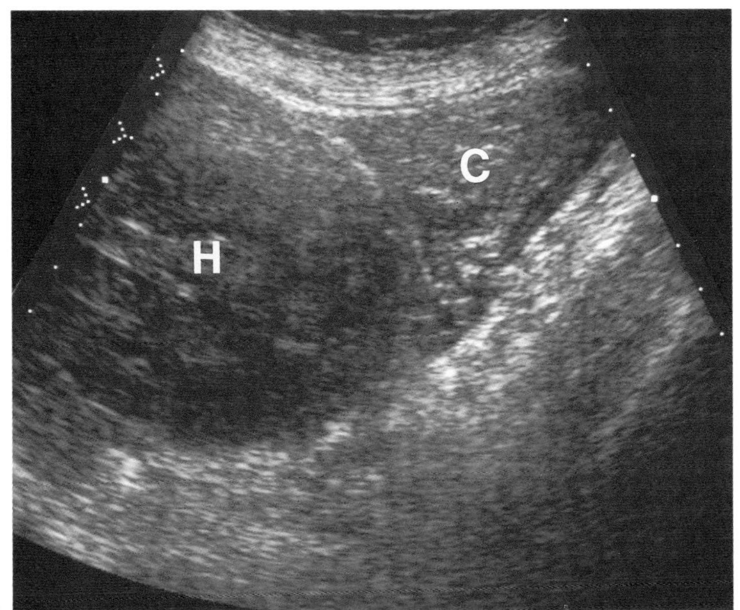

A

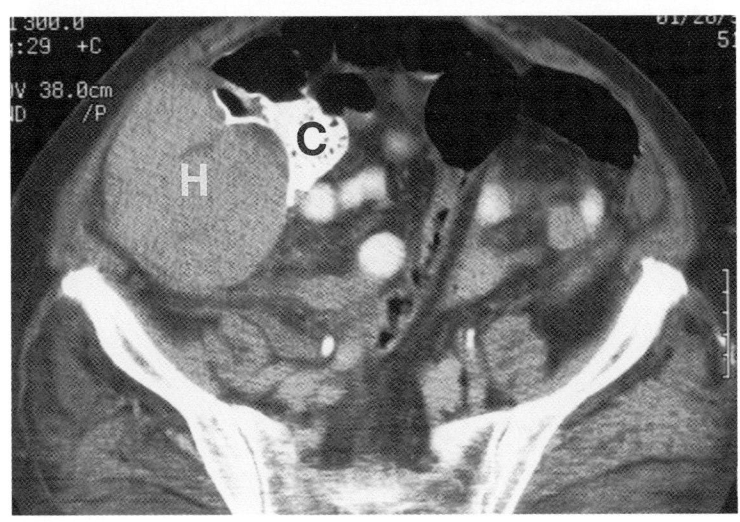

B

FIG. 1.57. Acute intramural hematoma of the cecum secondary to blunt trauma. **A:** Transverse scan of cecum (C) demonstrating large intramural hematoma (H). **B:** Corresponding CT scan demonstrates high-density intramural hematoma (H) of cecum (C).

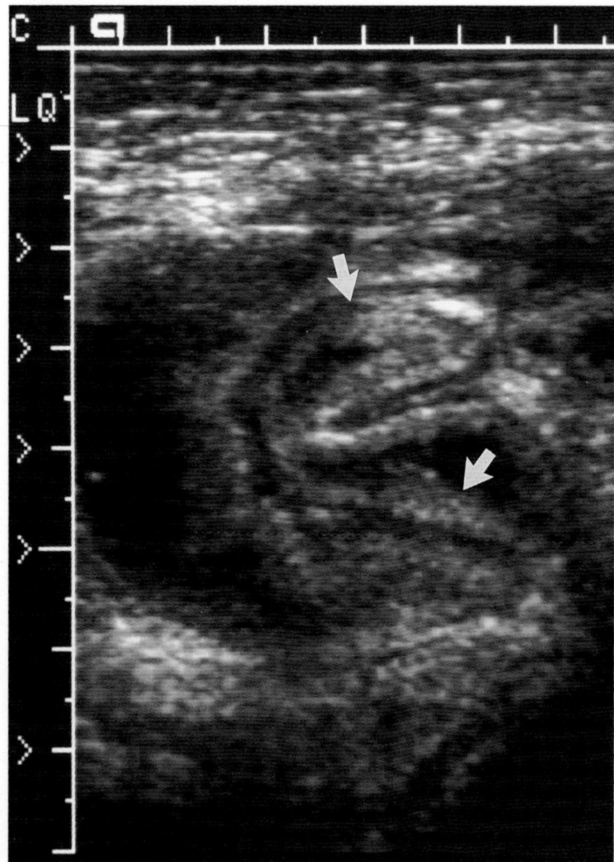

FIG. 1.58. Intramural hematoma of small bowel following blunt trauma. Note thickened echogenic walls of small bowel (*arrows*).

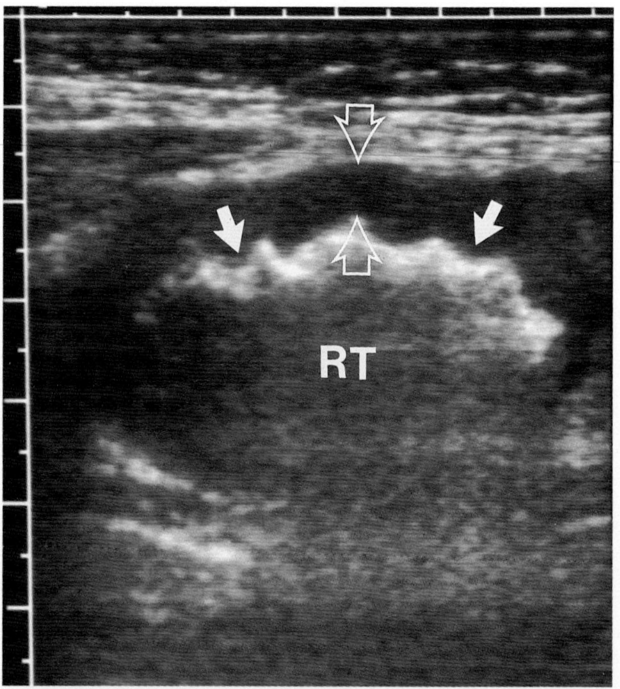

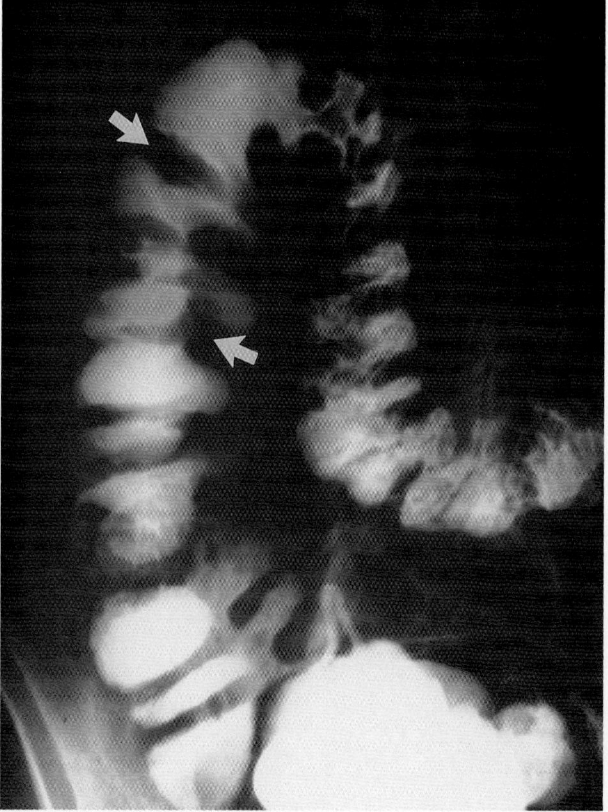

FIG. 1.59. Ischemic colitis of right colon. **A:** Transverse scan of right colon (RT). Note scalloping of submucosal line (*arrows*) and significant mural thickening (*open arrows*). **B:** Contrast enema demonstrates typical "thumbprinting" of submucosal hemorrhage from ischemic colitis (*arrows*).

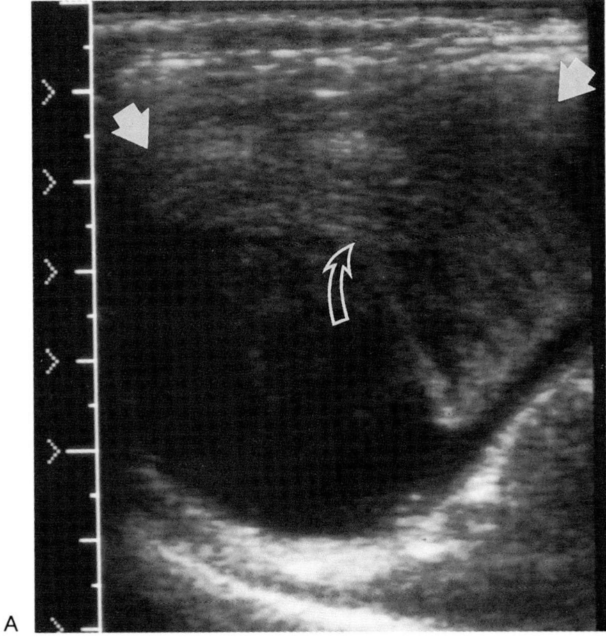

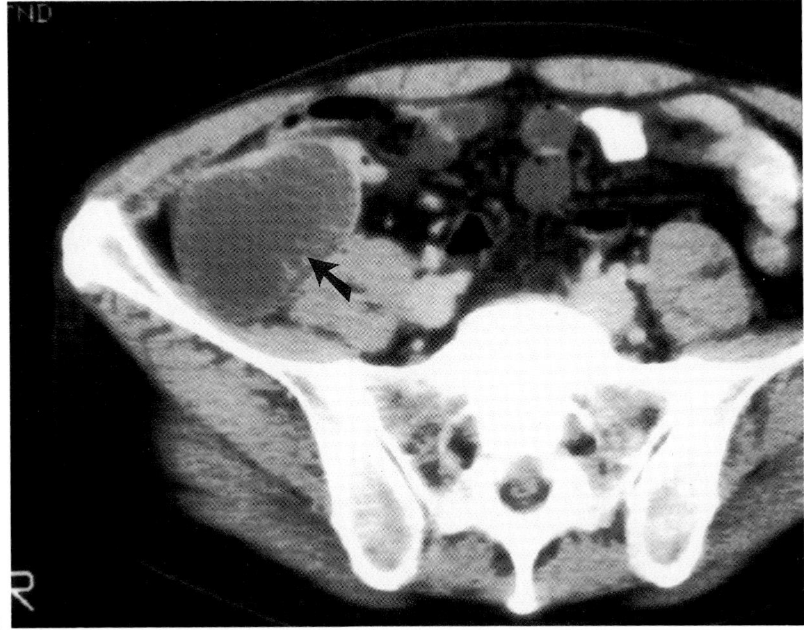

FIG. 1.60. Mucocele of the appendix. **A:** Transverse sonogram of cecal tip demonstrating well-defined complex cystic mass (*arrows*) representing mucocele of the appendix. Note echogenic layers of mucus within mass (*curved arrow*). **B:** Corresponding CT scan demonstrates low-density mucocele (*arrow*) at base of cecum.

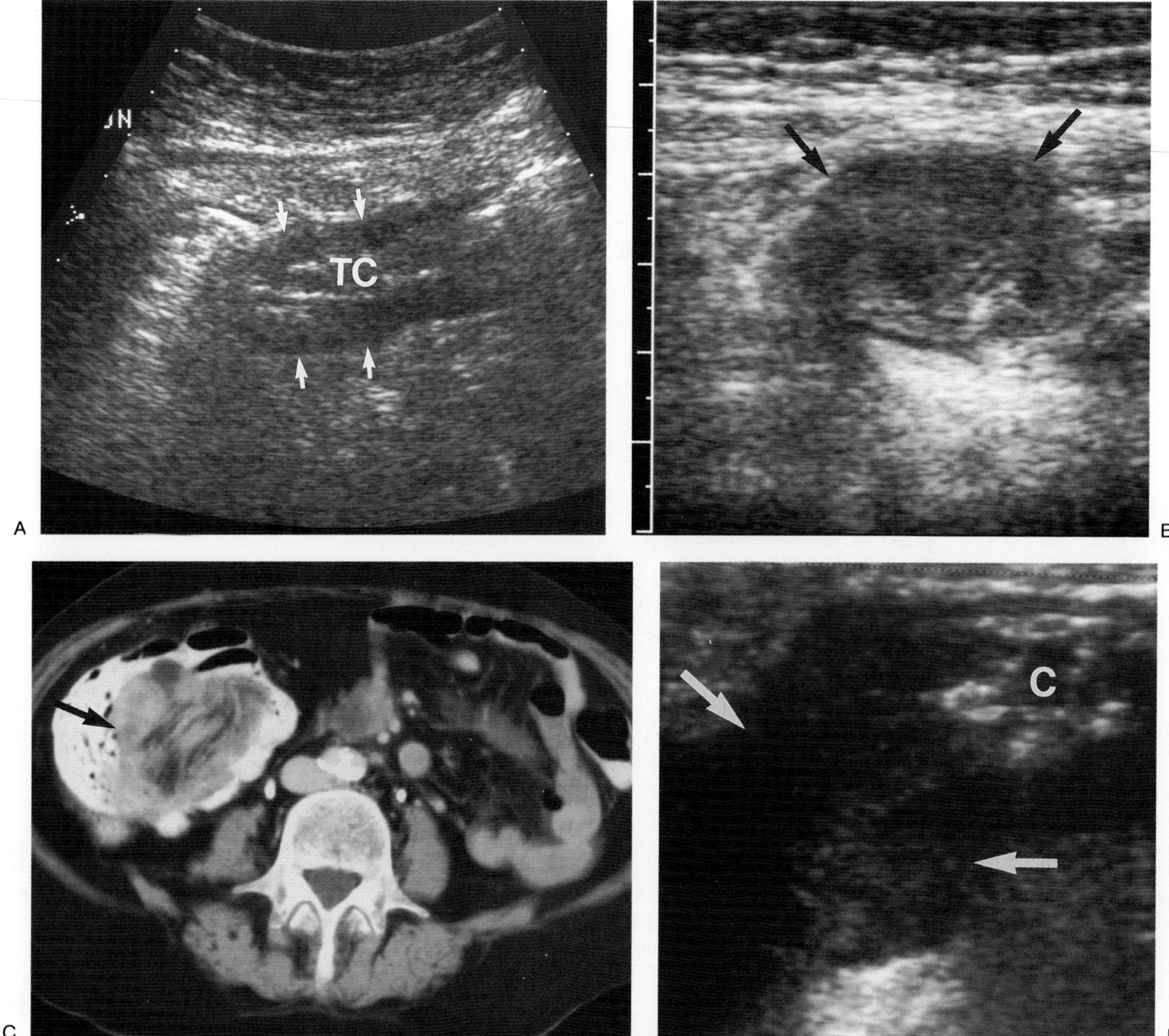

FIG. 1.61. Colon carcinoma in three patients discovered incidentally during screening sonogram for vague abdominal pain. **A:** Sagittal scan of transverse colon (TC) demonstrates hypoechoic carcinoma infiltrating bowel wall (*arrows*). **B:** In another patient, hypoechoic cecal carcinoma (*arrows*) is noted in right lower quadrant. **C:** Corresponding CT scan taken 2 days later demonstrates that the cecal mass (*arrow*) has intussuscepted into the right colon (*arrows*). **D:** In another patient, note cecal carcinoma (*arrows*) infiltrating wall of cecum (C).

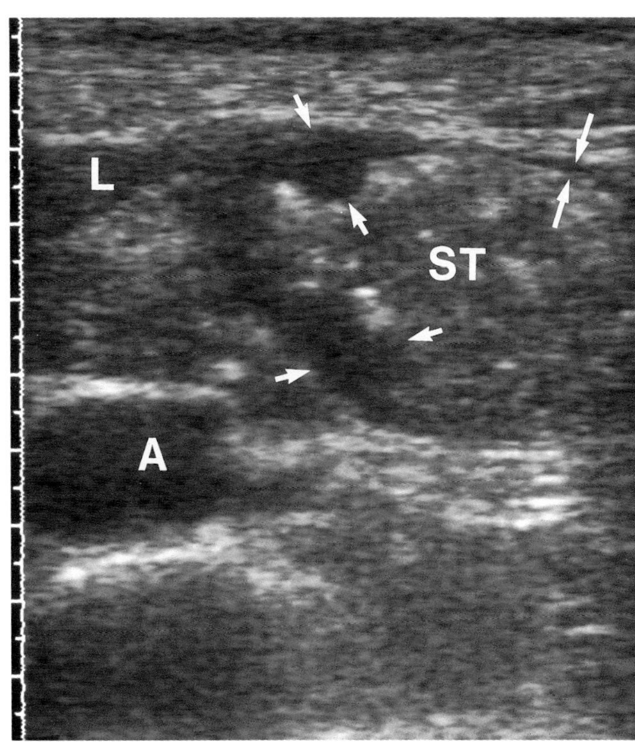

FIG. 1.62. Gastric carcinoma discovered incidentally during gallbladder sonogram. Transverse scan of distal stomach (ST) demonstrates hypoechoic tumor (*short arrows*) infiltrating distal antrum. Note normal wall thickness of more proximal stomach (*long arrows*). A, aorta; L, liver.

A

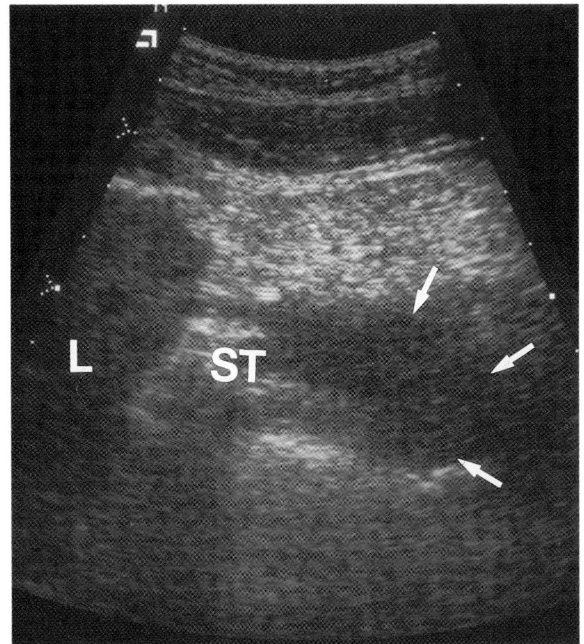

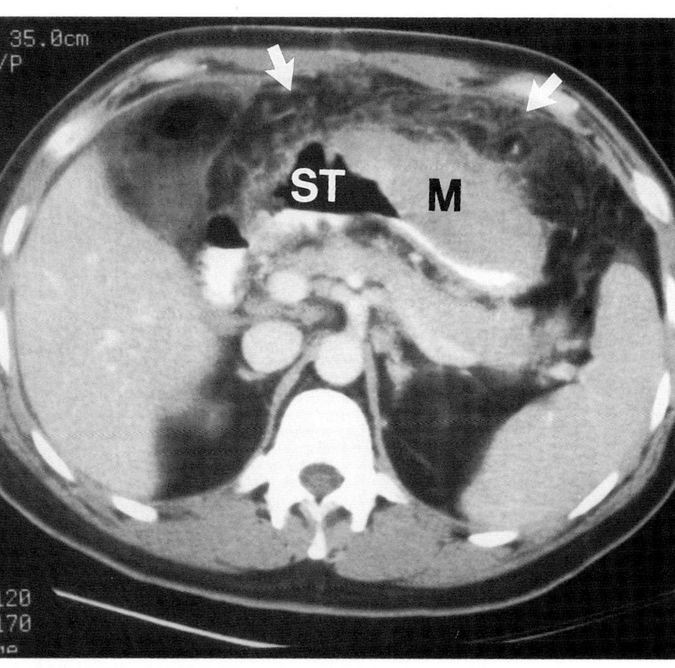

B

FIG. 1.63. Superiority of CT in defining infiltrating lesion of bowel wall. **A:** Transverse sonogram of stomach (ST) demonstrating vague hypoechoic mass (*arrows*). L, liver. **B:** Contrast CT scan clearly demonstrates infiltrating mass (M) within gastric wall. Biopsy revealed leukemic infiltration (chloroma). ST, stomach. Note soft tissue leukemic infiltration of gastrocolic ligament (*arrows*).

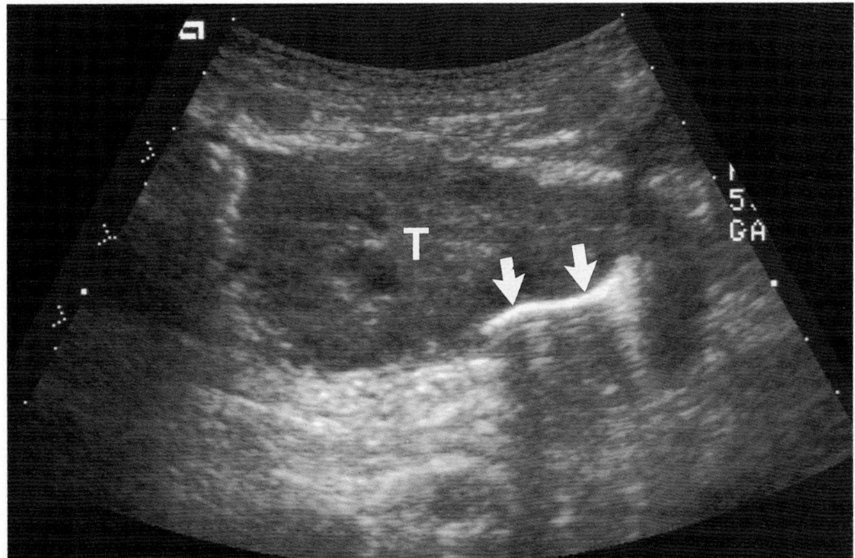

A

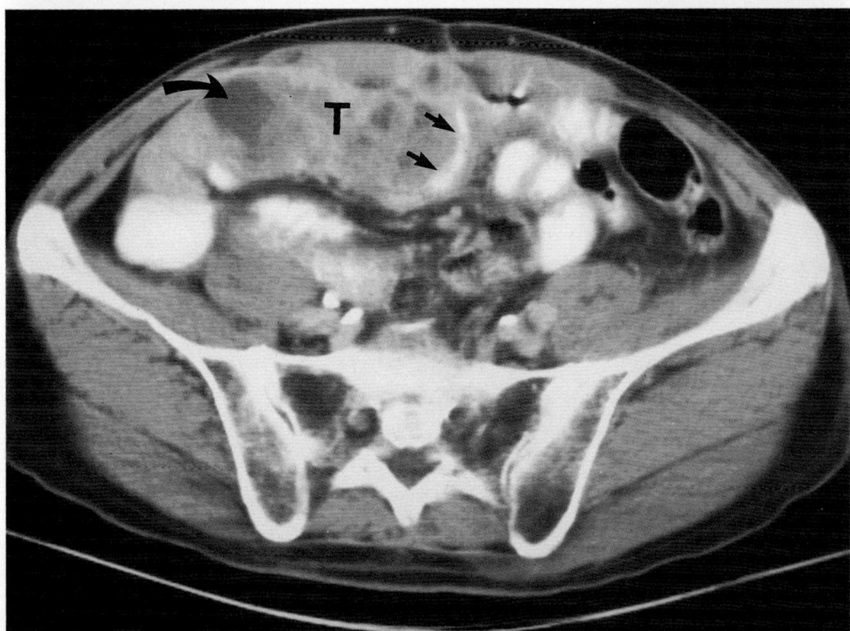

B

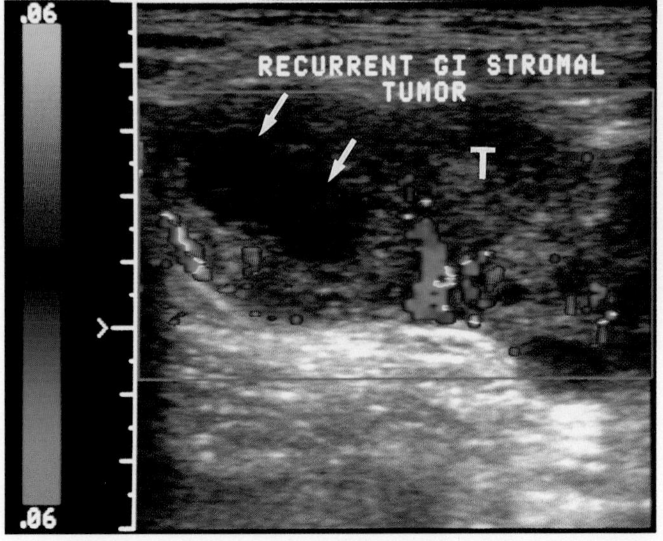

C

FIG. 1.64. Recurrent gastrointestinal stromal tumor (leiomyosarcoma). **A:** Transverse scan of right lower quadrant in a patient 8 months after resection of small bowel stromal tumor. Note large hypoechoic tumor (T) infiltrating ileum. Lumen of ileum can be identified by gas (*arrows*). **B:** Corresponding CT scan demonstrates lumen of ileum (*arrows*) outlined with oral contrast and large mural tumor with heterogeneous density (T). Note low-density areas of necrosis (*curved arrow*). **C:** Color Doppler sonogram reveals hypervascularity within tumor (T) as well as necrotic avascular area (*arrows*). Surgery revealed necrotic recurrent tumor.

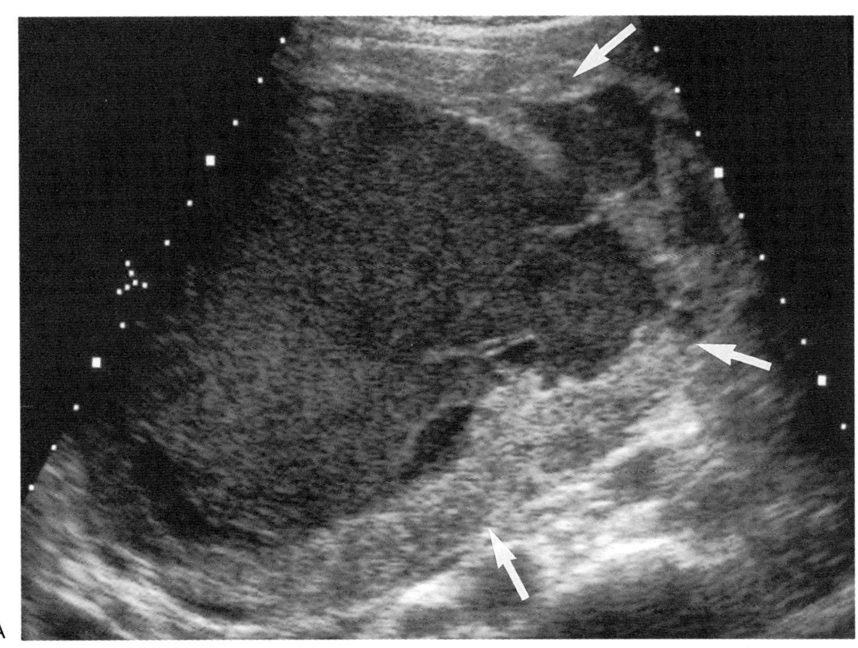

A

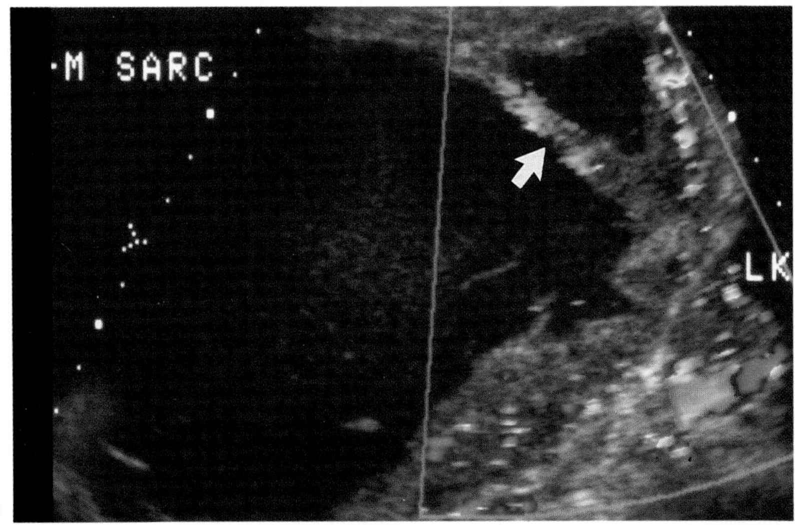

B

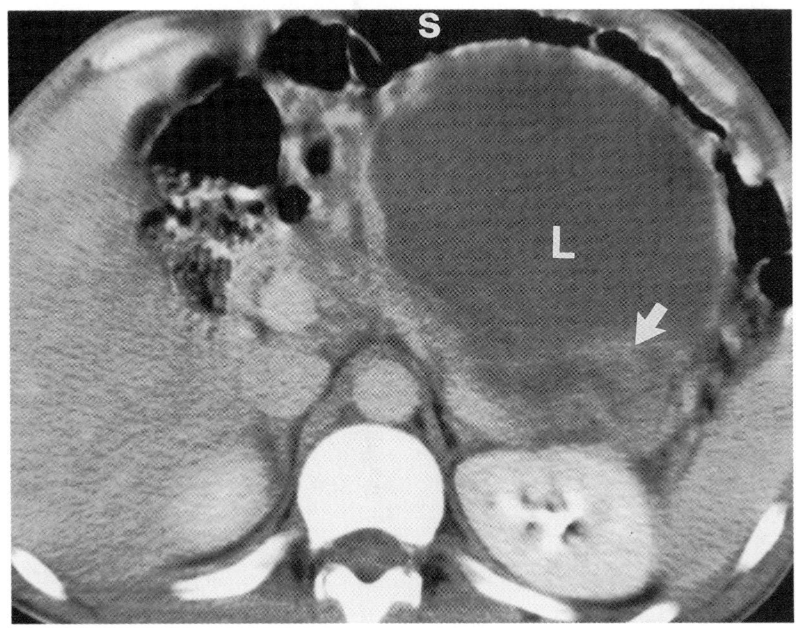

C

FIG. 1.65. Gastric stromal tumor (leiomyosarcoma). **A:** Sonogram of left upper quadrant demonstrates complex cystic mass (*arrows*). Note thickened wall of mass and septations. **B:** Color Doppler sonogram reveals increased blood flow (*arrow*) within septations. **C:** Contrast CT scan demonstrates cystic leiomyosarcoma (L) extending from stomach (S). Note solid components within the tumor (*arrow*).

produce marked mural thickening of the bowel wall, a polypoid nodular mass, or extensive ulceration within a bulky mass. Lymphoma is a relatively soft, pliable submucosal tumor. One characteristic feature of gastrointestinal lymphoma is the lack of obstruction (Figs. 1.66 to 1.68). This is in contrast to gastrointestinal carcinomas, which are scirrhous infiltrating lesions that circumferentially obstruct the bowel. In patients with AIDS there may be diffuse peritoneal involvement with lymphoma resulting in omental and peritoneal lymphomatous masses (Fig. 1.69).

Endoluminal sonography holds great promise for accurate local staging of esophageal, gastric, and colorectal tumors (28–30). This technique can readily define the five normal layers of the bowel wall. Superficial masses confined to the mucosa preserve the normal reflections of the submucosa and muscularis propria (Figs. 1.70 to 1.72). Deeply infiltrating malignant masses disrupt visualization of normal layers of the bowel wall. Bulky exophytic masses are characteristic of gastrointestinal stromal tumor (leiomyosarcoma) and lymphoma (Fig. 1.73). Deep mural invasion is diagnosed when there is widening and infiltration of the hypoechoic layer of the muscularis propria. Extrinsic masses such as mediastinal tumors or lymphadenopathy can be appreciated by endoluminal sonography of the esophagus and stomach (Figs. 1.74 and 1.75). Although diagnosis of distant liver metastases virtually always requires CT or conventional sonography, the main goal of endoluminal sonography is to determine the local depth of neoplastic invasion (Fig. 1.76).

Tio et al. (29) reported a 67 percent overall accuracy with endoluminal sonography in staging colorectal carcinoma. Tumor staging may be classified according to the tumor–node–metastasis (TNM) designation as follows: a T1 lesion is confined to the mucosa and submucosa; a T2 lesion invades through the muscularis propria; a T3 lesion invades the nonperitonealized fatty tissue (of the rectum) or subserosal and/or serosal layer of the colon; and a T4 lesion invades adjacent organs (i.e., bladder, prostate, uterus, vagina, major vascular structure) (29).

In some patients, regional lymph node metastases can be detected with endoluminal sonography. Preliminary work suggests that hyperechoic lymph nodes are often benign (29). However, hypoechoic lymph nodes are suspicious for malignancy (Fig. 1.76). Although lymph node metastases are rare in T1 lesions, Tio et al. (29) reported 30 percent of patients with T2 colorectal lesions to have lymph node metastases. Although some reports have suggested that lymph node metastases directly correlate with the degree of tumor infiltration, other studies do not corroborate this finding and thus all patients with T2 or greater lesions are likely at risk for lymph node metastases (29). However, both false-negative and false-positive diagnoses of lymph node metastases may occur with endoluminal sonography. It is likely that the development of endoscopic fine needle aspiration biopsy guided by sonography may facilitate diagnosis of nodal metastases.

Endosonography may also be useful in patients following surgery for rectal cancer to detect local recurrence. Recent reports suggest that in some patients endoluminal sonography is able to detect lesions that are not visible by proctoscopy alone (29). It may not be possible in all cases, however, to distinguish postoperative fibrosis from recurrent tumor, and therefore serial studies or biopsy may be required for accurate diagnosis.

Preliminary reports suggest that endoscopic sonography may be of considerable clinical value for staging of both esophageal and gastric carcinoma (Figs. 1.77 to 1.86). Comparison studies with CT suggest that endoluminal sonography is more accurate for local staging due to ability to directly visualize the layers of bowel wall. Ziegler et al. (79) reported an 89 percent accuracy for esophageal lesions without lymph node metastases and a 69 percent accuracy for lesions with lymph node metastases on endoluminal sonography. This compared to a 51 percent accuracy for CT staging for both groups of patients (79). The role in preoperative staging of gastric carcinoma remains controversial since virtually all these patients are treated with surgery regardless of the depth of mural invasion. This is due to the fact that, unless treated, many of these patients require surgery to treat gastrointestinal obstruction.

Endoluminal sonography is particularly valuable in assessing submucosal lesions of the gastrointestinal tract. These lesions do not disrupt the mucosal layer. Benign submucosal masses do not infiltrate or disrupt the muscularis propria. Gastric carcinoma rarely causes diffuse submucosal infiltration (Fig. 1.83). Lymphoma may also cause a bulky submucosal mass, as well as a large exophytic component (Fig. 1.86). Rarely, submucosal metastases from lymphoma, melanoma, Kaposi's sarcoma, or adenocarcinoma may be diagnosed with endoluminal sonography (Fig. 1.87).

REFERENCES

1. Meyers MA. *Dynamic radiology of the abdomen: normal and pathologic anatomy*, 3rd ed. New York: Springer-Verlag; 1988:27–48.
2. Federle MP, Jeffrey RB. Hemoperitoneum studied by computed tomography. *Radiology* 1983;148:187–192.
3. Federle MP, Crass RA, Jeffrey RB, Trunkey DD. Computed tomography in blunt abdominal trauma. *Arch Surg* 1982;117:645–650.
4. Siskind BN, Malat J, Hammers L, et al. CT features of hemorrhagic malignant liver tumors. *J Comput Assist Tomogr* 1987;11:766–770.
5. Jeffrey RB, Laing FC. Echogenic clot: a useful sign of pelvic hemoperitoneum. *Radiology* 1982;145:139–141.
6. Callen PW. Computer tomographic evaluation of abdominal and pelvic abscesses. *Radiology* 1979;131:171–175.
7. Korobkin M, Callen PW, Filly RA, Hoffer PB, Shimshak R, Kres-

(*text continues on page 69*)

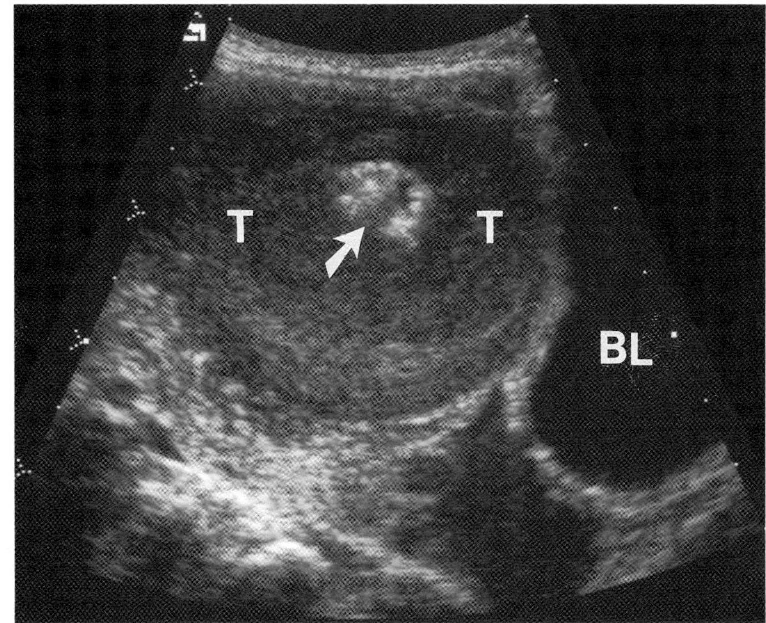

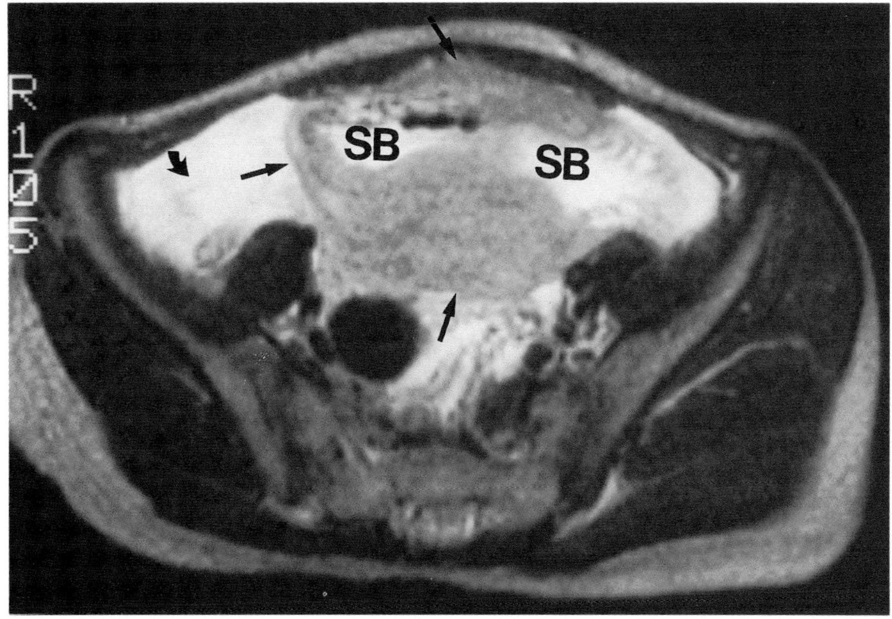

FIG. 1.66. Encasement of small bowel by non-Hodgkin's lymphoma without obstruction. **A:** Sagittal scan of pelvis demonstrating hypoechoic tumor (T) infiltrating but not obstructing small bowel lumen (*arrow*). BL, bladder. **B:** T2-weighted magnetic resonance image of pelvis demonstrating bulky lymphomatous mass (*arrows*) encasing small bowel. Note patent small bowel lumen (SB). Ascites (*curved arrow*) is noted.

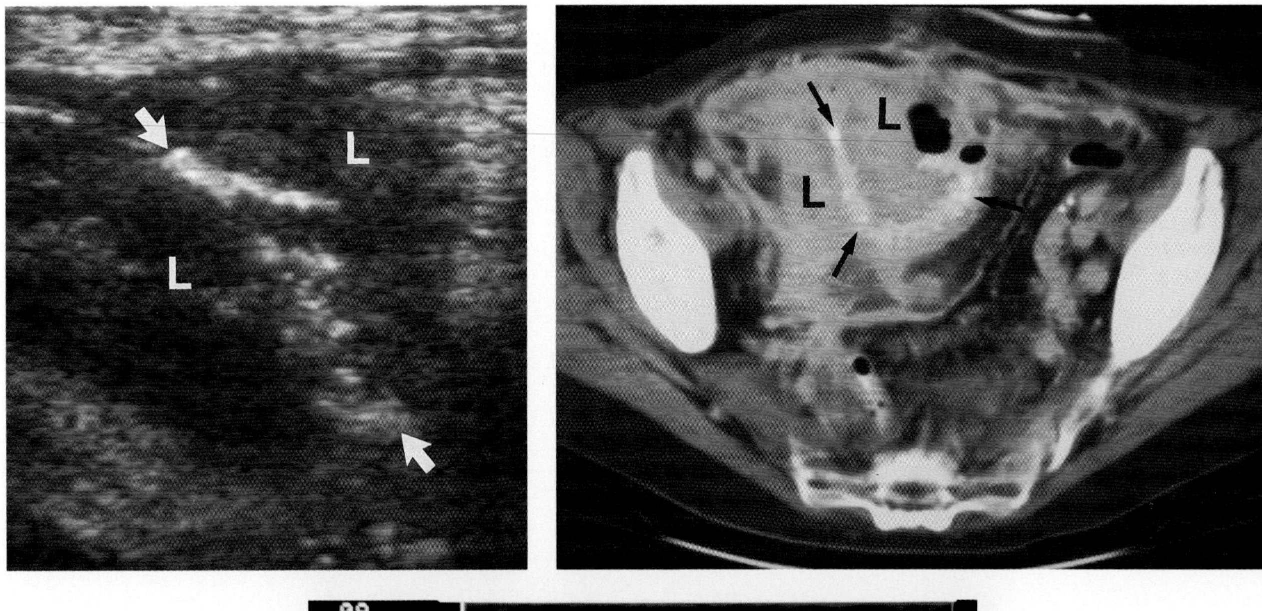

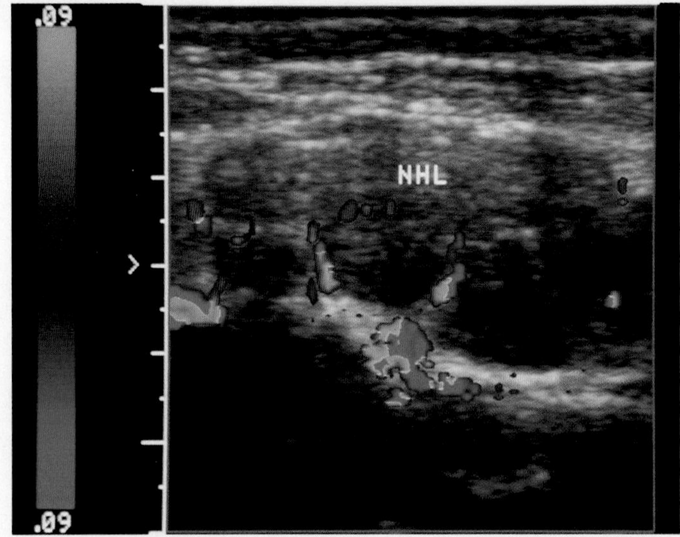

FIG. 1.67. Nonobstructing lymphoma of the small bowel. **A:** Transverse scan of right lower quadrant demonstrating hypoechoic lymphoma (L) infiltrating bowel wall. Note patent lumen (*arrows*). **B:** CT scan demonstrates oral contrast in lumen (*arrows*) of bowel loop involved with lymphoma (L). **C:** Color Doppler sonogram demonstrating intrinsic vascularity within the non-Hodgkin's lymphoma (NHL).

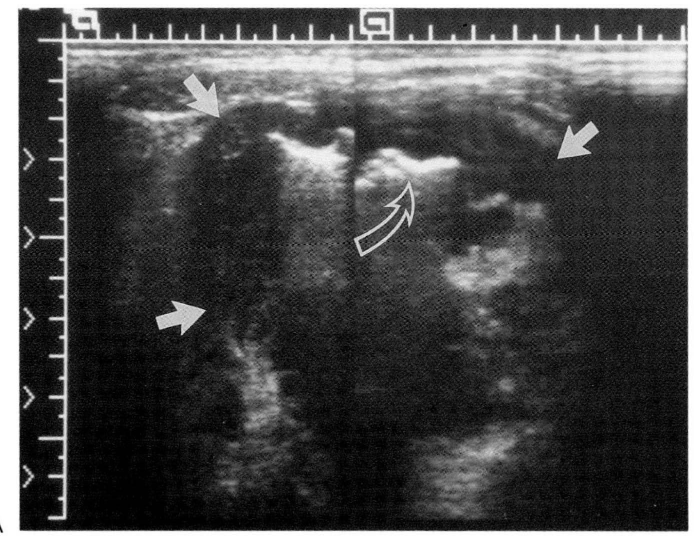

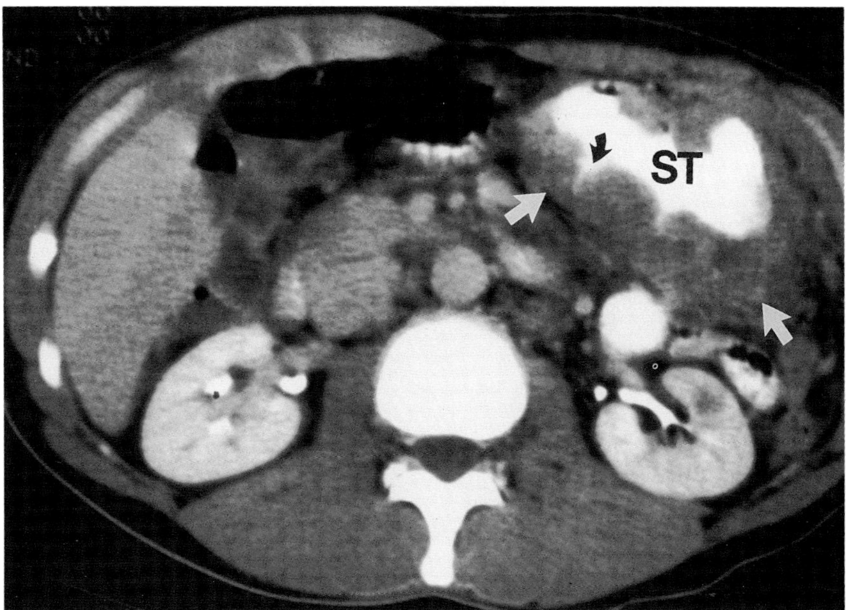

FIG. 1.68. AIDS-related gastric lymphoma. **A:** Sagittal scan of left upper quadrant demonstrates bulky hypoechoic gastric mass (*arrows*). Note gas within gastric lumen (*curved arrow*). **B:** CT scan demonstrates diffuse infiltration of stomach (ST) by bulky mass (*white arrows*). Note ulceration within mass (*curved arrow*).

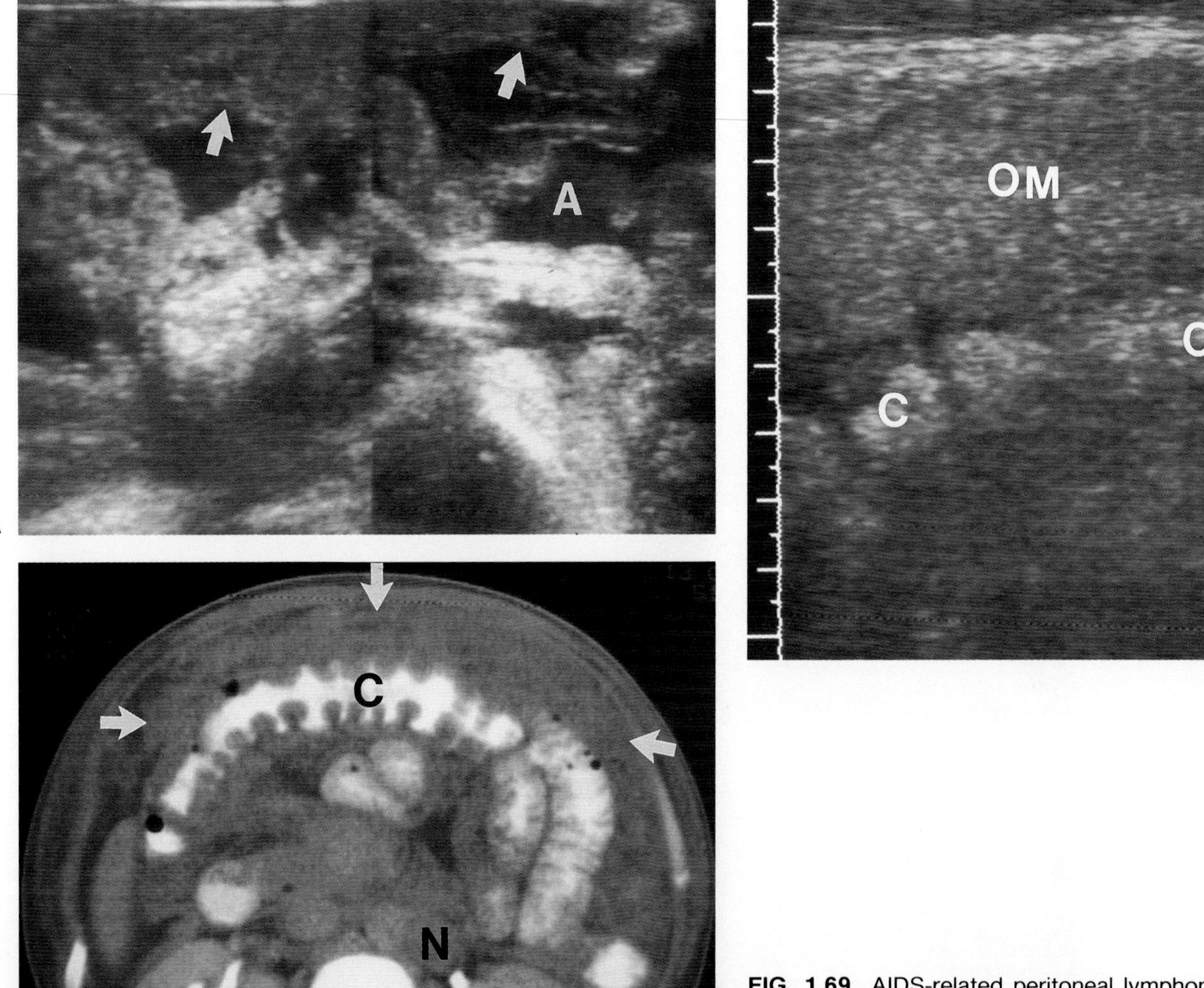

FIG. 1.69. AIDS-related peritoneal lymphomatosis in two patients. **A:** Transverse scan of midabdomen demonstrating lymphoma infiltrating omentum (*arrows*). Note associated ascites (A). **B:** In another patient, large omental mass (OM) is noted anterior to transverse colon (C). **C:** Contrast CT scan confirms omental involvement (*arrows*) anterior to transverse colon (C) as well as retroperitoneal adenopathy (N).

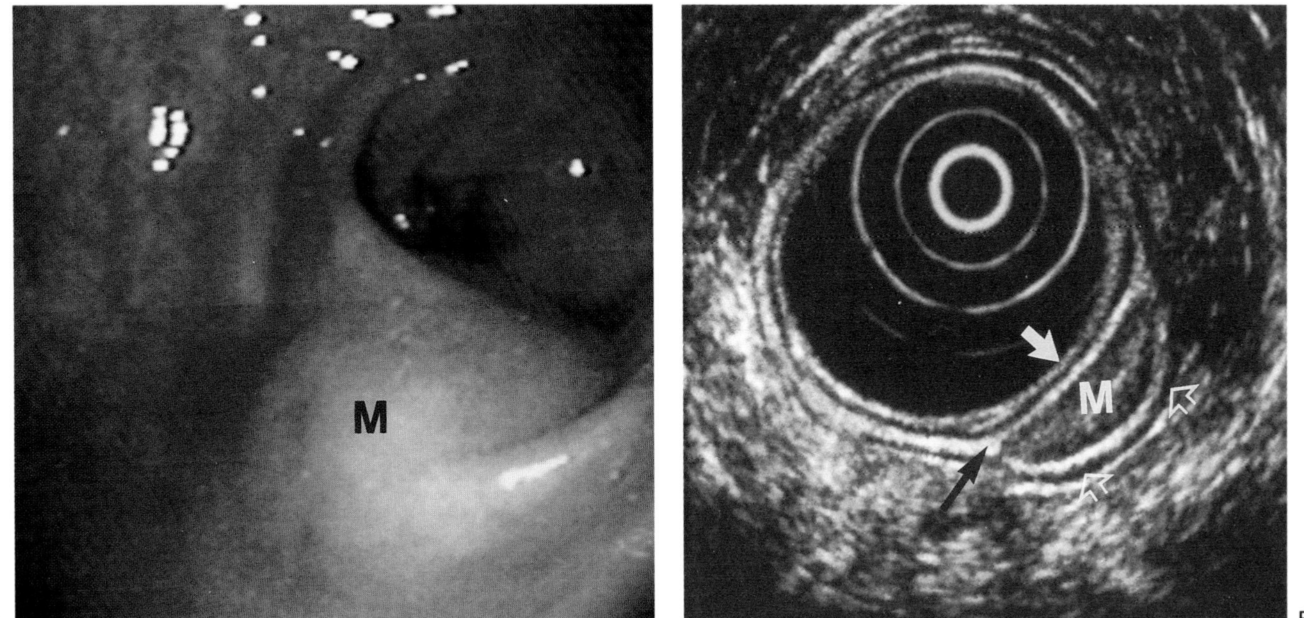

FIG. 1.70. Endoluminal sonography of benign intramural mass (leiomyoma). **A:** Endoscopy reveals bulging mass (M) with overlying normal mucosa in the body of the stomach. **B:** Endoluminal sonogram of mass (M) clearly demonstrating that the hypoechoic mass arises from echogenic submucosal layer (*black arrow*). Note normal mucosal reflection (*arrow*) and normal hypoechoic muscularis propria (*open arrow*). Biopsy revealed leiomyoma.

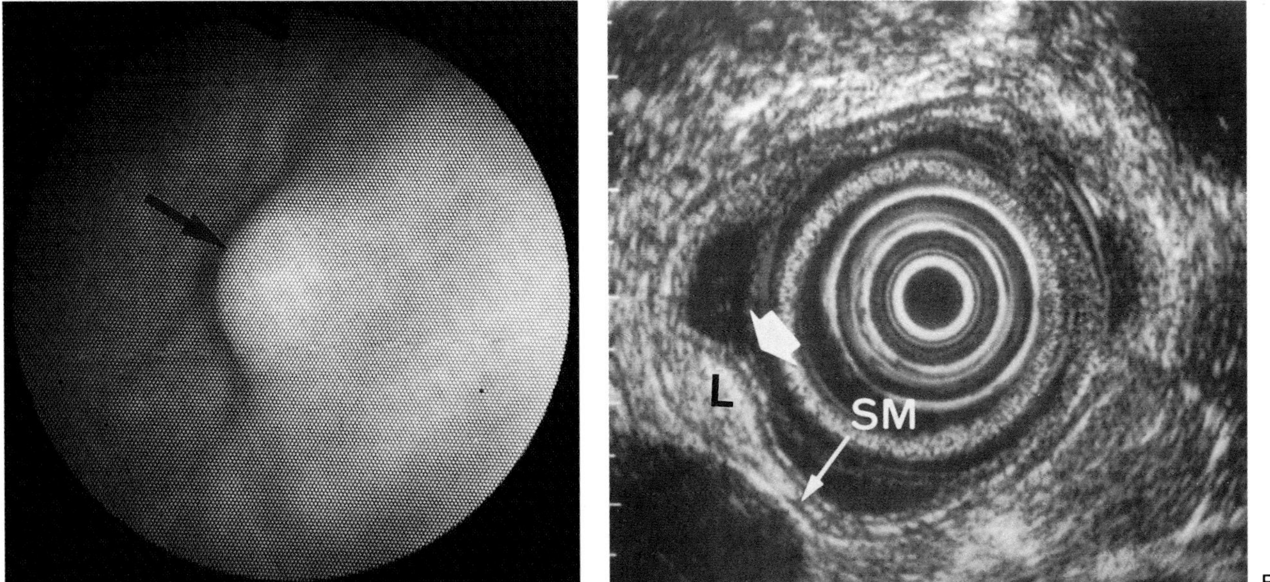

FIG. 1.71. Endoluminal sonography of benign intramural mass (gastric lipoma). **A:** Endoscopy demonstrates small mural mass (*arrow*) with overlying normal mucosa. **B:** Endoluminal sonogram demonstrates echogenic lipoma (L) within submucosal layer (SM). (Case courtesy of Jin Hong Kim, MD, Seoul, Korea.)

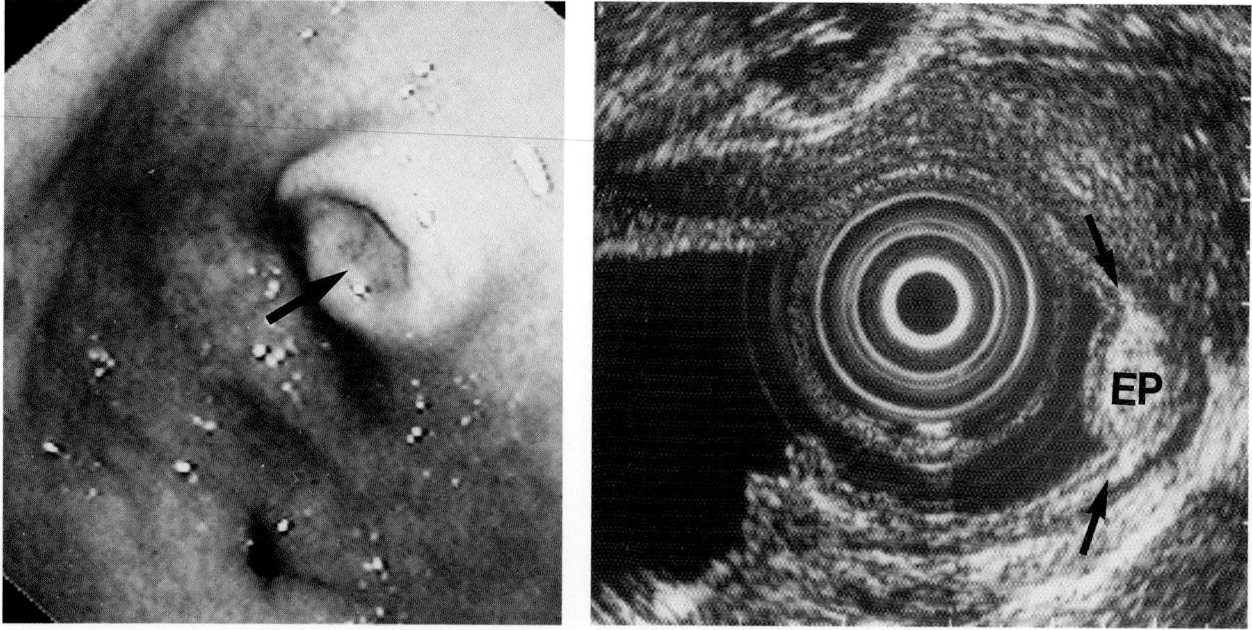

FIG. 1.72. Endoluminal sonography of benign intramural mass (ectopic pancreas). **A:** Endoscopy reveals umbilicated mass (*arrow*) in gastric antrum. **B:** Endoluminal sonogram reveals echogenic ectopic pancreas (EP) arising from submucosal layer (*black arrow*). (Case courtesy of Jin Hong Kim, MD, Seoul, Korea.)

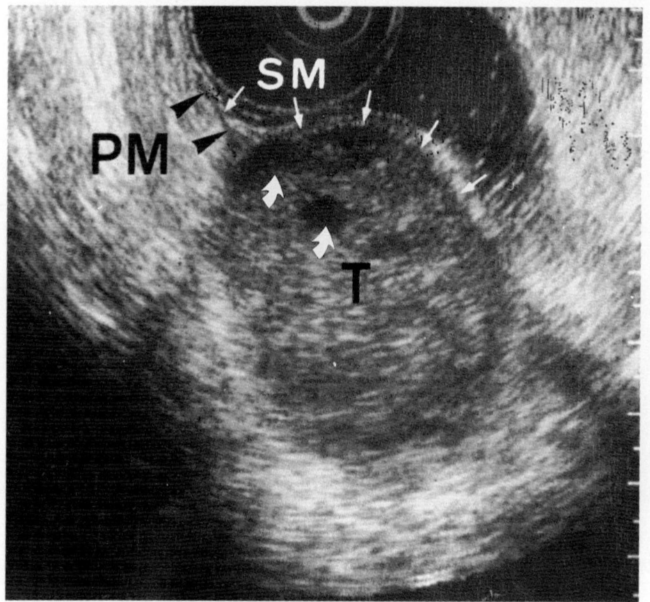

FIG. 1.73. Endoluminal sonography of exophytic intramural mass (gastric leiomyosarcoma or gastrointestinal stromal tumor). Endoluminal sonogram of stomach demonstrates large exophytic hypoechoic tumor (T) with areas of necrosis (*curved arrows*). Leiomyosarcoma is contiguous with muscularis propria (PM). Sm, submucosa. (Case courtesy of Jin Hong Kim, MD, Seoul, Korea.)

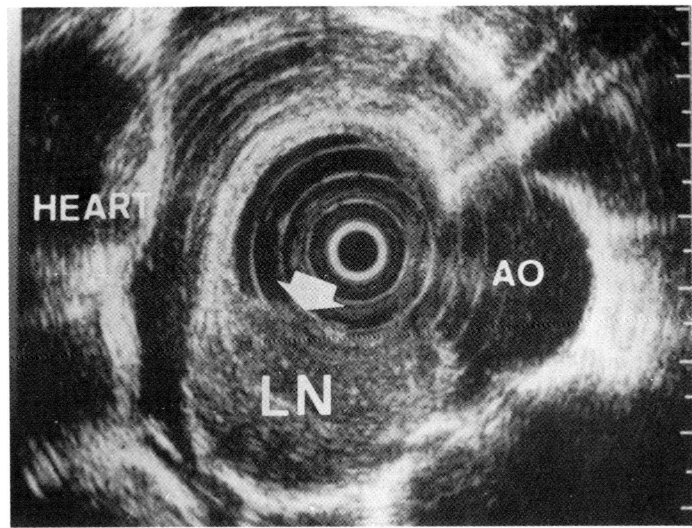

FIG. 1.74. Extrinsic lymph node mass demonstrated by endoluminal sonography of esophagus. Nodal mass (LN) is clearly demonstrated. AO, aorta. (Case courtesy of Jin Hong Kim, MD, Seoul, Korea.)

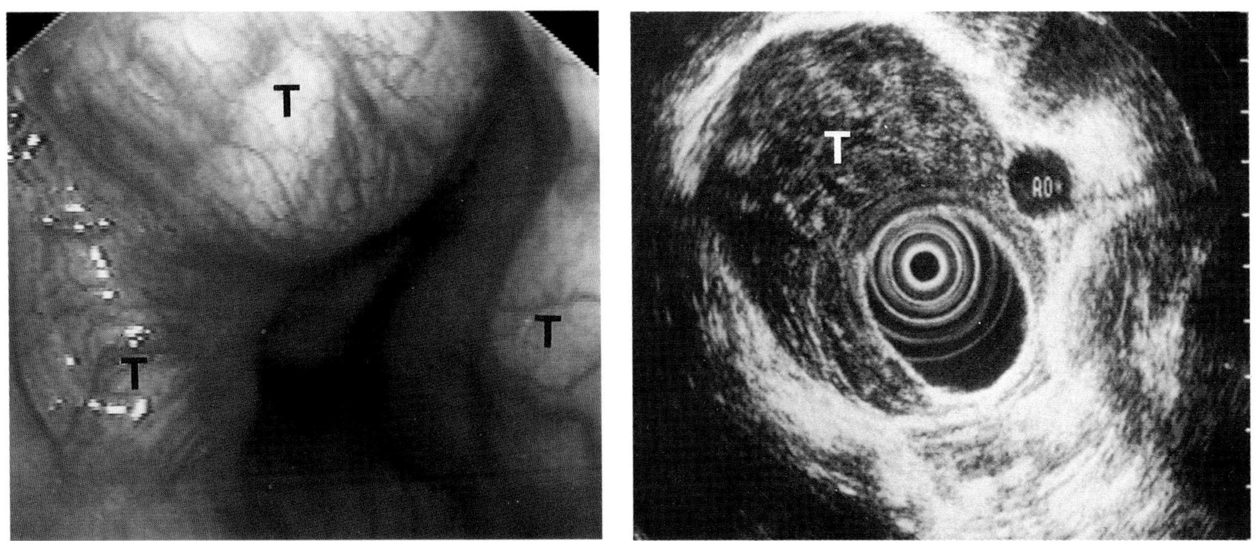

FIG. 1.75. Extrinsic impression on esophagus demonstrated by endoluminal sonography. **A:** Endoscopic view of esophagus demonstrating extrinsic impressions by mediastinal tumor (T). **B:** Endoluminal sonogram demonstrates bulky paraesophageal malignant mediastinal tumor (T). AO, aorta. (Case courtesy of Jin Hong Kim, MD, Seoul, Korea.)

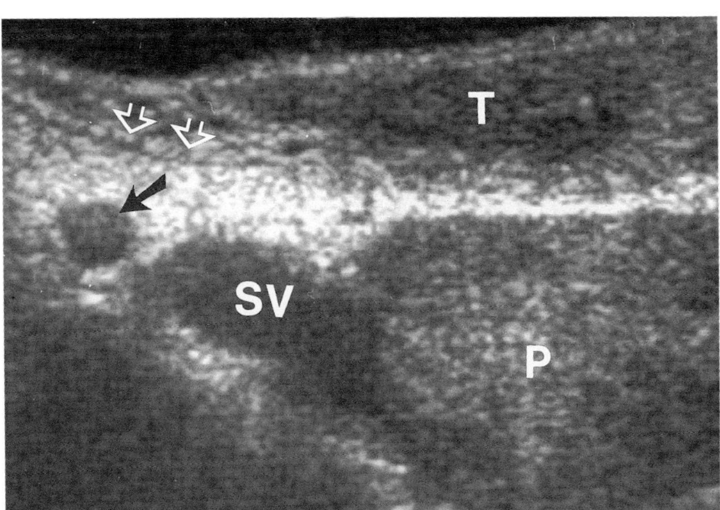

FIG. 1.76. Endoluminal sonography of infiltrating rectal cancer. Sagittal scan demonstrates hypoechoic tumor (T) deeply infiltrating rectal wall. Note disruption of serosal reflection. Normal serosal reflection noted by *open arrows*. Note hypoechoic perirectal lymph node metastasis (*black arrow*). P, prostate; SV, seminal vesicles.

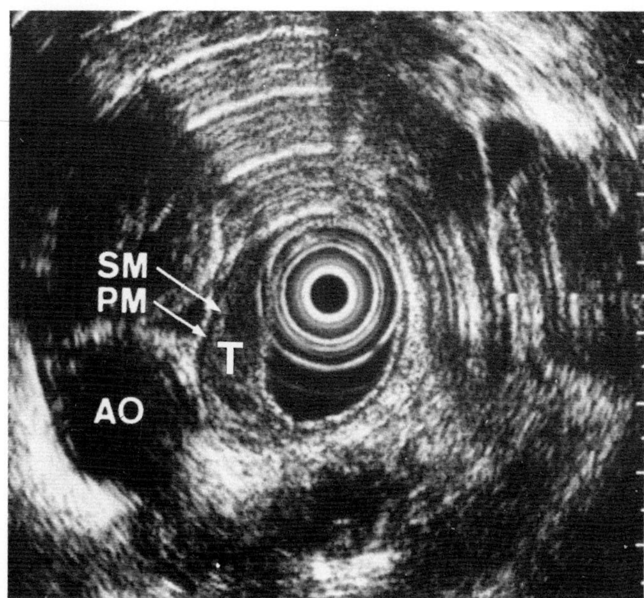

FIG. 1.77. Endoluminal sonography of early esophageal carcinoma. Note hypoechoic tumor (T) confined to submucosal (SM) layer. Note preservation of muscularis propria (PM). AO, aorta. (Case courtesy of Jin Hong Kim, MD, Seoul, Korea.)

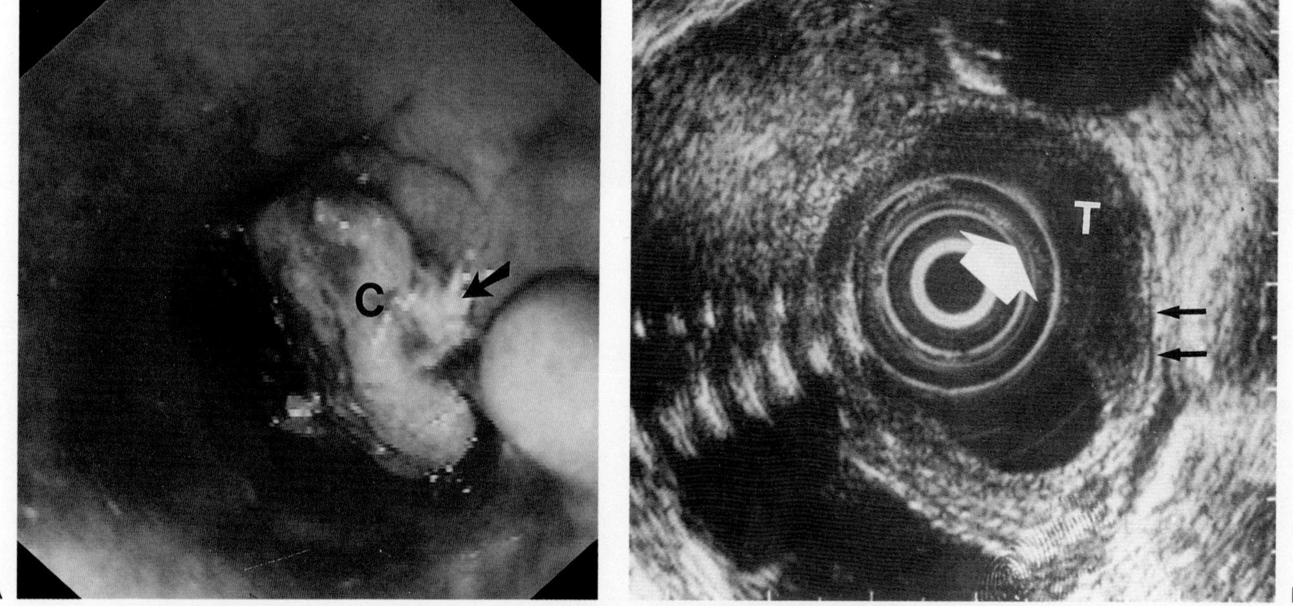

FIG. 1.78. Endoluminal sonography of advanced esophageal cancer. **A:** Endoscopic view of large nodular esophageal cancer (C) with ulceration (*arrow*). **B:** Endoluminal sonogram demonstrates infiltrating tumor (T). Portions of muscularis propria are preserved in one area (*black arrows*) but are absent throughout most of tumor. (Case courtesy of Jin Hong Kim, MD, Seoul, Korea.)

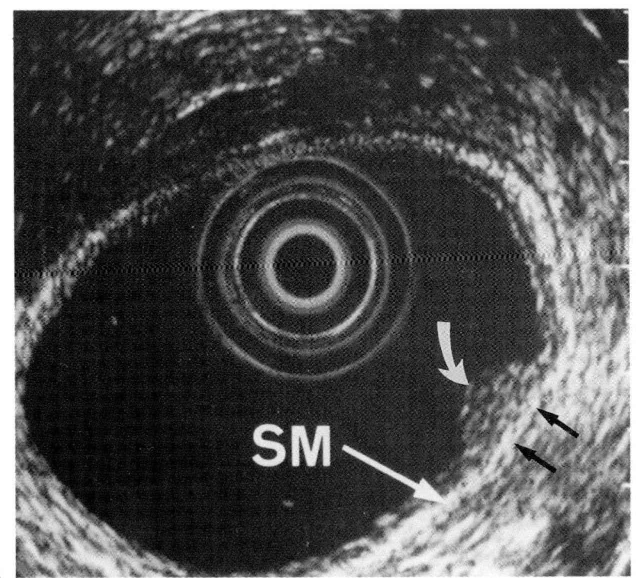

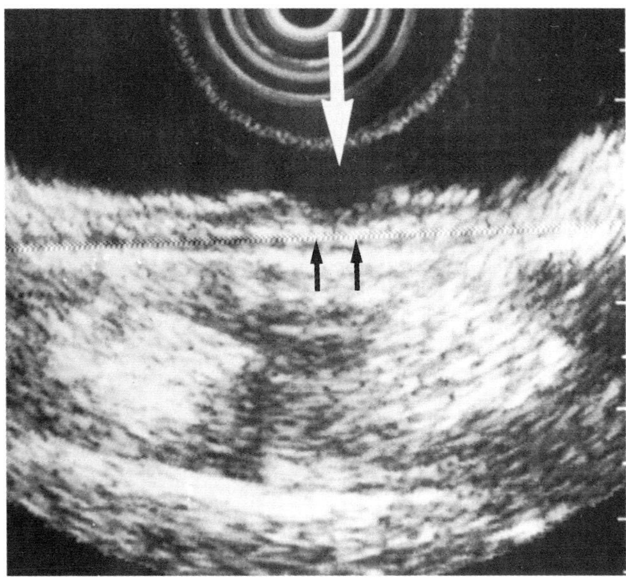

A B

FIG. 1.79. Superficial gastric carcinoma in two patients. **A:** Endoluminal sonogram demonstrates polypoid carcinoma (*curved arrow*) limited to mucosa. Note intact submucosa posterior to lesion (*black arrows*). SM, submucosa. **B:** In another patient, ulcerated lesion (*white arrow*) is noted with intact submucosa (*black arrows*). (Case courtesy of Jin Hong Kim, MD, Seoul, Korea.)

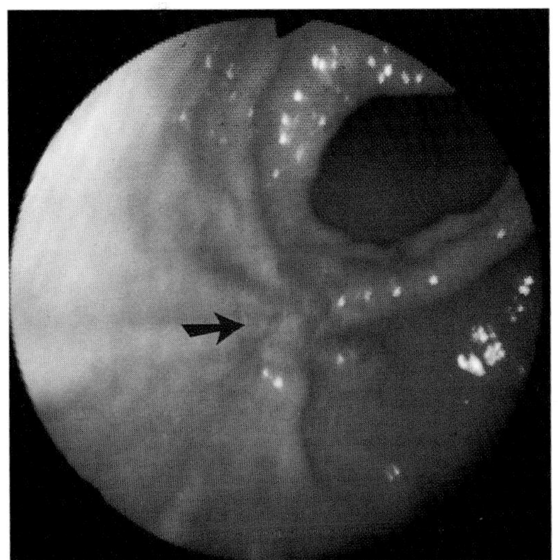

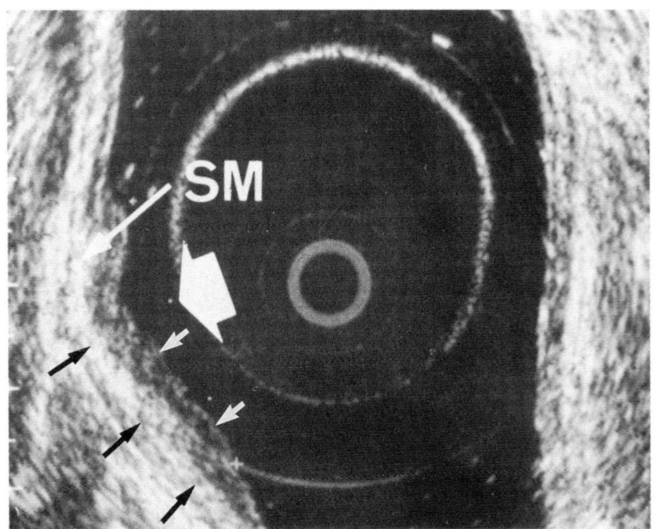

A B

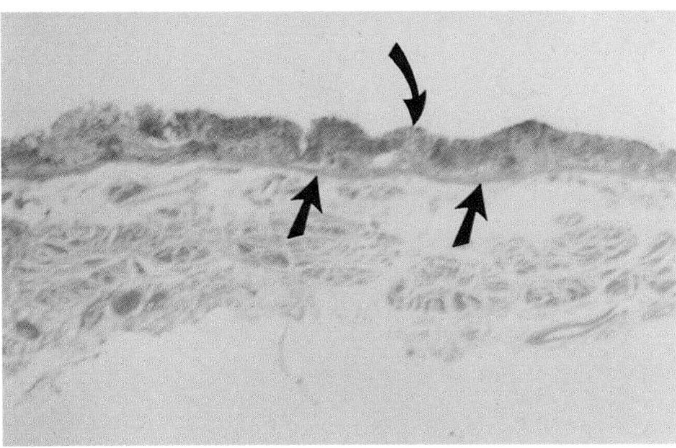

C

FIG. 1.80. Superficial gastric carcinoma. **A:** Endoscopy reveals depressed irregular lesion (*arrow*). **B:** Endoluminal sonogram demonstrating mucosal infiltration by superficial carcinoma (*white arrows*). Note intact submucosa (*black arrow*). SM, submucosa. **C:** Histologic specimen demonstrates carcinoma (*curved arrow*) confined to mucosa without infiltrating the submucosa (*arrows*). (Case courtesy of Jin Hong Kim, MD, Seoul, Korea.)

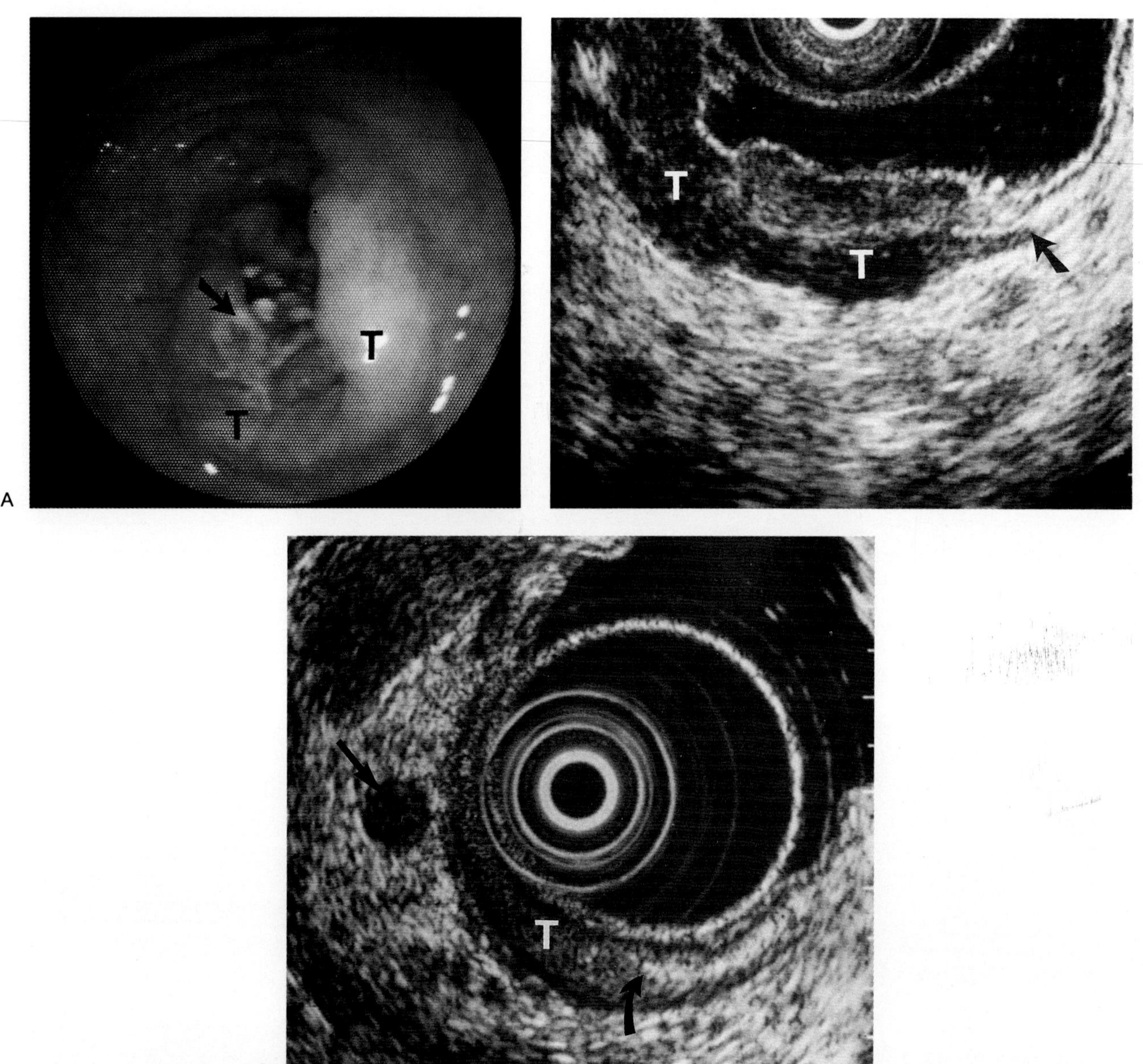

FIG. 1.81. Advanced gastric carcinoma in two patients. **A:** Endoscopic view of nodular antral tumor (T) with ulceration (*arrow*). **B:** Endoluminal sonogram demonstrates hypoechoic transmural tumor (T). Note site of interruption of submucosa. **C:** In another patient, deeply infiltrating tumor (T) destroys submucosa (*curved arrow*) and has regional nodal metastases (*curved arrow*). (Case courtesy of Jin Hong Kim, MD, Seoul, Korea.)

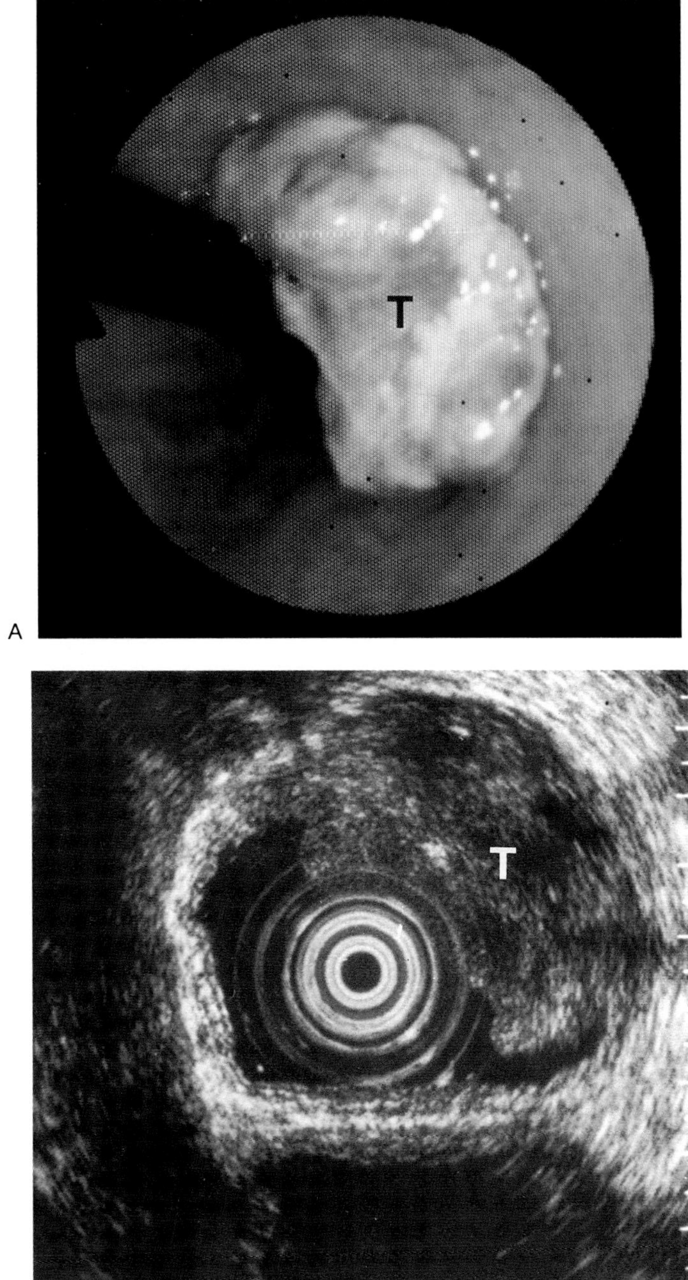

FIG. 1.82. Advanced gastric carcinoma. **A:** Endoscopy reveals fungating gastric tumor (T). **B:** Endoluminal sonogram demonstrates extensive transmural infiltration of bowel wall by tumor (T). (Case courtesy of Jin Hong Kim, MD, Seoul, Korea.)

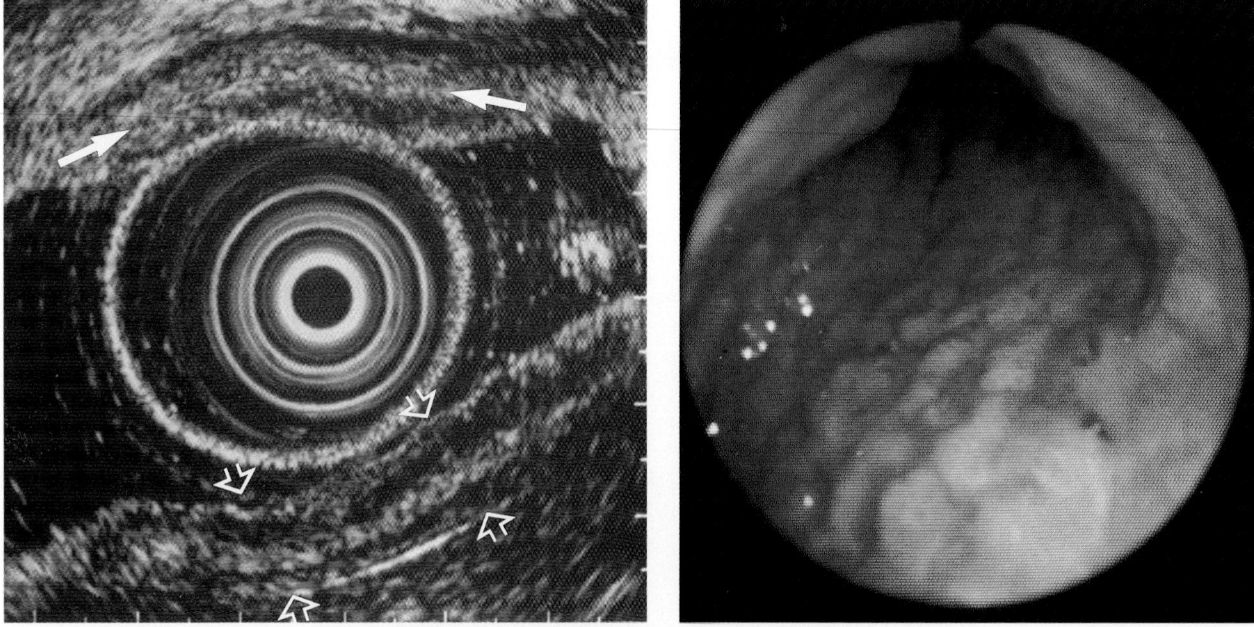

FIG. 1.83. Submucosal infiltration from gastric carcinoma. **A:** Endoluminal sonograms demonstrate marked mural thickening of gastric wall (*open arrows*) and echogenic tumor infiltration with widening of submucosal layer (*arrows*). **B:** Endoscopy reveals nodular edematous folds in body of stomach from submucosal infiltration. (Case courtesy of Jin Hong Kim, MD, Seoul, Korea.)

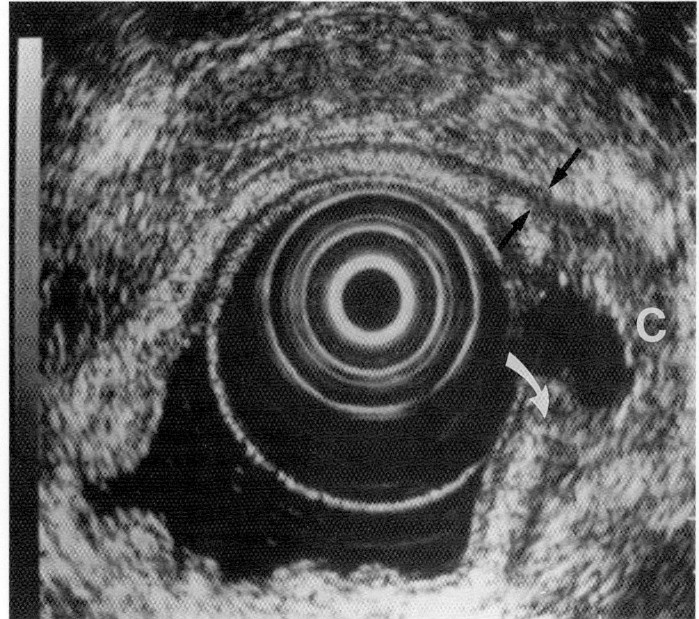

FIG. 1.84. Advanced gastric cancer. Endoluminal sonogram demonstrates deeply infiltrating carcinoma (C). Note widening and invasion of muscularis propria (*black arrows*) and abrupt termination of submucosal layer (*curved arrow*). (Case courtesy of Jin Hong Kim, MD, Seoul, Korea.)

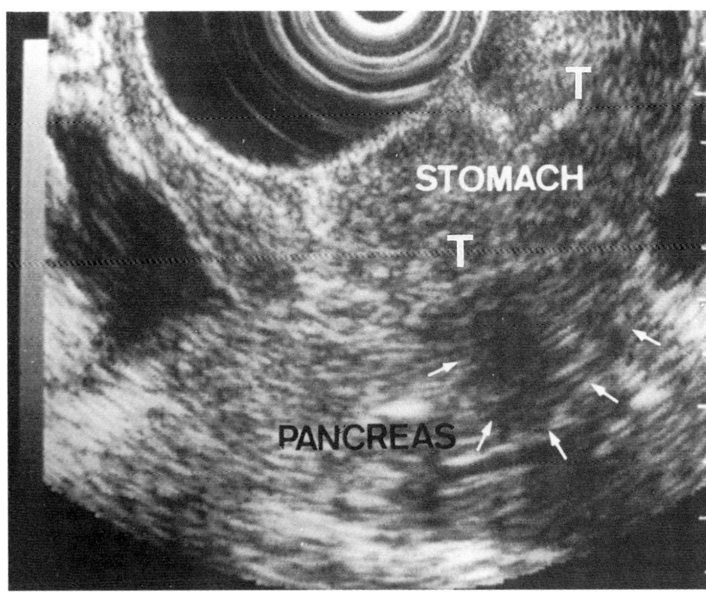

FIG. 1.85. Extragastric spread of gastric carcinoma. Endoluminal sonogram demonstrates bulky tumor (T) infiltrating stomach. Note hypoechoic tumor invading pancreas (*arrows*). (Case courtesy of Jin Hong Kim, MD, Seoul, Korea.)

A

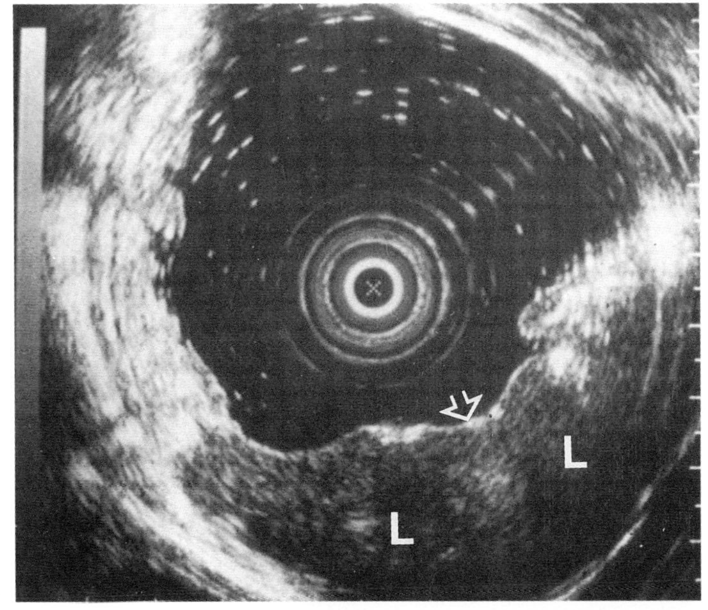

FIG. 1.86. Gastric lymphoma. **A:** Endoluminal sonogram demonstrating bulky submucosal lymphoma (L). Note preservation of mucosa (*open arrow*). **B:** Pathologic specimen demonstrates extensive infiltration by lymphoma. (Case courtesy of Jin Hong Kim, MD, Seoul, Korea.)

B

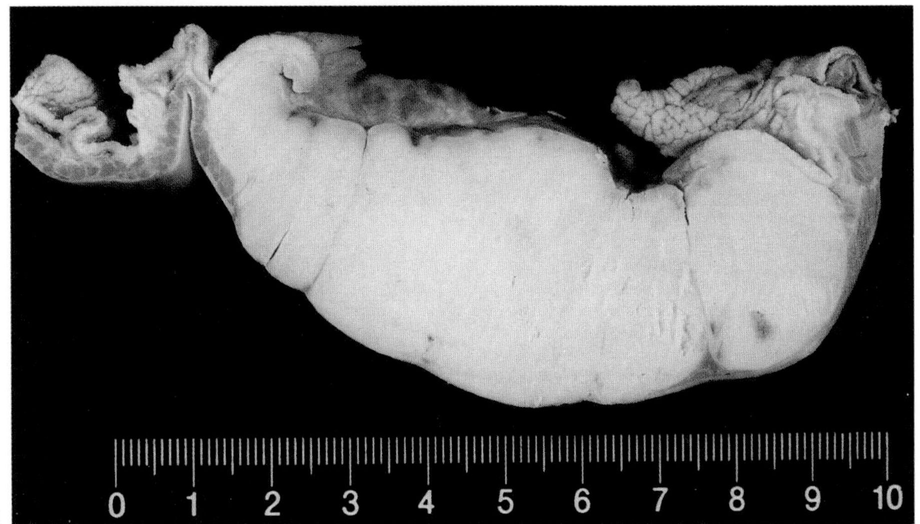

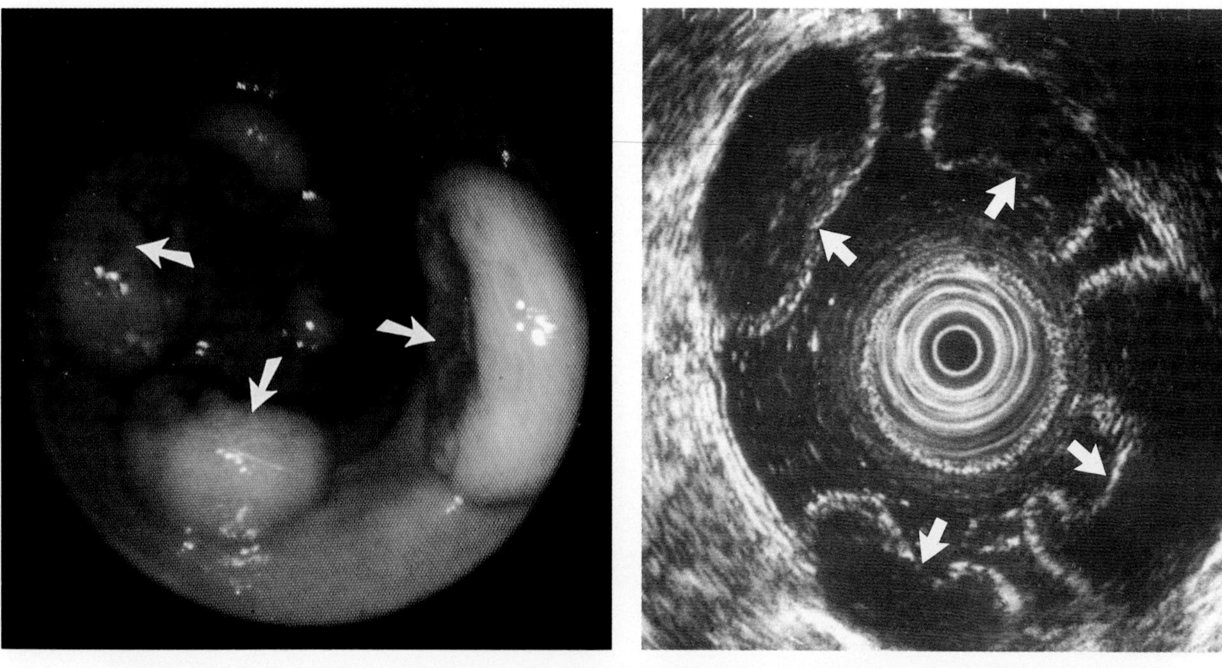

FIG. 1.87. Multiple submucosal gastric metastases. **A:** Endoscopy reveals multiple submucosal polypoid gastric lesions (*arrows*). **B:** Endoluminal sonogram demonstrates multiple submucosal metastases (*arrows*) from adenocarcinoma of unknown primary. (Case courtesy of Jin Hong Kim, MD, Seoul, Korea.)

sel HY. Comparison of computer tomography, ultrasonography and gallium-67 scanning in evaluation of suspected abdominal abscess. *Radiology* 1978;129:89–93.
8. Kuligowska E, Conners SK, Shapiro JH. Liver abscess: sonography in diagnosis and treatment. *AJR* 1982;138:253–257.
9. Kressel HY, Filly RA. Ultrasonographic appearance of gas-containing abscesses in the abdomen. *AJR* 1978;130:71–73.
10. Subramanyam BR, Balthazar EJ, Raghavendra BN, Horii SC, Hilton S, Naidich DP. Ultrasound analysis of solid-appearing abscesses. *Radiology* 1983;146:487–491.
11. Chiu LC, Schapiro RL, Yiu VS. Abdominal abscess I. Computed tomographic appearance, differential diagnosis and pitfalls in diagnosis. *CT* 1978;2:195–209.
12. Jeffrey RB. Abdominal abscesses: the role of CT and sonography. In: McGahan JP, ed. *Interventional ultrasound.* Baltimore: Williams & Wilkins; 1990:129–144.
13. Jeffrey RB, Federle MP, Tolentino CS. Periappendiceal inflammatory masses: CT-directed management and clinical outcome in 70 patients. *Radiology* 1988;167:13–16.
14. Jeffrey RB, Tolentino CS, Federle MP, Laing FC. Percutaneous drainage of periappendiceal abscesses: review of twenty patients. *AJR* 1987;149:59–62.
15. Borushok KF, Jeffrey RB, Laing FC, Townsend RR. Sonographic diagnosis of perforation in patients with acute appendicitis. *AJR* 1990;154:275–278.
16. Jeffrey RB, Nyberg DA, Bottles K, et al. Abdominal CT in acquired immunodeficiency syndrome. *AJR* 1986;146:7–13.
17. Jeffrey RB, Federle MP, Laing FC. Computed tomography of silent abdominal abscesses. *J Comput Assist Tomogr* 1984;8:67–70.
18. Wilson SR, Toi A. The value of sonography in the diagnosis of acute diverticulitis of the colon. *AJR* 1990;154:1199–1202.
19. Worlicek H, Lutz H, Heyder N, Matek W. Ultrasound findings in Crohn disease and ulcerative colitis: a prospective study. *J Clin Ultrasound* 1987;15:153–163.
20. Borgia G, Ciampi R, Nappa S, Vallone G, Marano I, Crowell J. Tuberculous mesenteric lymphadenitis clinically presenting as abdominal mass: CT and sonographic findings. *JCU* 1985;13:491–493.
21. Wu C-C, Chow K-S, Lü T-N, Huang F-T. Sonographic features of tuberculous omental cakes in peritoneal tuberculosis. *JCU* 1988;16:195–198.
22. Yeh HC. Ultrasonography of peritoneal tumors. *Radiology* 1979;133:419–424.
23. Yeh HC, Safer MK, Slater G, et al. Ultrasonography and computed tomography in pseudomyxoma peritonei. *Radiology* 1984;153:506–510.
24. Bluth EI, Merritt CRB, Sullivan MA. Ultrasonic evaluation of the stomach, small bowel, and colon. *Radiology* 1979;133:677–680.
25. Kimmey MB, Martin RW, Haggitt RC, Wang KY, Franklin DW, Silverstein FE. Histologic correlates of gastrointestinal ultrasound images. *Gastroenterology* 1989;96:433–441.
26. Puylaert JBCM. Acute appendicitis: US evaluation using graded compression. *Radiology* 1986;158:355–360.
27. Puylaert JBCM. Ultrasound for diagnosing appendicitis. *Br Med J* 1988;297:740–743.
28. Botet JF, Lightdale C. Endoscopic sonography of the upper gastrointestinal tract. *AJR* 1991;156:63–68.
29. Tio TL, Coene PPLO, van Delden OM, Tytgat GNJ. Colorectal carcinoma: preoperative TNM classification with endosonography. *Radiology* 1991;179:165–170.
30. Tio TL, Cohen P, Coene PP, Udding J, den Hartog Jager FCA, Tytgat GNJ. Endosonography and computed tomography of esophageal carcinoma: preoperative classification compared to the new (1987) TNM system. *Gastroenterology* 1989;96:1478–1486.
31. Jeffrey RB, Laing FC, Lewis FR. Acute appendicitis: high-resolution real-time US findings. *Radiology* 1987;163:11–14.
32. Abu-Yousef MM, Bleicher JJ, Maher JW, Urdaneta LF, Franken EA, Metcalf AM. High-resolution sonography of acute appendicitis. *AJR* 1987;149:53–58.
33. Jeffrey RB, Laing FC, Townsend RR. Acute appendicitis: sonographic criteria based on 250 cases. *Radiology* 1988;167:327–329.
34. Gaensler EHL, Jeffrey RB, Laing FC, Townsend RR. Sonography in patients with suspected acute appendicitis: value in establishing alternative diagnoses. *AJR* 1989;152:49–51.
35. Puylaert JBCM, Lalisang RI, van der Werf SDJ, Doornbos L. *Campylobacter* ileocolitis mimicking acute appendicitis: differentiation with graded-compression US. *Radiology* 1988;166:737–740.
36. Rioux M. Sonographic detection of the normal and abnormal appendix. *AJR* 1992;158:773–778.
37. Lee KH, Lim HK, Bae SH, Seo GS. Detection of appendicoliths in patients with acute appendicitis: comparative study with US and plain film, abstract. AFSUMB meeting Seoul, Korea, September 1992.
38. Kirshenbaum KJ, Warner JJ, Nadimpalli SR, Cavallino RP. Endometriosis of the right fallopian tube mimicking appendicitis on sonography. *J Ultrasound Med* 1990;9:57–59.
39. Puylaert JBCM. *Ultrasound of appendicitis and its differential diagnosis.* Berlin: Springer-Verlag; 1990:60–62.
40. Poljak A, Jeffrey RB, Kernberg M. The gas-containing appendix: potential sonographic pitfall in the diagnosis of acute appendicitis. *J Ultrasound Med* 1991;10:625–628.
41. Nghiem HV, Jeffrey RB. Acute appendicitis confined to the appendiceal tip: evaluation with graded compression sonography. *J Ultrasound Med* 1992;11:205–207.
42. Hulnick DH, Megibow AJ, Balthazar EJ, Naidich DP, Bosniak MA. Computed tomography in the evaluation of diverticulitis. *Radiology* 1984;152:491–495.
43. Johnson CD, Baker ME, Rice RP, Silverman P, Thompson WM. Diagnosis of acute colonic diverticulitis: comparison of barium enema and CT. *AJR* 1987;148:541–546.
44. Mueller PR, Saini S, Wittenburg J, et al. Sigmoid diverticular abscesses: percutaneous drainage as an adjunct to surgical resection in 24 cases. *Radiology* 1987;164:321–325.
45. Neff CC, vanSonnenberg E, Casola G, et al. Diverticular abscesses: percutaneous drainage. *Radiology* 1987;163:15–18.
46. Saini S, Mueller PR, Wittenberg J, Butch RJ, Rodkey GV, Welch CE. Percutaneous drainage of diverticular abscess: an adjunct to surgical therapy. *Arch Surg* 1986;121:475–478.
47. Blathazar EJ, Megibow AJ, Gordon RB, Hulnick D. Cecal diverticulitis: evaluation with CT. *Radiology* 1987;162:79–81.
48. Wilson SR, Toi A. The value of sonography in the diagnosis of acute diverticulitis of the colon. *AJR* 1990;154:1199–1202.
49. Parulekar SG. Sonography of colonic diverticulitis. *J Ultrasound Med* 1985;4:659–666.
50. Puylaert JBCM. *Ultrasound of appendicitis and its differential diagnosis.* Berlin: Springer-Verlag; 1990:81.
51. Puylaert JBCM. Mesenteric adenitis and acute terminal ileitis: US evaluation using graded compression. *Radiology* 1986;161:691–695.
52. Goldberg HI, Gore RM, Margulis AR, Moss AA, Baker EL. Computed tomography in the evaluation of Crohn disease. *AJR* 1983;140:277–282.
53. Fishman EK, Wolf EJ, Jones B, Bayless TM, Siegelman SS. CT evaluation of Crohn disease: effect on patient management. *AJR* 1987;148:537–540.
54. Casola G, vanSonnenberg E, Neff CC, Saba RM, Withers C, Emarine CW. Abscesses in Crohn disease: percutaneous drainage. *Radiology* 1987;163:19–22.
55. Millward SF, Ramsewak W, Fitzsimons P, Frost R, Tam P, Toi A. Percutaneous drainage of iliopsoas abscess in Crohn disease. *Gastrointest Radiol* 1986;11:289–290.
56. Lambiase RE, Cronan JJ, Dorfman GS, Paolella LP, Hass RA. Percutaneous drainage of abscesses in patients in Crohn disease. *AJR* 1988;150:1043–1045.
57. Orel SG, Rubesin SE, Jones B, Fishman EK, Bayless TM, Siegelman SS. Computed tomography vs. barium studies in the acutely symptomatic patient with Crohn disease. *J Comput Assist Tomogr* 1987;11:1009–1016.
58. Tedesco FJ. Pseudomembranous colitis: pathogenesis and therapy. *Med Clin North Am* 1982;66:655–664.
59. Merine D, Fishman EK, Jones B. Pseudomembranous colitis: CT evaluation. *J Comput Assist Tomogr* 1987;11:1017–1020.
60. Megibow AJ, Streiter ML, Balthazar EJ, Bosniak MA. Pseudomembranous colitis: diagnosis by computed tomography. *J Comput Assist Tomogr* 1984;8:281–283.
61. Goodman PC, Federle MP. Pseudomembranous colitis. *J Comput Assist Tomogr* 1980;4:403–404.

62. Bolondi L, Ferrentino M, Trevisani F, Bernardi M, Gasbarrini G. Sonographic appearance of pseudomembranous colitis. *J Ultrasound Med* 1985;4:489–492.
63. Downey DB, Wilson SR. Pseudomembranous colitis: sonographic features. *Radiology* 1991;180:61–64.
64. Parienty RA, Lepreux JF, Gruson B. Sonographic and CT features of ileocolic intussusception. *AJR* 1981;136:608–610.
65. Donovan AT, Goldman SM. Computed tomography of ileocecal intussusception: mechanism and appearance. *J Comput Assist Tomogr* 1982;6:630–632.
66. Curcio CM, Feinstein RS, Humphrey RL, Jones B, Siegelman SS. Computed tomography of entero-enteric intussusception. *J Comput Assist Tomogr* 1982;6:969–974.
67. Merine D, Fishman EK, Jones B, Siegelman SS. Enteroenteric intussusception: CT findings in nine patients. *AJR* 1987;148:1129–1132.
68. Mulvihill DM. Ultrasound findings of chronic intussusception in a patient with cystic fibrosis. *J Ultrasound Med* 1988;7:353–355.
69. Maglinte DDT, Fleischer AC, Chua GT, Kelvin FM. Sonography of appendiceal intussusception. *Gastrointest Radiol* 1987;12:163–165.
70. Swayne LC, Love MB. Computed tomography of chronic afferent loop obstruction: a case report and review. *Gastrointest Radiol* 1985;10:39–41.
71. Weissberg DL, Scheible W, Leopold GR. Ultrasonographic appearance of adult intussusception. *Radiology* 1977;124:791–792.
72. Alessi V, Salerno G. The "hay-fork" sign in the ultrasonographic diagnosis of intussusception. *Gastrointest Radiol* 1985;10:177–179.
73. Sauerbrei EE, Nguyen KT, Nolan RL. *Abdominal sonography*. New York: Raven Press; 1992:246–249.
74. Federle MP, Chun G, Jeffrey RB, Raynor R. Computed tomographic findings in bowel infarction. *AJR* 1984;142:91–95.
75. Clark RA. Computed tomography of bowel infarction. *J Comput Assist Tomogr* 1987;11:757–762.
76. Nichols DM. Computed tomography in acute mesenteric vein thrombosis. *J Comput Assist Tomogr* 1984;8:171–172.
77. Alpern MB, Glazer GM, Francis IR. Ischemic or infarcted bowel: CT findings. *Radiology* 1988;166:149–152.
78. Horgan JG, Chow PP, Richter JO, Rosenfield AT, Taylor KJW. CT and sonography in the recognition of mucoceles of the appendix. *AJR* 1984;143:959–962.
79. Ziegler K, Sanft C, Zeitz M, et al. Evaluation of endosonography in TN staging of oesophageal cancer. *Gut* 1991;32:16–20.

CHAPTER 2

The Liver

TECHNIQUE

The liver is best imaged with the patient in the supine and right anterior oblique positions, starting with 3- to 5-MHz curved linear or linear array transducers. A subcostal acoustic window should be used first, supplemented with intercostal scans. Sector or other small footprint transducers should be used to image areas inaccessible with other transducers. Scanning with 2 MHz may be required in echogenic highly attenuating livers, especially when Doppler information is sought. The liver surface (usually the ventral left lobe) should be evaluated for nodularity with a near-field optimized, 5- to 7-MHz linear array transducer. It is easier to appreciate subtle nodularity during real-time examination than on hard copy images. Care must be taken to scan with the transducer face parallel to the liver surface. Angulation may falsely simulate subtle nodularity.

Routine color flow imaging is useful in patients with suspected liver pathology. Initial scan parameters should be set for maximum sensitivity, so as to avoid missing unexpected flow abnormalities. Optimal color flow and spectral Doppler sonography of the liver generally requires relatively low-frequency (2 to 3 MHz) scanning and good acoustic access. A low (near 0 or 180 degrees) scan angle, where the blood flow is directly toward or away from the transducer, also facilitates flow detection. Sensitivity is enhanced by low wall filter and low pulse repetition frequency settings. Maximum power and gain settings, commensurate with an artifact-free image, are desirable. Larger effective sample volume and smaller color display areas may also enhance sensitivity.

Spectral Doppler and color flow settings optimized for sensitivity often result in artifact. "Flash" artifact—color related to tissue motion—and aliasing—"wrap around" artifacts resulting in ambiguous display of flow direction—are the most common. After an area of flow has been identified with high-sensitivity settings, parameters should be modified to better characterize flow. For example, increased wall filter and pulse repetition frequency yield less flash artifact and clear delineation of flow direction.

It is difficult to image the entire liver, even in the best circumstances. Difficult areas include the superficial liver above the costal margin, the left tip of the lateral segment of the left lobe, and the ventral subdiaphragmatic regions (1). Care should be taken to image the liver as completely as possible in all patients.

FOCAL LIVER DISEASE

Detection and analysis of focal liver lesions may be difficult and confusing. *All* standard noninvasive imaging modalities are insensitive detectors of focal hepatic disease. Controlled clinical trials that correlate image findings with surgical or autopsy findings yield individual lesion detection rates ranging from 38 to 66 percent for magnetic resonance imaging (MRI), delayed high dose computed tomography (CT), and dynamic incremental CT (2,3). Sensitivity problems are no surprise to radiologists experienced in hepatic imaging, since focal hepatic lesions are frequently missed with one modality, then detected with another (Fig. 2.1). Some studies have suggested that sonography is less sensitive than CT and MRI (4). Despite this, other studies show that modern sonography can perform well in detecting focal liver disease (5–7). Since all modalities are imperfect, there is no single "best test." The best approach is to use clinically tailored imaging strategies that take advantage of the strengths of CT, MRI, and sonography.

Hepatic sonography's main strengths are its ability to guide biopsy, to characterize common benign lesions (cysts, hemangiomas), its safety, and its low cost. Its weaknesses include inability to image the entire liver in some patients and inferiority to CT in detecting extrahepatic disease.

Sonography, like CT, can effectively guide biopsy.

(text continues on page 73)

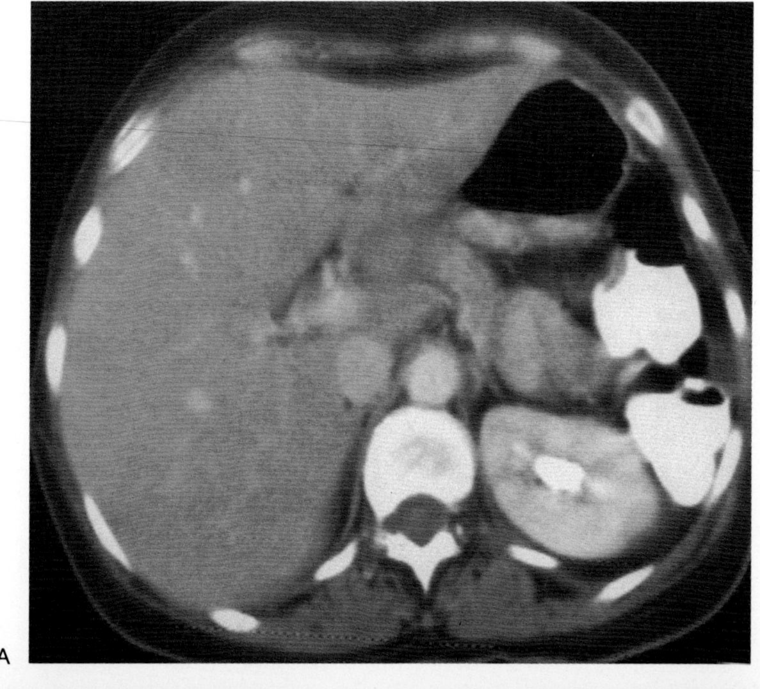

A

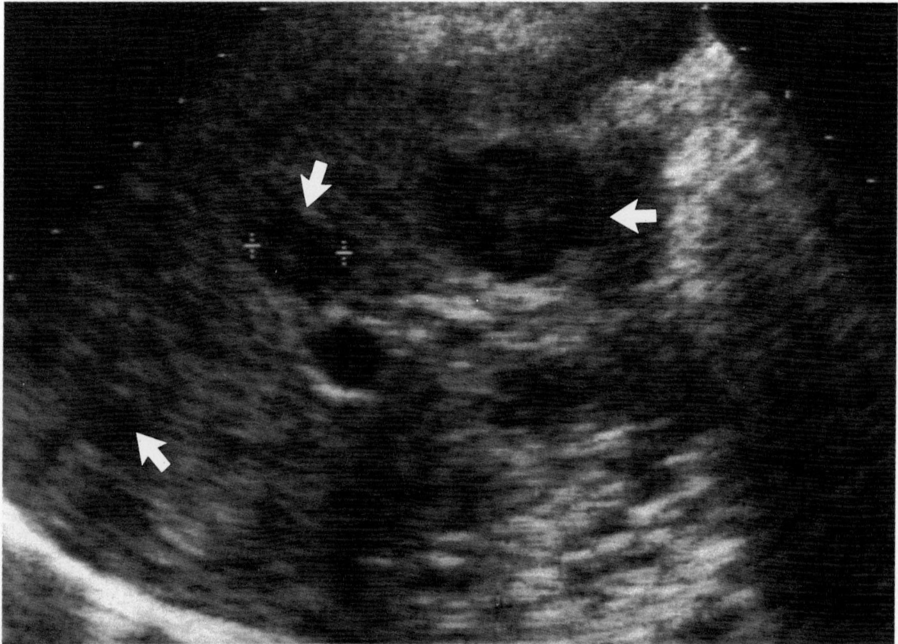

B

FIG. 2.1. Liver metastasis, invisible on CT. **A:** Pre- and postcontrast CT scans revealed no metastatic lesions in this patient with malignant fibrous histiocytoma. **B:** A transverse sonogram performed the same day revealed multifocal hepatic metastases (*arrows*). As all noninvasive liver imaging modalities are imperfectly sensitive, it is not unusual for one modality to detect lesions invisible on another. For this reason, selection of imaging modality should be dictated by the clinical situation.

Magnetic resonance imaging and nuclear medicine techniques lack this ability. In experienced hands, sonographically guided liver biopsy is often quicker and easier than CT guidance. Sonography directly visualizes the needle tip as it is placed in the lesion, facilitating biopsy of small lesions and lesions in uncooperative patients. Ultrasound guided biopsy is more efficient and cost effective, even when lesions are initially detected with some other modality.

Despite sonography's advantages, CT guided biopsy is often more popular with radiologists because it almost always shows needle location. Sonographic needle visualization often requires some experience. Visualization may be impossible when the liver is echogenic or when acoustic access is suboptimal. Newer sonographic techniques that enhance needle tip visualization and improved biopsy guides promise to make sonographically guided biopsies easier.

Sonography may be used to evaluate resectability of primary or metastatic liver tumors. Sonography's ability to image in any oblique plane often makes it superior to CT and MRI in localizing lesions to an anatomical hepatic segment. Sonography can guide biopsy of newly detected lesions that might preclude curative hepatic resection. If sonography indicates that a lesion is resectable, CT arterial portography is performed prior to surgery. Intraoperative sonography is currently the most sensitive means of detecting focal liver lesions (8,9). In many centers where hepatic resections are performed, intraoperative sonography is routine prior to resection (Figs. 2.2 and 2.3). When a questionable lesion is found intraoperatively, sonographically guided biopsy can be performed.

When liver abscess is suspected clinically, sonography is the preferred screening modality (6). Hepatic sonography can be used to screen for metastases, if extrahepatic staging is not needed. When an optimal sonographic exam cannot be obtained in an individual patient, CT should be performed. CT is also preferred when extrahepatic staging is required.

Unsuspected liver lesions are often found incidentally during sonography for extraneous indications. Depending on the sonographic findings and clinical setting, sonography can guide further evaluation or management, for example, percutaneous drainage, biopsy, or additional imaging. Sonography is often indicated to characterize focal liver lesions found with other modalities (Fig. 2.4).

Color flow sonography improves detection of focal lesions, especially anechoic or hypoechoic lesions. Hypoechoic lesions, such as cysts, are clearly identified adjacent to color-coded vessels (Fig. 2.5). Some tumors are more conspicuous because of increased flow compared to normal liver: focal nodular hyperplasia, most hepatocellular carcinomas, some metastases, and occasionally other masses (10–12). Increased tumor vascularity is rarely, if ever, the only sonographic finding. Focal hepatic lesions virtually always have associated grayscale abnormalities.

Doppler Analysis of Focal Liver Lesions

Recent advances in instrumentation have improved Doppler flexibility and sensitivity. The potential of both spectral and color flow sonography to enhance the analysis of focal liver lesions is one of the more interesting recent innovations in diagnostic sonography.

Taylor et al. (13) and Ohnishi and Nomura (14) evaluated focal liver lesions with spectral Doppler sonography. They found increased Doppler shifts in hepatocellular carcinoma, and lower shifts in other lesions. These results suggest the potential to differentiate among focal liver lesions by spectral Doppler analysis. Other observers have found it difficult to duplicate these results. The main technical difficulty lies in finding the tiny areas of arteriovenous (AV) shunting associated with high-frequency signal shift. The attempt to identify these small areas with spectral Doppler sonography may be very time consuming and hence impractical. In addition, high-frequency shifts may be found in other liver diseases, including chronic active hepatitis, cirrhosis, and alcoholic hepatitis. These Doppler signals should not cause confusion, as they are not associated with a mass.

Color flow pattern analysis of focal liver lesions is another interesting area of investigation. Hepatocellular carcinomas (HCCs) generally exhibit increased flow compared to normal liver (11). Tanaka et al. (10) described flow around the periphery and penetrating into the mass in 16 of 20 HCCs (Fig. 2.6). Intralesional flow was not detected in 15 patients with other focal liver lesions. Displacement of hepatic veins ("detour sign") (Fig. 2.7) was noted in two of four patients with metastatic disease. A small, spot-like area of flow was noted in three of six hemangiomas.

A recent study of 118 focal lesions, however, failed to confirm Tanaka's results. Significant overlap in the color flow patterns of hepatic neoplasms was noted (12). HCC (Figs. 2.8 and 2.9) had a higher prevalence of internal flow (76 percent) than metastasis (Figs. 2.10 and 2.11) (33 percent), but internal flow is not a specific finding. Flow within hemangiomas (Fig. 2.12) was seen in only 1 of 12 lesions.

Observing hypervascularity within a lesion makes HCC a more likely diagnosis. Most avascular lesions will be metastasis, not HCC. Even a hypervascular lesion is, in North America, slightly more likely to be a metastasis than HCC. This is so simply because metastases, despite their lower prevalence of internal color flow, are so much more frequent than HCC. Other lesions, notably focal nodular hyperplasia, also exhibit internal flow. A well-defined hyperechoic lesion is less likely to be hemangioma if there is internal flow; further imaging evaluation or biopsy should be performed. Further investigation is

(text continues on page 80)

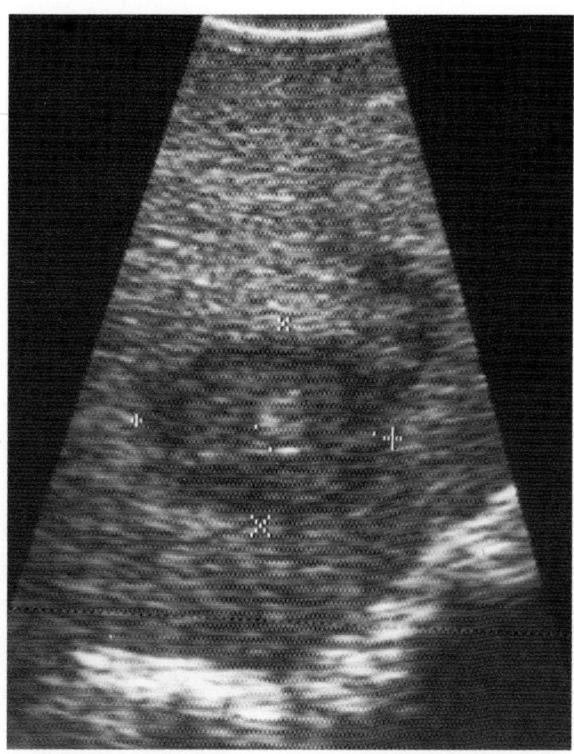

FIG. 2.2. Intraoperative sonogram, colon carcinoma metastasis. This intraoperative study reveals a well-defined target lesion that measures approximately 2 cm. This lesion was only questionably present on all preoperative imaging studies.

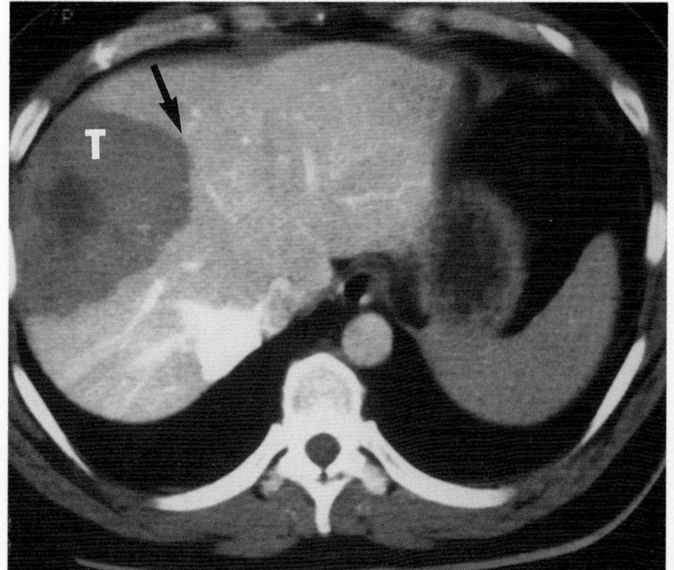

A

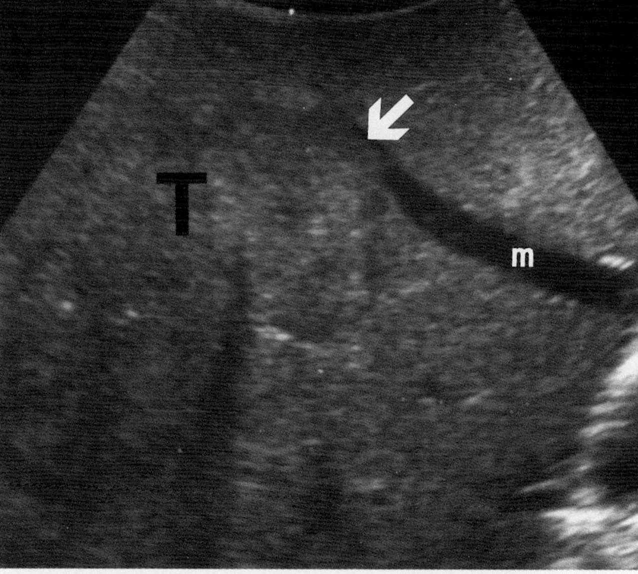

FIG. 2.3. Intraoperative sonogram, colon carcinoma. **A:** The preoperative CT arterial portography image reveals a large tumor mass (T) that is near the middle hepatic vein (*arrow*). **B:** The intraoperative sonogram reveals invasion of the middle hepatic vein (*arrow*). This is important information, significantly affecting the approach to surgical resection. m, middle hepatic vein; T, tumor mass.

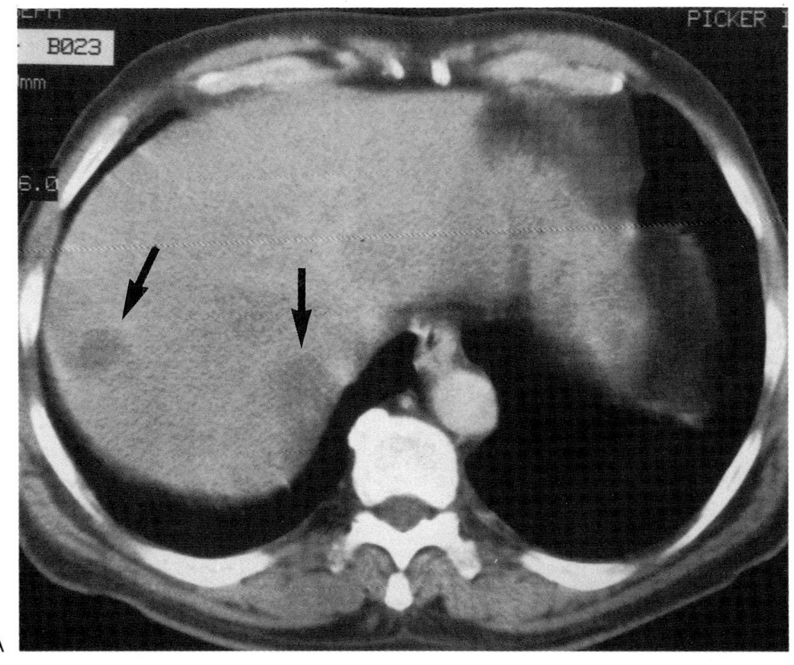

A

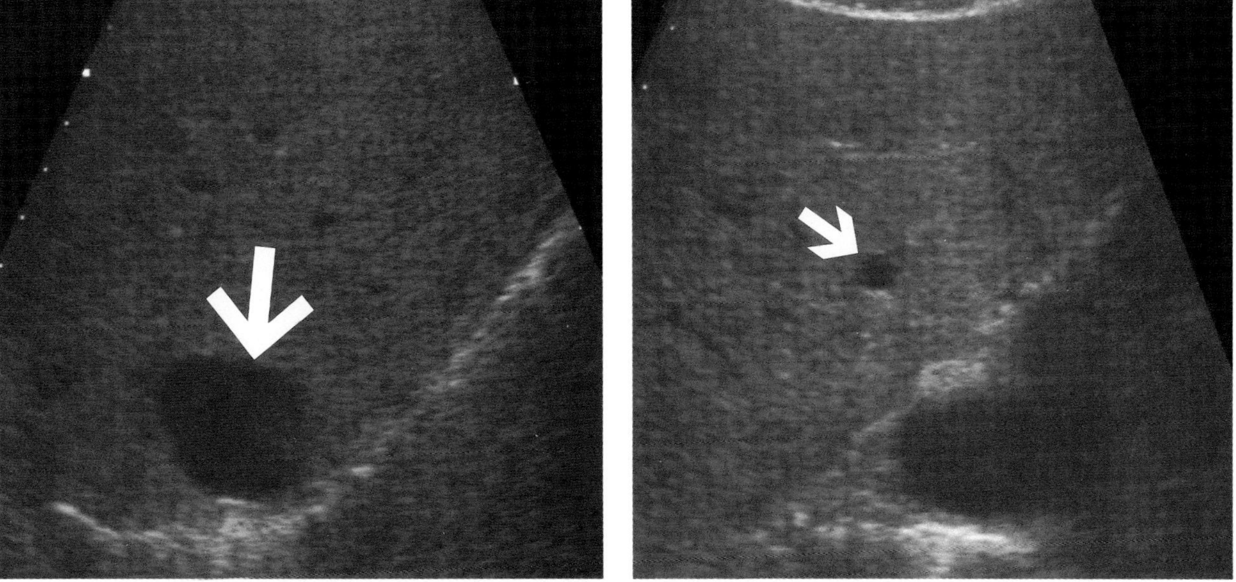

B C

FIG. 2.4. Lung carcinoma, CT equivocal for metastasis. The CT scan (**A**) in this patient with lung carcinoma reveals low attenuation areas (*arrows*) suspicious for metastasis. Transverse sonograms through the dome of the liver (**B**) and the left lobe (**C**) reveal that the lesions detected by CT are, in fact, cysts (*arrows*). Sonography is often useful to characterize lesions that are detected on other imaging modalities.

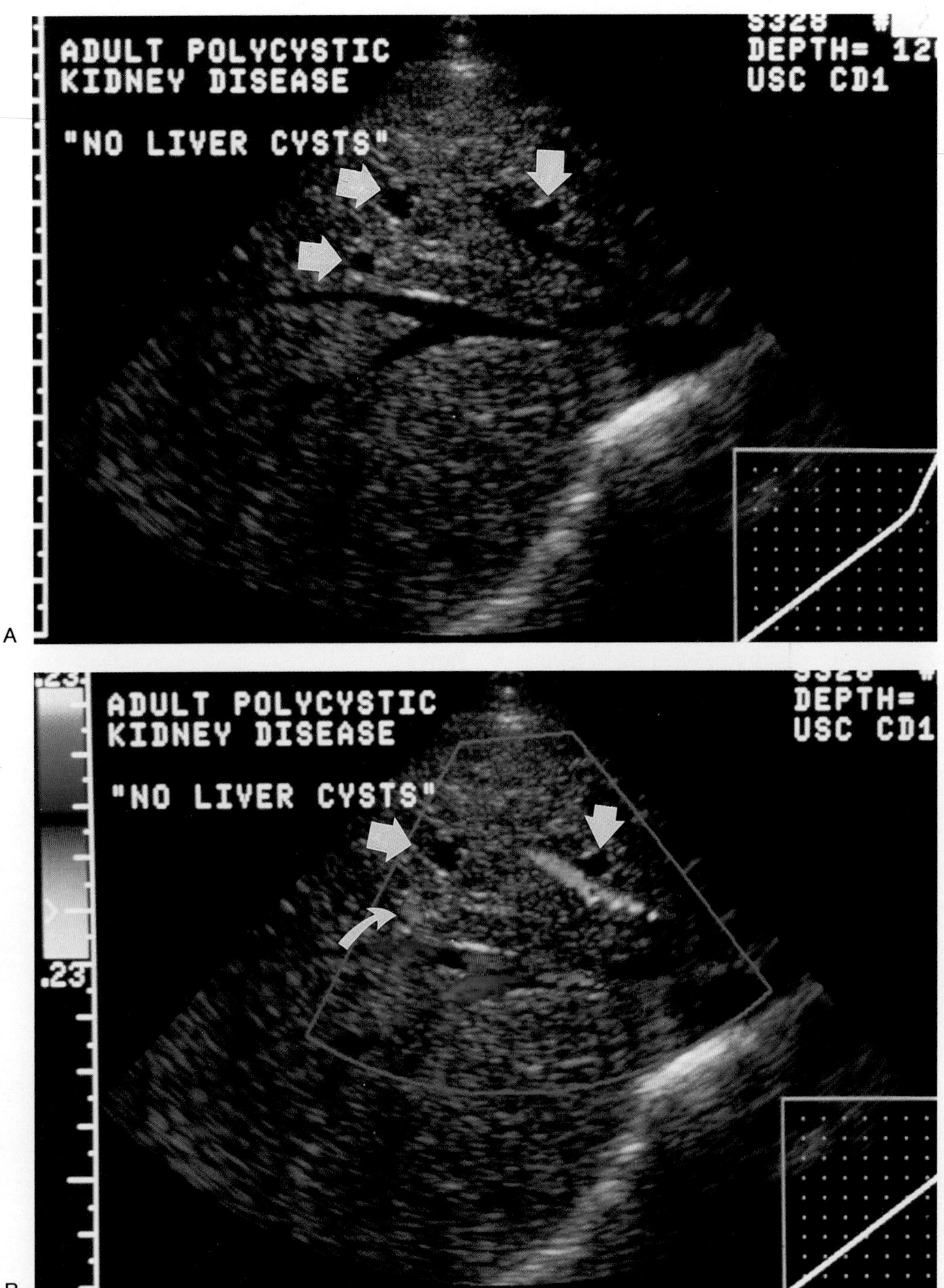

FIG. 2.5. Hepatic cysts detected only with color Doppler sonography. In this patient with renal (autosomal dominant) polycystic disease, preliminary grayscale examination revealed no liver cysts. This grayscale (**A**) and color Doppler (**B**) image pair demonstrates several small anechoic areas suggestive of cysts (*arrows*). On color Doppler, one of these (*curved arrow*) is a vascular structure, while the other two are cysts (*arrows*). Color Doppler, by highlighting flow, facilitates detection of low echogenicity hepatic lesions such as these small cysts. Tiny cysts like these are often only detected using color flow sonography. They are dismissed as small vessels on grayscale exam.

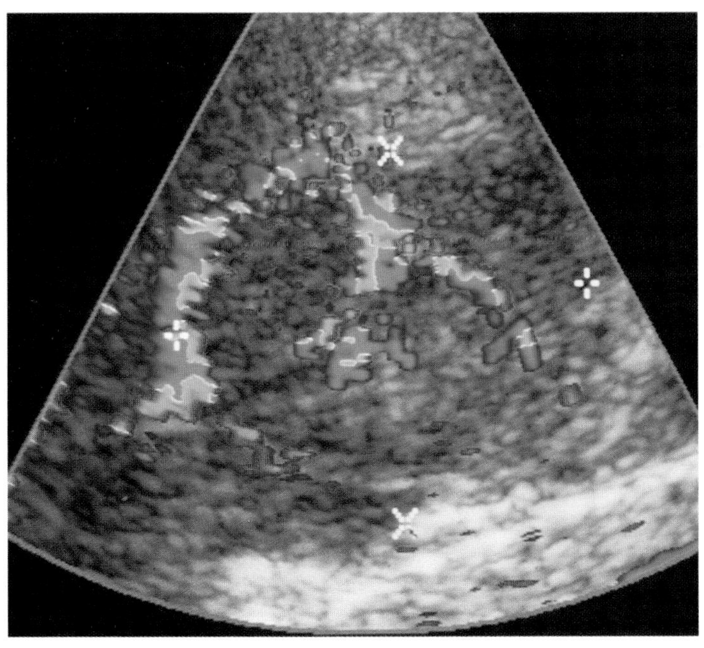

FIG. 2.6. HCC color Doppler "basket" sign. Transverse color Doppler sonogram of small HCC nodule reveals flow at the periphery and penetrating into the mass. Internal flow can be detected in approximately 75 percent of HCCs, but in only 33 percent of metastases. This is an example of Tanaka's "basket sign."

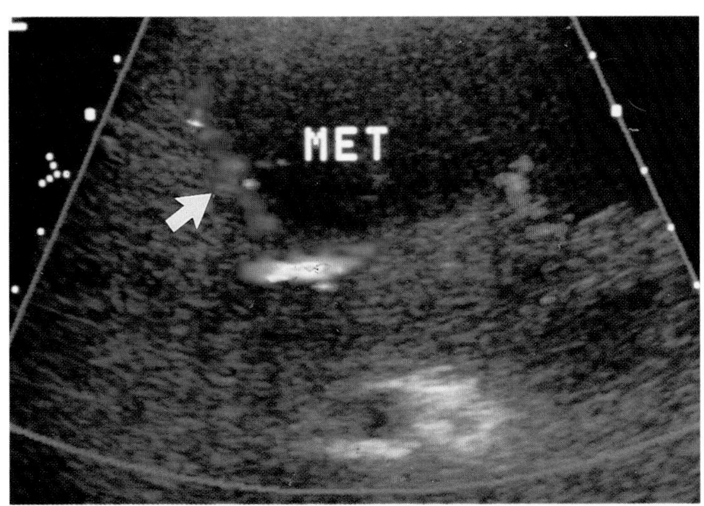

FIG. 2.7. Hepatic metastasis, color flow detour sign. Transverse oblique color Doppler sonogram through the liver reveals a metastasis (MET) from malignant melanoma. The metastasis displaces a color-coded vein (*arrow*). This pattern, venous displacement with no internal flow, is Tanaka's "detour sign," a sign she described as characteristic of metastatic focal liver lesions.

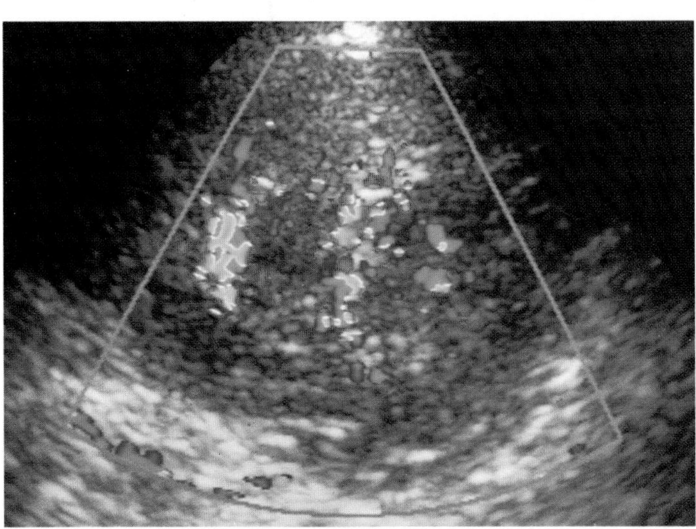

FIG. 2.8. HCC internal flow. Transverse sonogram of the left lobe shows increased flow in this HCC nodule. Internal flow is demonstrated by color flow imaging in about three-quarters of HCCs.

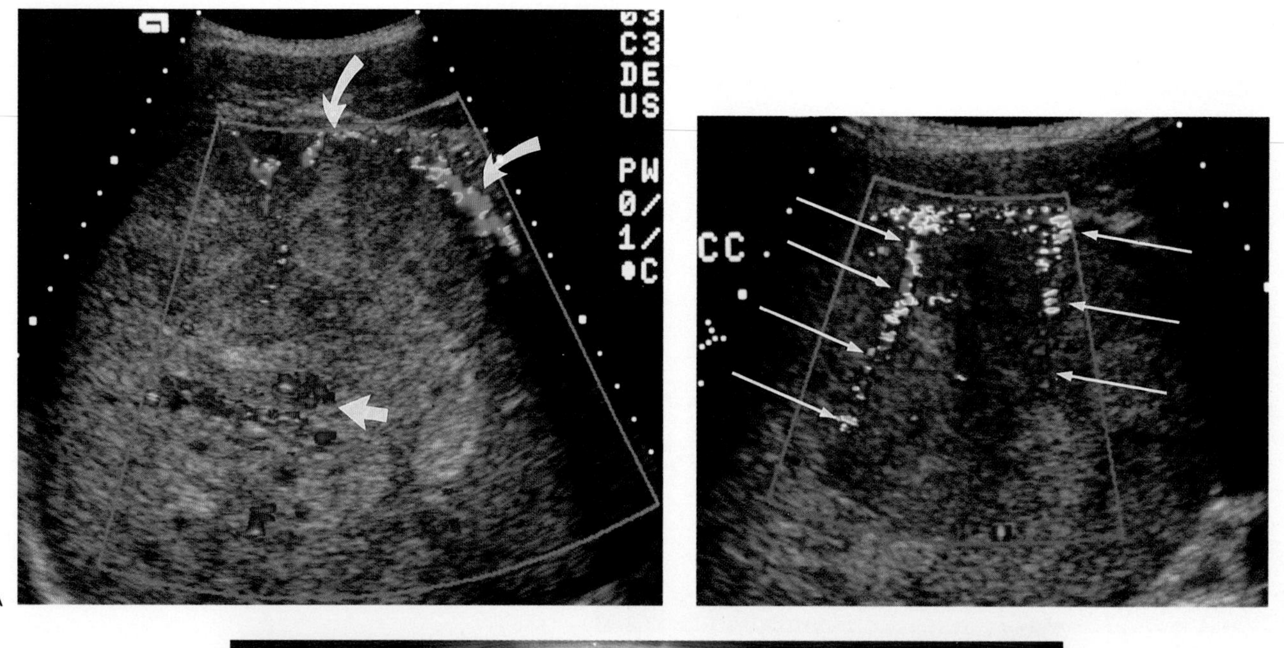

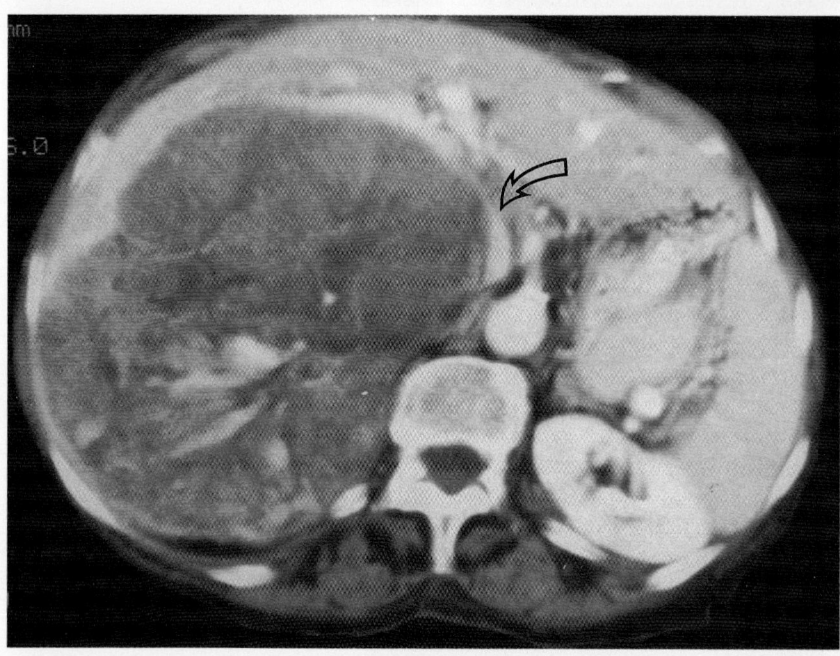

FIG. 2.9. Large HCC. Longitudinal (**A**) and transverse (**B**) color Doppler sonograms show internal flow (*arrow*) and a displaced middle hepatic vein (*curved arrow*). Note the radial flow from the periphery of the lesion down into the interior portion of the tumor (*thin arrows*). The dynamic contrast-enhanced CT scan (**C**) shows similar findings. The inferior vena cava (*curved open arrow*) is displaced medially. Tumoral flow with color Doppler sonography is not related to lesion size. Many large lesions exhibit little or no internal flow, while some small lesions are markedly hypervascular on color flow sonography.

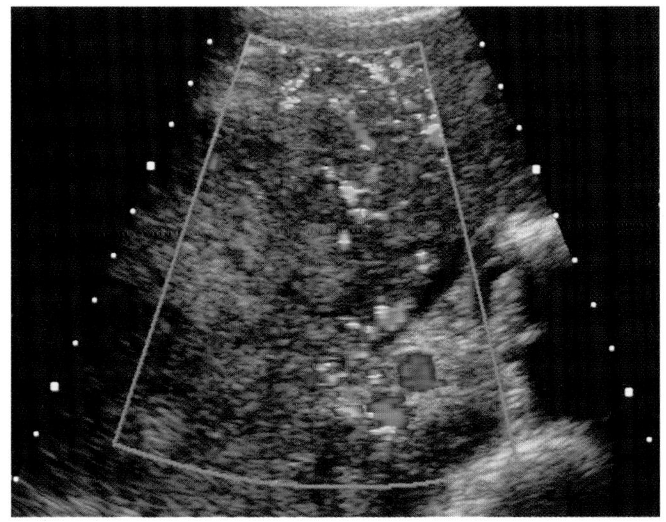

FIG. 2.10. Hepatic metastasis with internal flow. Transverse color Doppler sonogram reveals internal flow in this hepatic metastasis from nasopharyngeal carcinoma. Although most hepatic metastases do not have internal flow on color Doppler sonography, approximately one-third do. Although internal HCC has internal color flow much more frequently (75 percent) than metastasis (33 percent), metastases with internal flow are encountered at least as often because metastatic lesions are so much more common than HCC.

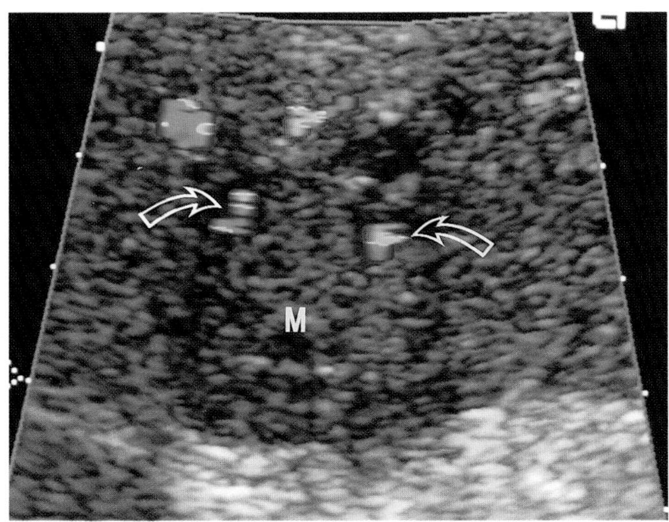

FIG. 2.11. Hepatic metastasis, internal flow. Transverse color Doppler sonogram shows a small amount of internal flow (*curved open arrows*) in this metastasis (M) from gastric carcinoma. In many instances, flow within hepatic metastasis is less than that seen in HCC. Despite this, distinction between HCC and metastasis based on differences in color flow is impossible, as both may have markedly increased internal flow compared to the normal liver (see Fig. 2.8).

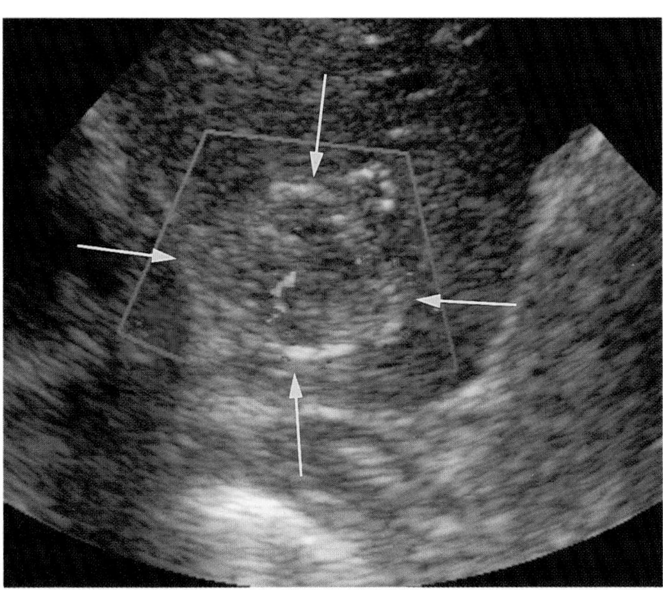

FIG. 2.12. Hemangioma with internal flow on color Doppler. Oblique sonogram of a biopsy proved hemangioma (*thin arrows*) with internal color flow. Flow was identified in only one of 12 hemangiomas in Nino-Murcia's recent series (12). When flow is detected within a lesion that has the grayscale appearance of hemangioma, further evaluation is indicated. See Fig. 2.38.

needed to clarify the usefulness of color Doppler sonography (CDS) in evaluating focal liver lesions.

Image Findings in Common Liver Lesions

Sheila Sherlock, the renowned English hepatologist, has stated "focal (liver) lesions can be divided into two classes: those that one wishes had never been seen and those that are clinically significant" (15). The most common insignificant lesions are cysts and hemangiomas, often discovered incidentally. Common significant lesions include metastasis, hepatocellular carcinoma (HCC), and liver abscess. Focal nodular hyperplasia, a clinically insignificant lesion, and hepatic adenoma, which may have adverse clinical consequences, are less frequent examples of this dichotomy.

Simple Hepatic Cysts

Simple cysts, usually considered congenital, are better described as developmental, since their prevalence increases with age. In a large series, cysts were found in fewer than 1 percent of patients less than 60 years old, but in 3 to 7 percent of older patients (16). Thus other diseases should be considered when a cyst is found in a young patient: hepatic polycystic disease, renal (autosomal dominant) polycystic kidney disease, von Hippel–Lindau disease, and conditions simulating simple cysts, such as echinococcal disease, residua from trauma or infection, and cystic neoplasia.

Simple hepatic cysts are usually solitary, have a thin epithelial lining, and contain serous fluid. Their size varies from less than 1 cm to more than 20 cm in diameter. Simple cysts are four times more common in females. Symptoms are rare but may occur from mass effect, rupture, hemorrhage, or infection (17).

Most liver cysts are easily diagnosed with sonography, CT, or MRI. Simple cysts are usually round or oval. The classic sonographic findings of a well defined, echo-free lesion with good through transmission and an imperceptible wall are well known (Figs. 2.5, 2.13, and 2.14). Thin septations are frequent and should not suggest a different diagnosis (Fig. 2.15). Thicker septations are generally a sign of a complicated cyst (Figs. 2.16 and 2.17) or of a cystic neoplasm. Sonography is usually the best method to evaluate cysts. With CT, the attenuation of small cysts may be higher than that of water (partial volume phenomenon) and may not fulfill CT diagnostic criteria (Fig. 2.4). Because of their distinctive sonographic features, cysts rarely simulate clinically significant lesions.

Hepatic Polycystic Disease

Hepatic polycystic disease is characterized by multiple liver cysts varying in number from a few to many. The cysts are lined with bile duct epithelium but do not communicate with the ducts (Fig. 2.18). Extensive involvement may cause symptomatic hepatomegaly. The cysts tend to be more numerous peripherally, although diffuse involvement may occur. Complications, rupture, infection (Fig. 2.19), and hemorrhage (Fig. 2.20) may cause pain or other symptoms (18). Liver insufficiency occurs only occasionally and late (19), even though little normal parenchyma may be apparent in extensively involved livers. Gene analysis suggests that hepatic polycystic disease and renal (autosomal dominant) polycystic disease result from the same genetic defect (19); inheritance is autosomal dominant. About one-half of patients have renal cysts. Sonographic findings include multiple, often contiguous, simple cysts. Irregular shape and septa are common. Hemorrhage or infection may cause debris-like echoes within one or more cysts (Figs. 2.19 and 2.20).

Von Meyenberg's complex is a rare disorder characterized by multiple small cystic hamartomas of the bile ducts (Fig. 2.21). It may result in multiple liver cysts that may be detected on images.

Other Cystic Lesions

Acquired cysts may occur as a result of trauma (18,20) (Figs. 2.22 and 2.23) or infection (18,21) (Fig. 2.24). Neoplasms that simulate simple cysts are unusual; metastases from squamous cell carcinoma, sarcomas, and cystic adenocarcinomas occasionally do this.

Hepatobiliary cystadenoma is a rare neoplasm probably arising from bile duct epithelium. It is more common in women. Sonographically, these lesions are predominantly multicystic with varying amounts of solid tissue (Figs. 2.25 to 2.27). Tumors that have significant solid areas are usually of the mesenchymal type and have greater malignant potential (22–24).

Hydatid disease is a severe and common parasitic disease in which humans are the accidental intermediate hosts of *Echinococcus* tapeworms. The liver is the most frequently involved organ. Sonographic findings vary; several inconsistent classification systems have been proposed (25–28). A spectrum of sonographic findings from purely cystic to solid appearing pseudotumors (Fig. 2.28) occurs. Internally, wavy bands of delaminated endocyst (the "water lily" sign) (Fig. 2.29) may be noted (29). Daughter cysts, sometimes surrounded by echogenic debris ("matrix") (Fig. 2.29) are frequent. Calcifications, varying from tiny to massive, are often present and more sensitively detected by CT (Figs. 2.30 and 2.31) (26). Calcification probably correlates with cyst maturation and aging (27). A densely calcified cyst usually indicates a dead, inactive lesion. Previously considered contraindicated, percutaneous drainage and treatment have recently been described (30,31).

(*text continues on page 92*)

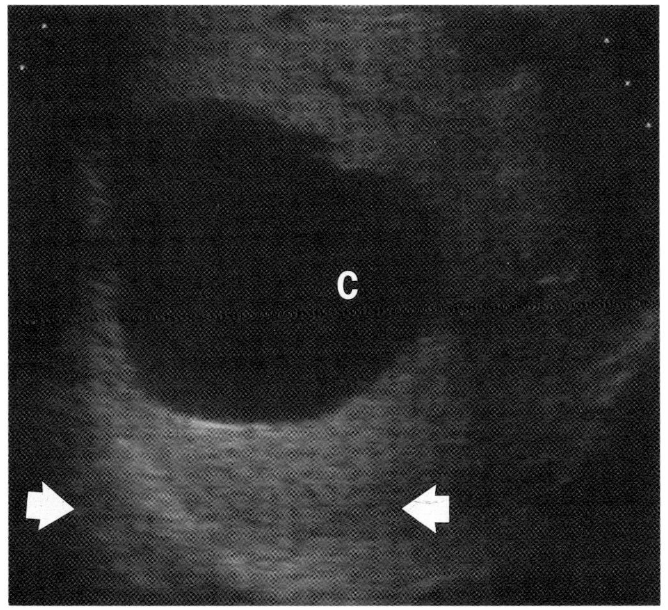

FIG. 2.13. Large simple cyst. Transverse sonogram of right lobe of the liver. An echo-free, well-defined lesion with imperceptible walls and good through transmission (*arrows*) allows confident diagnosis of simple cyst. No further evaluation is needed. C, cyst.

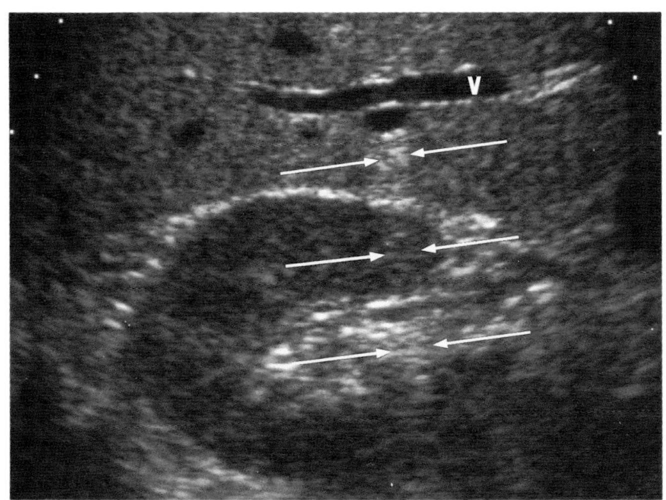

FIG. 2.14. Tiny simple cyst. Transverse sonogram of the right lobe of the liver reveals a tiny, less than 1 cm, simple cyst of the liver that fulfills the classic sonographic criteria. Note the distal enhanced through transmission (*thin arrow*). Most millimeter-sized cysts, such as this, lack through transmission. This cyst, similar in size to an adjacent portal vein (V), was detected only with the use of color flow sonography, like the cyst illustrated in Fig. 2.5.

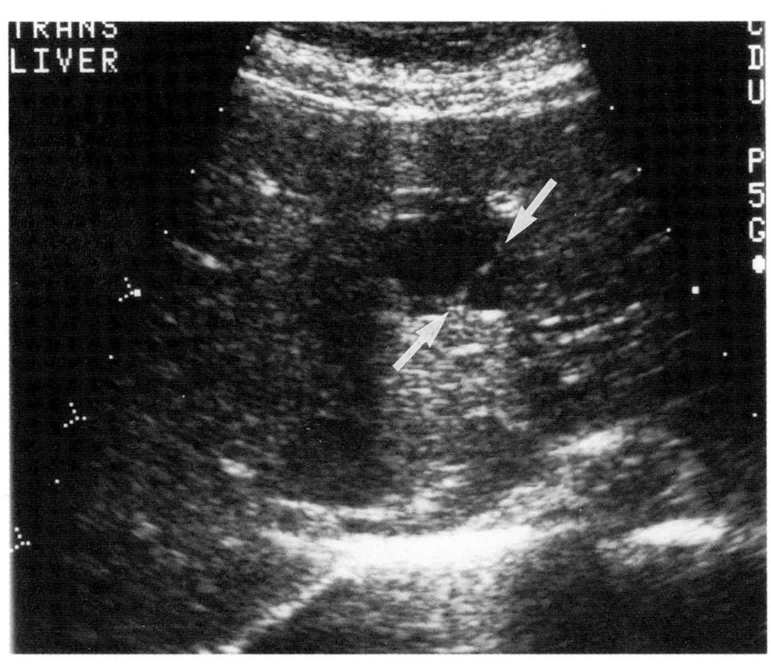

FIG. 2.15. Simple cyst with thin septation. Transverse sonogram of the left lobe of the liver. Thin septations, as noted here (*arrow*), do not remove an otherwise classic cyst from the simple cyst category.

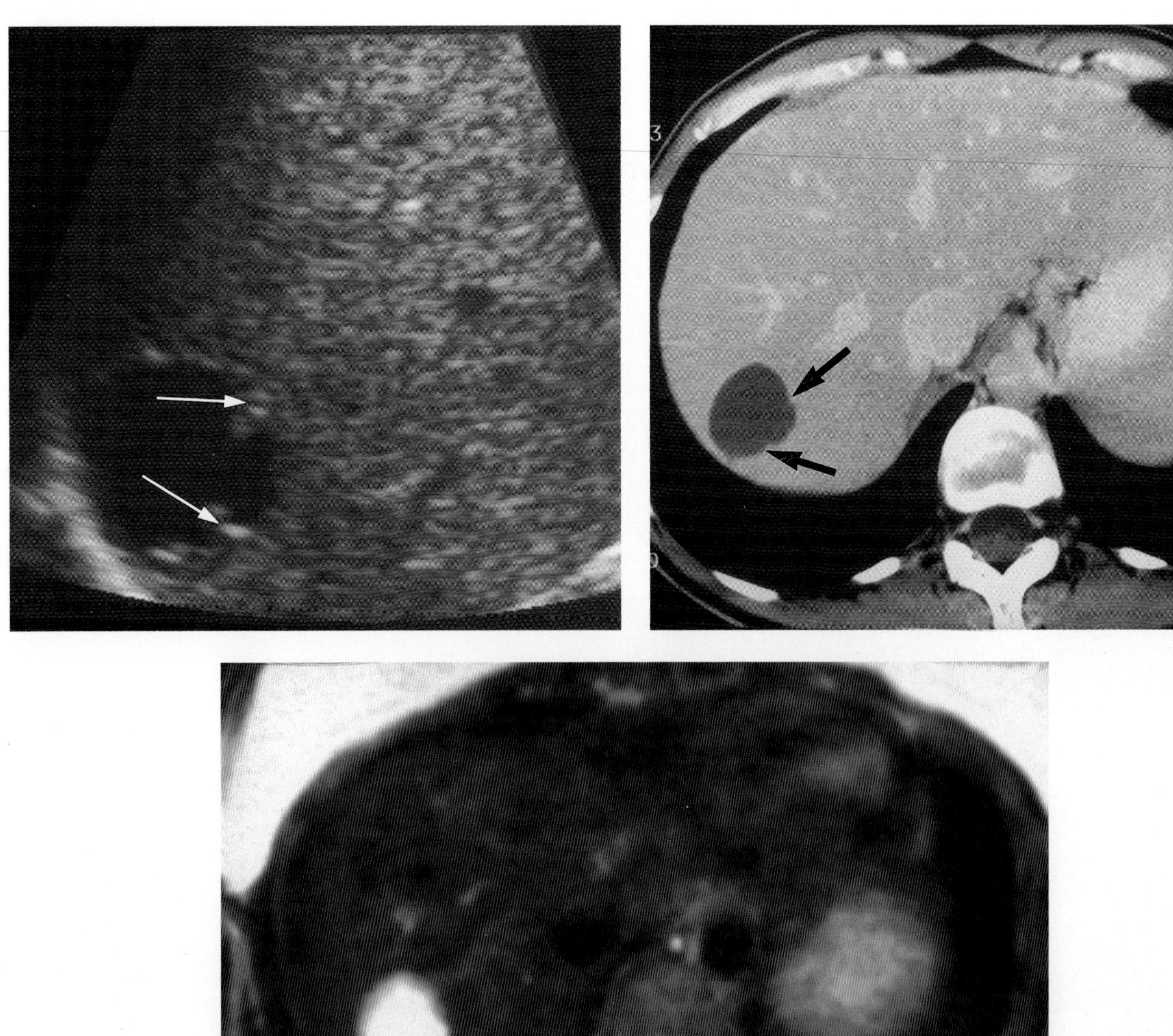

FIG. 2.16. Simple cyst with mildly thickened septations. Transverse sonogram (**A**) of the right lobe of the liver reveals slightly thickened septations (*arrows*) within an otherwise classic simple cyst. Minimal irregularities are also noted on the CT scan (**B**) and T2-weighted MRI (**C**). This lesion did not fulfill the classic criteria for simple cyst on images because of these mildly thickened septations and the irregularities noted on the other imaging modalities. Histologically, this lesion was a simple cyst.

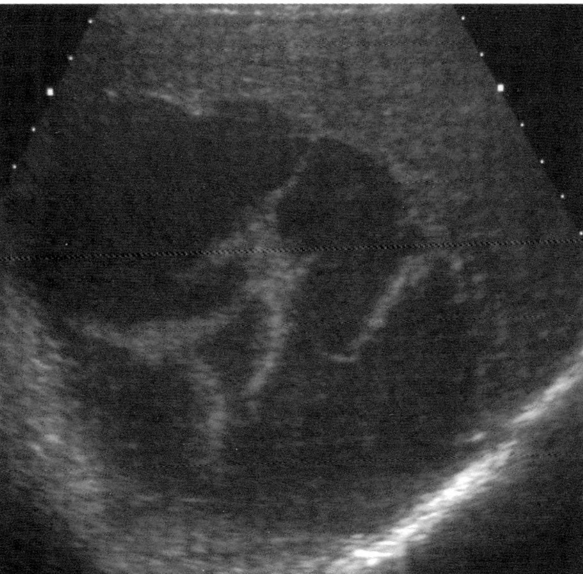

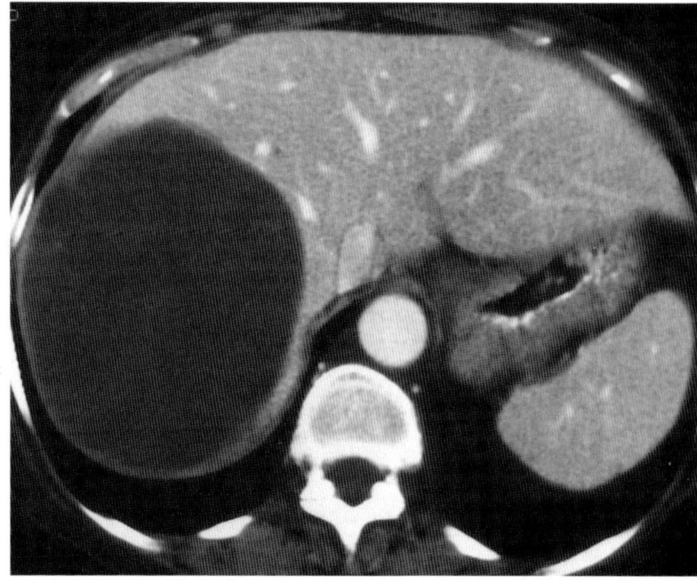

B

FIG. 2.17. Large hemorrhagic cysts with thickened septations. **A:** This transverse sonogram of the right lobe reveals a hypoechoic lesion with lobular margins, internal echoes, and thick septations. These findings may occur in either a complicated simple cyst, such as this, or other lesions, such as cystic neoplasms. **B:** The CT scan does not show the internal features of the lesion as well as the ultrasound. Ultrasound typically reveals the internal architecture of cystic lesions more clearly than CT.

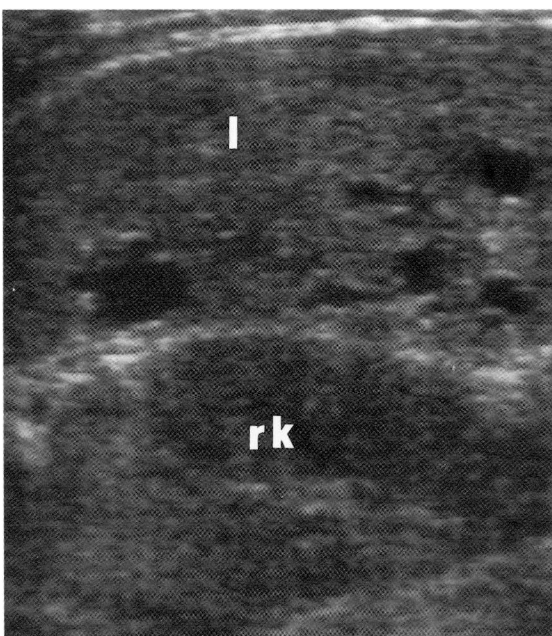

A

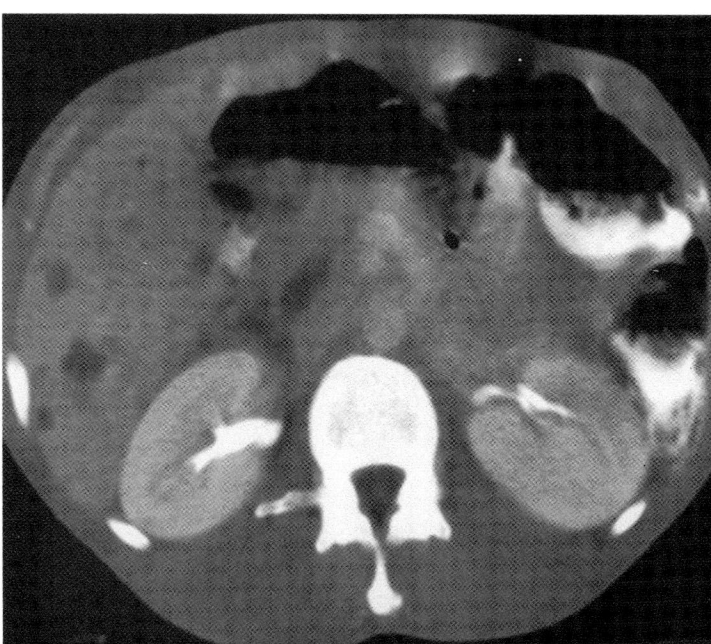

B

FIG. 2.18. Hepatic polycystic disease. **A:** Transverse sonogram of the right lobe of the liver reveals multiple, somewhat irregular cysts. **B:** Similar lesions are detected on the CT scan. Cysts in polycystic disease are often more irregular than simple cysts. rk, right kidney; l, liver.

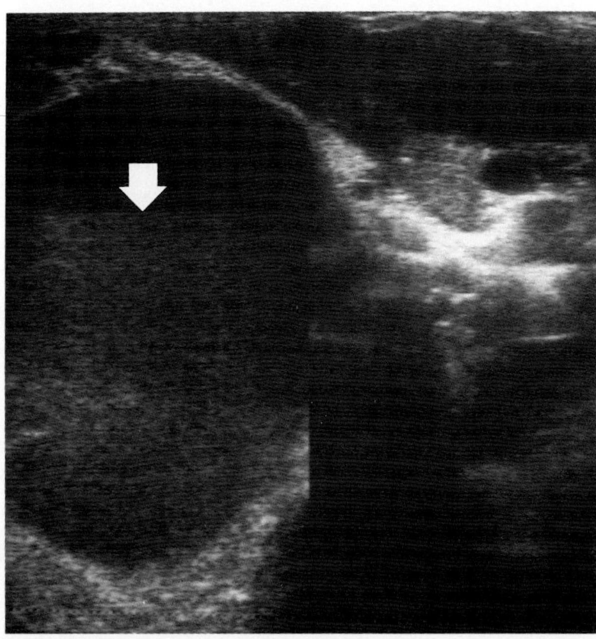

FIG. 2.19. Hepatic polycystic disease, infected cyst. Transverse composite sonogram reveals multiple liver cysts. One large liver cyst has a debris fluid level (*arrow*), indicative of infection in this febrile patient. Hemorrhagic cysts can also have this sonographic appearance. Detection of focal tenderness over a debris-filled cyst often allows the sonographer to distinguish the symptomatic cyst from other debris-filled cysts.

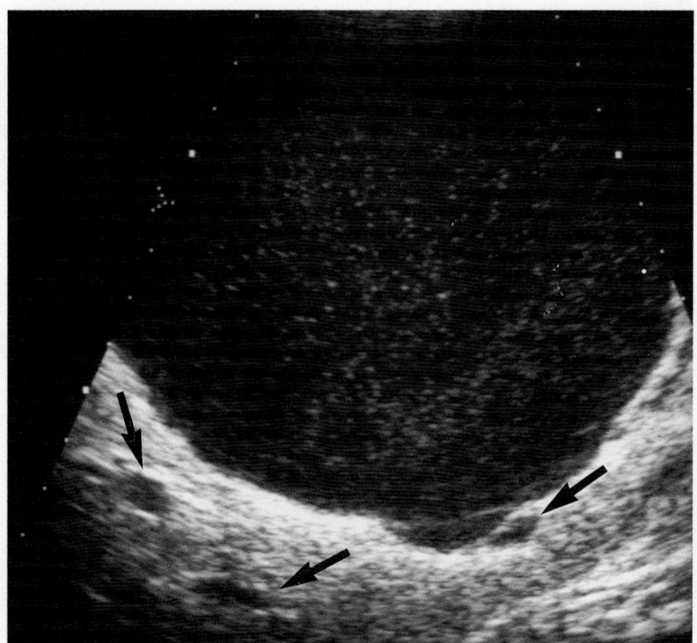

FIG. 2.20. Hepatic polycystic disease, hemorrhagic cyst. Longitudinal sonogram through the right lobe of the liver reveals a huge debris-filled cyst in a patient with hepatic polycystic disease. The patient complained of intermittent pain over this cyst. Aspiration showed "crankcase" fluid compatible with old hemorrhage. Note the other small cysts (*arrows*) in the adjacent hepatic parenchyma.

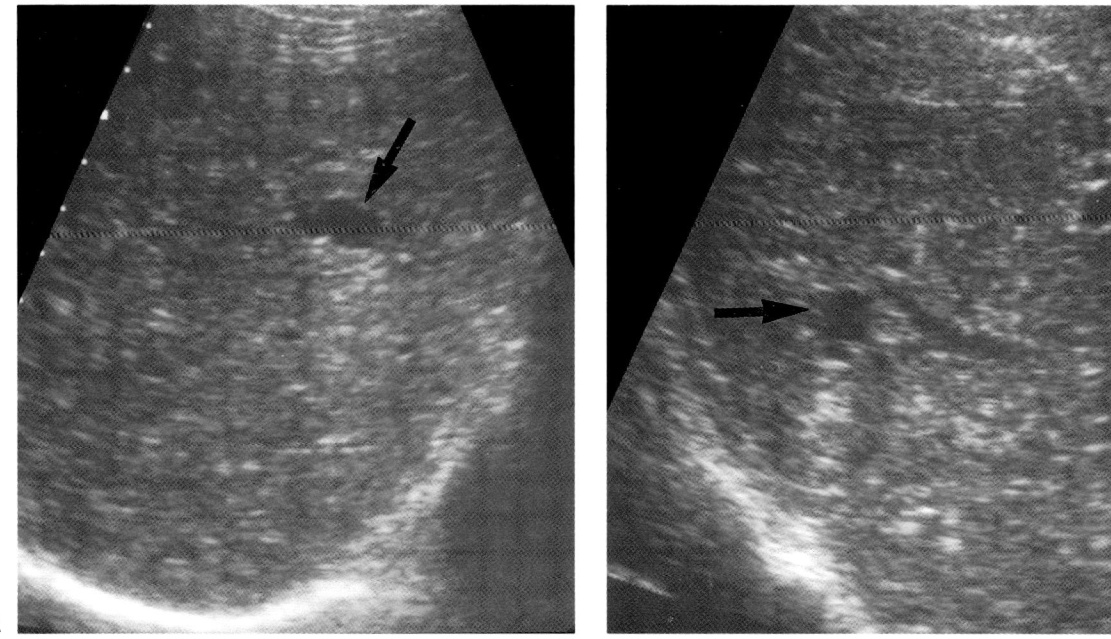

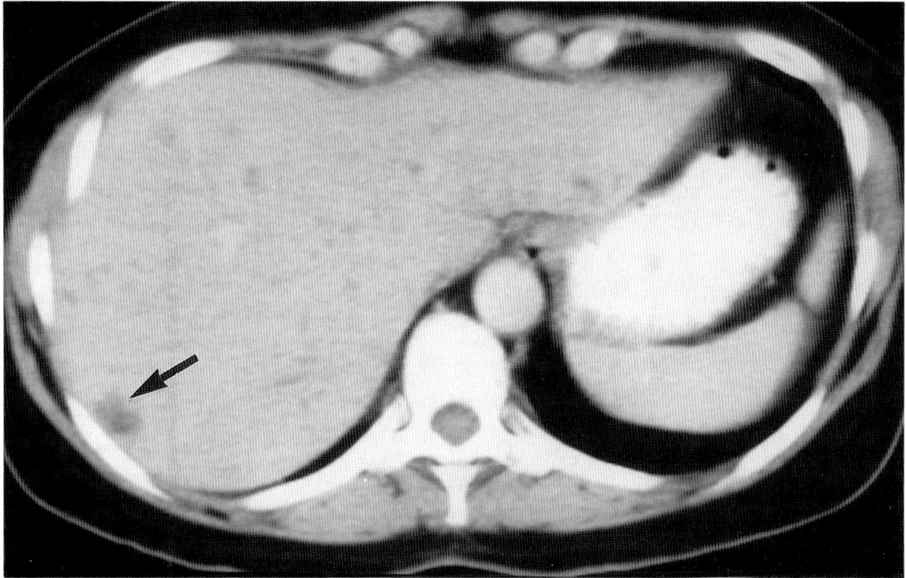

FIG. 2.21. Von Meyenberg's complex. Transverse oblique (**A**) and longitudinal oblique (**B**) sonograms reveal two different small, slightly irregular, cysts (*arrows*) that exhibit increased through transmission deep to the cyst. Also noted is distorted parenchymal architecture with areas of increased and decreased echogenicity representing smaller cysts that are less well resolved individually. The CT scan (**C**) reveals one of these larger cysts (*arrow*), as well as multiple smaller cysts throughout the liver. Von Meyenberg's complex is a rare disorder characterized by multiple small cystic bile duct hamartomas. Most of the cysts are too small to be resolved by either CT or sonography, but larger cysts, such as the ones imaged here, are often visible.

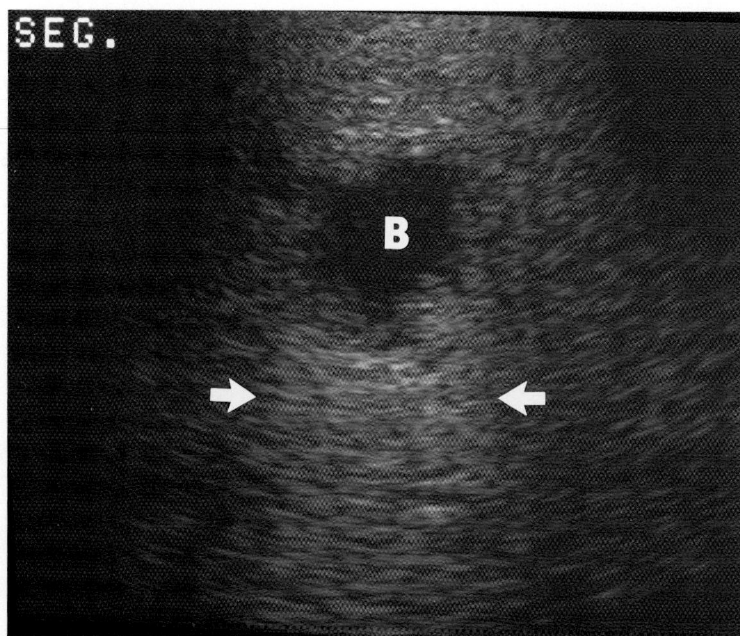

FIG. 2.22. Post-traumatic hepatic biloma. Transverse image of the right lobe reveals an ill-defined hypoechoic biloma (B), with through transmission (*arrows*). Post-traumatic bilomas occur when there is a persistent disruption of the biliary tree after hepatic injury.

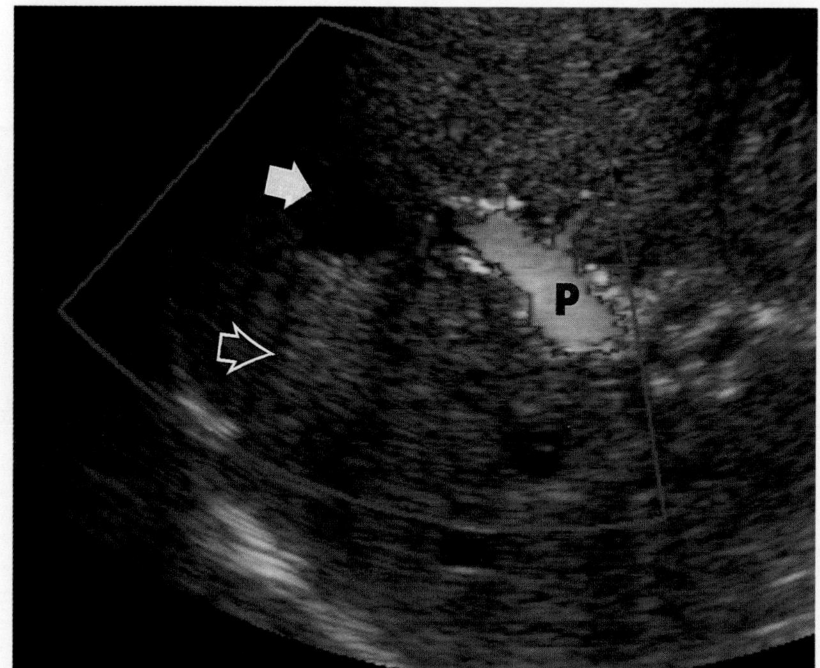

FIG. 2.23. Post-traumatic biloma. Oblique transverse color Doppler sonogram through the right lobe of the liver reveals a small, approximately 2-cm post-traumatic biloma (*arrow*). Note the distal sonic enhancement deep to the lesion (*open arrow*). Prominent through transmission, as noted here, should suggest the possibility of a bile-filled lesion. This patient presented with pain 5 weeks subsequent to hepatic injury. Post-traumatic bilomas generally require no therapy, although percutaneous drainage can be curative when indicated. They typically arise in a region of persistent bile duct injury. Clinical presentation usually occurs 4 to 6 weeks after injury, as in this case. P, right portal vein.

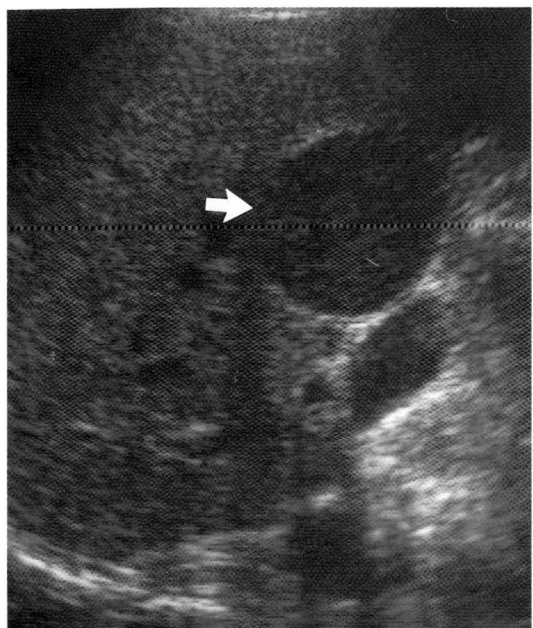

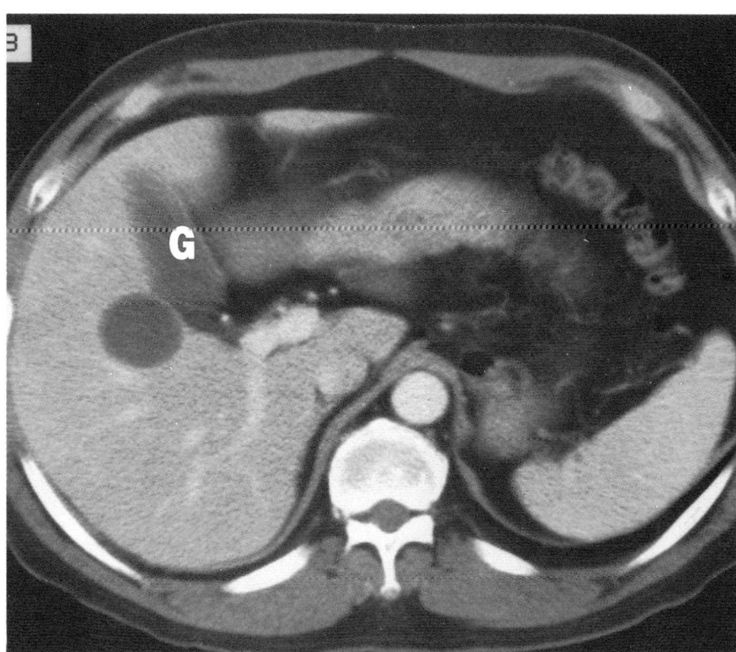

A B

FIG. 2.24. Postinflammatory cyst. **A:** Oblique transverse sonogram reveals a well-defined hypoechoic spherical lesion (*arrow*) with through transmission deep to the lesion. This is an image obtained 6 weeks after the patient had been treated for a pyogenic liver abscess in this location. **B:** A CT scan also reveals the spherical lesion adjacent to the gallbladder (G). This fluid-filled, predominantly cystic lesion represents a residual abnormality after successful treatment of a liver abscess. Residual abnormality is not unusual. Lesions that simulate simple cysts may result and persist for the remainder of the patient's life. Debris-filled cysts, such as this, also occur. Of course, successfully treated abscesses may also resolve with little or no residua.

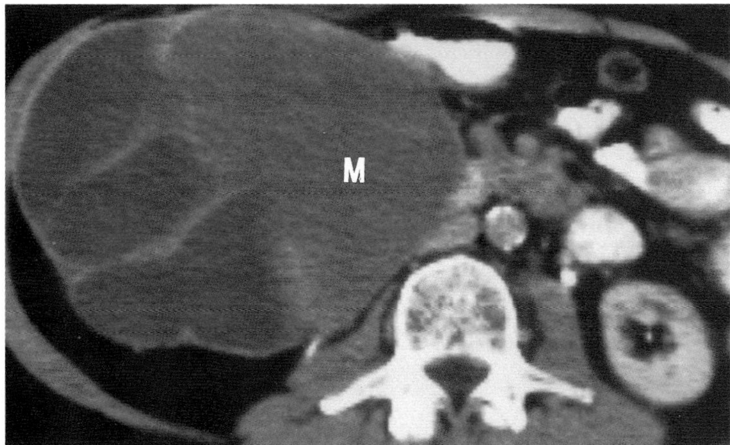

A

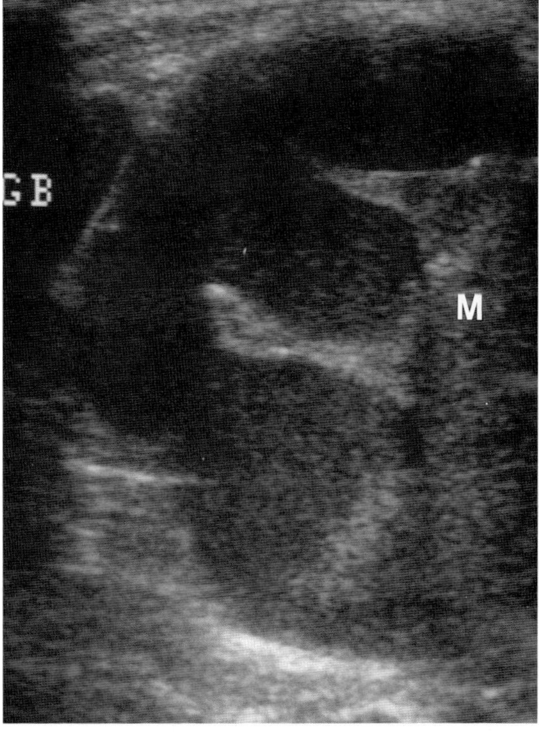

B

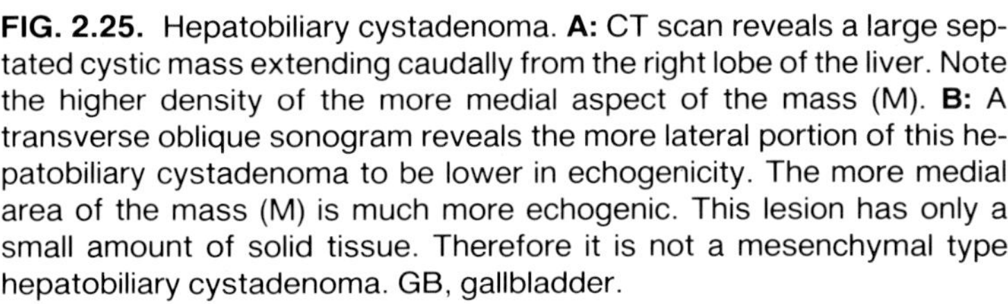

FIG. 2.25. Hepatobiliary cystadenoma. **A:** CT scan reveals a large septated cystic mass extending caudally from the right lobe of the liver. Note the higher density of the more medial aspect of the mass (M). **B:** A transverse oblique sonogram reveals the more lateral portion of this hepatobiliary cystadenoma to be lower in echogenicity. The more medial area of the mass (M) is much more echogenic. This lesion has only a small amount of solid tissue. Therefore it is not a mesenchymal type hepatobiliary cystadenoma. GB, gallbladder.

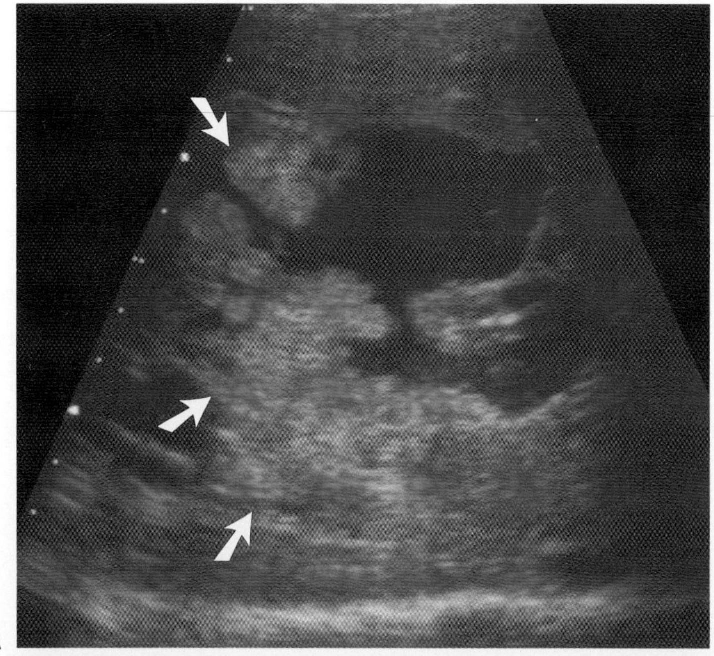

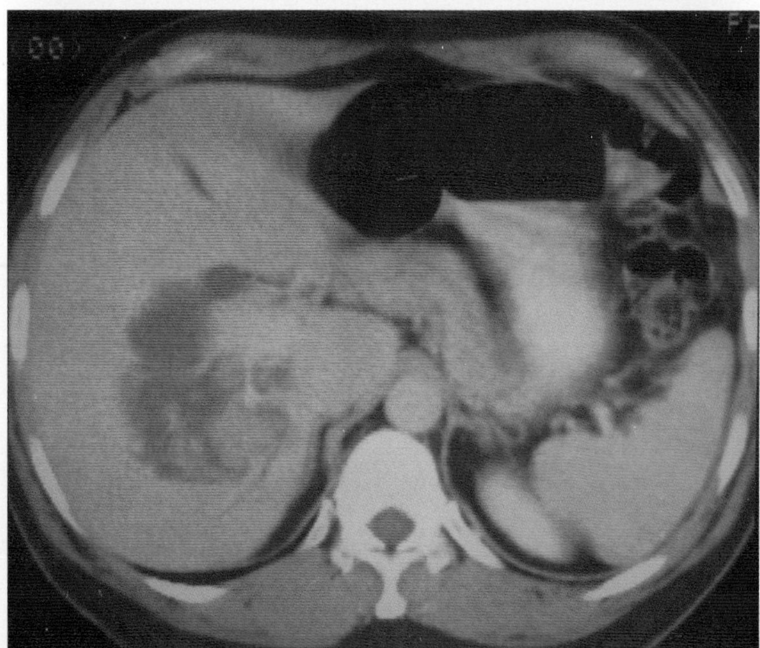

FIG. 2.26. Mesenchymal hepatobiliary cystadenoma. **A:** Transverse sonogram reveals a cystic mass with large internal soft tissue regions (*slanted arrows*). **B:** A CT scan reveals similar features. Hepatobiliary cystadenomas with more solid components, as seen here, are called mesenchymal hepatobiliary cystadenomas. This variant has greater malignant potential.

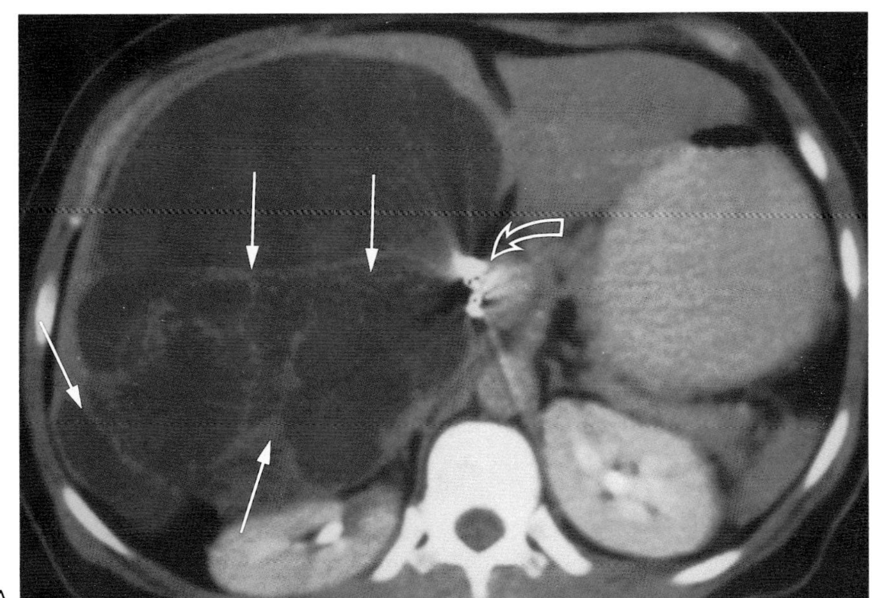

FIG. 2.27. Mesenchymal hepatobiliary cystadenoma. **A:** The CT scan reveals a large lesion with internal septations (*arrows*). Vascular clips (*open curved arrow*) are from a previous incomplete resection. **B:** The transverse sonogram in the cephalic area of the liver reveals multiple septations (*arrows*). **C:** A more caudal transverse sonogram reveals cystic and solid components, typical of a mesenchymal hepatobiliary cystadenoma. RK, right kidney.

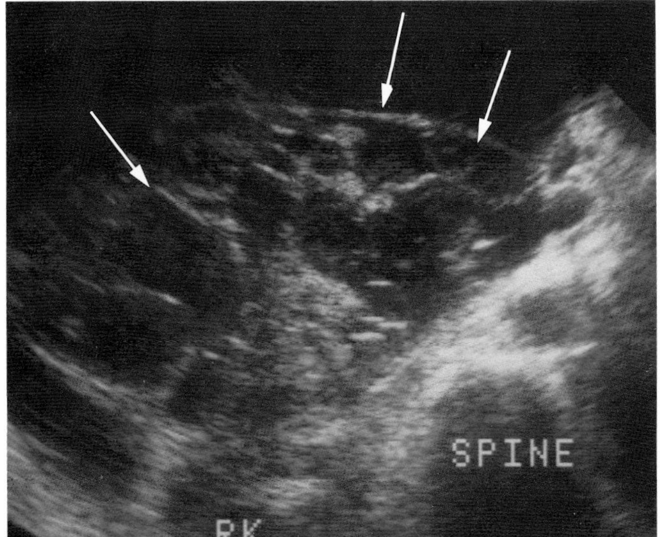

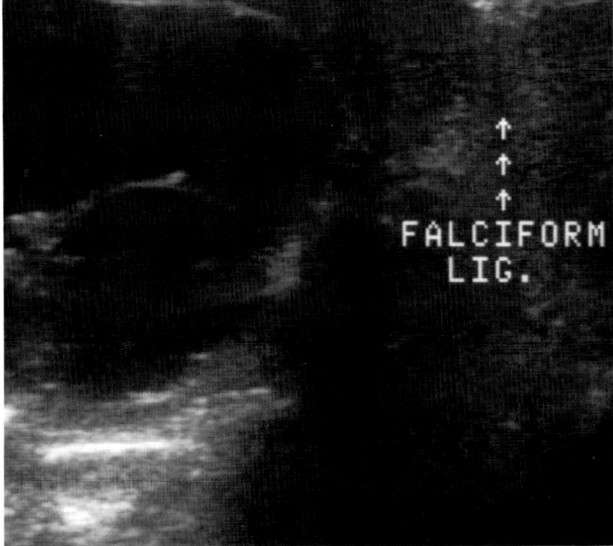

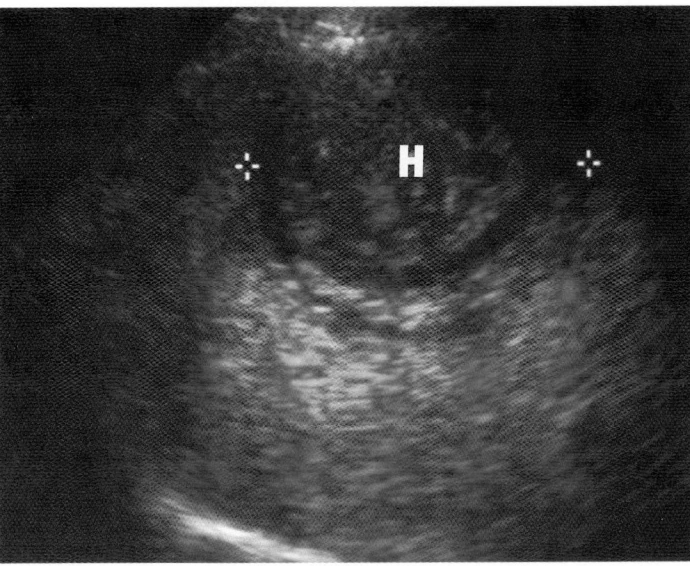

FIG. 2.28. Hydatid disease of the liver. This transverse oblique sonogram of the liver reveals a hydatid cyst (calipers—H) that is predominantly filled with echoes. A spectrum of sonographic findings occurs with hepatic hydatid disease, ranging from purely cystic to solid appearing pseudotumors, as noted here.

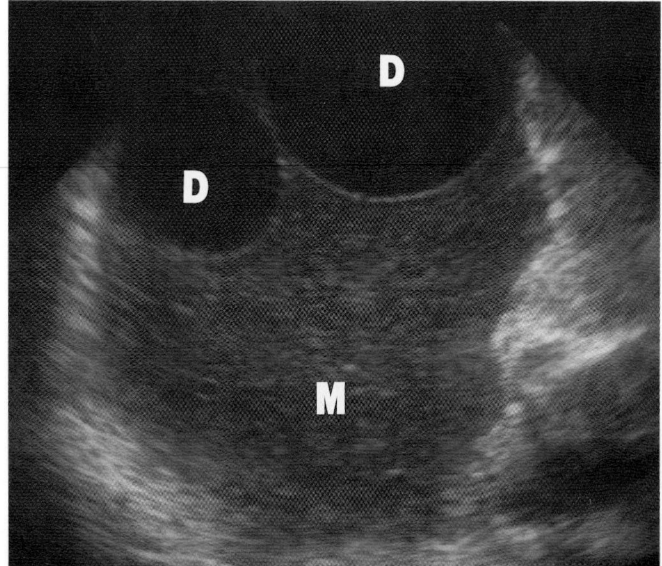

A

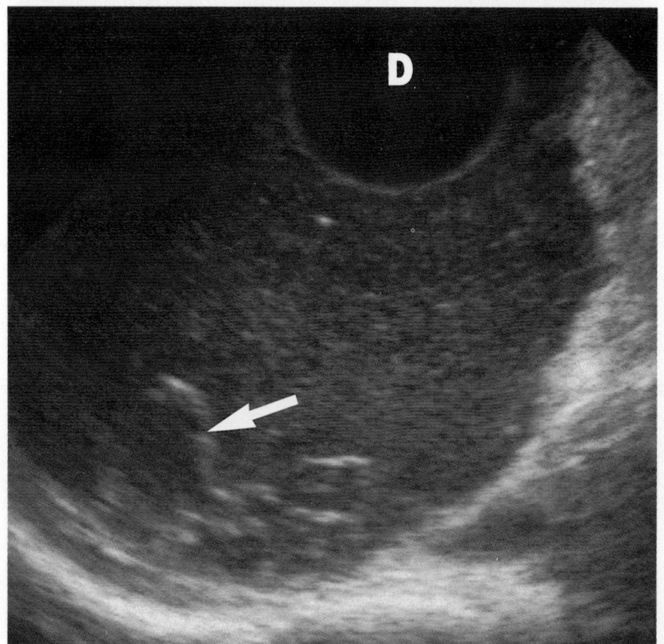

B

FIG. 2.29. Hepatic hydatid disease, daughter cysts, "water lily sign." **A:** Transverse sonogram near the dome of the liver reveals a large hydatid cyst with two well-defined anechoic daughter cysts (D). The higher echogenicity material within the main cyst dorsal to the daughter cysts is called matrix (M). **B:** The longitudinal sonogram reveals one of the daughter cysts (D). Curvilinear delaminated endocyst (*arrow*), lying in a dependent position dorsally within the cyst (*arrow*), results in the "water lily sign." **C:** CT scan reveals a smaller hydatid cyst in the left lobe (*curved arrow*). It is more difficult to appreciate the daughter cyst in the main right lobe cyst on CT than sonography. The matrix (M) is of slightly higher attenuation than the fluid within the daughter cyst.

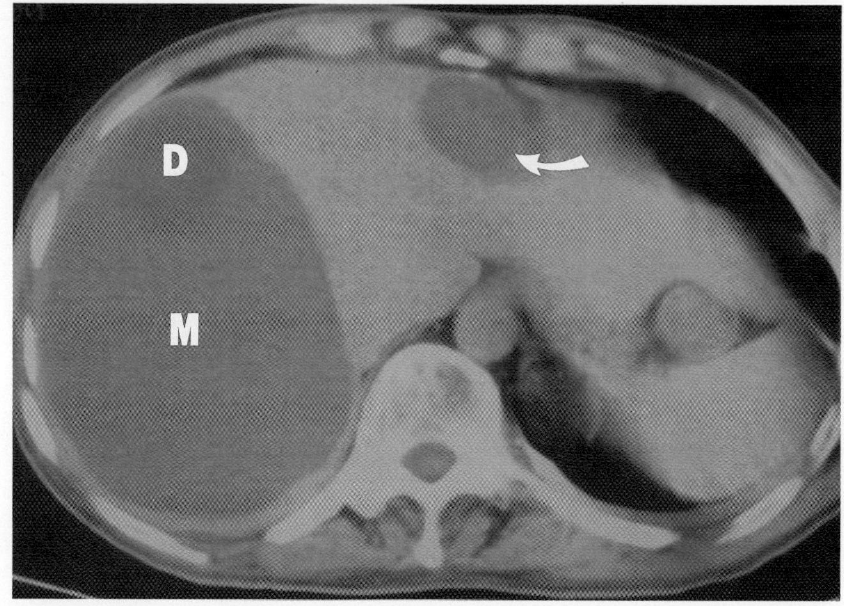

C

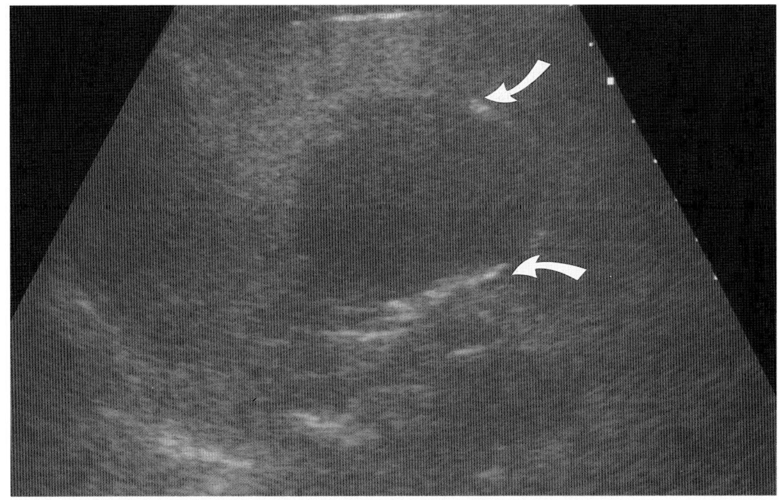

FIG. 2.30. Calcified hydatid cyst. Oblique transverse sonogram through the right lobe of the liver. This predominantly hypoechoic hydatid cyst has some peripheral nonshadowing mural calcifications (*curved arrows*). CT is a more sensitive means of detecting calcifications in a hydatid cyst than sonography. Calcification such as this generally indicates a dead, inactive cyst.

A

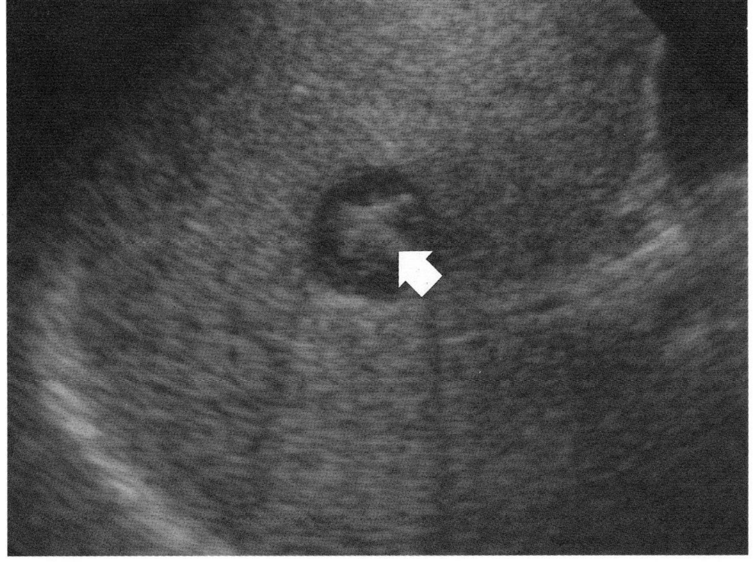

B

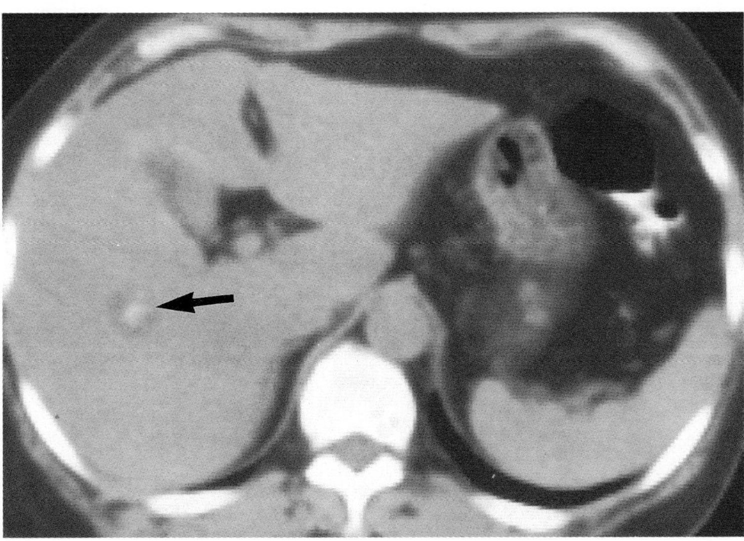

FIG. 2.31. Small calcified hydatid cyst. **A:** Transverse sonogram reveals a predominantly cystic lesion with through transmission. **B:** The internal echogenic material is calcified (*arrow*), as demonstrated by the CT scan. The manifestations of hepatic hydatid disease are extremely variable. In this patient, the diagnosis was unsuspected clinically and on the images. A biopsy was performed. The diagnosis of hydatid disease was made when a tapeworm scolex was seen on the aspirate. There were no adverse effects after biopsy.

Cavernous Hemangioma

Cavernous hemangioma is the most common benign hepatic neoplasm with a prevalence of 1 to 4 percent. Hemangiomas are more common in females (32,33). Clinical symptoms are very rare. Rupture with hemorrhage and thrombocytopenia from intralesional thrombosis have been reported. Large hemangiomas can cause symptoms from mass effect (32). Sonographic findings are often classic (see later discussion). Despite this, hemangiomas must often be evaluated further to exclude more significant lesions, especially in patients with malignancy. The sonographic appearance of hemangiomas overlaps enough with the appearance of significant lesions to make definitive distinction difficult or impossible in many patients.

Small hemangiomas are usually echogenic and well defined and often exhibit enhanced through transmission (34) (Fig. 2.32). Larger hemangiomas frequently diverge from this pattern. Mixed echogenicity lesions (Figs. 2.33 and 2.34) and even hypoechoic hemangiomas may occur (Figs. 2.35 and 2.36). One ironic impact of the better images produced by newer ultrasound systems is that internal inhomogeneity and even peripheral halos may be imaged in what would have previously been a "classic" hemangioma (Fig. 2.37). An interesting intraoperative finding reported by Choji et al. (35) was decreased internal echogenicity in hemangiomas when compressed.

Spectral Doppler signals equivalent to normal liver parenchyma have been described in cavernous hemangiomas (13). In our experience, color Doppler sonography reveals internal flow in fewer than 10 percent of hemangiomas (Figs. 2.12 and 2.38) (12). This is less than reported by Tanaka et al. (10), who detected "spot" flow (tiny dots of flow) in three of six hemangiomas. A normal hepatic vessel may be encompassed by a hemangioma.

Typical small hemangiomas in a patient without evidence of malignancy should be evaluated with color flow imaging. If no flow is found, the patient should be followed by ultrasound in 3 to 4 months, although one might also reasonably argue that no follow-up is required. Hemangiomas rarely change on serial exams (36). Lesions exhibiting flow on color flow imaging or those in patients with malignancy should be evaluated further. ^{99m}Tc-tagged red blood cell (RBC) blood pool SPECT scanning may be valuable for single lesions larger than 3 cm in diameter (Figs. 2.34 and 2.38) and T2-weighted MRI for smaller or multiple lesions. CT and MRI may fail to identify small (<1 cm) hemangiomas detected with ultrasound.

Biopsy is a reasonable and safe way to evaluate hemangiomas (33,37), provided skilled cytologic consultation is available. To minimize the risk of postbiopsy hemorrhage, the needle path should always interpose normal liver between the capsule and the lesion. Generally, needles no larger than 21 gauge should be used for fine-needle biopsy of suspected hemangioma.

Hepatic Metastasis

In the United States, metastatic disease is by far the most common clinically significant focal liver lesion. Metastases are 18 to 20 times more common than hepatocellular carcinoma (HCC) and produce symptoms 10 times more frequently. In one large autopsy series, 38 percent of all patients with carcinoma had hepatic metastases. The most common liver metastases originate from—in decreasing order—lung, colon, pancreas, breast, and stomach carcinomas (32). The highest prevalence of metastasis occurs with gallbladder, pancreas, colon, and breast carcinoma; the lowest with prostate carcinoma (17).

Metastatic disease is multifocal in approximately 90 percent of patients. Virtually any sonographic appearance may occur in liver metastasis. Metastatic lesions, whether diffuse or focal, are usually inhomogeneous (Figs. 2.39 to 2.43). Hypoechoic halos are common (Figs. 2.40 and 2.44). Target or bull's eye patterns with varying rings of hypo- and hyperechogenicity are common (Figs. 2.45 to 2.47). Hypoechoic rims may comprise liver parenchyma or tumor (38,39). An ill-defined infiltrative lesion with focal nodularity is another fairly frequent pattern. Metastases that simulate simple cysts or classic appearing hemangiomas are uncommon. Predominantly fluid-filled, presumably necrotic metastases occur most frequently with squamous cell carcinoma, sarcomas, and ovarian and testicular carcinoma (Figs. 2.48 to 2.50). Calcified lesions, especially arising from mucinous adenocarcinoma, may occur (Figs. 2.50 to 2.53). CT is a more sensitive detector of this type of calcification. Biliary obstruction may occur (Fig. 2.54). Although sonographic appearance is a poor predictor of the primary tumor, certain patterns are suggestive. Large to moderate sized hyperechoic metastases should suggest the possibility of a colonic primary (Fig. 2.55). Lesions with fluid–fluid levels (representing intralesional necrosis and hemorrhage) are often found with metastatic leiomyosarcoma (Fig. 2.56).

Metastasis and HCC may be impossible to distinguish clinically or sonographically. When the diagnosis is unclear clinically or when a definitive diagnosis is required, sonographically guided biopsy should be performed. Invasion of the portal or hepatic veins suggests hepatocellular carcinoma, rather than metastasis. Even though portal venous invasion in metastatic disease has been reported in as many as 8 percent of patients (40,41), our experience suggests a lower prevalence (Fig. 2.57).

About one-third of metastases have identifiable internal color (Figs. 2.10 and 2.11) flow (versus three-quarters of HCCs) (Figs. 2.6, 2.8, and 2.9). About 40 per-

(*text continues on page 106*)

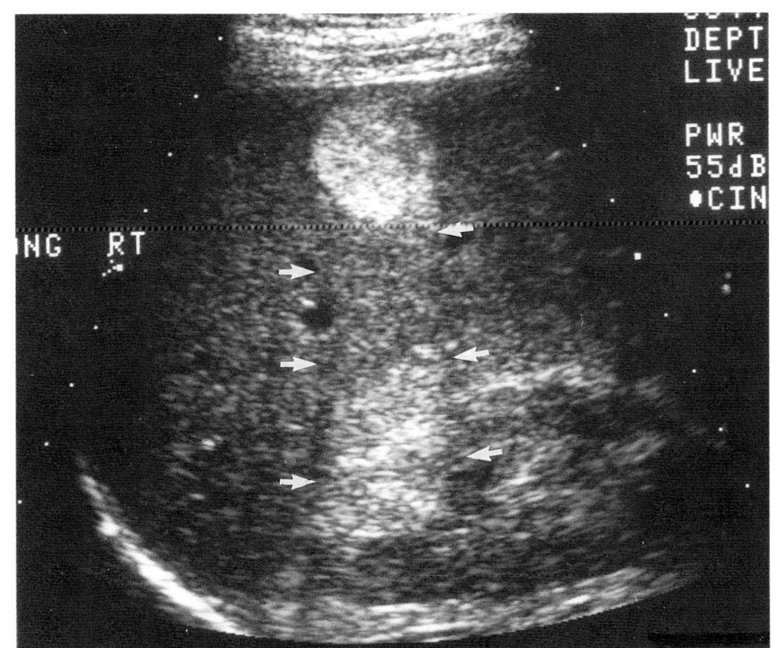

FIG. 2.32. Small hepatic hemangioma, classic sonographic findings. This longitudinal sonogram reveals a small, approximately 2-cm hemangioma that has classic sonographic findings. Small hemangiomas are usually echogenic and well defined. They often exhibit enhanced through transmission, as noted here (*small arrows*).

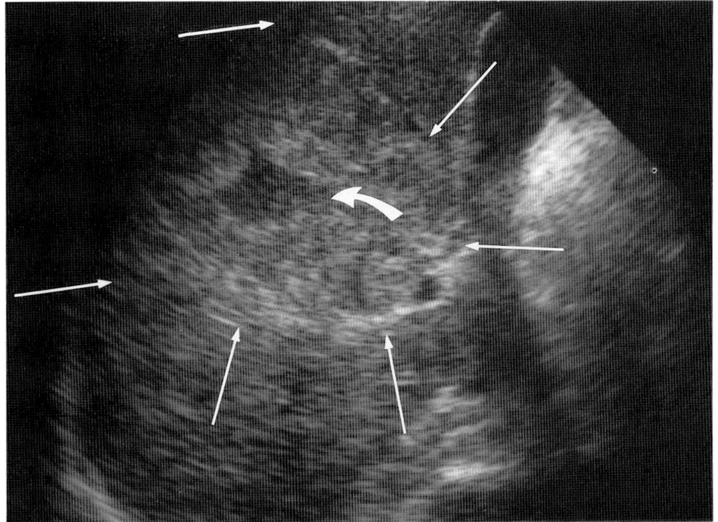

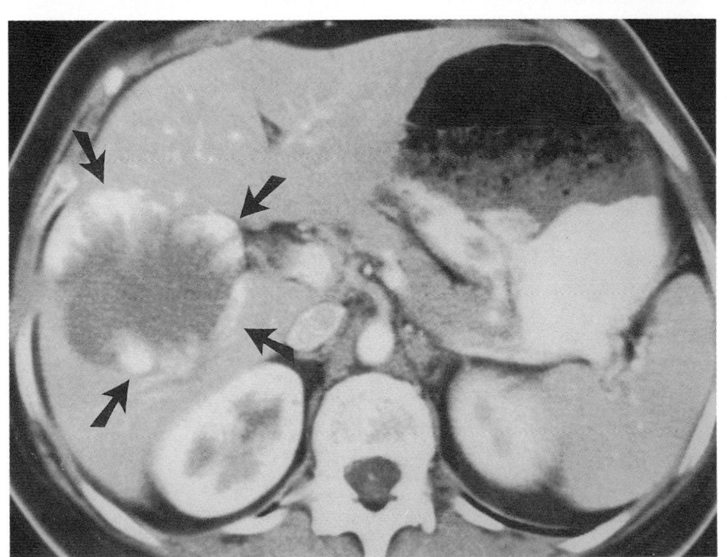

FIG. 2.33. Atypical hepatic hemangioma, mixed echogenicity. **A:** Transverse sonogram reveals a large hemangioma (*thin arrows*) with mixed echogenicity and a central isoechoic region (*curved arrow*). Most of the lesion's periphery consists of a thin echogenic rim. **B:** Dynamic contrast-enhanced (CE) CT scan reveals intense lobular peripheral enhancement (*slanted arrows*), a finding typical of hemangioma on CECT.

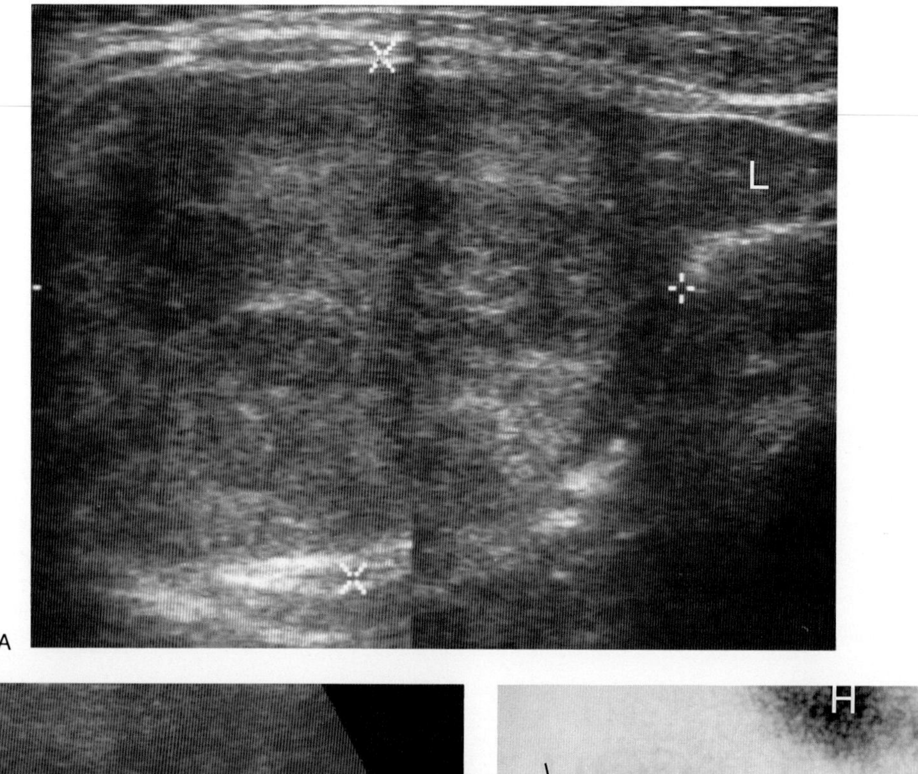

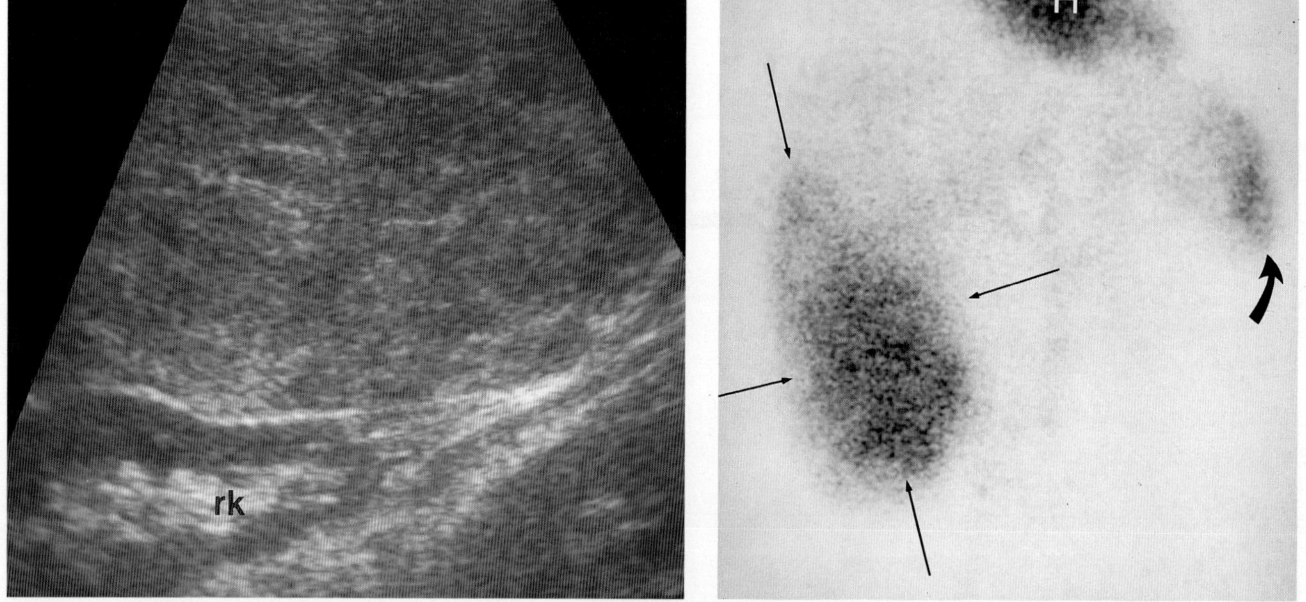

FIG. 2.34. Huge hepatic hemangioma. **A:** Composite transverse sonogram reveals a gigantic mixed echogenicity, predominantly hyperechoic, right lobe hemangioma (calipers). Note the normal left lobe (L) of the liver. **B:** The longitudinal sonogram reveals internal heterogeneity, usual in large hemangiomas. Note the indentation on the right kidney (rk). **C:** A technetium-tagged RBC blood pool scan reveals increased uptake in the right lobe hemangioma (*thin arrows*). A small amount of uptake is noted in the spleen (*curved arrow*). The heart (H) is at the upper portion of the image.

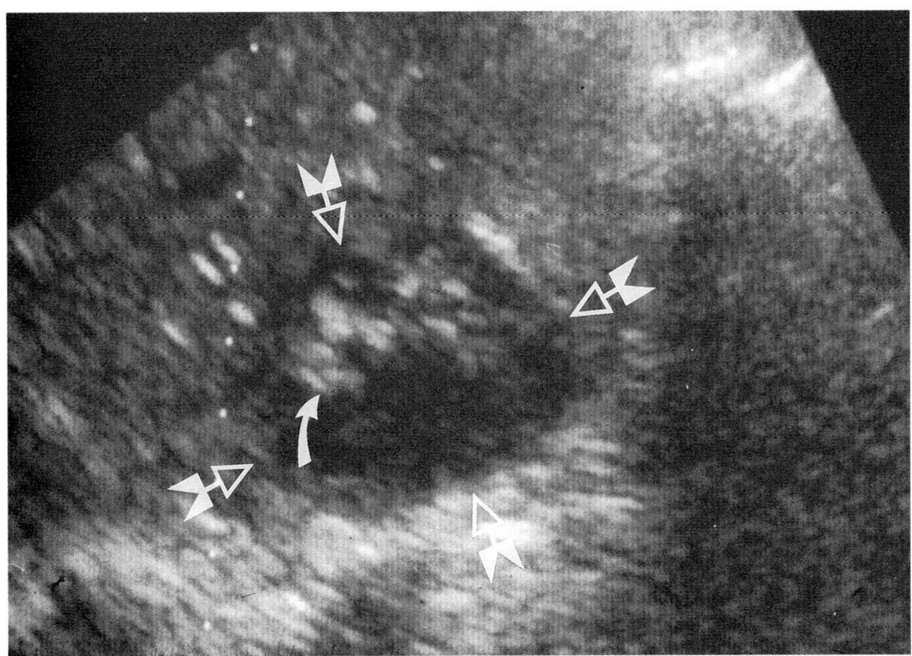

FIG. 2.35. Predominantly hypoechoic hepatic hemangioma. Longitudinal sonogram reveals a 5-cm, predominantly hypoechoic hemangioma (*tailed arrows*). Some small internal hyperechoic areas are seen (*curved arrow*). As hemangiomas become larger, their sonographic appearance often diverges from the classic homogeneously hyperechoic pattern.

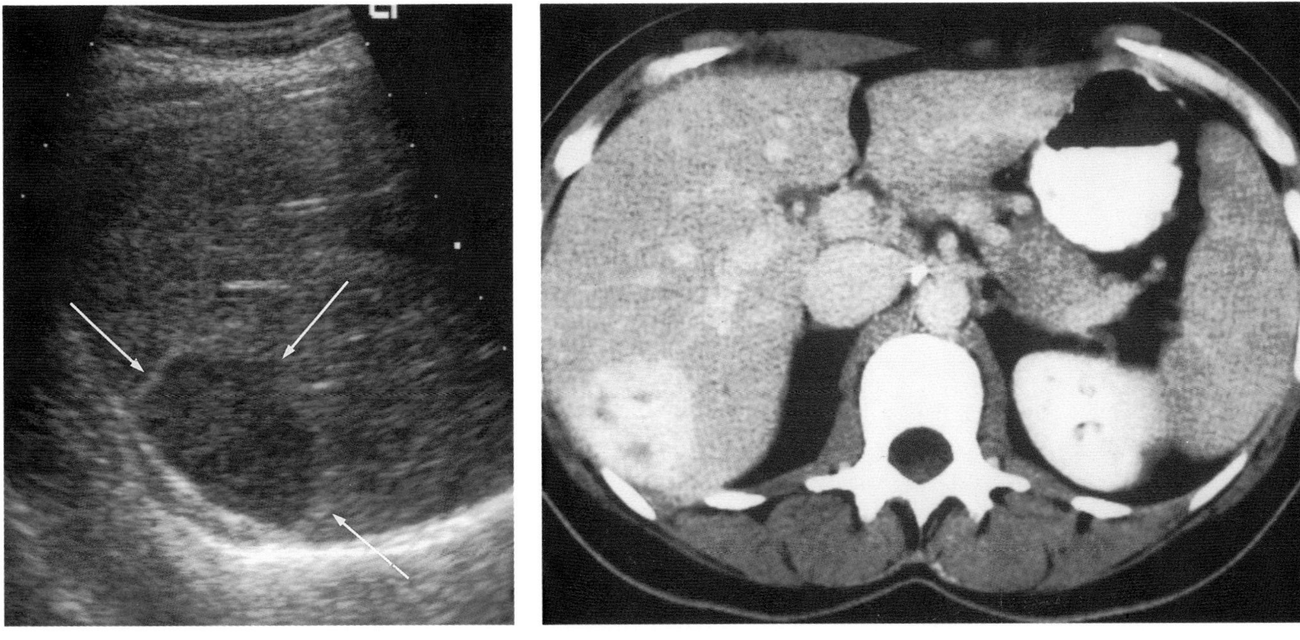

FIG. 2.36. Hypoechoic hemangioma. **A:** Oblique sonogram of the cephalic right lobe demonstrates a well-defined, slightly hypoechoic mass with a partial echogenic rim (*thin arrows*). **B:** This hemangioma, atypical sonographically, has a classic contrast-enhanced CT pattern. Homogeneous high attenuation of the lesion with small central low-attenuation areas is seen in this mid-to-late phase dynamic contrast-enhanced CT (*arrows*). This high-attenuation "fill-in" CT pattern is seen at a later phase on sequential CT scans than the peripheral enhancement noted in Fig. 2.33.

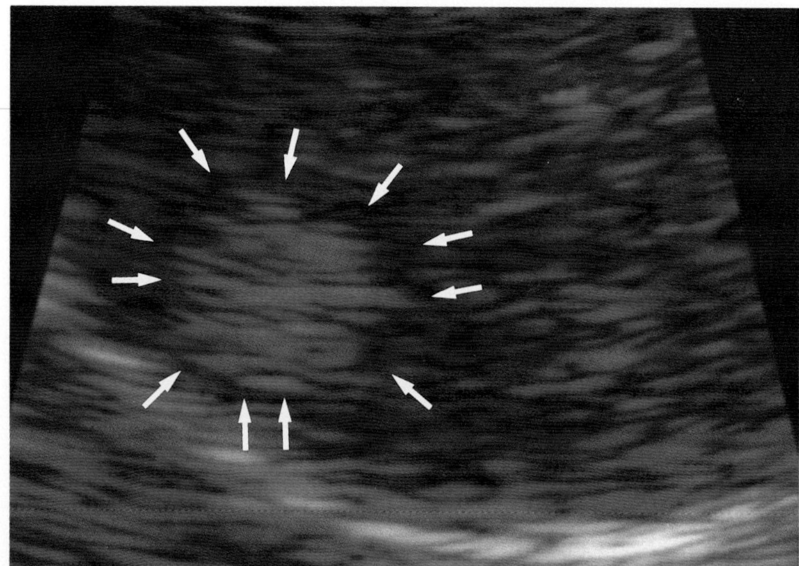

FIG. 2.37. Small hemangioma, faint hypoechoic halo. Transverse oblique sonogram of right lobe of the liver. This small hemangioma exhibits the classic "pattern" except for a faint hypoechoic halo (*arrows*). Newer ultrasound systems reveal findings such as internal inhomogeneity and peripheral halos in lesions that would probably have been "classic" hemangiomas had they been imaged on older generation sonographic systems.

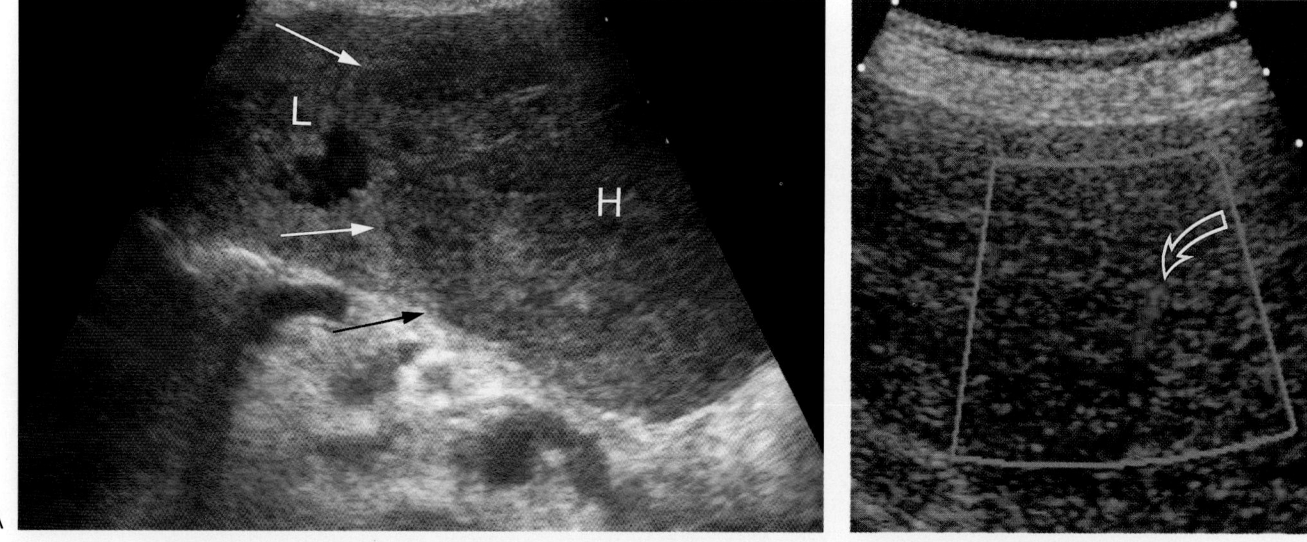

FIG. 2.38. Huge left lobe hemangioma. **A:** Transverse sonogram of the left lobe reveals a large hemangioma (H, *thin arrows*) that is hypoechoic compared to the more normal liver (L). **B:** A transverse color flow sonogram of the lesion reveals a small amount of flow within the mass (*open arrow*), reflecting low-velocity blood flow within the lesion. **C:** Despite the slow flow within the lesion itself, a transverse color Doppler sonogram in the region of the left portal vein shows rapid and massive aberrant blood flow around the hemangioma (H). Multiple enlarged peripheral feeding arteries are detected (*arrows*). Blood draining from the hemangioma exits via the left portal vein (pv) and its branches (*curved arrows*). The surprising and rare finding of portal vein flow reversal is noted. **D:** Findings typical of hemangioma are shown on an anterior blood pool scan with marked uptake in the huge left lobe hemangioma (*arrows*). **E:** The T2-weighted MRI revealed increased signal intensity (*white area*) suggestive of hemangioma. G, gallbladder. Because of the atypical image features and an inconclusive biopsy, the lesion was resected.

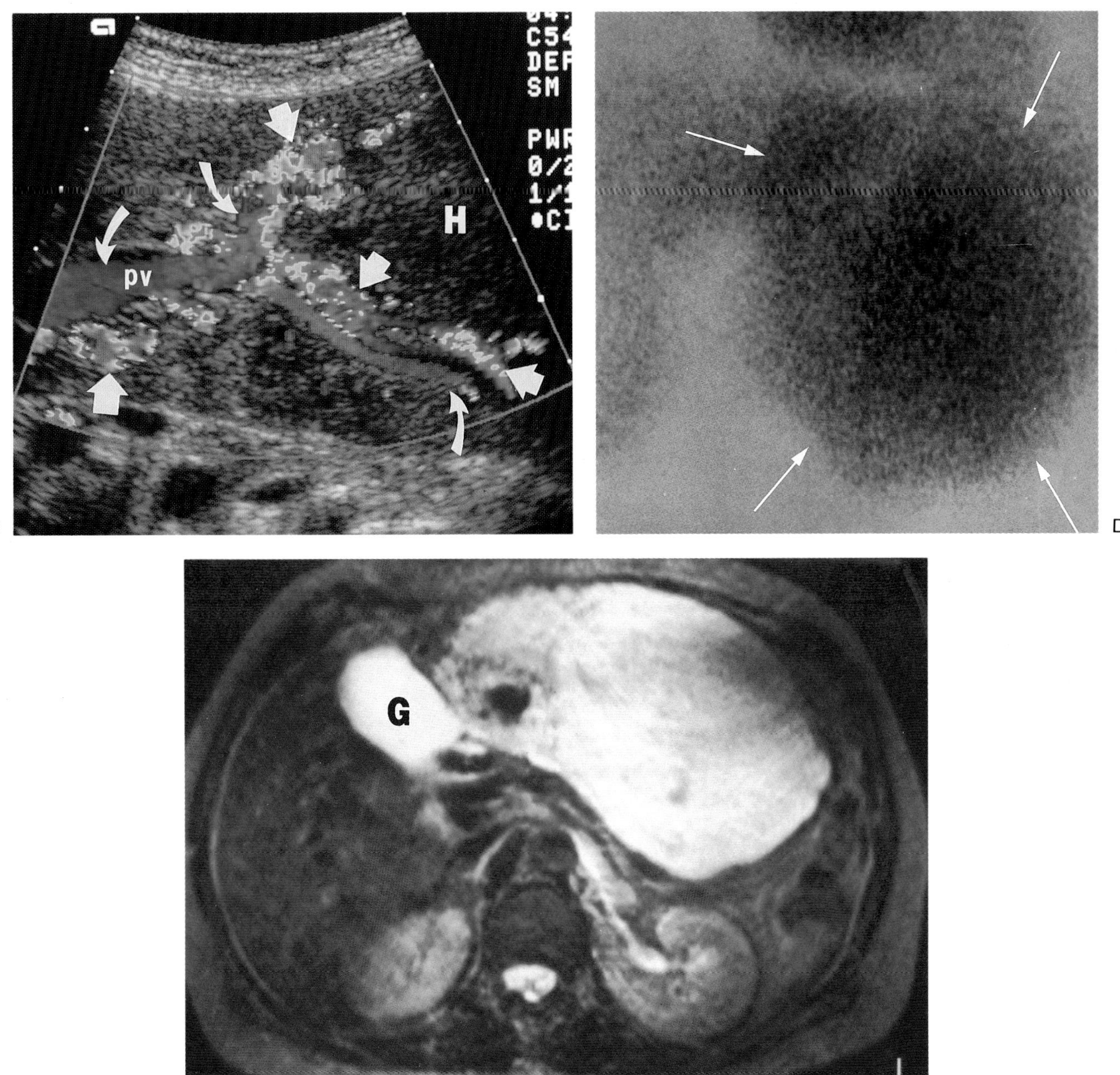

FIG. 2.38. *Continued.*

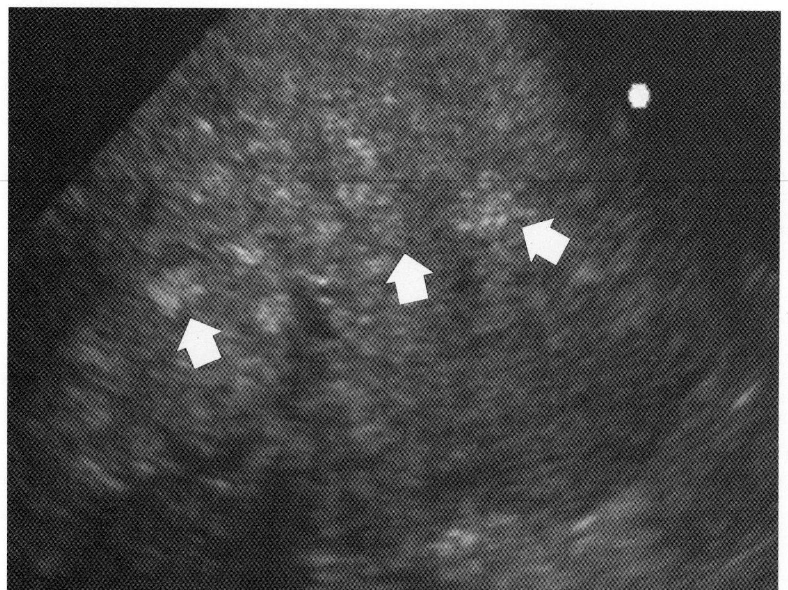

FIG. 2.39. Diffuse metastasis, colon carcinoma. This transverse sonogram reveals parenchymal inhomogeneity with focal areas of increased echogenicity (*arrows*) indicative of diffuse metastasis.

A

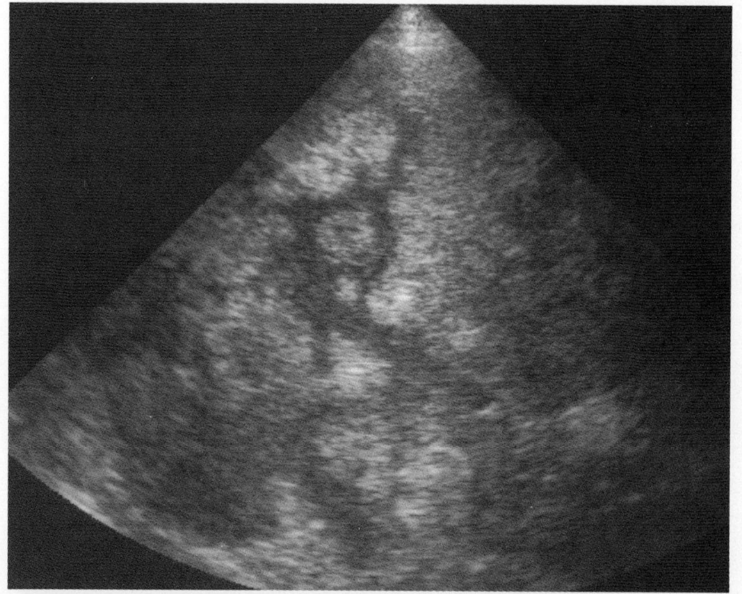

B

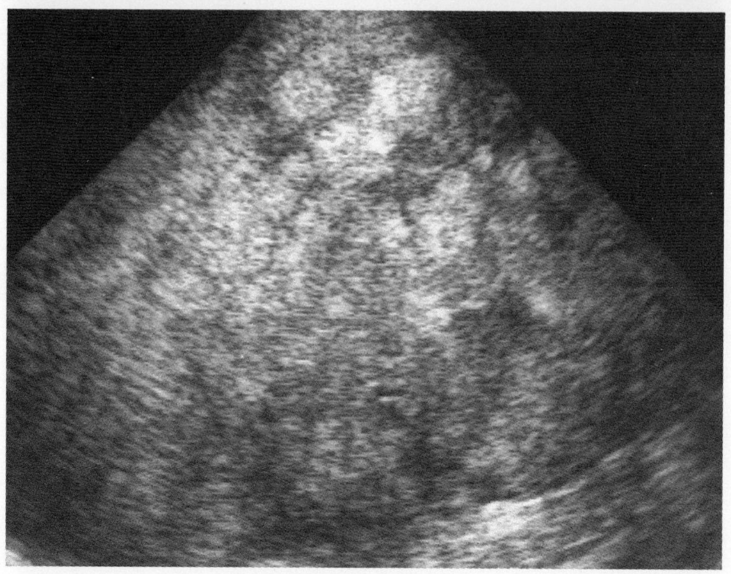

FIG. 2.40. Diffuse metastases with focal lesions, colon carcinoma. Transverse (**A**) and longitudinal (**B**) hepatic images reveal diffuse hepatic metastases. Note that many of the echogenic tumor nodules are surrounded by hypoechoic halos.

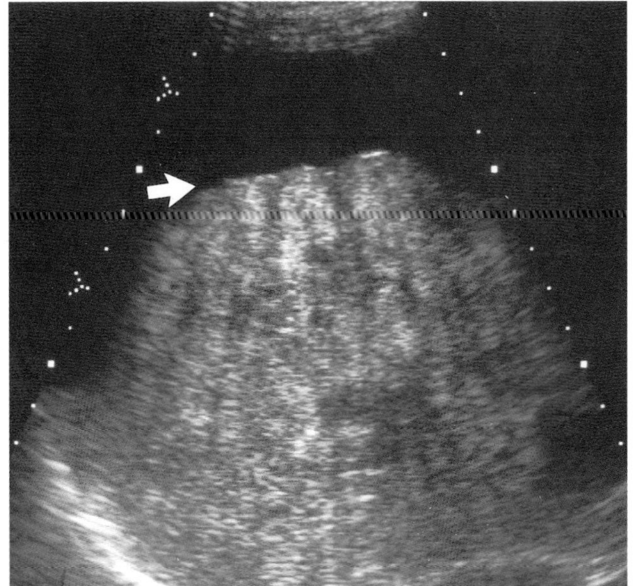

FIG. 2.41. Diffuse hepatic metastasis, breast carcinoma. Transverse sonogram of the liver. There is diffuse metastasis throughout the liver. Ascites highlights the nodular liver surface (*arrow*) caused by subcapsular metastases.

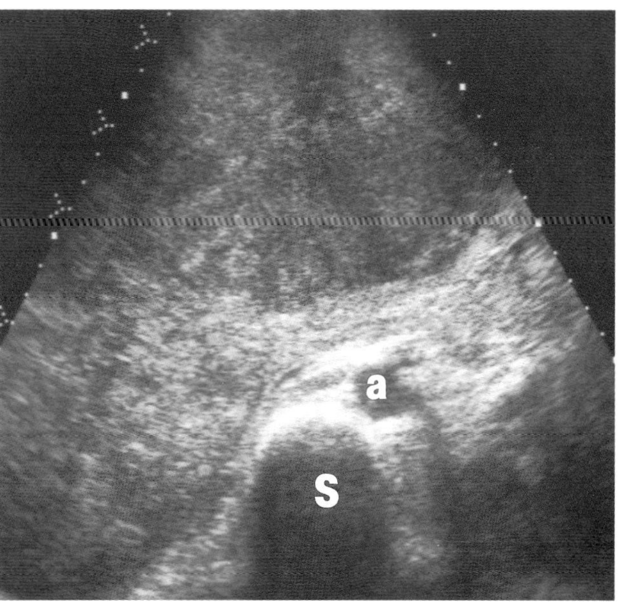

FIG. 2.42. Large focal liver metastasis, nasopharyngeal carcinoma. Transverse sonogram reveals a large metastasis that primarily involves the left lobe (*arrows*). Note the inhomogeneous, palisaded interior of the lesion. a, aorta; S, spine.

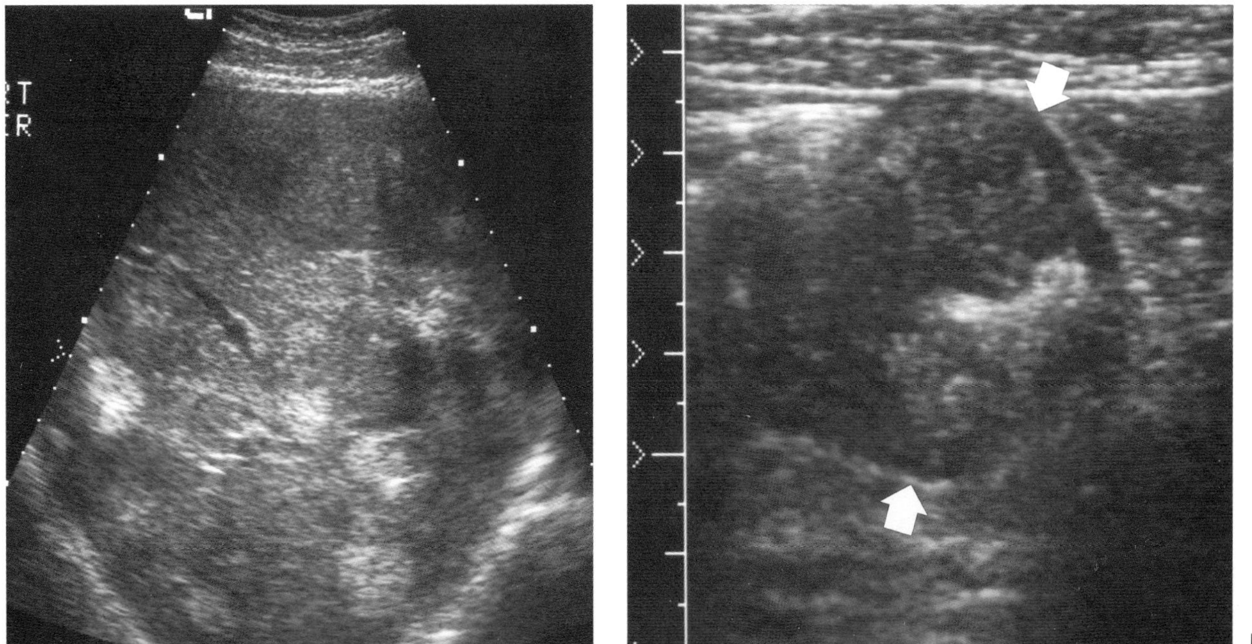

FIG. 2.43. Colon carcinoma, multifocal hepatic metastases. **A:** Transverse sonogram of the right lobe reveals multifocal involvement throughout the liver. Echogenic and hypoechoic lesions are present. The normal architecture of the liver is distorted. **B:** An oblique high-resolution sonogram in the right abdomen reveals the primary colon carcinoma (*arrows*).

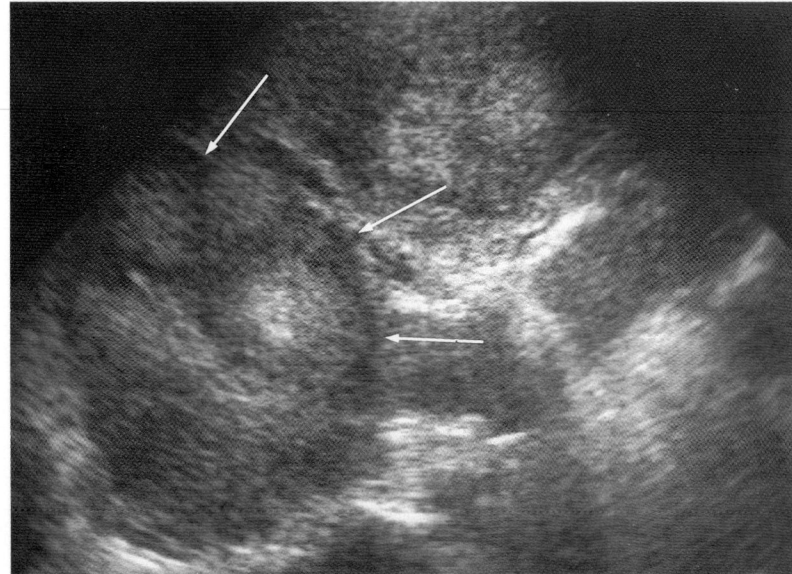

FIG. 2.44. Liver metastases, hypoechoic halos. Transverse sonogram of the right lobe reveals multifocal metastases from leiomyosarcoma. Note the hypoechoic halo (*thin arrows*) around the echogenic metastatic nodules.

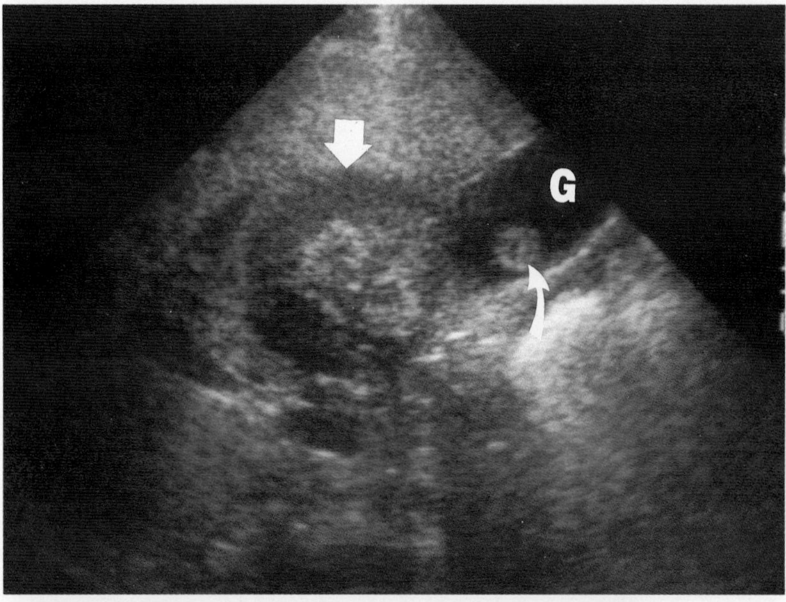

FIG. 2.45. Liver metastasis, target pattern. Longitudinal sonogram reveals a target pattern metastasis from colon carcinoma (*arrow*). This lesion is contiguous to the gallbladder (G), which contains a stone (*curved arrow*).

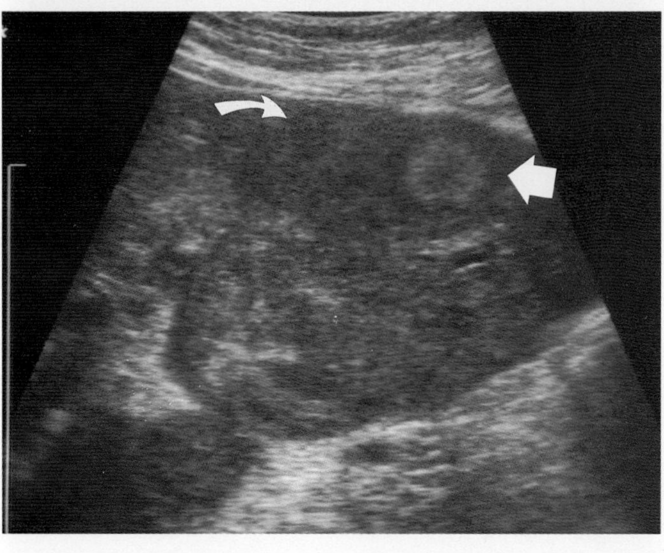

FIG. 2.46. Bull's eye metastasis. Longitudinal sonogram of the left lobe of the liver reveals multiple metastases from gastric carcinoma. A prominent bull's eye lesion (*arrow*) is noted. Other lesions including subtle hypoechoic (*curved arrow*) and diffuse echogenic lesions are noted.

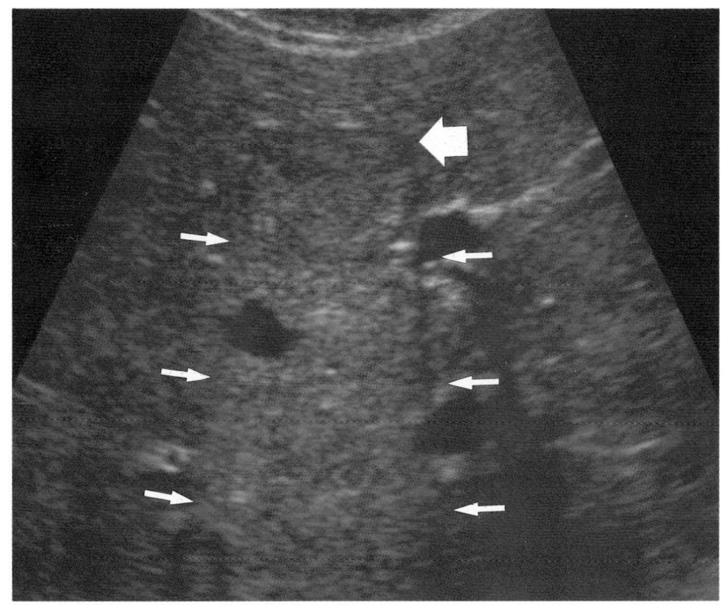

FIG. 2.47. Bull's eye metastasis with through transmission. Transverse sonogram through the medial segment of the left lobe reveals a mildly hypoechoic bull's eye pattern metastasis (*arrow*). Prominent through transmission is noted deep to this lesion (*small arrows*).

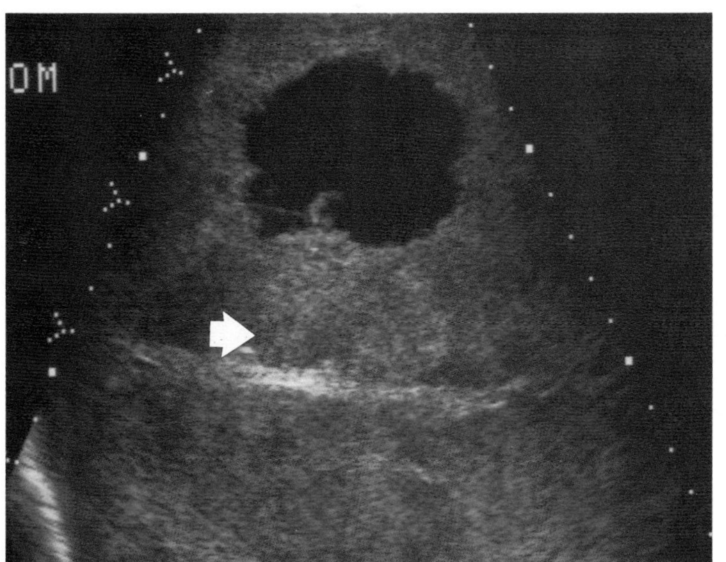

FIG. 2.48. Cystic metastasis, nasopharyngeal carcinoma. This oblique transverse sonogram through the right lobe reveals a predominantly cystic metastasis with through transmission (*arrow*). The irregular walls of this lesion make distinction from simple cyst easy, as did the presence of other metastases in other parts of the liver.

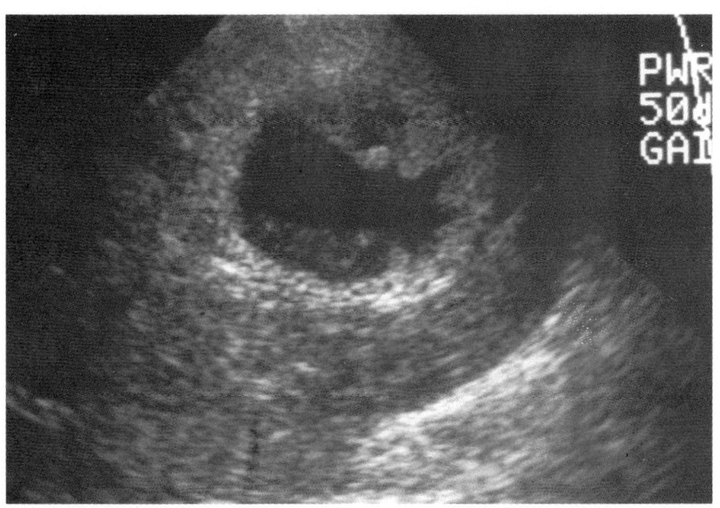

FIG. 2.49. Mixed pattern metastasis, bronchial carcinoid. Oblique sonogram reveals a mixed echogenicity metastasis with a central anechoic area. Predominantly cystic metastases like this are unusual.

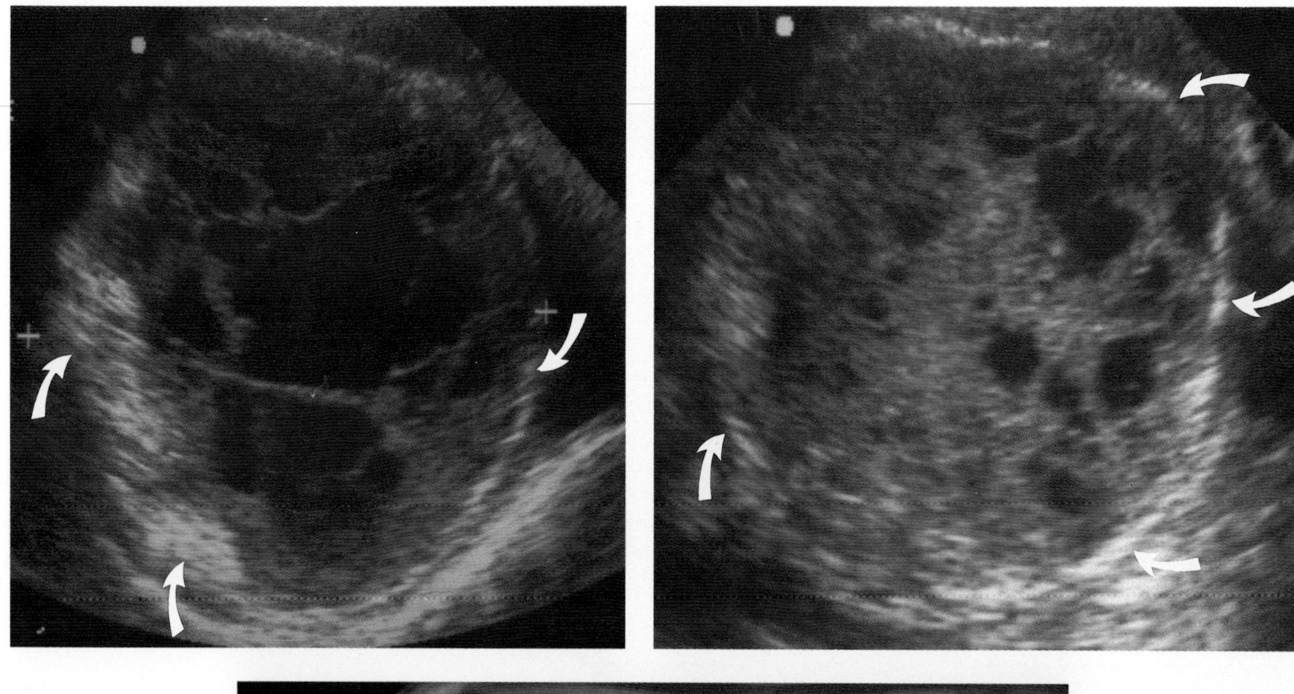

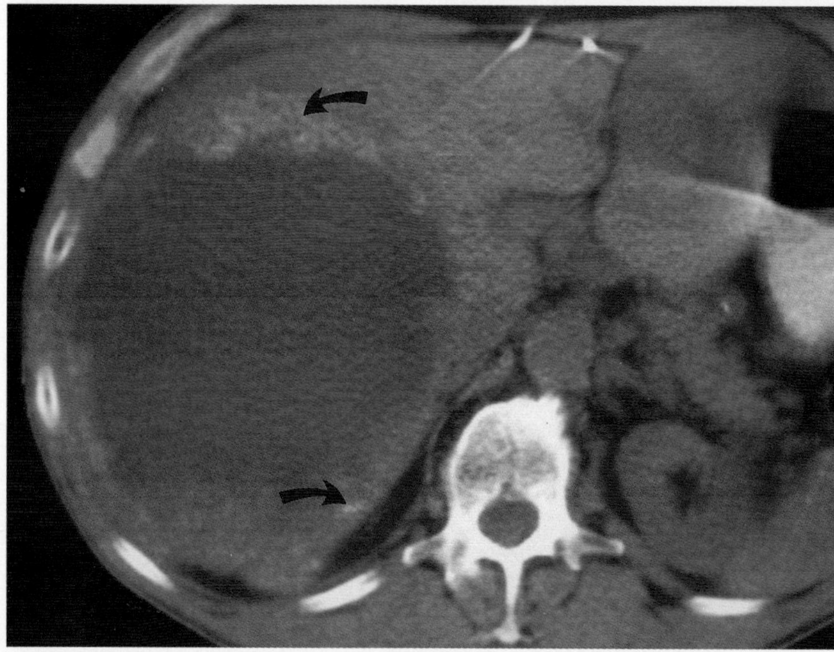

FIG. 2.50. Mixed echogenicity, mainly cystic hepatic metastasis. Transverse sonograms (**A, B**) show a mixed solid/cystic mass with peripheral hyperechoic echoes (*curved arrows*) that prove calcified on CT scan (**C**). This is a large metastasis from mucinous colon carcinoma. Generally, sonography shows the internal structure of a cystic mass better than CT.

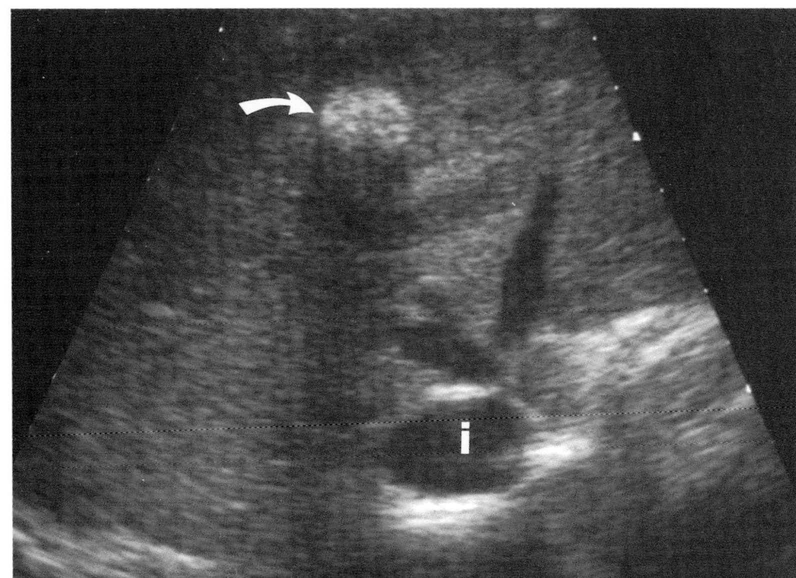

FIG. 2.51. Calcified metastasis, prostate carcinoma. Transverse sonogram at the level of the hepatic veins reveals a densely calcified shadowing metastasis (*curved arrow*). Metastasis from prostate carcinoma to the liver is unusual. i, inferior vena cava.

A

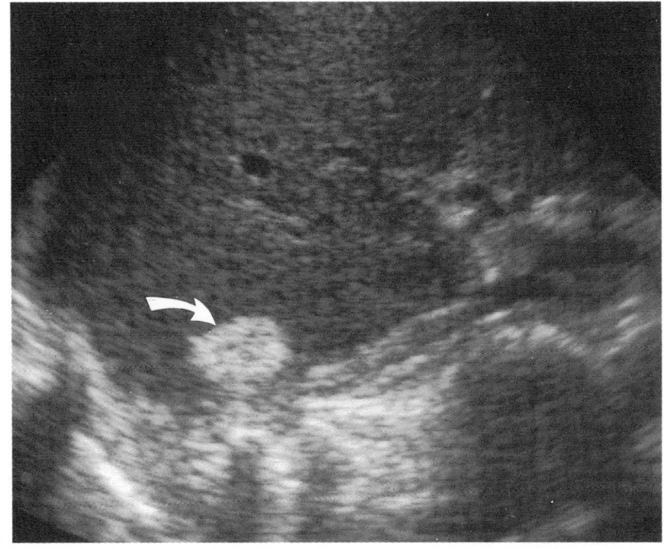

FIG. 2.52. Calcified metastasis, ovarian carcinoma. Transverse sonogram (**A**) through the upper right lobe of the liver reveals a discrete echogenic metastasis (*curved arrow*) that is shown to be calcified on CT scan (**B**). CT is more sensitive to calcification than sonography.

B

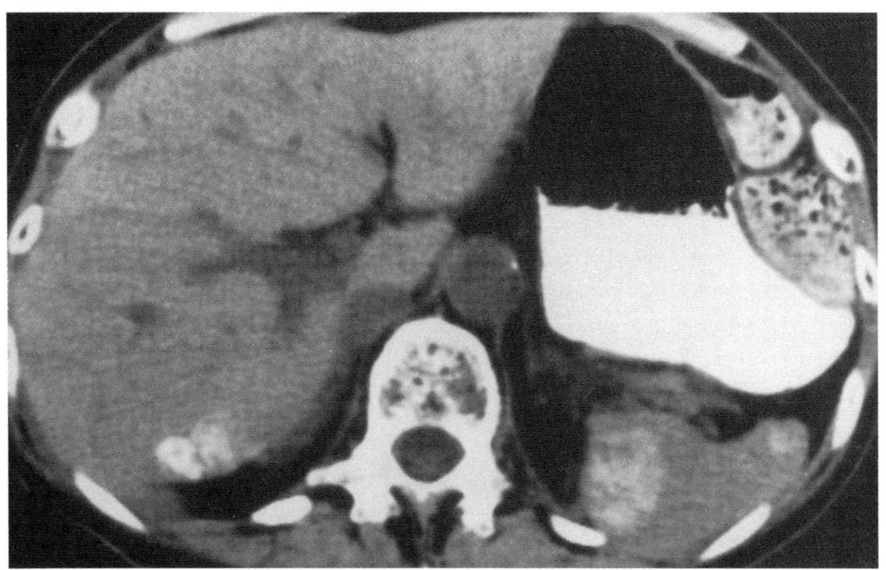

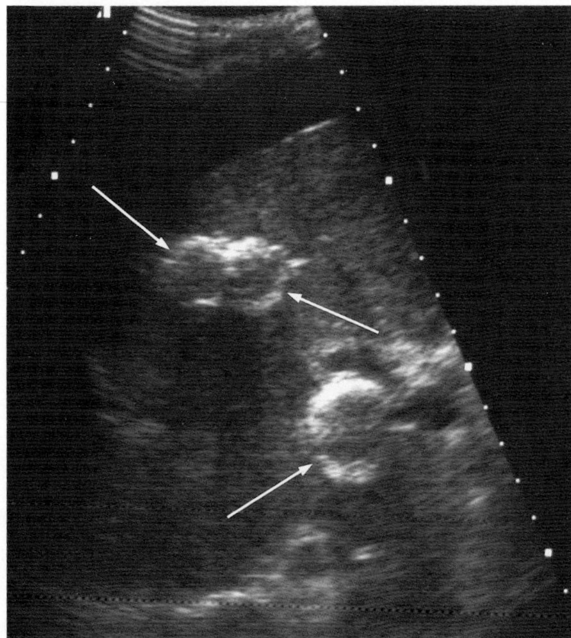

FIG. 2.53. Metastases with calcified margins. Transverse sonogram in the upper abdomen reveals peripherally calcified metastases (*arrows*) from gastric carcinoma. Mucin-secreting tumors such as gastric carcinoma have a propensity to calcify.

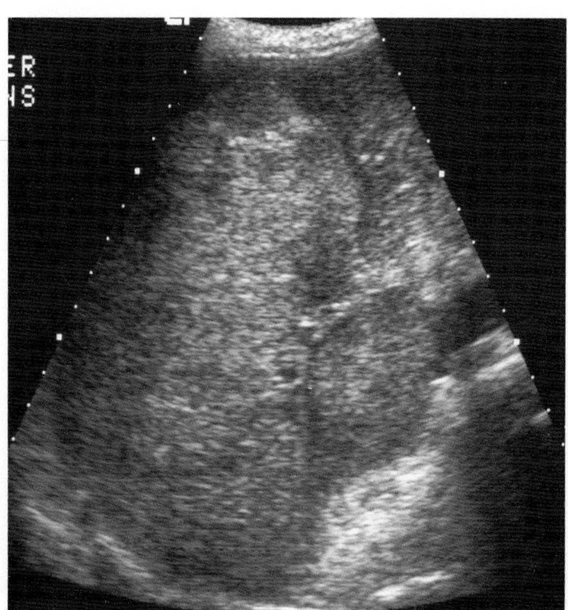

FIG. 2.55. Large echogenic metastasis, colon carcinoma. Transverse sonogram of the right lobe reveals multiple large, predominantly hyperechoic hepatic metastases. There is no specific pattern of metastasis that allows a reliable diagnosis of the primary of origin. Despite this, large to moderate size hyperechoic metastasis should suggest a colonic primary.

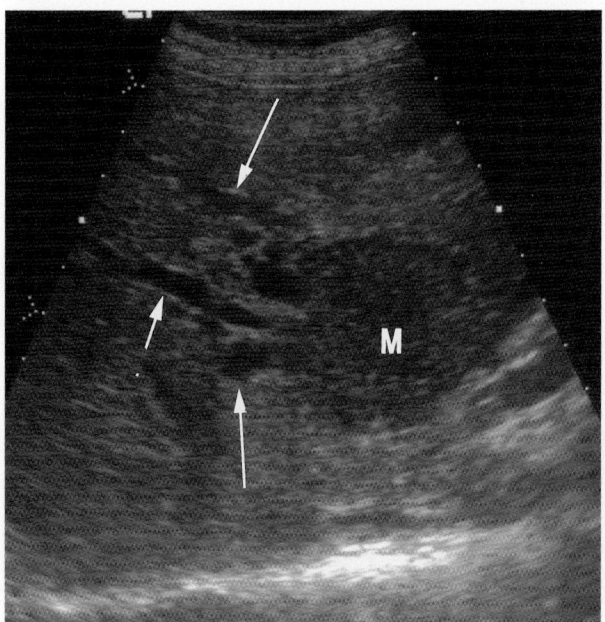

FIG. 2.54. Portal metastasis with bile duct obstruction. Metastasis to the region of the porta often causes biliary obstruction, as noted here. This hypoechoic metastasis (M) is impossible to differentiate on images from a primary cholangiocarcinoma. (See Fig. 2.79.) *Thin arrows,* dilated ducts.

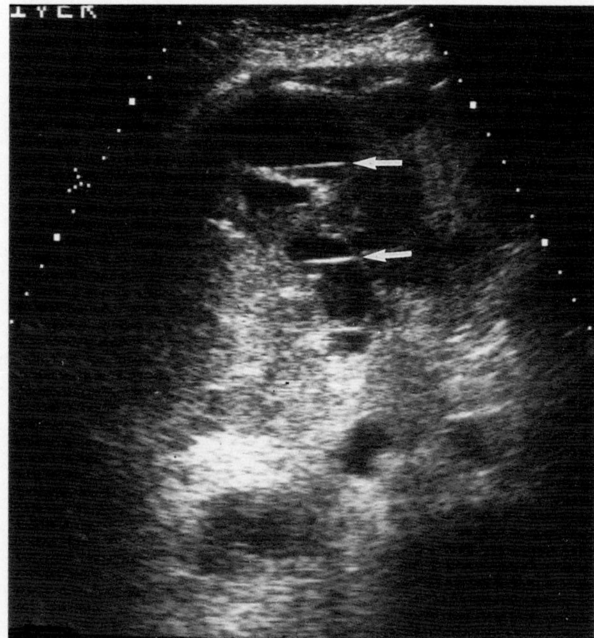

FIG. 2.56. Fluid–fluid levels in metastatic leiomyosarcomas. Transverse sonogram of the right lobe of the liver reveals discrete fluid–fluid levels (*small arrows*) in necrotic hepatic metastases. This finding, while not definitive, should suggest a primary leiomyosarcoma.

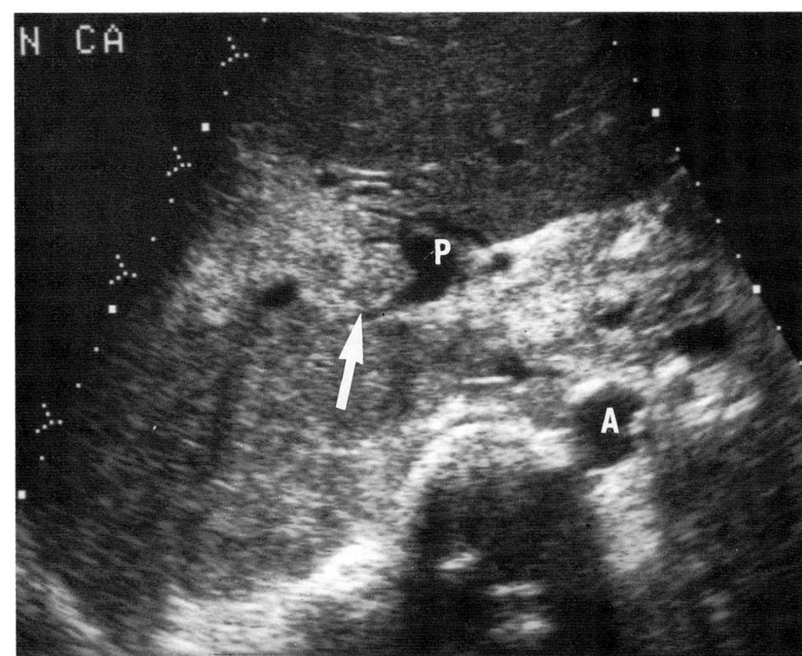

FIG. 2.57. Metastasis invades the portal vein. Transverse sonogram shows an echogenic hepatic metastasis from colon carcinoma. The proximal portion of the left portal vein (P) is invaded (*arrow*). On color flow sonography, a tiny persistent flow channel was identified. Portal vein invasion by metastasis is unusual. Venous invasion by HCC is more frequent. A, aorta.

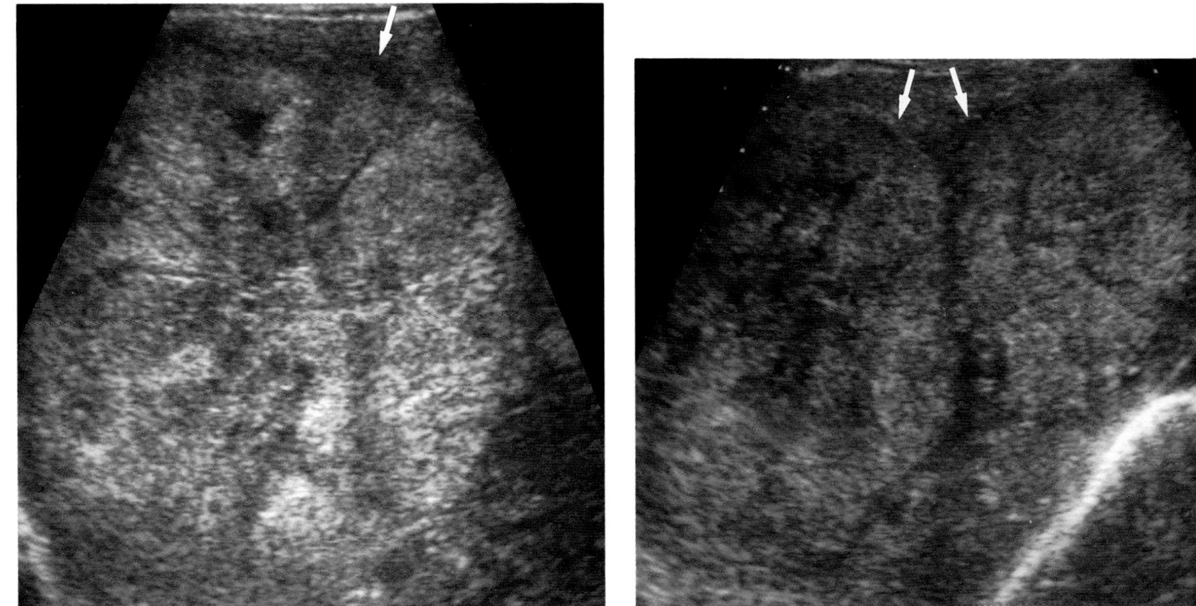

FIG. 2.58. Multifocal HCC. Transverse images of the right lobe of the liver (**A, B**) reveal multiple palisaded masses with a hypoechoic rim (*small arrows*). Multifocal HCC is impossible to differentiate on images from metastatic disease.

cent have an adjacent displaced vessel (Tanaka's detour sign) (Fig. 2.7) (12).

Hepatocellular Carcinoma

Hepatocellular carcinoma (HCC) is the commonest primary liver cancer, comprising 80 percent in the United States. It is much less common than hepatic metastases. It typically occurs in middle aged and elderly individuals. HCC is the most common primary or metastatic liver malignancy in certain parts of Southeast Asia and sub-Saharan Africa (17).

In the United States, 85 percent of HCCs occur in patients with cirrhosis or precirrhotic conditions. Hepatitis-B-related cirrhosis has the highest prevalence of hepatocellular carcinoma, almost 40 percent at autopsy. Although alcoholic cirrhosis-related HCC has a lower prevalence (10 percent of autopsied patients), it is by far the commonest type of cirrhosis leading to HCC in the United States, accounting for 52 percent in one series (32). Other types of cirrhosis may also predispose to hepatocellular carcinoma, including hemochromatosis (10 to 20 percent of patients) and hepatitis C. HCCs arising in normal livers (15 percent) tend to occur in younger patients and to be single, well-defined lesions, not multifocal.

Sonography is a sensitive and integral component of HCC screening programs in high-prevalence countries. Screening generally consists of serologic testing for alpha fetoprotein and/or hepatitis-B surface antigen, coupled with liver sonography (42,43). Sonographic findings in HCC are variable. It is difficult to distinguish advanced HCC from metastatic disease (Figs. 2.58 to 2.61). This is less of a problem in screening programs, where small HCCs are often detected. Small HCCs (smaller than 5 cm) have more uniform sonographic findings; as many as 75 percent are diffusely hypoechoic (42,43) (Fig. 2.62). In screening situations, adenomatous hyperplastic nodules may simulate small HCCs (Fig. 2.63). These regenerative nodules are probably premalignant. As HCCs grow, they tend to develop hypoechoic peripheral rims (44). With further progression, lesions become more numerous and heterogeneous (Fig. 2.64). Some HCCs, even small lesions, undergo fatty metamorphosis (Fig. 2.65) (45,46), causing increased echogenicity and potential confusion with hemangioma. Vascular invasion is common and should suggest the diagnosis of HCC, although other tumors occasionally also invade veins (40,41). HCC invades portal veins more frequently than hepatic veins (Figs. 2.66 to 2.69). Invasion of the inferior vena cava is common (Fig. 2.70). Occasionally, tumor thrombus extends into the heart (Fig. 2.71). Rarely, bile duct invasion may occur (Fig. 2.72). Edge shadowing, caused by reflection and refraction, may be seen more commonly in HCC than in other hepatic neoplasms (Fig. 2.73).

Fibrolamellar HCC, which accounts for 2 percent of hepatocellular carcinoma, but 25 to 50 percent of HCC in young adults, is typically a single, well-circumscribed lesion in an otherwise normal liver. Fibrolamellar HCC is clinically and pathologically distinct from other forms of HCC (47,48). These tumors tend to have a lobulated margin and variable echogenicity ranging from prominently hyperechoic to hypoechoic (Fig. 2.74). Other features include a "central scar" (Fig. 2.75) and a high prevalence of calcification. A central scar is nonspecific and may occur in other types of HCC (Fig. 2.76) and other lesions including focal nodular hyperplasia, hemangiomas, and adenomas (49). Calcification also occurs in other histologic types of HCC (Fig. 2.77).

On occasion, HCC may rupture, causing catastrophic hemorrhage and hemoperitoneum (Fig. 2.78) (50). Acute onset of peritoneal fluid or sudden hypotension in an HCC patient should suggest this possibility. Sonographically guided percutaneous injection of absolute alcohol has been used to treat HCC (51,52).

Cholangiocarcinoma

Cholangiocarcinomas arise from the bile ducts, accounting for about 10 percent of all primary liver cancers. Cholangiocarcinoma is associated with hemochromatosis, ulcerative colitis, Caroli disease, and choledochal cyst (32,53). Cholangiocarcinoma has two forms, peripheral cholangiocarcinoma (PCC) and hilar cholangiocarcinoma (Klatskin tumor) (54,55). In the United States, PCC is three times more common than hilar cholangiocarcinoma. In Japan, hilar and peripheral cholangiocarcinoma occur in equal numbers (32). PCC is usually a large tumor, while hilar cholangiocarcinoma presents earlier with ductal obstruction and jaundice. Hilar cholangiocarcinoma is usually not associated with a large mass (see Chapter 3). Hemochromatosis is associated with both PCC (9 percent of patients) and HCC (18 percent of patients).

The sonographic findings in PCC are variable, some reporting predominantly hypoechoic (56) (Fig. 2.79) and others predominantly hyperechoic lesions (57). Hilar cholangiocarcinoma is more difficult to image than PCC, as extraductal masses are usually small or nonexistent. CT is generally superior to sonography in demonstrating masses in hilar cholangiocarcinoma (58,59), but CT and sonography are comparable in determining the level of biliary obstruction.

Liver Abscess

Worldwide, pyogenic liver abscesses are less common than amebic abscesses. In the United States, pyogenic abscesses occur more frequently. Pyogenic liver abscesses are usually a complication of some other condition, of-

(*text continues on page 119*)

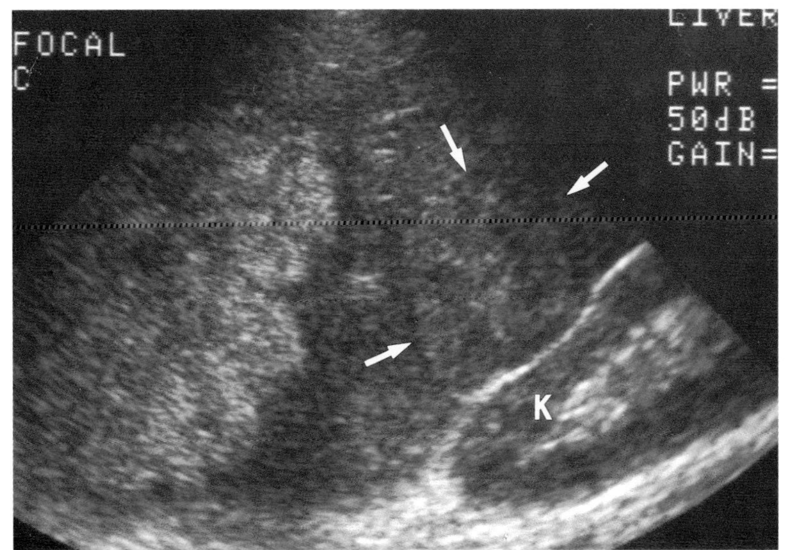

FIG. 2.59. Multifocal HCC. Longitudinal sonogram through the right lobe of the liver reveals two separate nodules of HCC. Each has different features. The larger lesion is lobulated and hyperechoic while the smaller nodule (*arrows*) is nearly isoechoic. Note how the smaller lesion indents the right kidney (K).

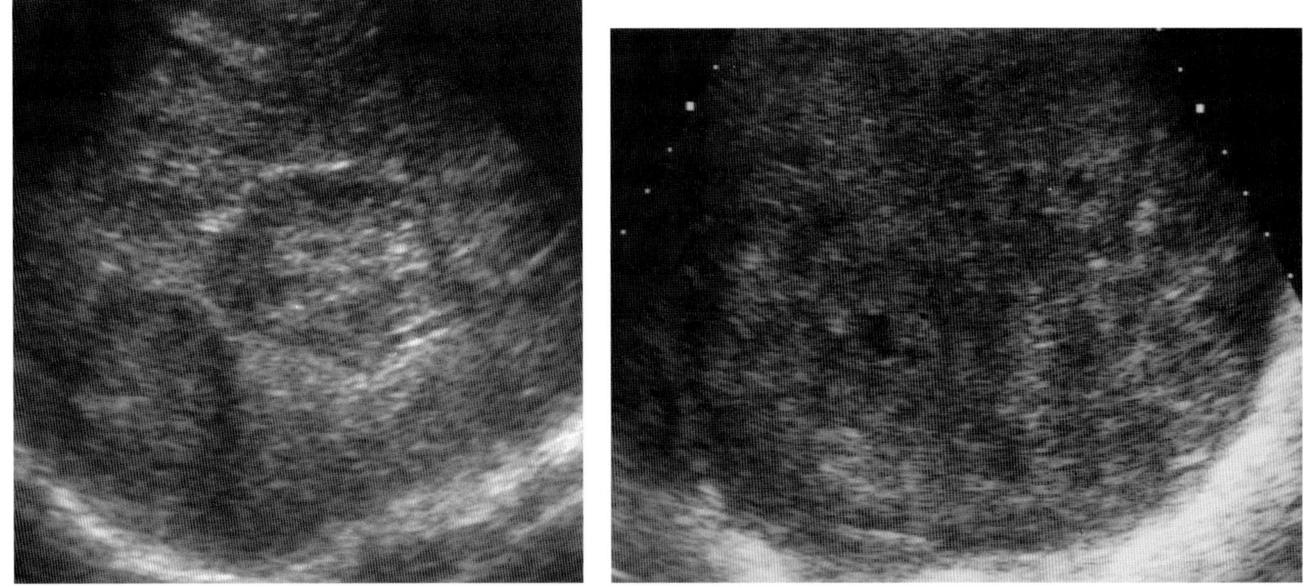

FIG. 2.60. Multifocal HCC. Transverse (**A**) and longitudinal (**B**) sonograms reveal a multifocal HCC that is sonographically indistinguishable from metastatic disease. Eighty-five percent of HCCs are multifocal and thus difficult to distinguish from metastases. This patient was successfully resected by an extended right lobectomy (trisegmentectomy).

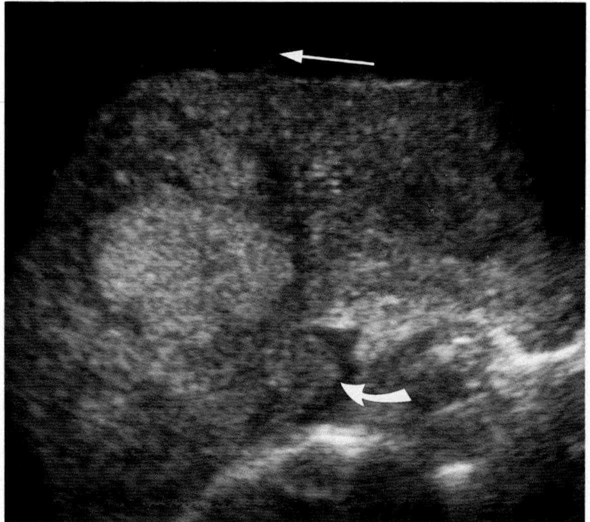

FIG. 2.61. Multifocal HCC. This transverse sonogram reveals a multifocal HCC that encompasses virtually the entire liver. The falciform ligament (*arrow*) is outlined by ascites. Note invasion of the inferior vena cava (*curved arrow*).

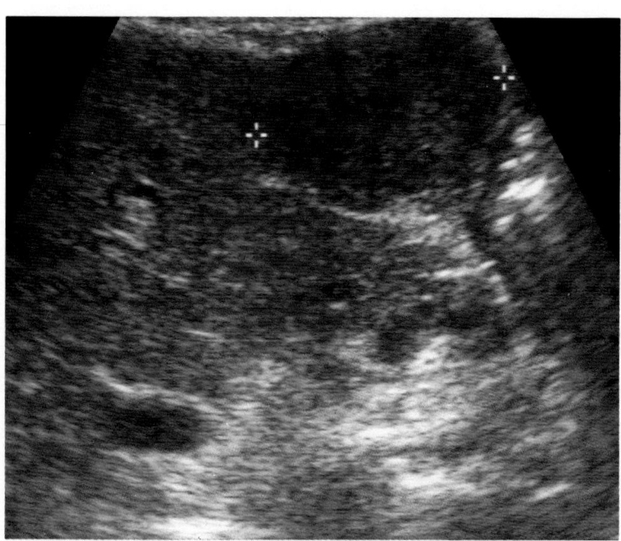

FIG. 2.62. Small hypoechoic HCC. Transverse sonogram of the left lobe of the liver. This hypoechoic 5-cm HCC (calipers) arose in a patient with hepatitis B. Of HCCs smaller than 5 cm, 75 percent are hypoechoic.

A

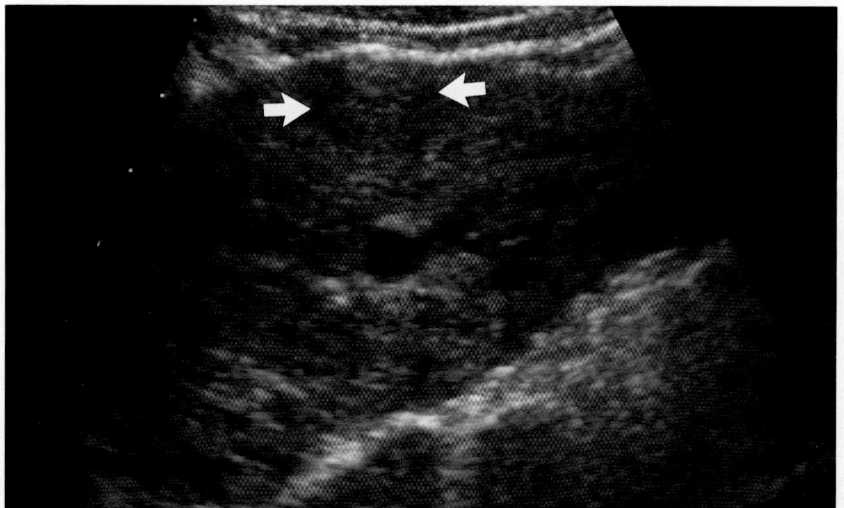

B

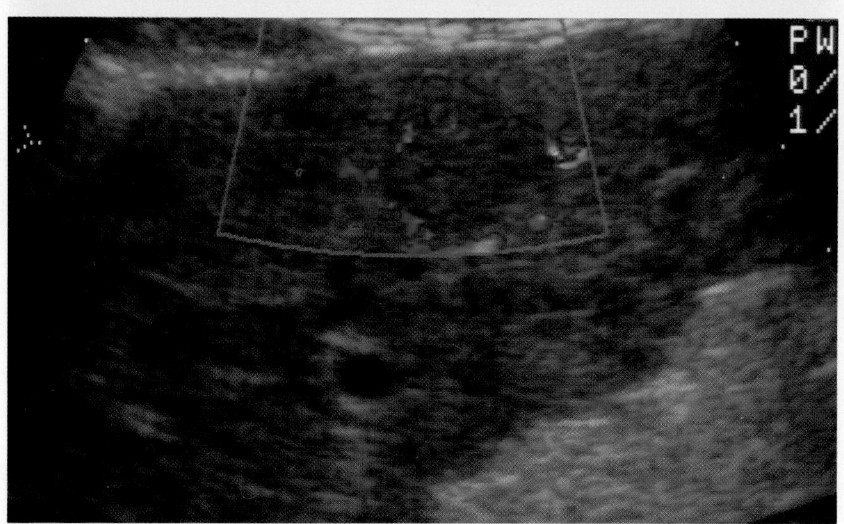

FIG. 2.63. Adenomatous hyperplastic nodule with internal flow. **A:** The longitudinal grayscale sonogram reveals a subtle 1.5-cm nodule (*tailed arrows*). This lesion was detected on a sonogram requested because of slightly elevated alpha fetoprotein and a history of chronic liver disease related to hepatitis B. **B:** The longitudinal color Doppler sonogram revealed internal flow. At surgery, this proved to be an adenomatous hyperplastic nodule. This is a regenerative lesion that may be a precursor to HCC.

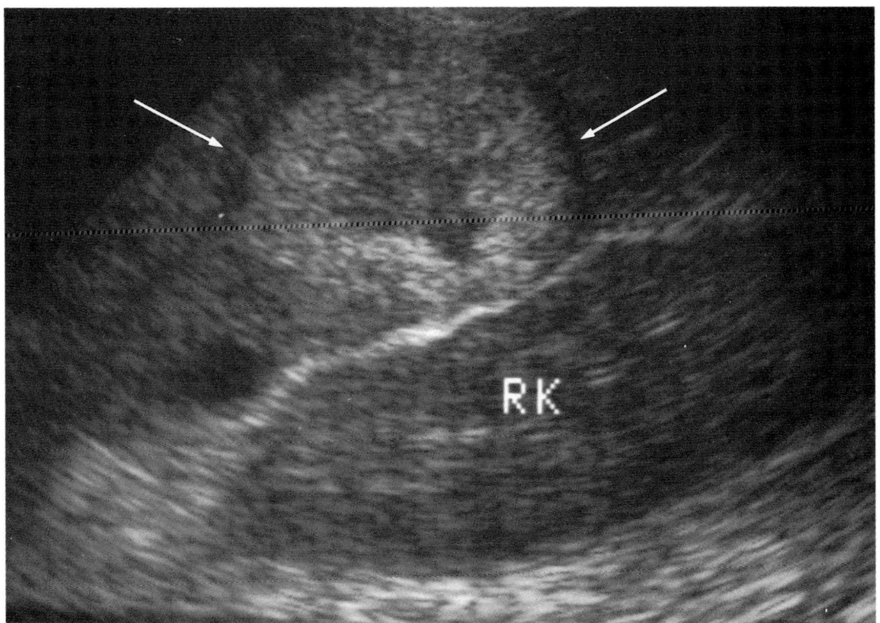

FIG. 2.64. HCC—target pattern. Longitudinal sonogram, right lobe of the liver. As HCCs grow, their sonographic pattern becomes extremely variable. This lesion indents the right kidney (RK) and has a "target" appearance with a thin hypoechoic pseudocapsule (*small arrows*).

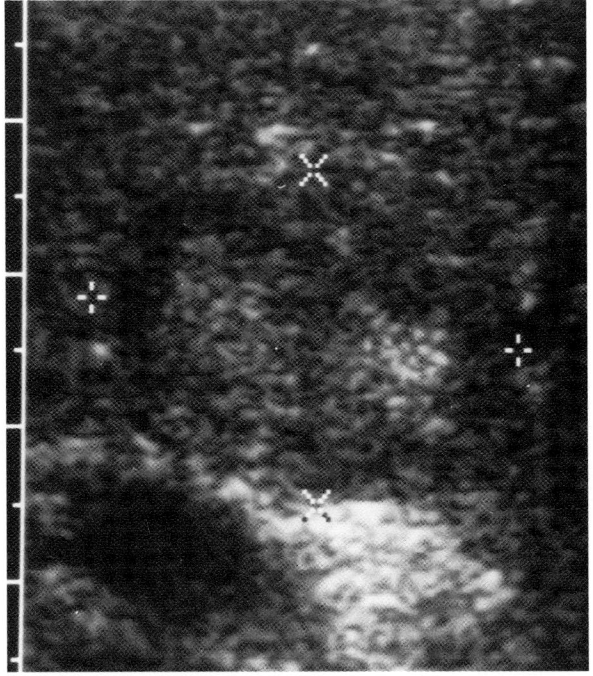

FIG. 2.65. Fatty infiltration of small HCC. Oblique transverse sonogram of the left lobe of the liver shows a 2-cm HCC (calipers), which is predominantly hyperechoic centrally. Pathologically, there was extensive fatty infiltration in this lesion.

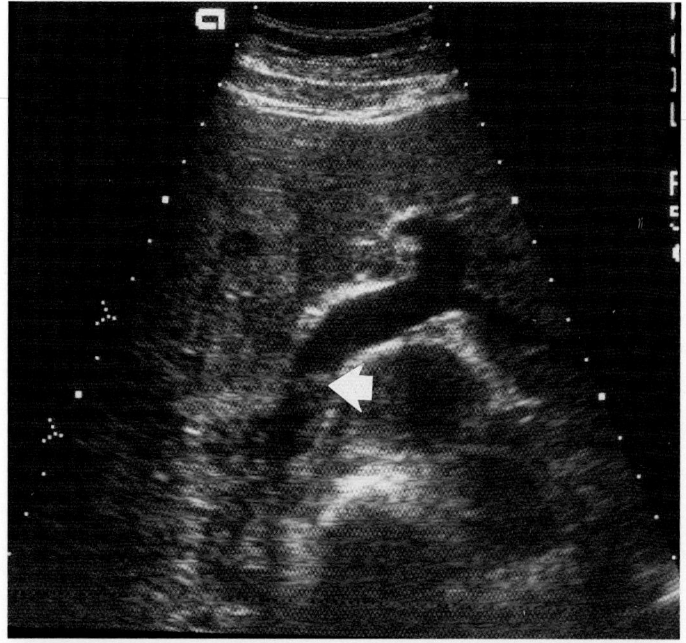

A

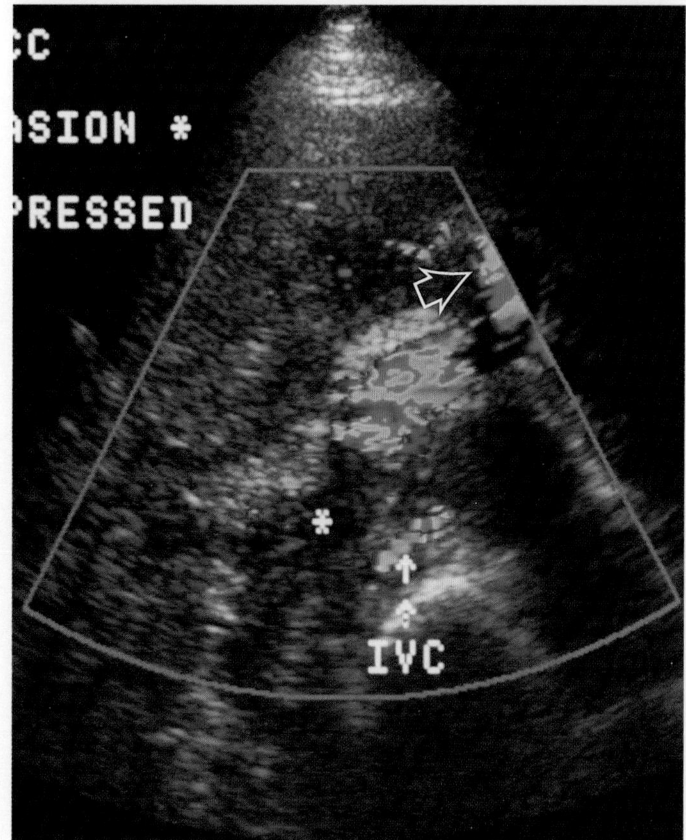

B

FIG. 2.66. HCC invades right portal vein. **A:** Transverse sonogram of the left and right portal vein. A large, predominantly right-sided HCC invades the right portal vein (*arrow*). **B:** The transverse color Doppler sonogram at this level confirms invasion of the right portal vein (*) and shows color flow in the uninvolved left portal vein (*open arrow*). The inferior vena cava (IVC) is compressed but not invaded. MRI had previously been interpreted as showing IVC invasion.

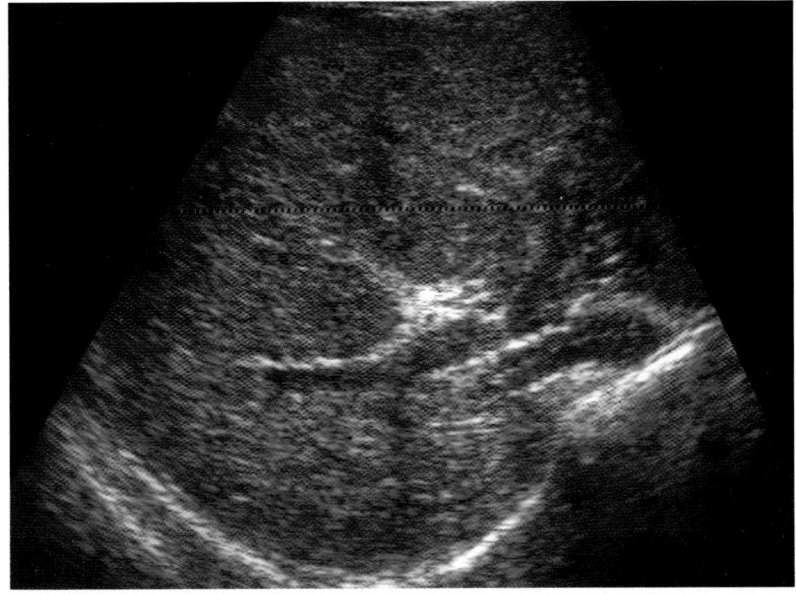

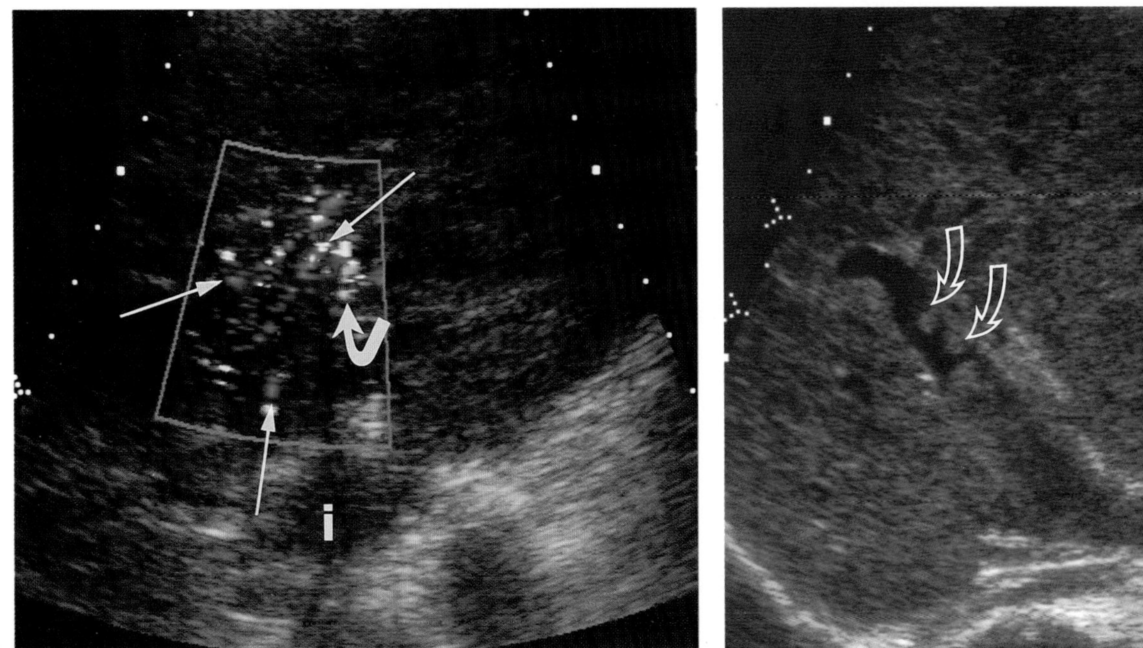

FIG. 2.67. Threads and streaks sign, HCC. **A:** Transverse sonogram shows diffuse abnormality throughout the liver, indicative of an infiltrative, multifocal HCC. Note the parenchymal inhomogeneity. **B:** Transverse color Doppler sonogram of the left portal vein shows linear vascular flow (*small arrows*), coursing through the tumor thrombus that completely fills the left portal vein. This finding is comparable to the angiographic sign of linear flow within portal venous tumor thrombus, the "threads and streaks" sign. A hepatic artery (*curved arrow*) is noted next to the tumor-filled left portal vein. **C:** Transverse sonogram of the right portal vein reveals nodular tumor invasion (*curved open arrows*). i, inferior vena cava.

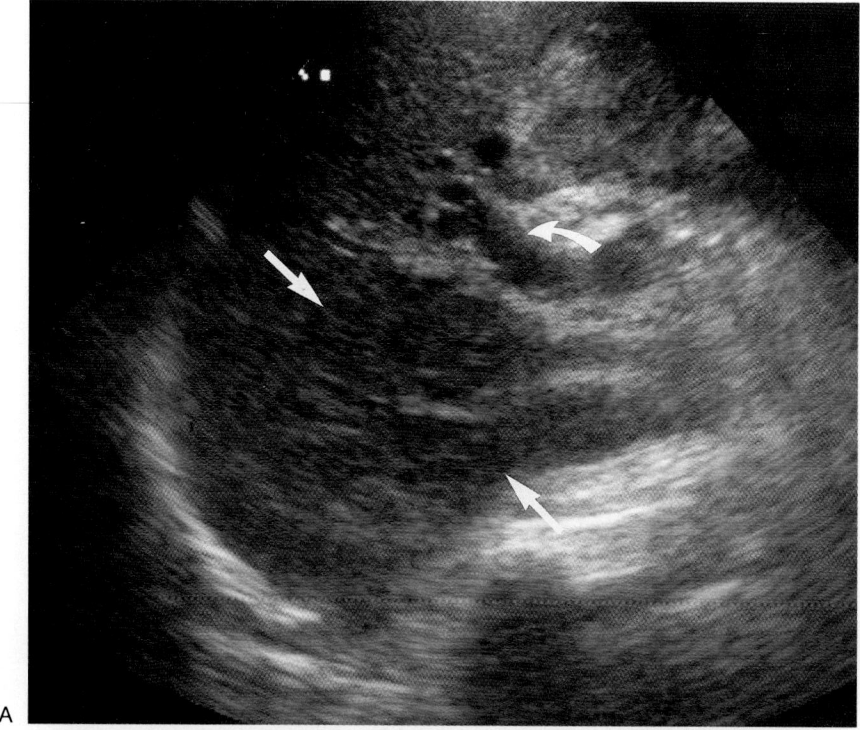

A

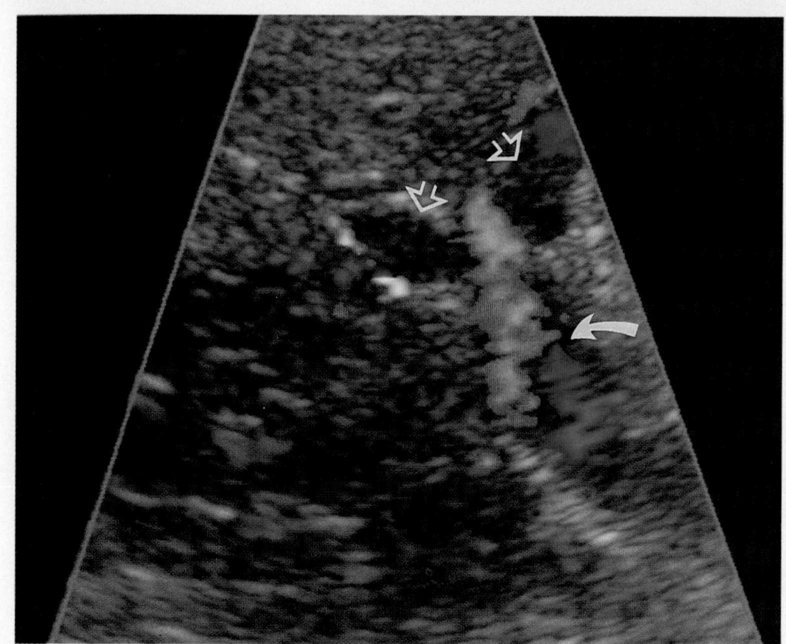

B

FIG. 2.68. HCC invades the right portal vein. **A:** Transverse grayscale sonogram reveals a large right lobe HCC (*arrows*). It is unclear on this grayscale image whether the right portal vein (*curved arrow*) is invaded. In fact, it appears there are more echoes in the main portion of the right portal vein than in its branches. **B:** Enlarged color Doppler sonogram reveals that the main portal vein (*curved arrow*) is not invaded. Rather, the anterior and posterior segmental branches of the right portal vein (*open arrows*) are involved with tumor. Color Doppler sonography not only allows a more confident diagnosis of venous invasion, but it also is very useful in delineating the extent of involvement.

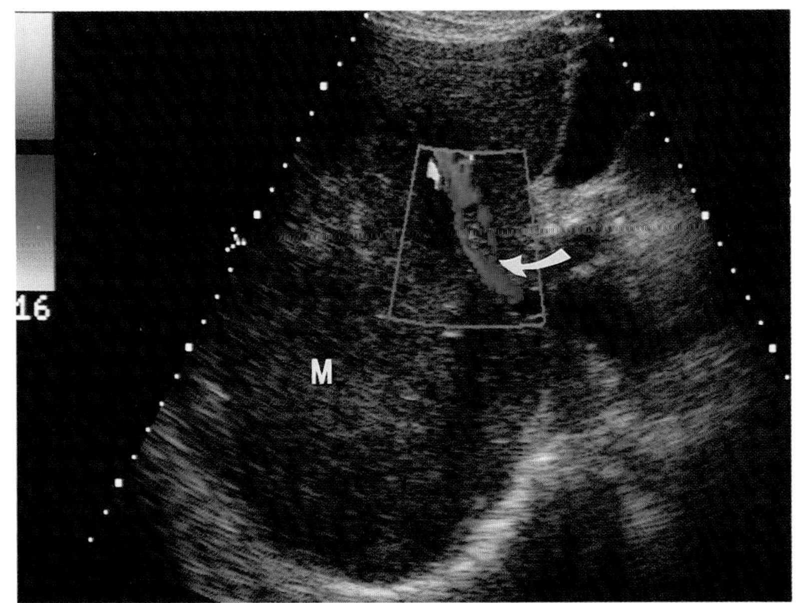

FIG. 2.69. HCC, middle hepatic vein invasion. A transverse color Doppler sonogram through the middle hepatic vein reveals a partially occluding thrombus (*curved arrow*) outlined by color-coded flow. There is a large right-sided HCC. M, mass. Color Doppler sonography's ability to precisely display flow allows precise delineation of lesions such as this partially occluding thrombus. Detailed flow information such as this is essentially impossible to obtain with any other means.

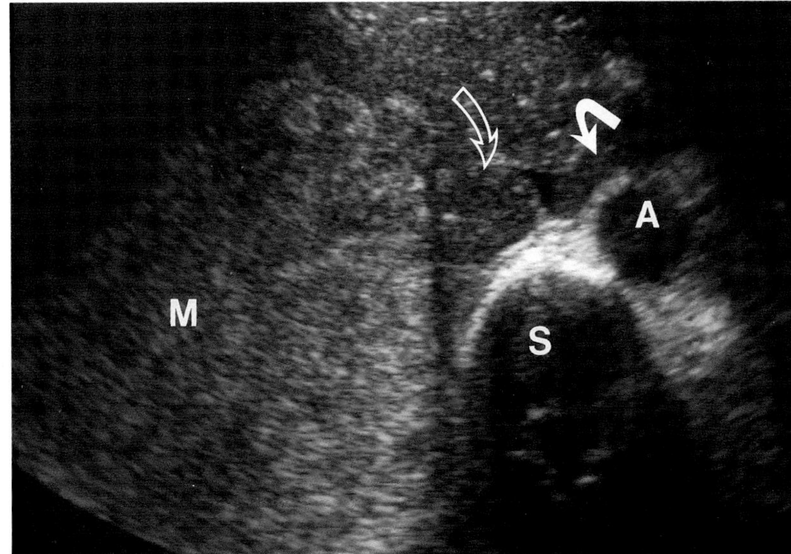

A

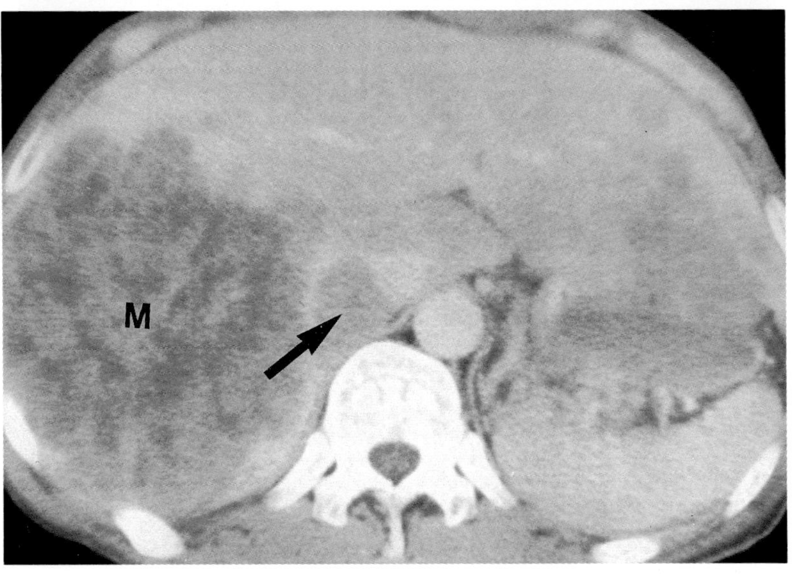

B

FIG. 2.70. HCC, IVC invasion. **A:** A transverse sonogram in the upper portion of the liver reveals a large tumor mass (M) related to HCC. There is invasion of the IVC (*open curved arrow*). Also noted is invasion of the left hepatic vein (*sharply curved arrow*), leaving only a small area of patency in the IVC. **B:** The CT scan reveals partial occlusion of the IVC (*arrow*). The left hepatic vein invasion was not detected by CT. S, spine; A, aorta.

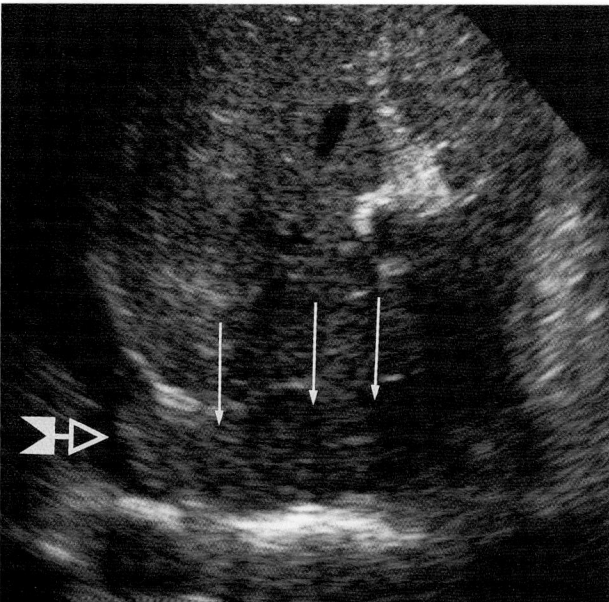

FIG. 2.71. HCC invades the heart. Longitudinal sonogram reveals tumor thrombus extending from the IVC (*thin arrows*) into the right atrium (*tailed arrow*). Cardiac invasion is an infrequent but grave complication of HCC.

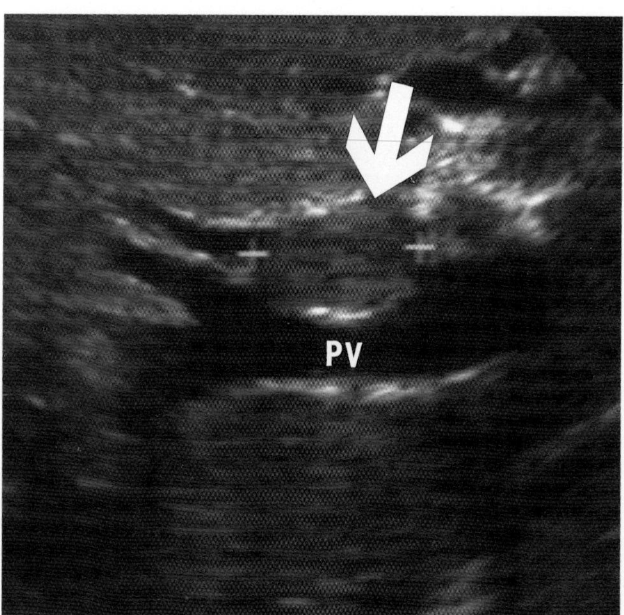

FIG. 2.72. HCC invades the common bile duct. Transverse oblique sonogram in the region of the porta hepatis. In this patient with HCC, invasion of the bile duct (*arrow*) is seen ventral to the portal vein (PV). Although venous invasion is far more frequent, HCC occasionally invades the bile ducts.

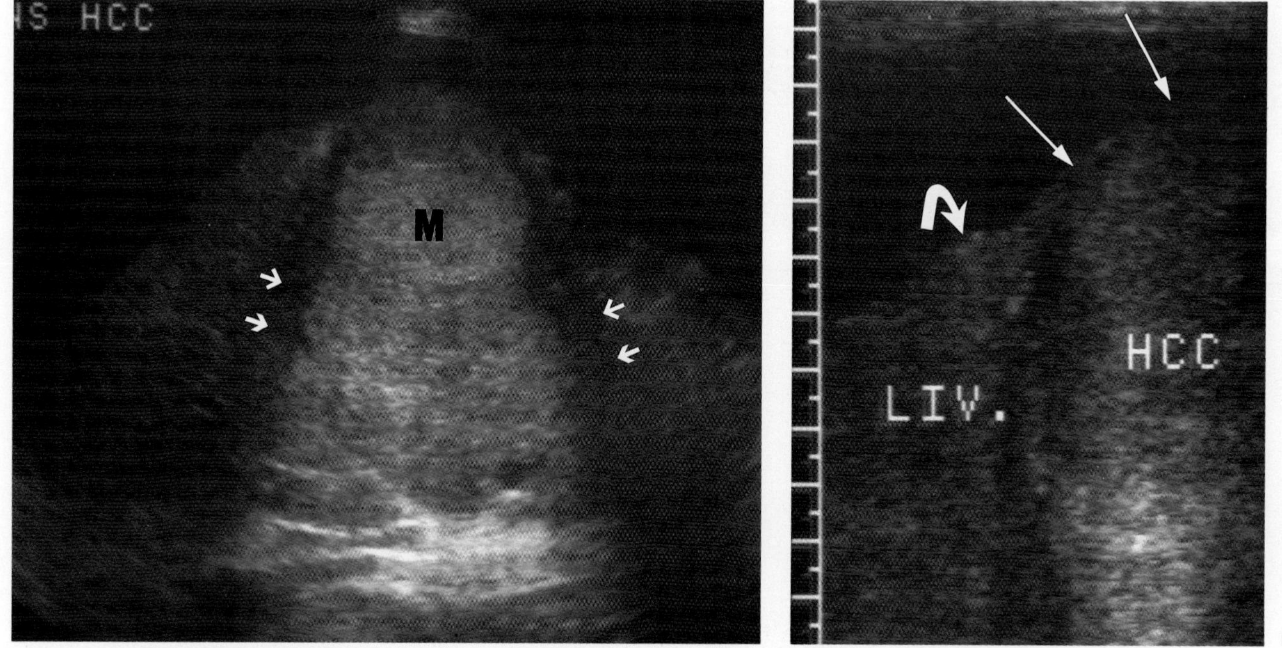

FIG. 2.73. HCC with prominent edge shadowing. Transverse sonograms of the liver (**A, B**). Prominent edge shadowing (*arrows*) is noted at the periphery of the mass (M). Edge shadows are caused by reflection and refraction occurring at curved boundaries between tissues with different acoustic impedance. HCCs often result in more prominent edge shadowing than other hepatic neoplasms. The linear array image (**B**) reveals a nodular liver surface (*curved arrow*) caused by cirrhosis. The neoplasm has a smooth surface that is easily identified through the ascites (*arrows*).

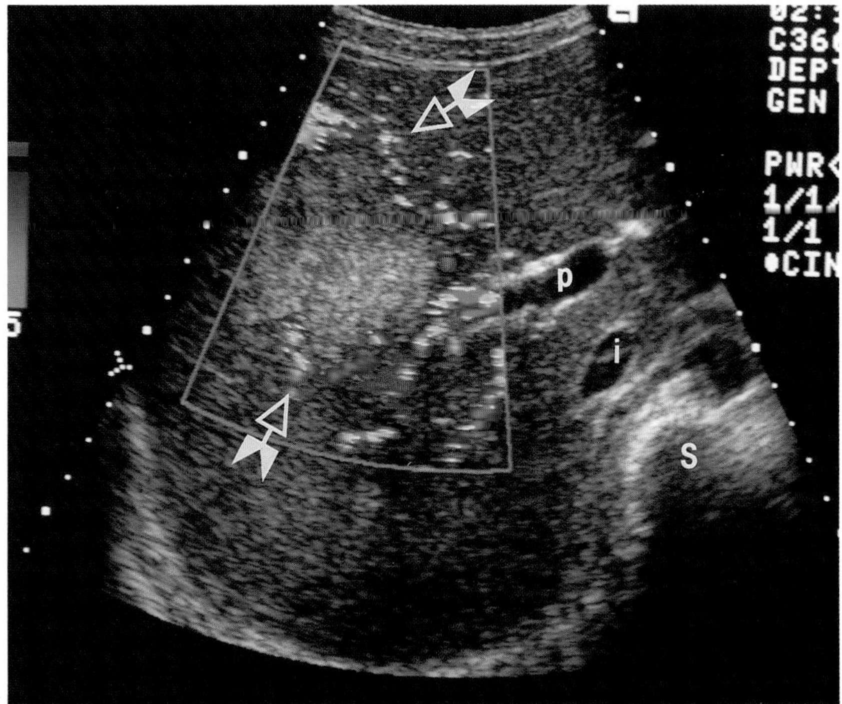

FIG. 2.74. Fibrolamellar HCC. Transverse color Doppler sonogram shows prominent flow (*tailed arrows*) around the periphery of this predominantly echogenic lesion. These areas of vascularity were hypoechoic on grayscale, but no discrete vessels were identified. This lesion lacked both a central scar and calcification, two frequent features of fibrolamellar HCC. P, right portal vein; S, spine; i, inferior vena cava.

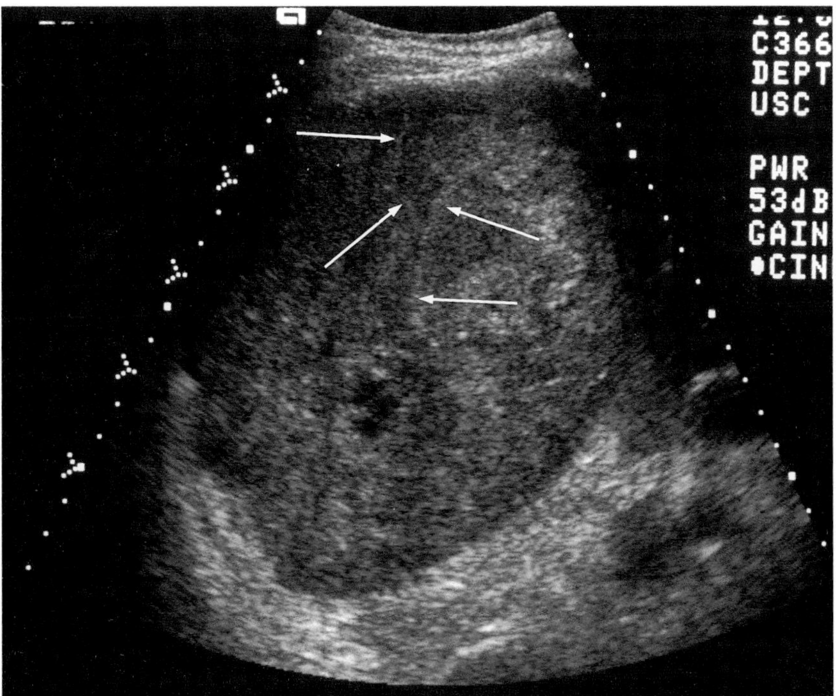

FIG. 2.75. Fibrolamellar HCC. Transverse sonogram through the right lobe of the liver reveals a large lesion that has a central scar (*thin arrows*). Presence of a large single lesion is typical of fibrolamellar HCC. Central scars are often present. The central scar pattern is not specific for this histology of HCC. It also occurs in other types of liver neoplasm. Calcification, often found in fibrolamellar HCC, is not present in this patient.

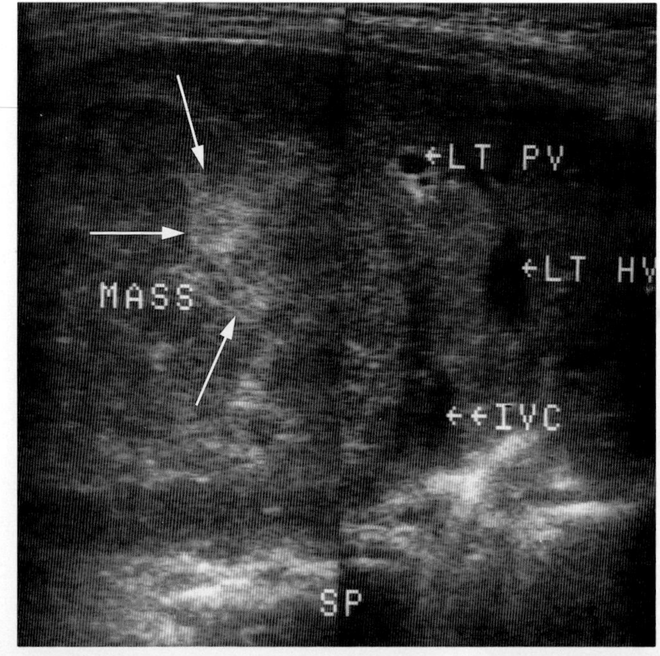

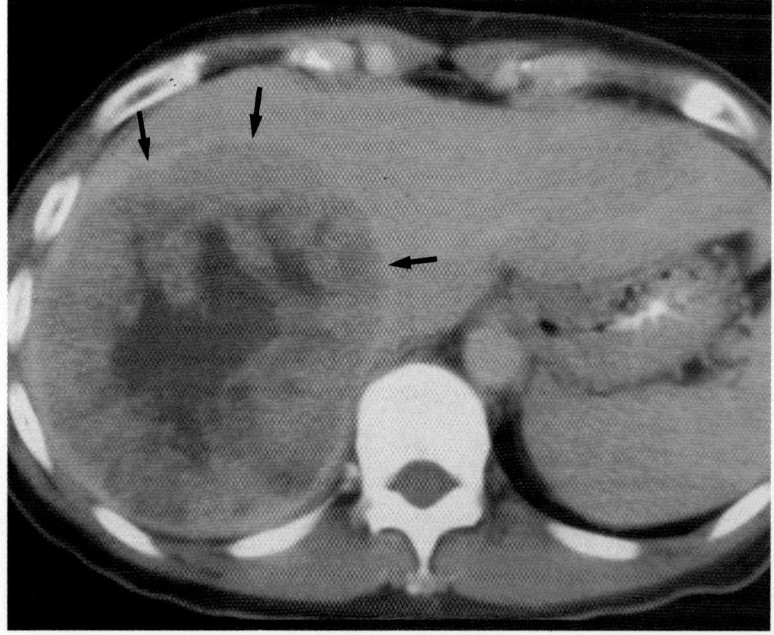

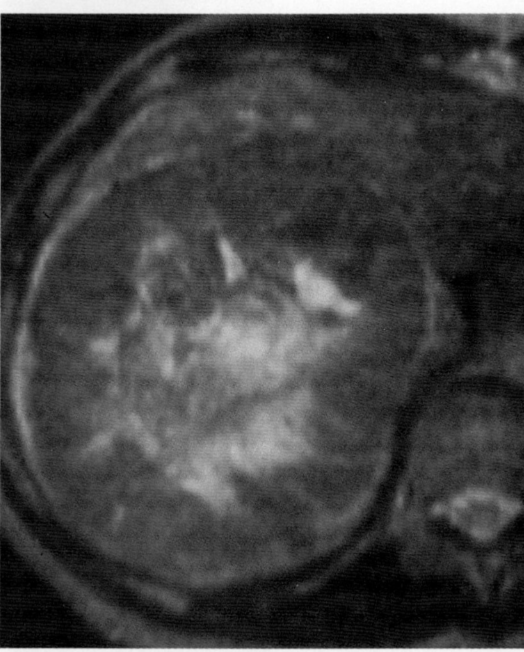

FIG. 2.76. HCCs with "central scar." **A:** Transverse composite sonogram revealed a large heterogeneous mass with a central stellate echogenic area (*thin arrows*) within the mass. The HCC displaced the IVC to the left. **B:** The contrast-enhanced CT scan reveals an enhancing pseudocapsule (*small arrows*) and a nonenhancing central low-attenuation region. **C:** T2-weighted MRI shows high signal in the central region. Despite the "central scar," this was not a fibrolamellar HCC. IVC, inferior vena cava; LT PV, left portal vein; LT HV, left hepatic vein; SP, spine.

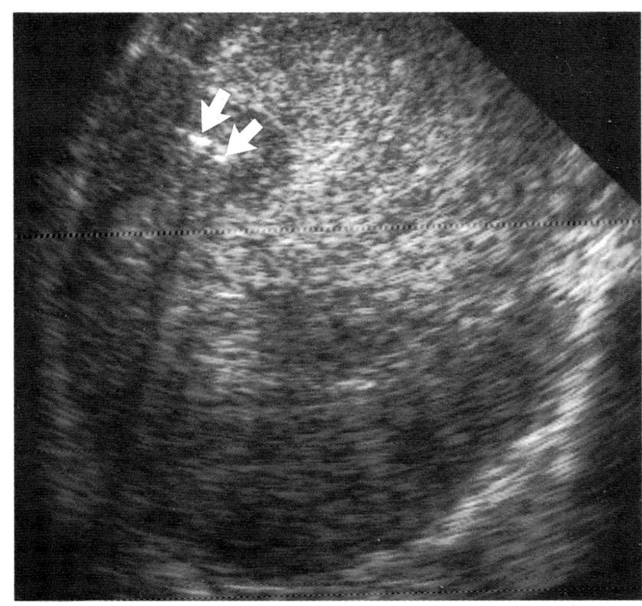

FIG. 2.77. Calcification in HCC. Transverse oblique sonogram through the right lobe of the liver. There are several small calcifications (*arrows*) within this large HCC. Although fibrolamellar HCC has a high prevalence of calcification, it is not the only histologic type of HCC that exhibits calcification visible on images. This HCC is of the usual histology. It is not a fibrolamellar HCC.

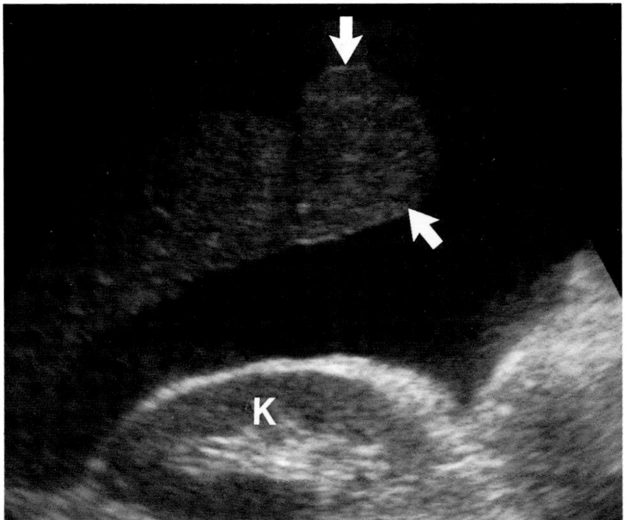

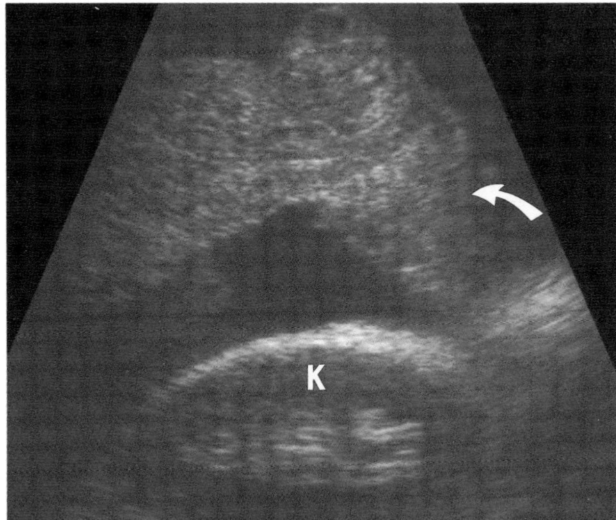

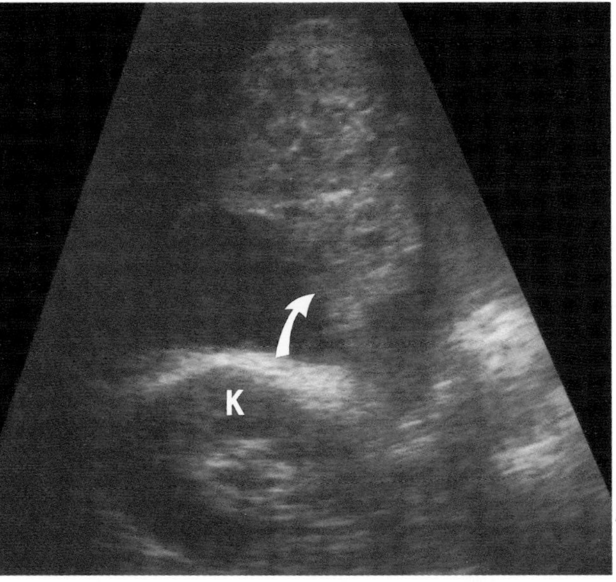

FIG. 2.78. Hemoperitoneum related to ruptured HCC. Longitudinal (**A**) sonogram reveals a HCC at the tip of the right lobe of the liver (*arrows*). K, right kidney. Two days later, the patient developed sudden hypotension and a falling hematocrit. Repeat longitudinal (**B**) and transverse (**C**) sonograms show fresh clot (*curved arrow*) originating from the HCC. The hemorrhage was stopped by therapeutic embolization. Rupture and hemorrhage, causing hemoperitoneum, are fairly common complications of peripheral HCCs.

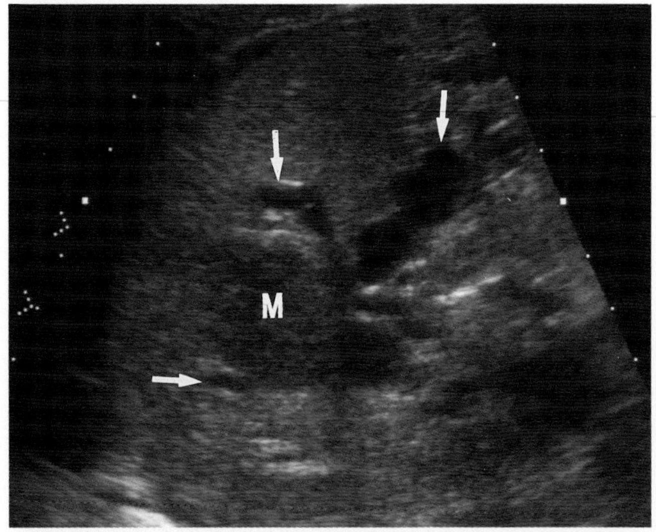

FIG. 2.79. Peripheral cholangiocarcinoma. Longitudinal oblique sonogram through the left lobe of the liver. There is a several centimeter hypoechoic mass (M) that is associated with bile duct obstruction (*arrows*). Peripheral cholangiocarcinoma not infrequently presents with relatively large masses such as this. Hilar cholangiocarcinoma is often more difficult to image than peripheral cholangiocarcinoma, as the patients present with biliary obstruction before a large mass has developed. Cholangiocarcinoma may be indistinguishable from other malignant lesions of the liver including HCC and metastasis (see Fig. 2.54).

A

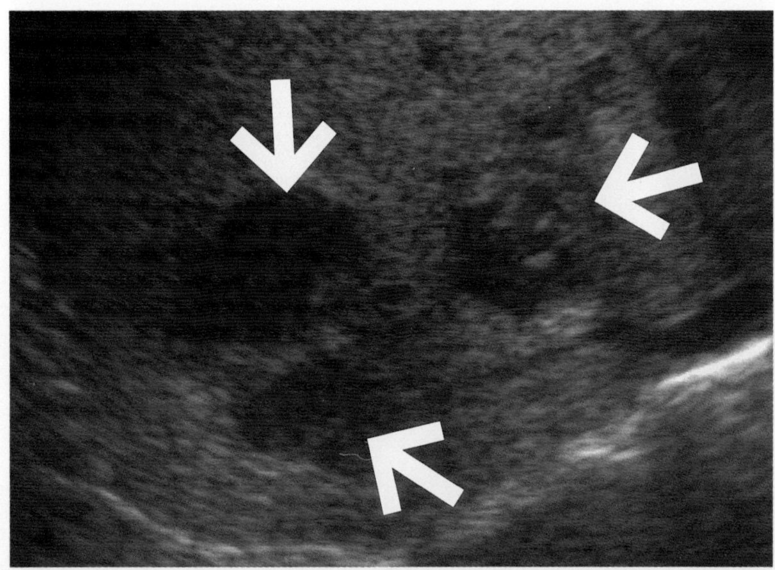

B

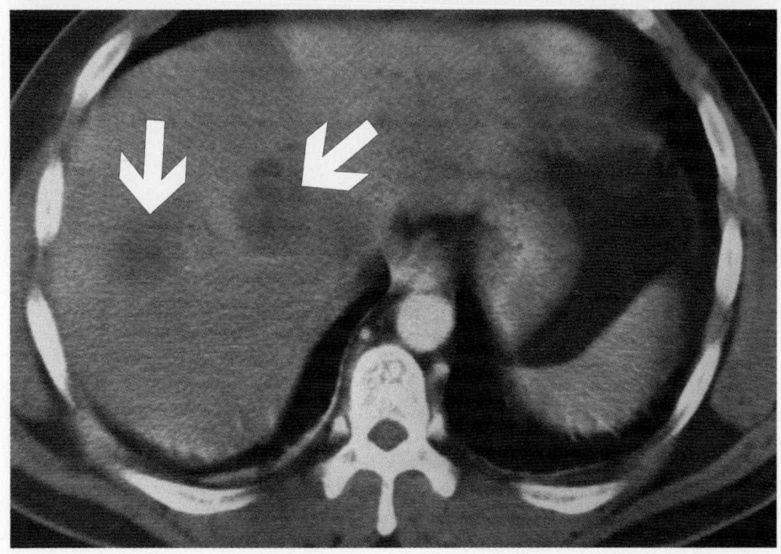

FIG. 2.80. Hepatic abscess, septic portal venous thrombosis (pylephlebitis). **A:** Transverse sonogram of the right lobe of the liver reveals several predominantly hypoechoic, ill-defined abscesses (*arrows*) that were related to septic thrombosis of the portal vein in a patient with bacterial gastroenteritis. **B:** The CT scan reveals the same abscesses (*arrows*). Septic venous portal thrombosis (pylephlebitis) usually results from ascending infection via the portal system, usually a bacterial gastrointestinal infection. Despite the associated venous thrombosis, no special anticoagulant therapy is necessary. Conventional antibiotic and percutaneous abscess drainage therapy suffices to cure these patients.

ten occurring in older or immunocompromised patients. Common predisposing conditions include cholecystitis, bile duct obstruction, gastrointestinal infections, trauma, and surgery. Septic portal venous thrombosis (pylephlebitis) may lead to liver abscess (Fig. 2.80) but usually resolves on standard therapy, without anticoagulation (Fig. 2.81) (60). *Escherichia coli* is the commonest pathogen, but aerobic and anaerobic organisms are both frequent. Approximately 50 percent of all pyogenic liver abscesses are polymicrobial. The clinical features of pyogenic liver abscess are variable and, surprisingly, symptoms are often mild and vague (6). Sonographically, pyogenic liver abscesses have a variable appearance (61). Typical features include irregular margins and a primarily hypoechoic mass (Figs. 2.82 and 2.83). Irregular areas of increased echogenicity are frequent (Fig. 2.84). On occasion, a diffusely hyperechoic appearance may be noted, related to microbubbles from gas-forming organisms (Fig. 2.85). Diffuse microabscesses, often associated with biliary obstruction, cause a confusing sonographic pattern of increased irregular hepatic echogenicity (Fig. 2.86). Clusters of small, low echogenicity lesions may also be noted (Fig. 2.87), usually caused by coliform bacteria (62). Chronic pyogenic abscess may sometimes occur (Fig. 2.88).

Percutaneous image-guided abscess drainage has replaced surgery as the primary treatment for pyogenic liver abscesses. Multiple loculations should not preclude percutaneous drainage, as virtually all abscesses that appear multiloculated can be successfully drained with one catheter (63). Antibiotics alone may be curative in smaller (<5 cm) abscesses.

Amebic liver abscess is the most common nonenteric complication of amebiasis. It is very common worldwide but uncommon in the United States. Amebic liver abscess generally prompts the patient to seek medical attention with acute symptoms of fever and right upper quadrant pain; it is a primary complaint. This is different from pyogenic liver abscesses, which often cause an indolent presentation and usually occur as a complication related to some other primary disease. Amebic liver abscess should be suspected when a patient in a high-risk population presents with image findings compatible with the diagnosis. High-risk populations include recent immigrants from endemic areas, patients living in poor sanitary conditions, and human immunodeficiency virus (HIV) positive patients.

Amebic liver abscesses tend to have a round or oval shape and hypoechoic appearance with fine, homogeneous, low-level echoes throughout (Figs. 2.89 to 2.91). These findings are somewhat unusual for pyogenic liver abscess. Nevertheless, image findings alone are rarely sufficient to distinguish amebic from pyogenic liver abscesses (Fig. 2.92); clinical and epidemiologic information is needed to differentiate them (64). Amebic liver abscess can have sonographic patterns that are bizarre, including diffuse increased echogenicity, debris levels, and prominent heterogeneity.

When it is unclear clinically if an abscess is amebic or pyogenic, percutaneous diagnostic aspiration should be performed (necessary in 15 percent of patients in our institution). In contrast to pyogenic liver abscesses, percutaneous drainage of amebic liver abscess is rarely indicated (65). Therapeutic aspiration provides no objective benefit when compared to the use of oral amebicidals alone (66).

Fungal microabscess may have a distinctive sonographic appearance. Candidiasis, occurring in HIV and other immunocomprised patients, causes multifocal hypoechoic lesions typically smaller than 2 cm (Figs. 2.93 and 2.94). Internal echogenic foci may produce a target or "wheel within a wheel" appearance (Fig. 2.95) (67,68). Echogenic lesions and lesions larger than 2 cm are much less common.

Tuberculosis, usually a miliary process that causes hepatic heterogeneity (69), can occasionally cause focal hypoechoic masses that may calcify (70,71). Echogenic calcified masses may also occur (72) (Fig. 2.96). On occasion, the liver is affected by other fungal infections (Fig. 2.97).

Focal Nodular Hyperplasia/Liver Cell Adenoma

Focal nodular hyperplasia (FNH) and liver cell adenoma (LCA) are rare benign liver tumors; both are more common in females. LCA is clearly associated with the use of oral contraceptives; FNH may be weakly associated (17,32). FNH is a clinically insignificant lesion. LCA can cause morbidity and mortality because of hemorrhage (Fig. 2.98) and, occasionally, malignant degeneration. At one time, the estimated annual incidence in long-term oral contraceptive users was 3 to 4 per 100,000 (17). Some believe current lower dose oral contraceptives may cause fewer adenomas. Other factors that predispose to liver cell adenoma include glycogen storage diseases, androgen administration, tyrosinemia, glacactosemia, diabetes, and cirrhosis (32). FNH is less well encapsulated pathologically than LCA. There are no proven cases in which FNH has become malignant.

The sonographic features of FNH and LCA are variable. There is a tendency for focal nodular hyperplasia to be more homogeneous than liver cell adenoma. FNH often has mildly increased echogenicity compared with normal parenchyma (Fig. 2.99), whereas LCAs are usually hypoechoic and more inhomogeneous (73–75). These patterns are variable (Fig. 2.100) and cannot be relied on to distinguish these lesions. FNH may exhibit a "central scar" (76), a nonspecific finding also seen in other hepatic lesions, both benign and malignant (49).

Distinction between FNH and LCA is sometimes possible with technetium sulfur colloid liver spleen scan-

(*text continues on page 133*)

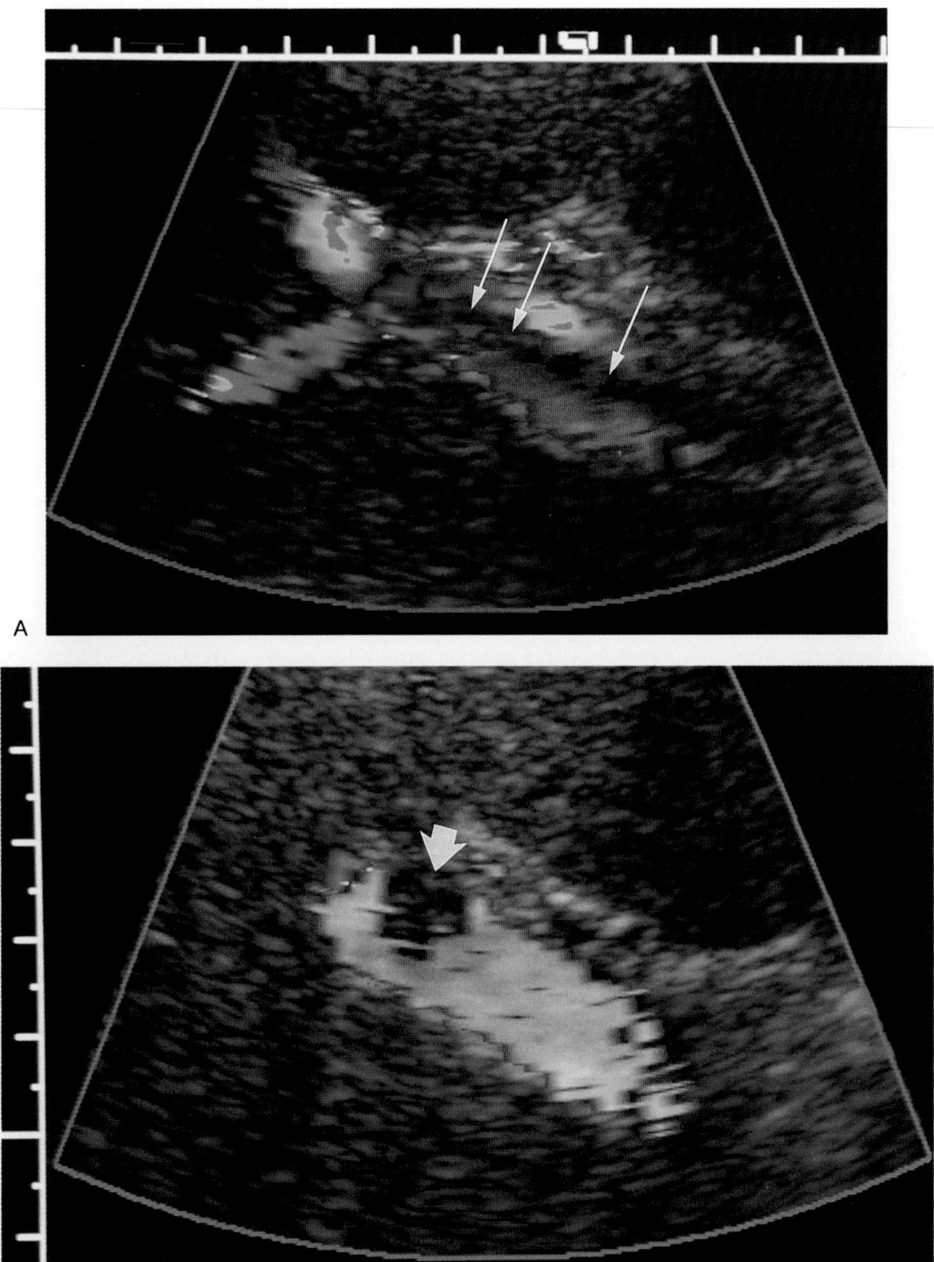

FIG. 2.81. Pylephlebitis, right portal vein. **A:** A transverse color Doppler sonogram of the right portal vein reveals clot (*thin arrows*) running down the middle of the partially thrombosed channel. This is septic portal venous thrombosis (pylephlebitis) in a patient with appendicitis. **B:** A follow-up color Doppler sonogram performed 9 days later shows almost total resolution of the thrombus. There is a small nodular residual clot (*arrow*). Follow-up study 2 weeks subsequent to this (not shown), revealed complete resolution. This patient developed a liver abscess (not shown), a frequent concomitant of septic portal venous thrombosis. Resolution of the clot related to pylephlebitis, as noted here, generally occurs without the use of anticoagulants. Antibiotics alone generally suffice for therapy.

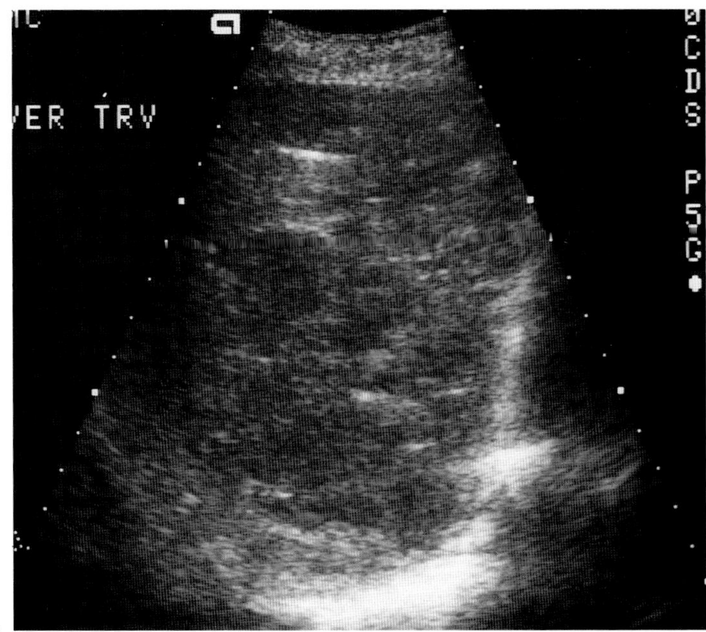

A

FIG. 2.82. Pyogenic liver abscess. **A:** Transverse sonogram through the right lobe of the liver shows a mottled, ill-defined, primarily hypoechoic liver abscess. Several small areas of increased echogenicity are noted (*arrows*). **B:** The CT scan shows a more well-defined lesion. Poor definition is typical for pyogenic liver abscesses on sonography. Often, CT reveals a better defined lesion.

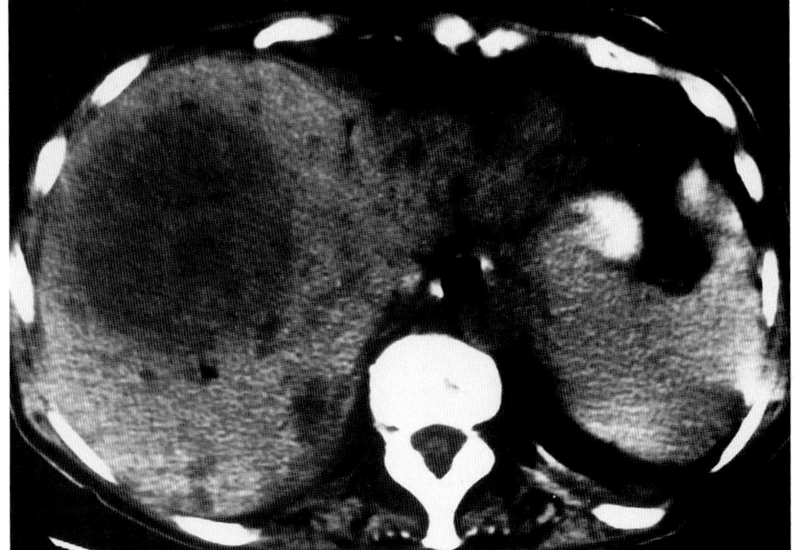

B

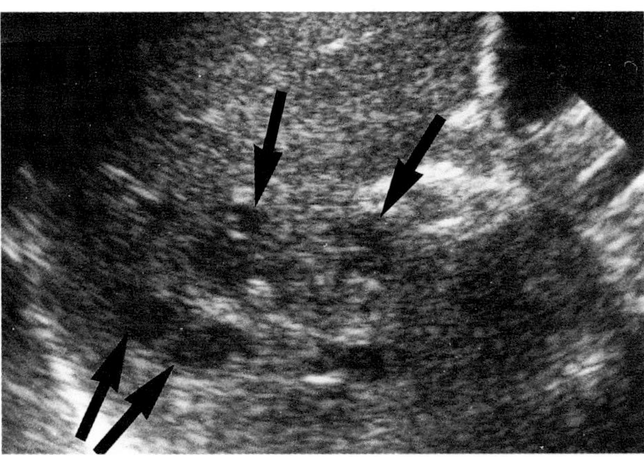

FIG. 2.83. Pyogenic liver abscess. Longitudinal sonogram through the right lobe of the liver. This ill-defined pyogenic liver abscess shows multiple focal low-echogenicity areas (*arrows*) within the poorly defined liver abscess. It is difficult or impossible to identify the border of this pyogenic liver abscess on sonography. Ill-defined margins are a typical sonographic finding for pyogenic liver abscess.

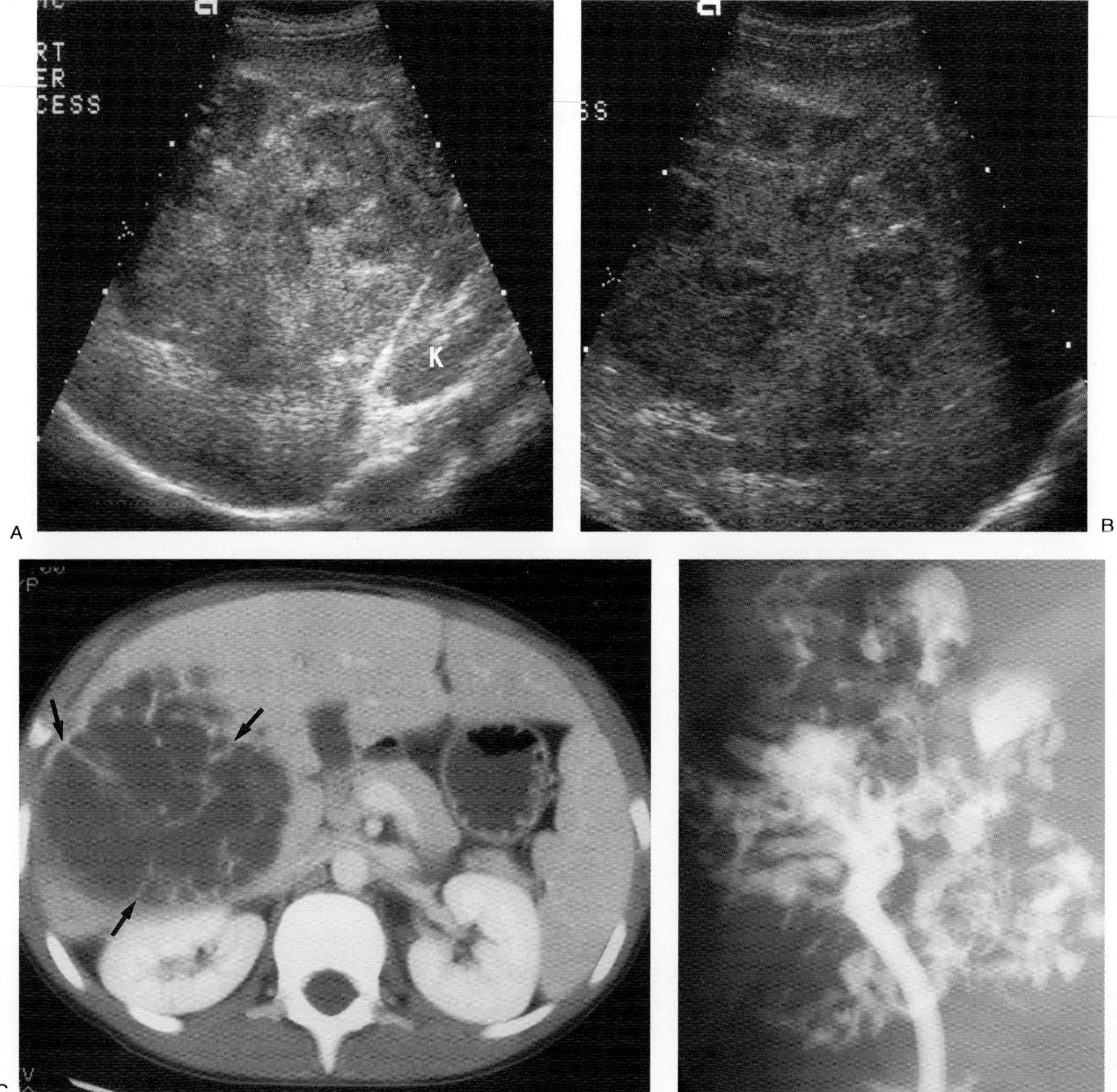

FIG. 2.84. Pyogenic liver abscess. **A:** Longitudinal sonogram shows a large, moderately well-deformed pyogenic liver abscess that has hypoechoic and hyperechoic internal characteristics. K, right kidney. **B:** The transverse sonogram of the right lobe reveals the heterogeneous lobulated architecture. **C:** CT scan shows the lobulated architecture and also multiple linear septa-like areas of higher attenuation (*arrows*). **D:** The abscessogram after percutaneous drainage reveals the multilocular nature of this abscess. Even multilocular abscesses can often be drained successfully with one catheter.

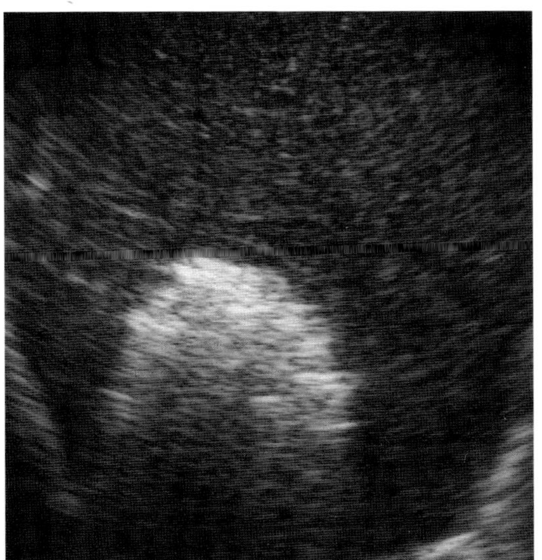

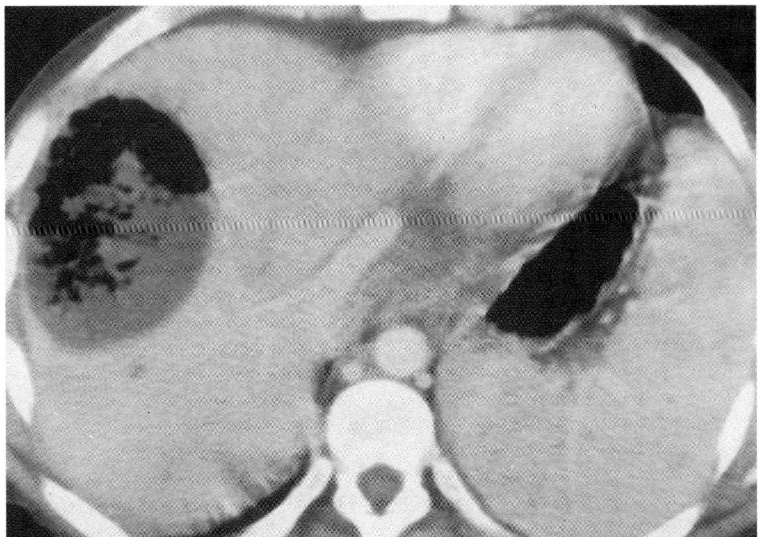

A B

FIG. 2.85. Gas-containing pyogenic liver abscess. **A:** Transverse sonogram through the right lobe of the liver. This abscess, which contains a large amount of gas that creates distal acoustic shadowing, was caused by gas-forming *E. coli* organisms. **B:** The CT scan shows the gas within the lesion.

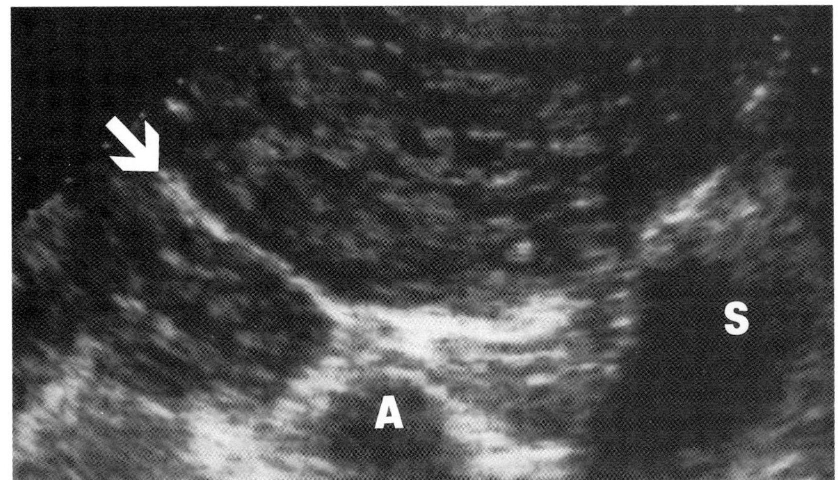

A

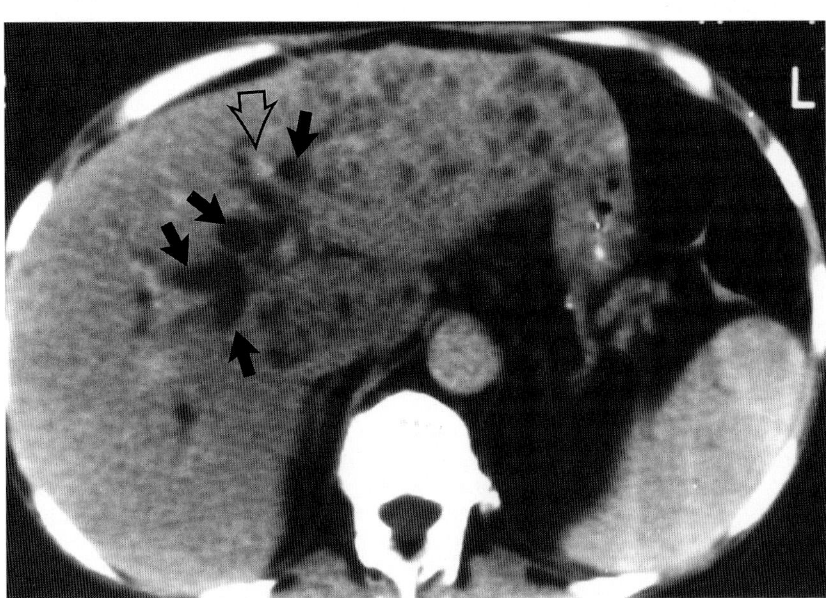

B

FIG. 2.86. "Cholangitic" liver abscess, confusing ultrasound pattern. **A:** Transverse sonogram through the left and caudate lobes of the liver shows multiple areas of increased and decreased echogenicity. These are multiple tiny microabscesses. This pattern may cause confusion with metastatic disease, especially as it is often related to malignant obstruction. Because of the association with biliary obstruction and infection, these microabscesses are often called "cholangitic" abscesses. Note the fissure for the ligamentum venosum (*arrow*) that separates the left and caudate lobes. A, aorta; S, stomach. **B:** The CT scan also reveals the multifocal low-attenuation areas throughout the caudate and left lobes. Note the dilated bile ducts (*black arrows*). *Open arrow,* left portal vein.

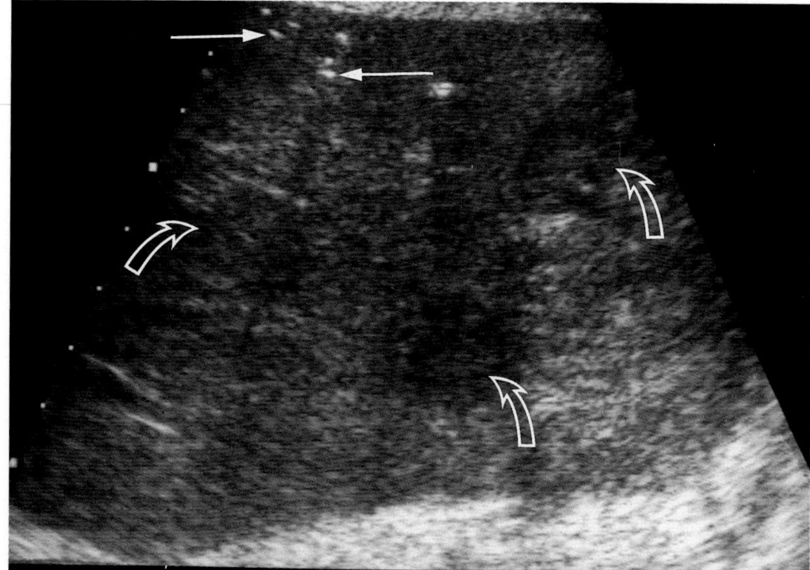
A

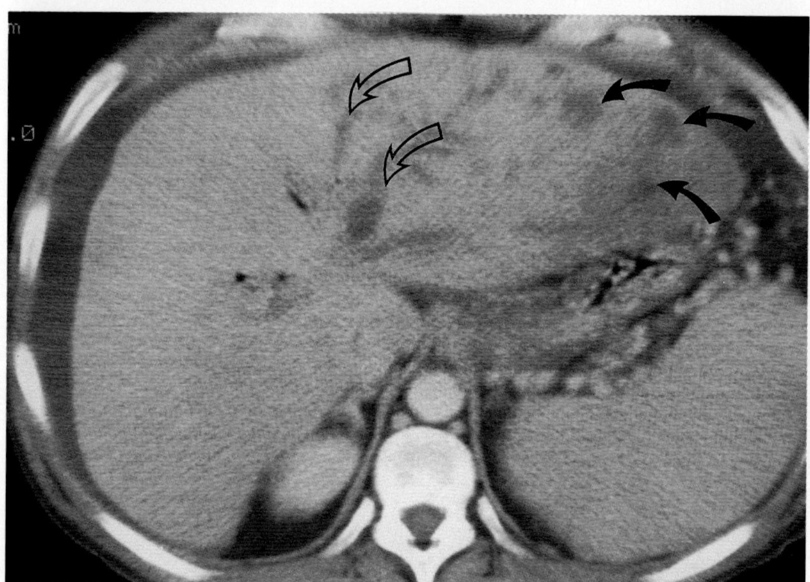
B

FIG. 2.87. "Cholangitic" abscesses, biliary obstruction. **A:** Transverse sonogram of left lobe of the liver. Multiple, subtle, very poorly defined, predominantly hypoechoic abscesses (*open curved arrows*) are present. Air in bile ducts is noted (*thin arrows*). **B:** The CT scan reveals the abscesses (*curved arrows*) as well as biliary dilatation (*open curved arrows*). Microabscesses proximal to a biliary obstruction are often called "cholangitic" abscesses. This patient had biliary obstruction caused by recurrent pancreatic carcinoma.

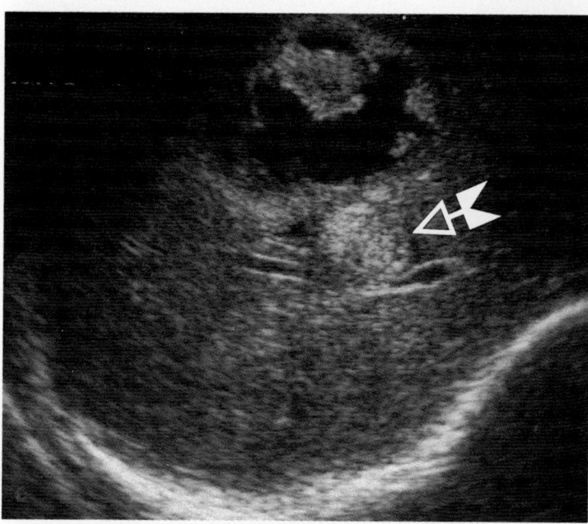

FIG. 2.88. Chronic pyogenic liver abscess, superinfected metastasis. Transverse sonogram through the right lobe of the liver reveals a fairly well-defined chronic pyogenic liver abscess in a patient with metastatic pancreatic carcinoma. Superinfected metastases such as this are difficult to treat. Percutaneous abscess drainage and antibiotics usually result in a reasonably good response. No malignant material was retrieved from this lesion. Note the focal hyperechoic metastasis (*tailed arrow*) dorsal to the chronic abscess.

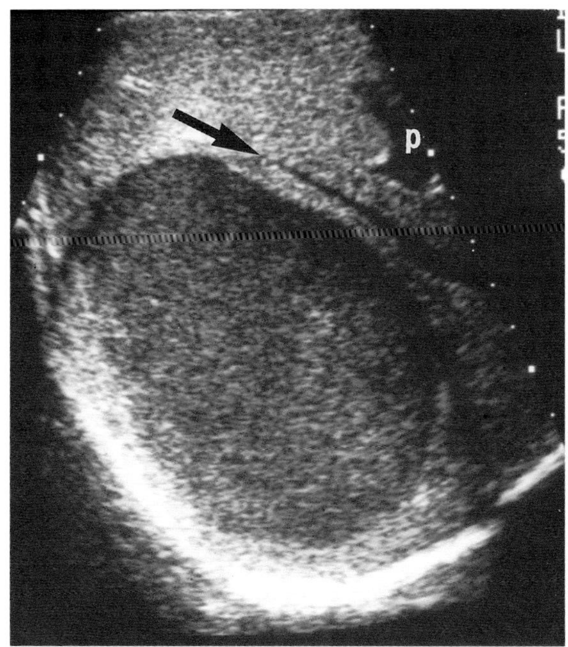

FIG. 2.89. Amebic liver abscess. Oblique transverse image through the right lobe of the liver. This large, 10 × 12 cm amebic abscess is well defined and predominantly hypoechoic throughout. This pattern is distinct from that present with most pyogenic liver abscesses, which are poorly defined and hetrogeneous. P, left portal vein; *arrow*, middle hepatic vein.

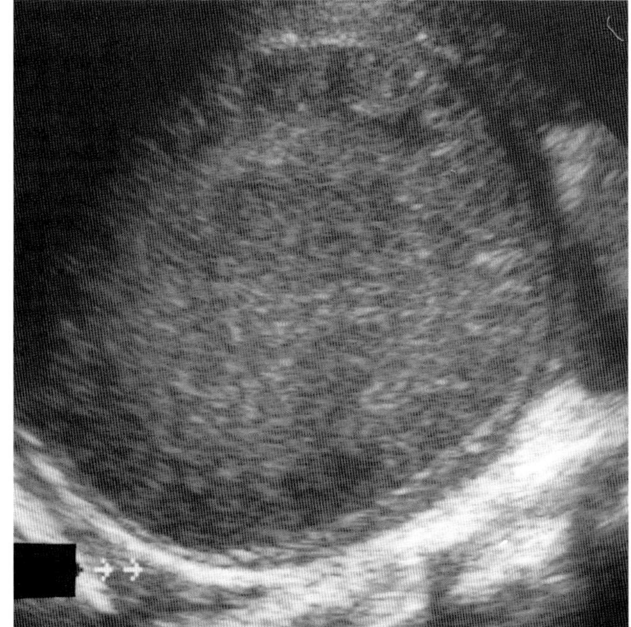

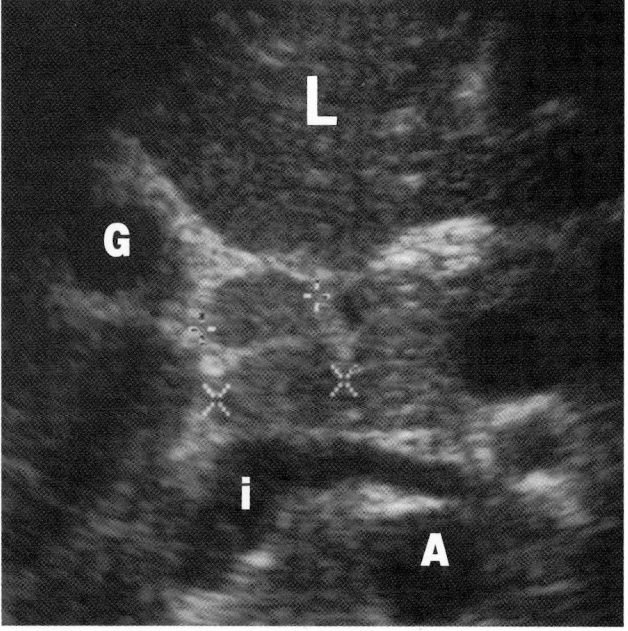

FIG. 2.90. Amebic liver abscess, pleural effusion, lymphadenopathy. **A:** Longitudinal oblique sonogram reveals a large amebic liver abscess with a palisaded peripheral zone. This lesion is hypoechoic compared to normal liver parenchyma but is internally inhomogeneous. Note the small sympathetic pleural effusion (*arrows*). **B:** A transverse sonogram through the porta hepatis reveals two slightly enlarged lymph nodes (calipers). Lymphadenopathy is unusual in patients with amebic liver abscess. L, liver; A, aorta; G, gallbladder; i, IVC.

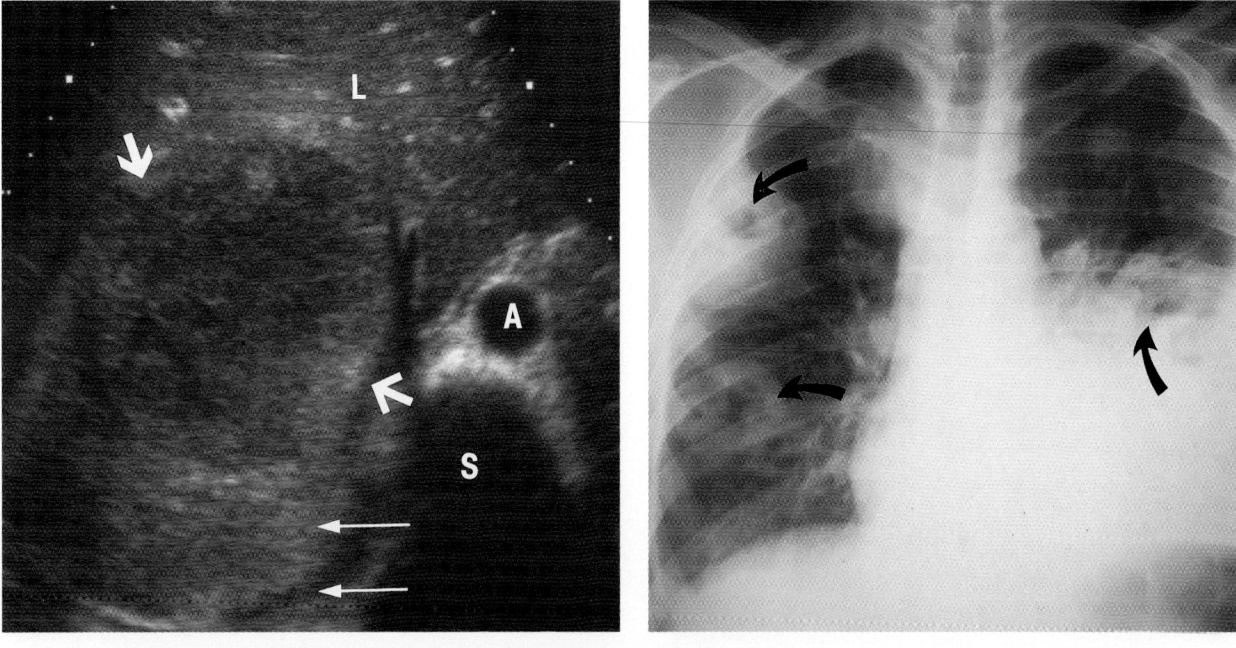

FIG. 2.91. Amebic liver abscess with metastatic pulmonary amebiasis. **A:** Transverse sonogram through the right lobe of the liver shows a somewhat atypical amebic liver abscess. There are some peripheral areas of isoechogenicity (*arrows*) in the predominantly hypoechoic lesion. Note the through transmission (*thin arrows*). L, liver; S, spine; A, aorta. **B:** The chest radiograph shows bilateral pleural disease and multiple pulmonary nodules, some of which are cavitating (*curved arrows*). Direct invasion through the diaphragm into the pleural space and lung is not unusual in patients with amebic liver abscess. Hematogeneous spread to the lungs, as present in this patient, is quite rare.

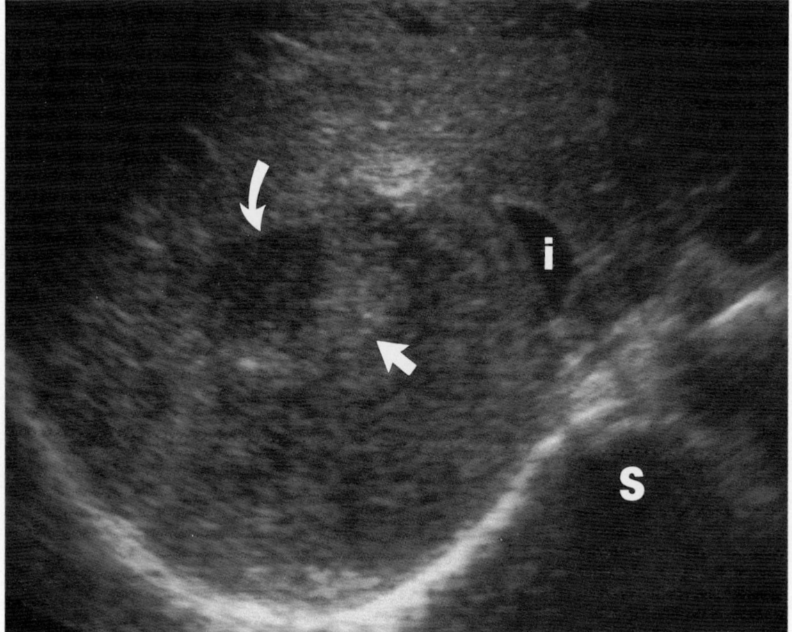

FIG. 2.92. Amebic liver abscess, atypical pattern. Transverse sonogram through the right lobe of the liver shows a very poorly defined amebic liver abscess. Note the medial displacement of the IVC (i) by the abscess. The mixed internal increased (*arrow*) and decreased (*curved arrow*) echogenicity, coupled with the poorly defined margins, are more typical of pyogenic than amebic liver abscess. S, spine.

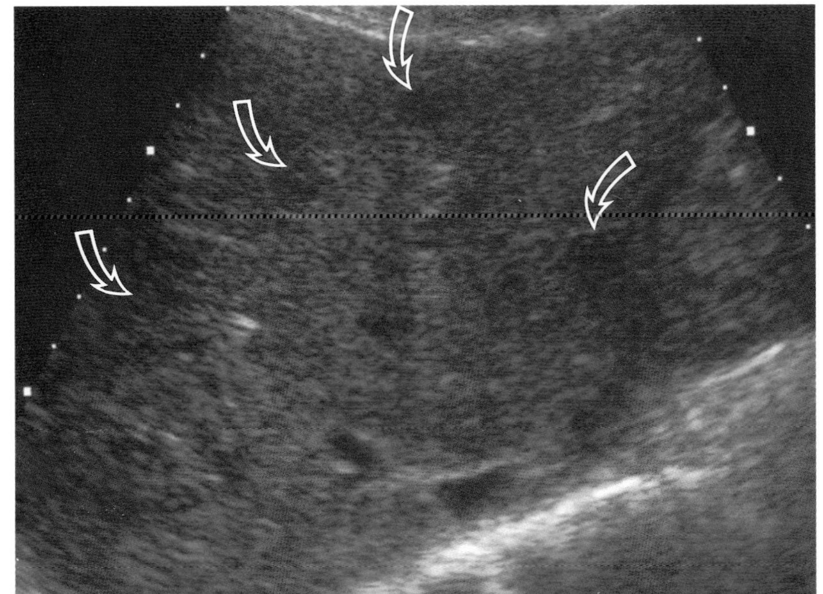

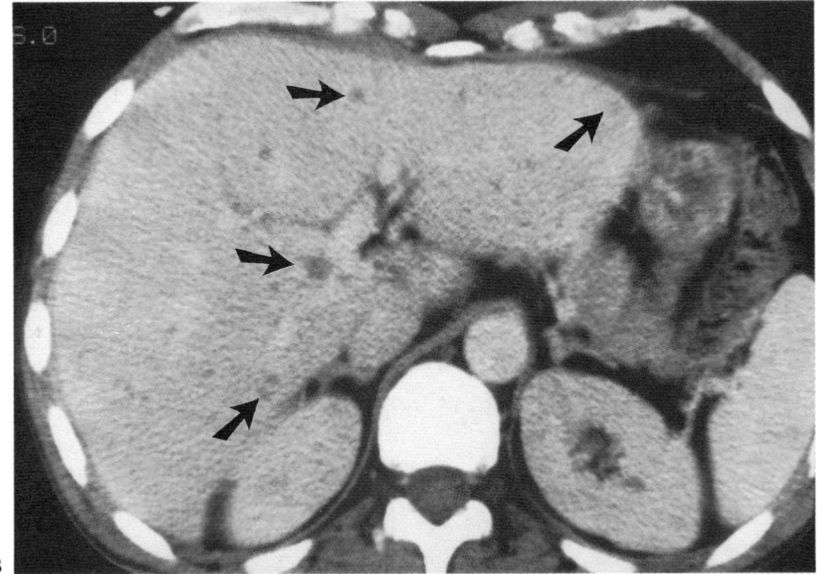

FIG. 2.93. *Candida* microabscesses. **A:** Transverse sonogram through the left lobe of the liver reveals multiple subtle, poorly defined, less than 1-cm microabscesses (*open curved arrows*). **B:** The CT scan, with its improved contrast resolution from intravenous contrast administration, shows the multiple small lesions (*slanted arrows*) more clearly. *Candida* microabscesses such as these may be subtle or even inapparent on sonograms. These microabscesses usually occur in patients who have a lymphoproliferative disorder or are otherwise immunocompromised. This is a patient with acute myelogenous leukemia.

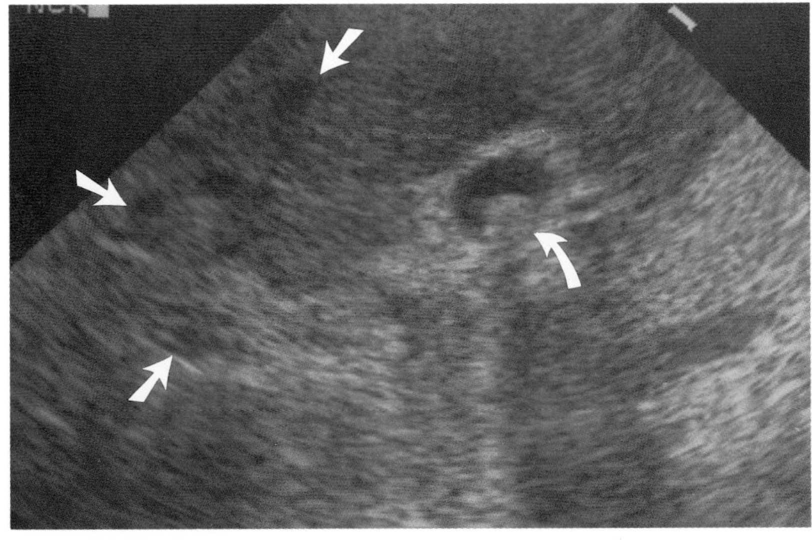

FIG. 2.94. *Candida* microabscesses. This transverse sonogram shows multiple small hypoechoic *Candida* microabscesses that measure less than 1 cm in size (some indicated by *slant tail arrows*). Note the gallstone (*curved arrow*).

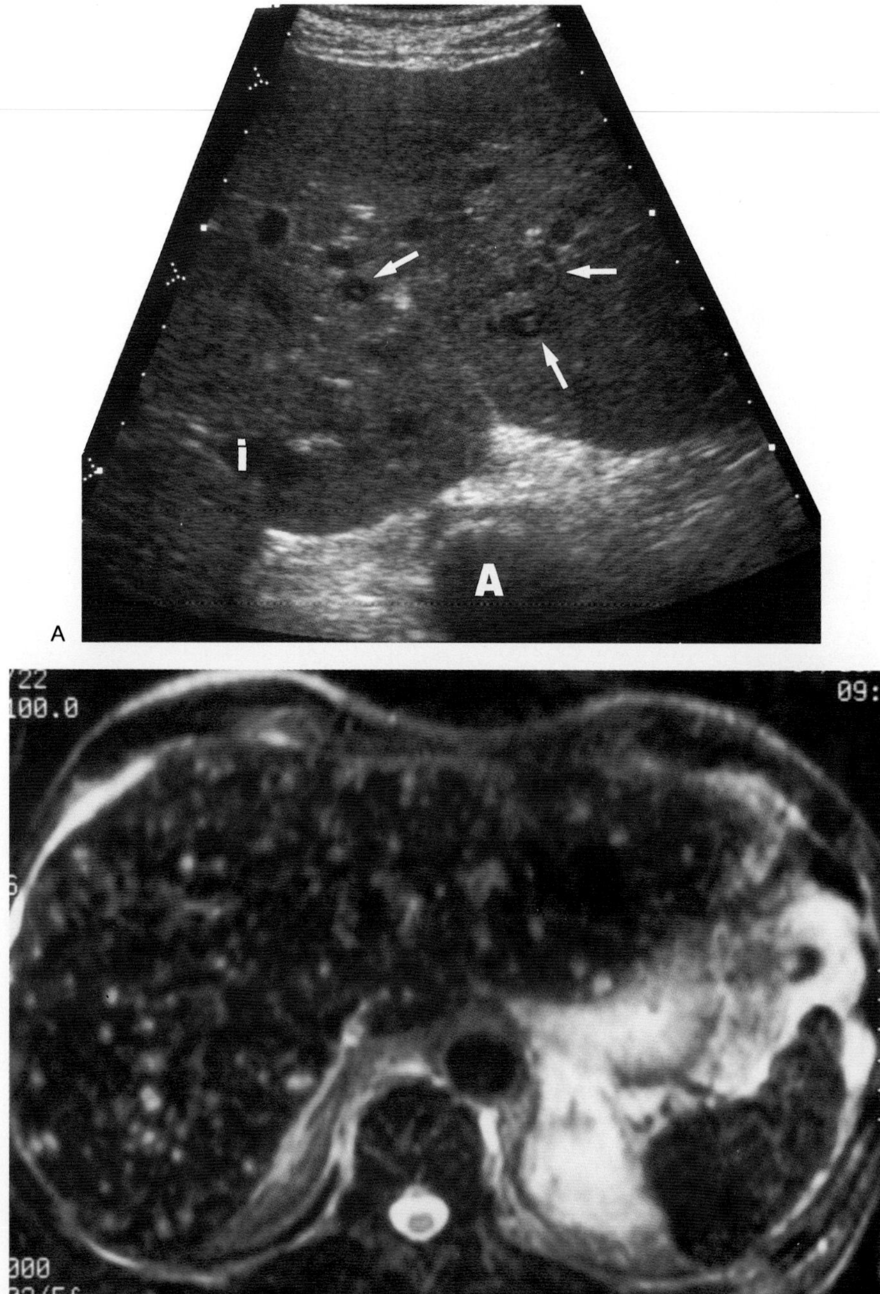

FIG. 2.95. Hepatic candidiasis, "Wheel within wheel" pattern. **A:** Transverse sonogram through the left and caudate lobes of the liver reveals multiple small *Candida* abscesses with central hyperchoic areas (some indicated by *thin arrows*). While this "wheel within wheel" pattern is considered classic, it is not universally present (see Figs. 2.89 and 2.90). **B:** On the T2-weighted MRI, the abscesses appear as small white areas of increased signal intensity. A, aorta; i, IVC.

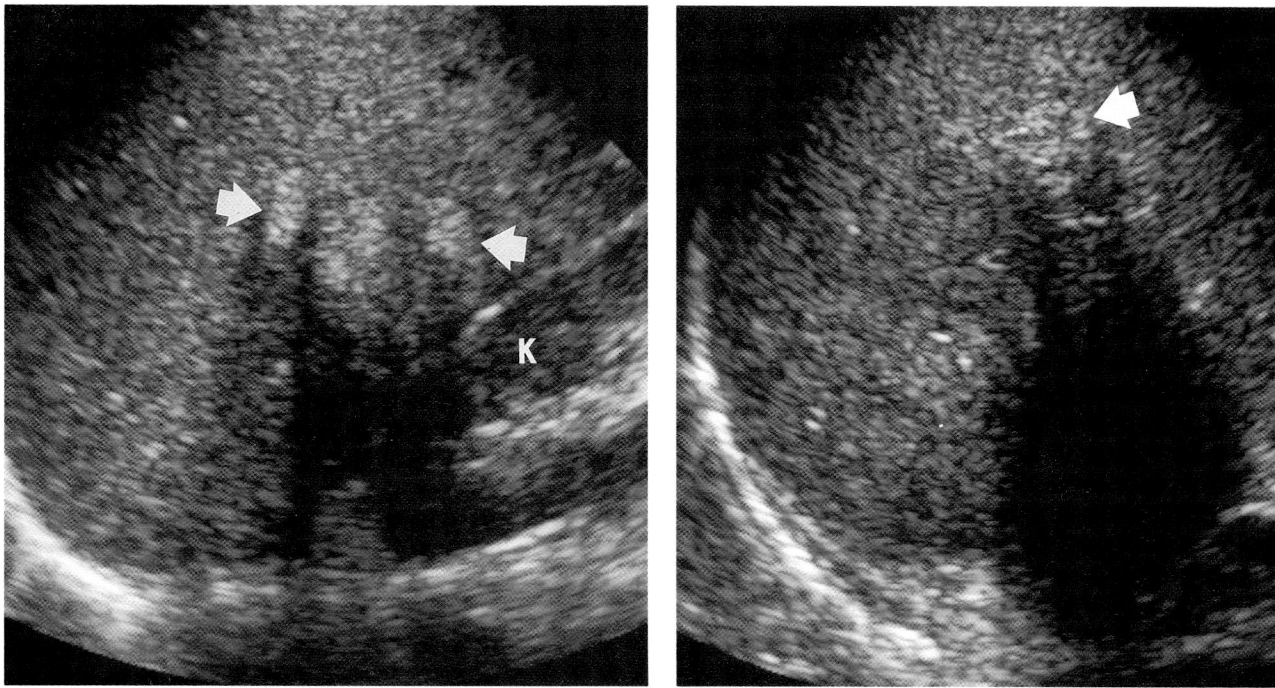

FIG. 2.96. Chronic hepatic tuberculosis. **A:** Longitudinal sonogram through the right lobe of the liver reveals dense echogenic calcifications (*arrows*) that engender shadowing. **B:** A transverse sonogram shows similar findings. Dense calcified masses like this, while not diagnostic, suggest chronic hepatic hepatobiliary tuberculosis in patients with longstanding tuberculosis. K, right kidney.

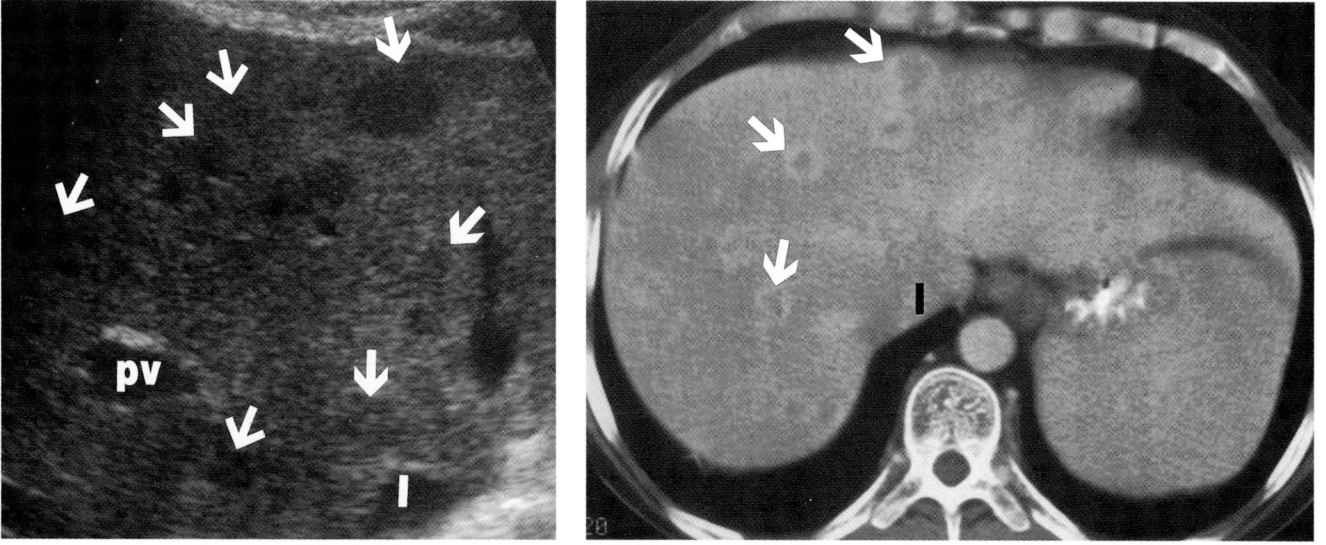

FIG. 2.97. Hepatic aspergillosis. **A:** The transverse sonogram of the junction of the left and right lobes of the liver reveals multiple hypoechoic abscesses (*arrows*) caused by aspergillosis. **B:** The CT scan revealed pronounced rim-enhancing lesions that were slightly decreased in attenuation centrally (*arrows*). I, inferior vena cava; PV, right portal vein.

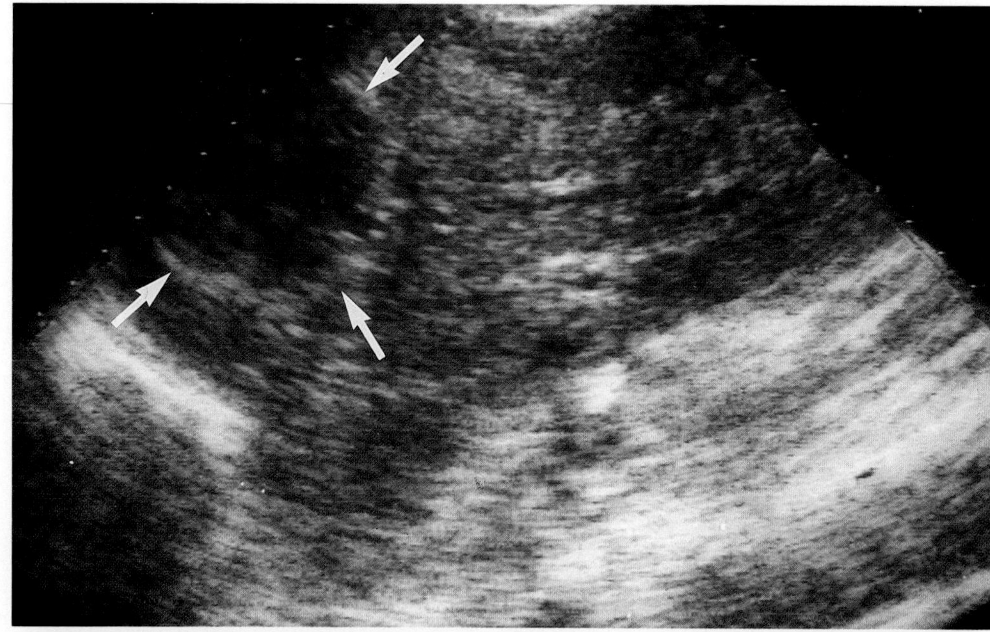
A

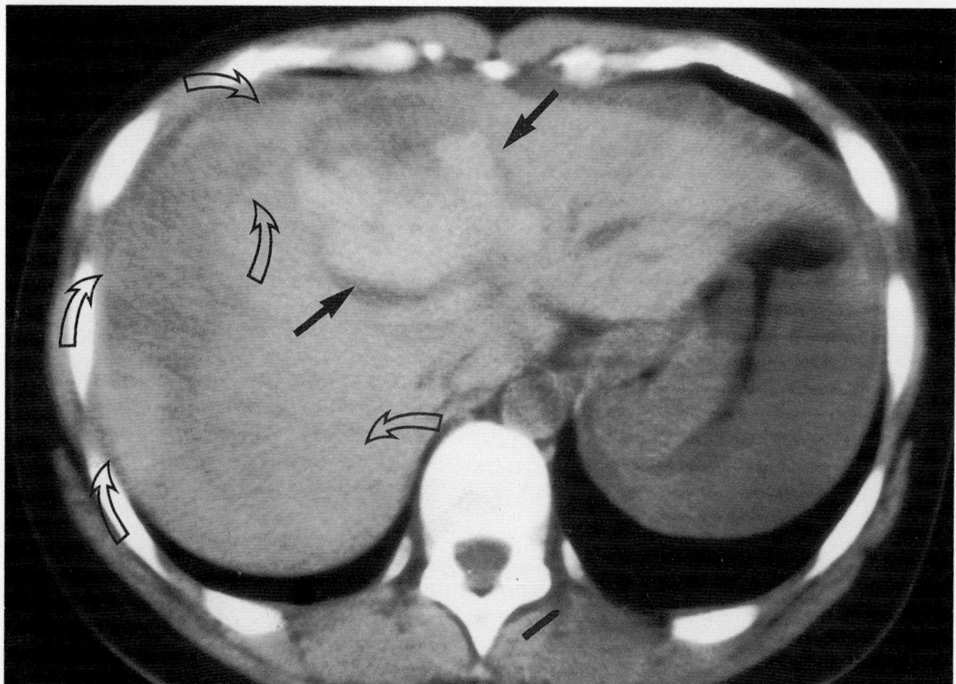
B

FIG. 2.98. Hemorrhage from a liver cell adenoma. **A:** Longitudinal sonogram reveals a hypoechoic liver lesion that proved to be a liver cell adenoma (*arrows*). The parenchymal inhomogeneity surrounding the lesion was caused by intraparenchymal hemorrhage. **B:** The CT scan shows fresh intralesional hemorrhage (*arrows*) more clearly, as areas of high attenuation. An older hematoma is noted laterally as a region of mixed attenuation (*curved open arrows*). Liver cell adenoma, although a rare lesion, is clinically significant because life-threatening hemorrhage can occur. Rarely, a malignant lesion can arise in an adenoma.

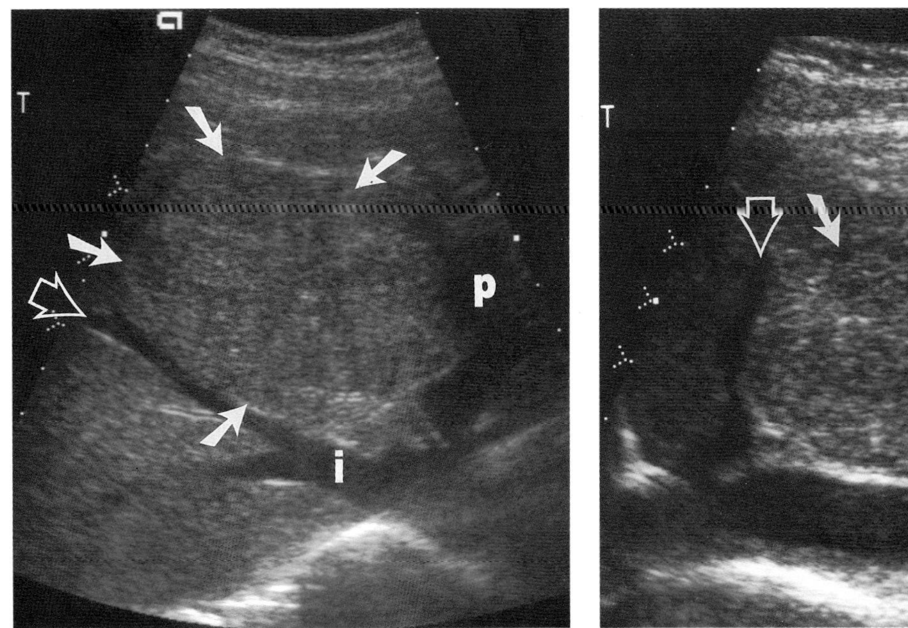

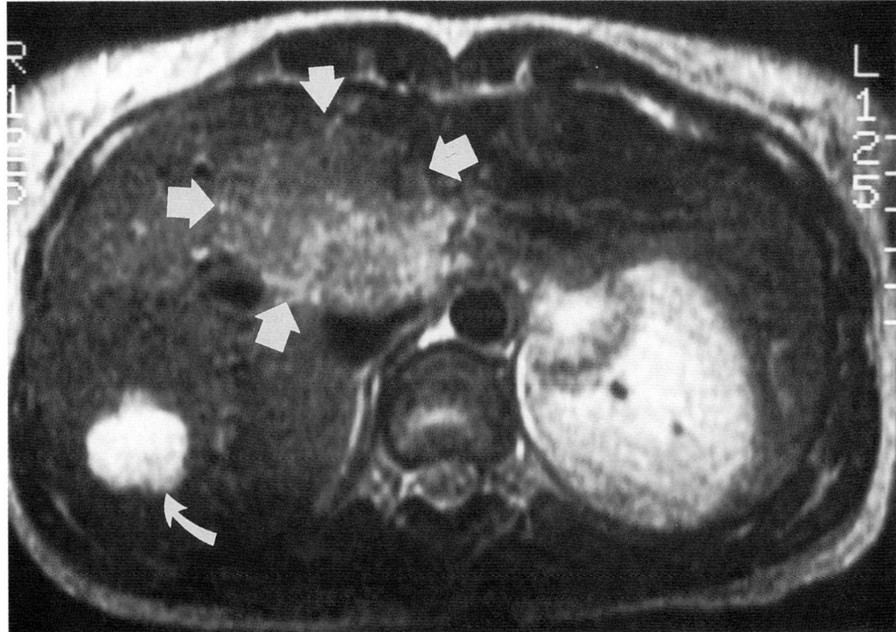

FIG. 2.99. Focal nodular hyperplasia. The transverse (**A**) and longitudinal (**B**) sonograms reveal this 6-cm FNH lesion (*slant tailed arrows*) as slightly increased in echogenicity compared to normal hepatic parenchyma. The main reason the lesion is detectable is the mass effect it produces; it displaces hepatic (*open arrow*) and portal veins (P). The lesion (*arrows*) is subtle on the T2-weighted MRI (**C**). Note the high signal intensity hemangioma (*curved arrow*). FNH is often subtle on images because it consists of cells very much like normal hepatocytes. i, inferior vena cava.

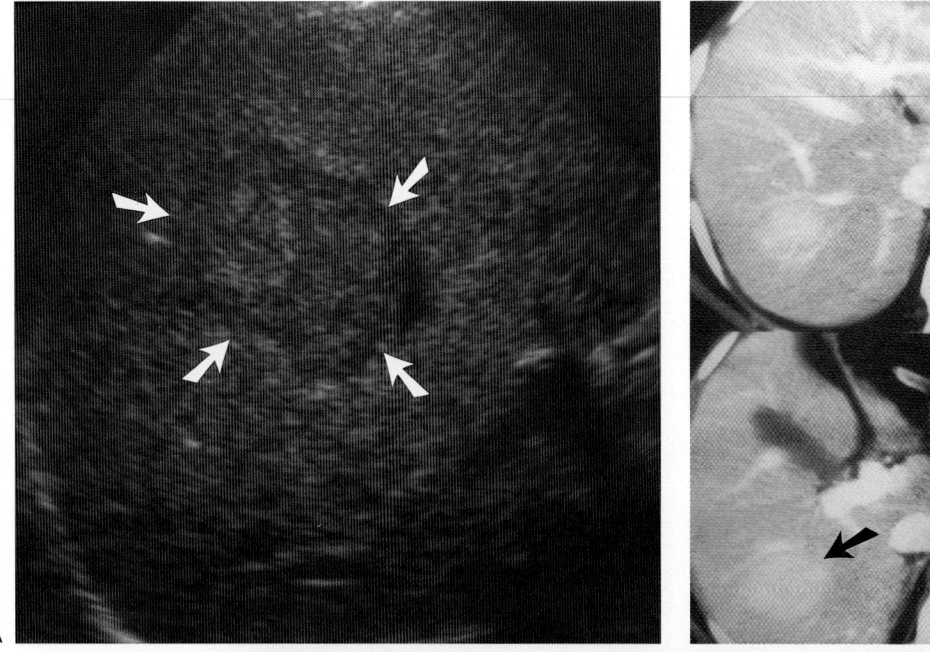
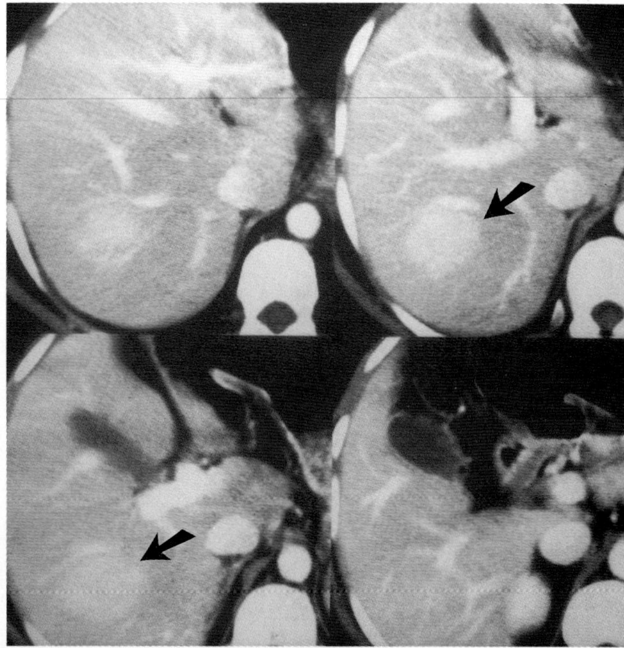
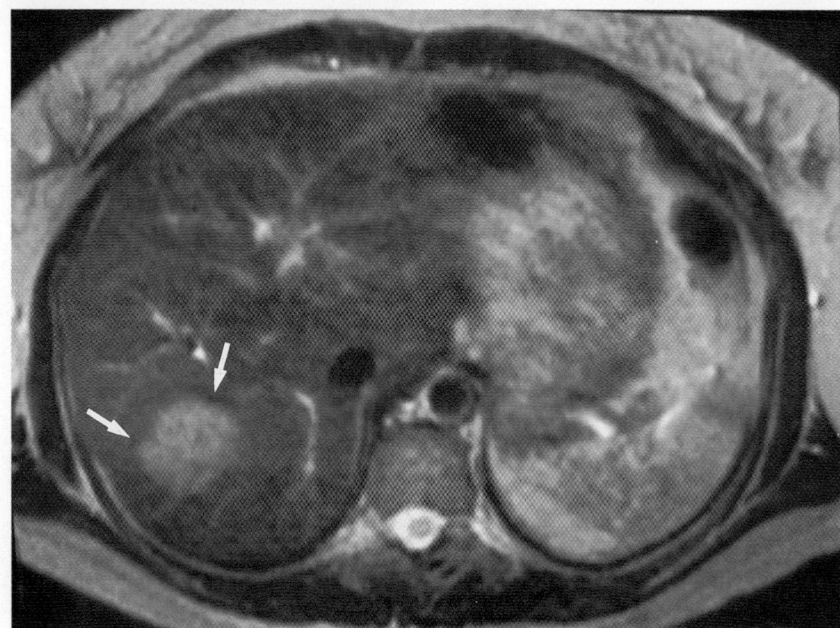

FIG. 2.100. Focal nodular hyperplasia. **A:** Transverse sonogram through the right lobe of the liver reveals an essentially isoechoic mass that is visible mainly because of its hypoechoic rim (*arrows*). **B:** A collage from a dynamic contrast-enhanced CT scan reveals a hyperdense lesion (*arrow*). **C:** The T2-weighted MRI reveals a slightly increased signal intensity lesion with a subtle lower signal intensity rim (*small arrows*). Findings on images are rarely sufficient to differentiate FNH from hepatic adenoma. For that matter, differentiation from other focal lesions is also impossible, based on the images alone. History and laboratory data suggestive of a benign lesion help limit the differential diagnosis.

ning. FNH can be confidently diagnosed when the liver exhibits normal or increased uptake (73) (Fig. 2.101). On color flow imaging, FNH usually has markedly increased flow (Fig. 2.101). This hypervascularity, related to hepatic AV fistulas, may also cause enlarged hepatic arteries and veins (Fig. 2.101). FNH may have a color flow pattern of vessels radiating peripherally from a central feeding artery, similar to conventional arteriographic findings in FNH (Fig. 2.102). Color flow sonographic findings in LCA have not been described.

Other Focal Liver Lesions

Hepatic lymphoma and leukemia are usually microscopic and only occasionally cause sonographically detectable focal liver lesions. Although autopsy series reveal liver involvement in more than half of Hodgkin's and lymphoma patients, only about 5 percent have identifiable abnormalities (77), probably because involvement is usually infiltrative or micronodular. When present, anechoic or hypoechoic lesions are the rule (Figs. 2.103 and 2.104), but lesions with increased echogenicity (77), target lesions, and large confluent geographic hypoechoic masses also occur (78,79). HIV related B-cell lymphomas cause more frequent and conspicuous focal lesions than other lymphomas (Fig. 2.105).

Chloroma of the liver, a focal lesion caused by myelogenous leukemia, has been described in a case report (80) as hypoechoic with a central echogenic spot. We have noted a single patient with four well-defined echogenic chloromas, which simulated hemangioma (Fig. 2.106).

Adenomatous hyperplastic nodules (AHNs) in cirrhotic livers (regenerating nodules) are premalignant lesions that are rarely visible with sonography because of their small size and composition similar to normal liver (Fig. 2.63) (81–83). Recently, more frequent detection of AHNs has been reported (81). AHNs, which are typically hypoechoic and have a thin echogenic rim (81,82), may be difficult to distinguish from small HCCs.

Hepatic sarcomas are rare. Angiosarcomas related to thorotrast or vinyl chloride are more frequent in males (17). Undifferentiated embryonal sarcoma is usually a large, internally inhomogeneous mass (84) (Fig. 2.107). Hepatobiliary embryonal rhabdomyosarcoma (sarcoma botryoides) is a rare sarcoma that involves both the liver and bile ducts. It often has grape-like protuberances into the ducts (Fig. 2.108).

Hepatic epithelioid hemangioendothelioma (EHE) is a rare vascular tumor, sometimes classified as a sarcoma, that has a variable but often protracted clinical course (85,86). Sonographically, EHE may be nodular or confluent. It tends to be hypoechoic compared to normal liver. Hypertrophy of the spared normal liver may occur.

Hepatoblastoma is the commonest symptomatic liver tumor in children less than 5 years old. Sonographically, these masses are usually inhomogeneous, mainly hyperechoic lesions that may have hypoechoic or anechoic areas; calcification may be noted (87).

Intrahepatic extramedullary hematopoiesis may cause inhomogeneous, mainly hypoechoic masses (88,89). Mesenchymal hamartoma of the liver is usually a large, mainly cystic mass with septa of variable thickness and solid internal components (90,91). Infantile hepatic hemangioma is usually single, predominantly hypoechoic, and solid (92).

Intrahepatic hematomas may cause sonographically visible masses. While trauma causes most hematomas (Fig. 2.109), spontaneous hematomas may occur (Fig. 2.110).

HIV Infection

Infection with the human immunodeficiency virus (HIV) causes a spectrum of disease, part of which is the rather arbitrarily defined acquired immunodeficiency syndrome (AIDS). The liver is often involved by neoplasm (non-Hodgkin's lymphoma, Kaposi's sarcoma [KS]) or by opportunistic infection (e.g., mycobacterial, amebic, fungal). Sonographic findings of uncertain cause, such as decreased periportal echogenicity, may occur.

High and intermediate grade HIV-related B-cell lymphomas often cause focal, usually hypoechoic masses (Fig. 2.105) that may exhibit increased peripheral color flow (Fig. 2.111). Hodgkin's lymphoma, while not an HIV-related lymphoma, may also present with advanced disease and focal parenchymal lesions. These findings are distinct from other lymphomas that only occasionally cause focal abnormalities. Kaposi's sarcoma usually infiltrates the liver, causing little or no sonographic abnormality. Focal hypoechoic (Fig. 2.112) or mixed echogenicity (Fig. 2.113) masses occur occasionally. Increased periportal echogenicity may be noted (93,94) (Fig. 2.114).

Successful suppression of clinical *Pneumocystis carinii* pneumonia (PCP) by aerosolized pentamidine has improved survival in HIV patients. Disseminated *Pneumocystis carinii* infection (DPC), which appears to have little clinical significance, may result in striking abnormality in the liver, as well as in lymph nodes and other parenchymal organs. Multiple microcalcifications, often imaged much more clearly sonographically than with CT, may give a "starry sky" pattern (Fig. 2.115) (95,96). While suggestive of DPC, this pattern may also occur with either mycobacterial (Fig. 2.116) or cytomegalovirus (CMV) infection (97). On occasion, larger calcifications or hypoechoic lesions may occur.

HIV-infected patients are at higher risk for other opportunistic infections, especially *Candida albicans,* which usually causes small hypoechoic lesions, often

(*text continues on page 143*)

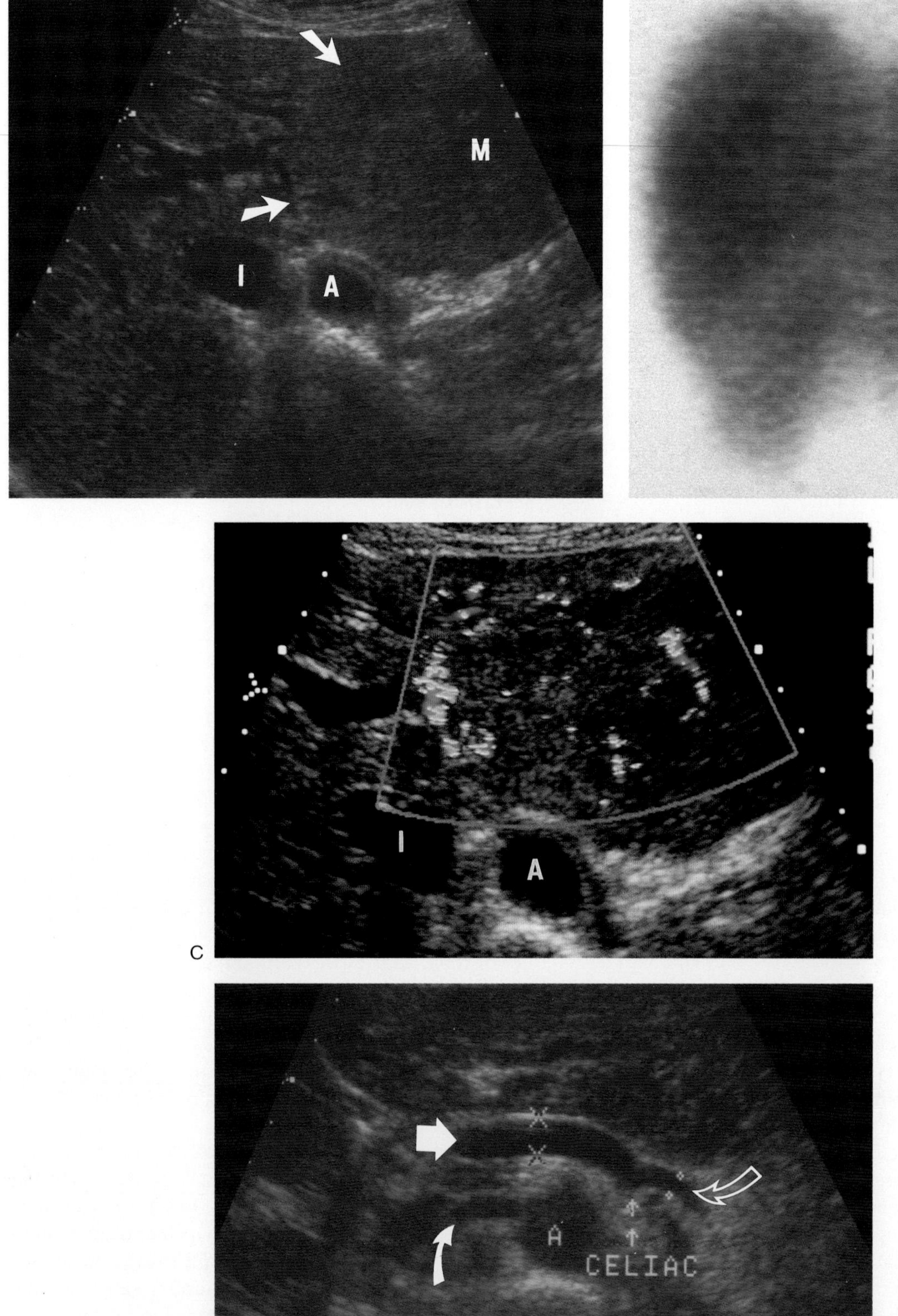

FIG. 2.101. Focal nodular hyperplasia. **A:** A transverse sonogram through the liver reveals an essentially isoechoic FNH mass (M, *arrows*) in the left lobe that is detectable mainly because of the mass effect it causes. **B:** A technetium sulfur colloid liver spleen scan reveals mottled uptake (*arrow*), rather than a cold defect. This radionuclide uptake strongly suggests the diagnosis of FNH. **C:** A transverse color Doppler sonogram of the left lobe shows marked hypervascularity compared to the normal liver. **D:** A transverse sonogram through the celiac axis reveals an enlarged common hepatic artery (*arrow*). The hepatic artery is enlarged because of the increased arterial flow to the FNH lesion. Contrast the enlarged common hepatic artery with the normal size splenic (*curved open arrow*) and right renal (*curved arrow*) arteries.

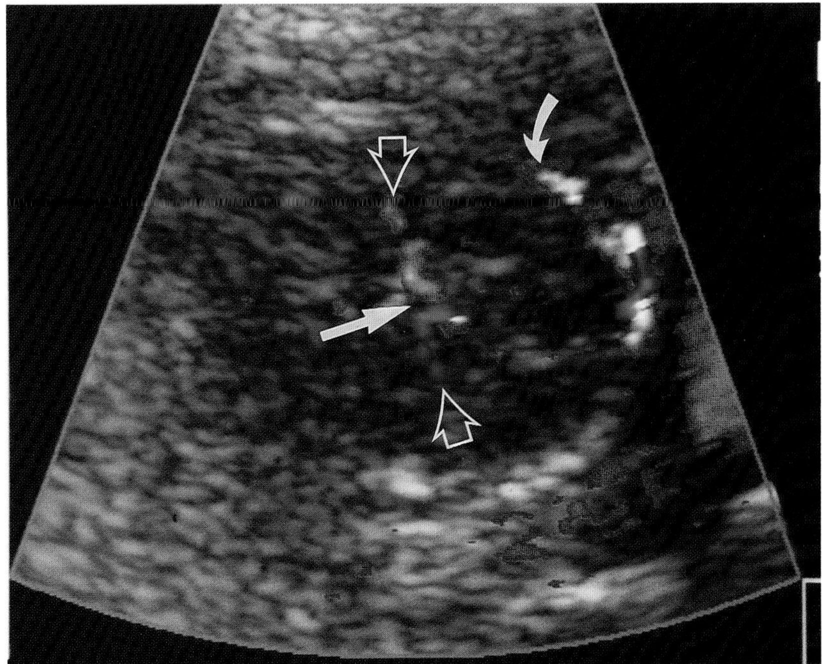

FIG. 2.102. Focal nodular hyperplasia. This 3-cm FNH lesion demonstrates radial flow from a central vessel (*arrow*) out toward the periphery of the lesion (*open arrow*). Flow along the margin of the FNH lesion is also present (*curved arrow*).

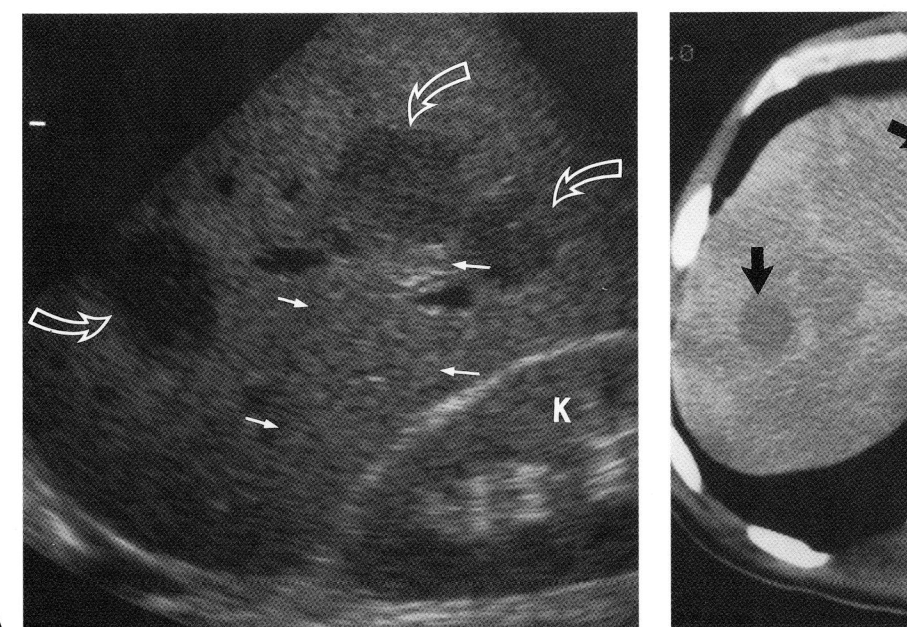

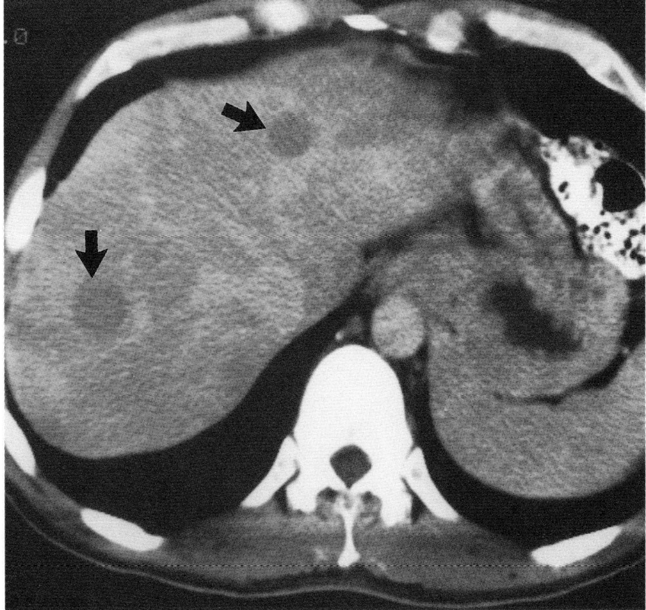

FIG. 2.103. Focal hepatic non-Hodgkin's lymphoma. **A:** Longitudinal sonogram through the right lobe of the liver reveals three primarily hypoechoic, well-defined lesions (*open curved arrows*). Minimal through transmission (*thin arrows*) is noted deep to one lesion. **B:** The CT scan also reveals relatively low-attenuation lesions (*arrows*). Hypoechoic lesions with varying levels of internal echogenicity are typical for both Hodgkin's and non-Hodgkin's lymphoma. On occasion, anechoic lesions that simulate cysts can be present. K, right kidney.

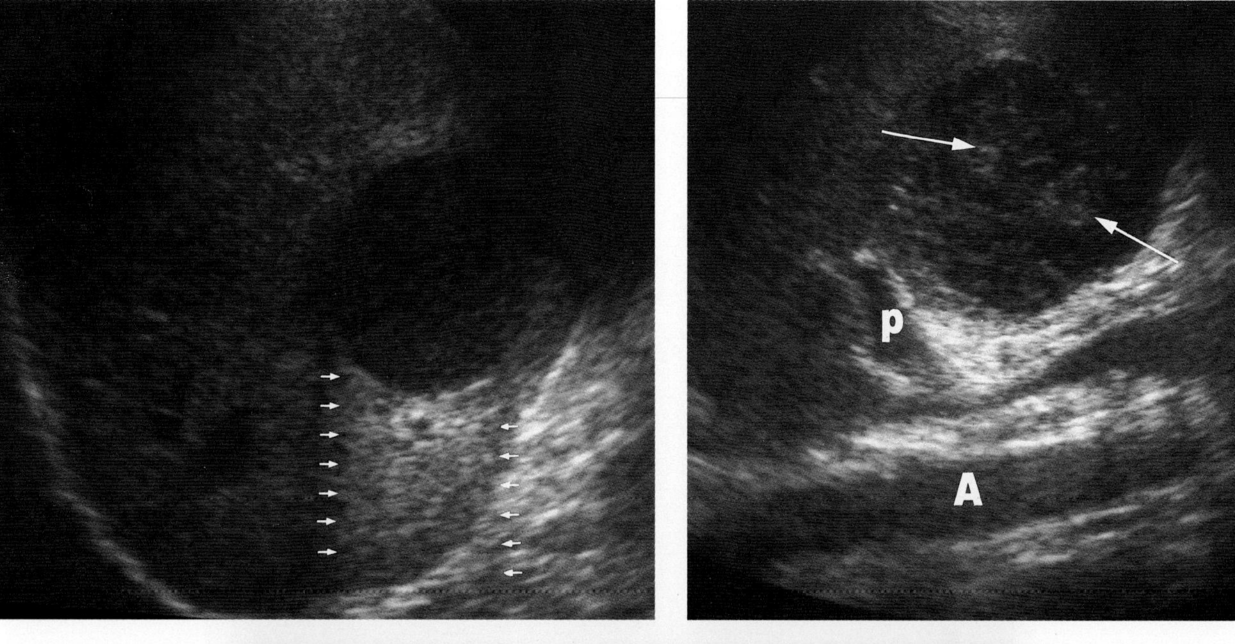

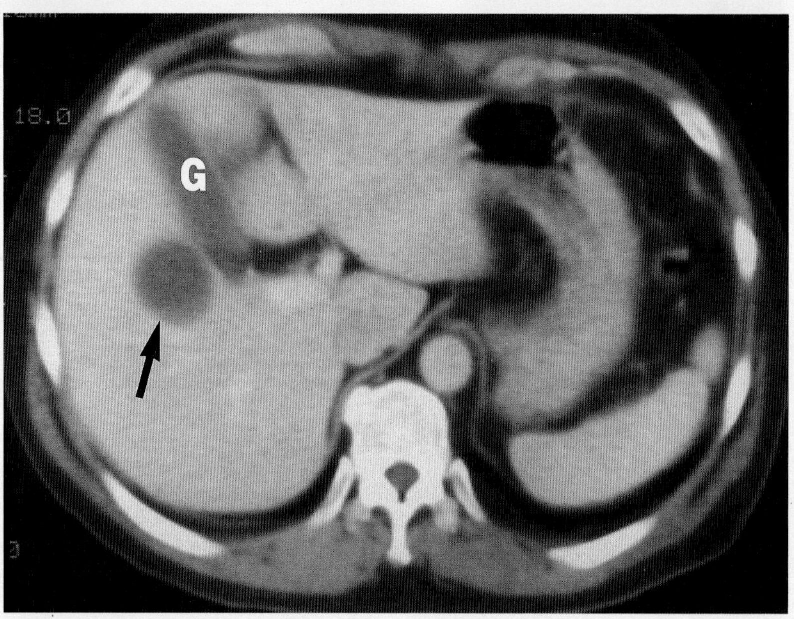

FIG. 2.104. Focal hepatic Hodgkin's lymphoma. **A:** Transverse oblique sonogram through the right lobe of the liver reveals a well-defined hypoechoic lesion with prominent through transmission (*tiny arrows*). **B:** Another focal lesion with mixed echogenicity is noted on a longitudinal sonogram through the left lobe of the liver. This lesion has some areas of increased echogenicity (*thin arrows*). **C:** A contrast-enhanced CT scan demonstrates the well-defined right lobe lesion (*arrow*). G, gallbladder. Focal hepatic lesions are unusual in Hodgkin's and non-Hodgkin's lymphoma. They are present in only about one-tenth of all patients with lymphomatous involvement of the liver. A, aorta; p, left portal vein.

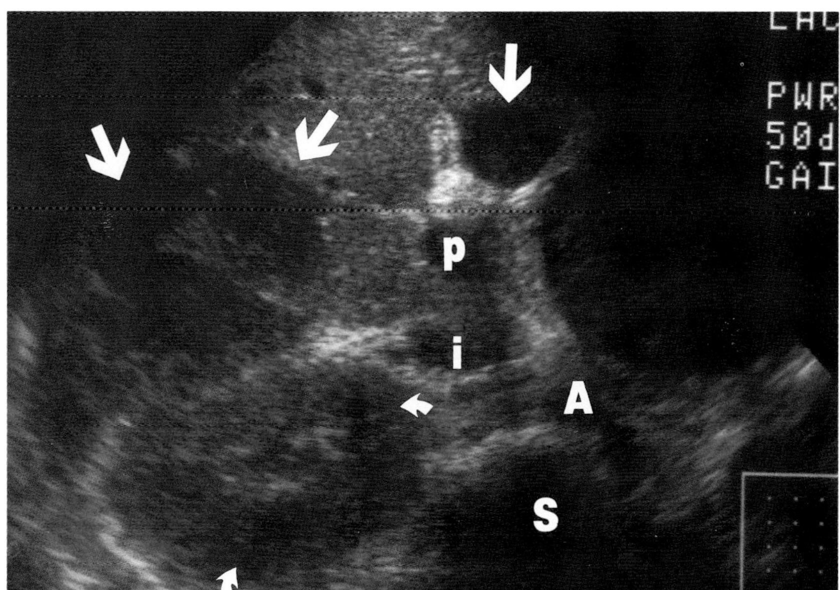

A

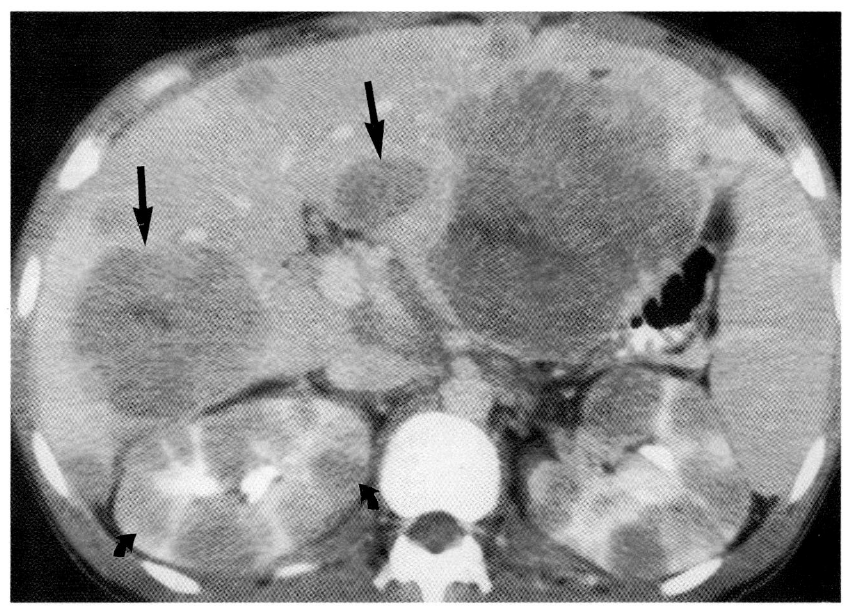

B

FIG. 2.105. AIDS-related lymphoma of the liver. **A:** Transverse sonogram through the liver reveals multiple hypoechoic liver lesions (*arrows*). **B:** The same lesions are shown on the CT scan. Renal lesions (*small curved arrows*) are present but are shown to better advantage on the CT scan. S, spine; A, aorta; i, inferior vena cava; p, left portal vein.

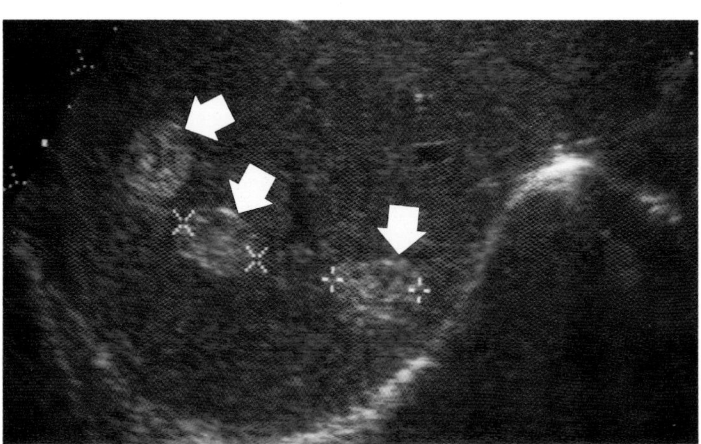

FIG. 2.106. Focal hepatic chloromas. Transverse sonogram through the right lobe of the liver. Chronic myelogenous leukemia may result in focal deposits of abnormal lymphoproliferative cells in any organ in the body. In this patient, multiple hepatic chloromas were present. These three echogenic lesions (*arrows*) had an appearance similar to that generally seen with hemangioma. Two other lesions (not shown) elsewhere in the liver had similar patterns.

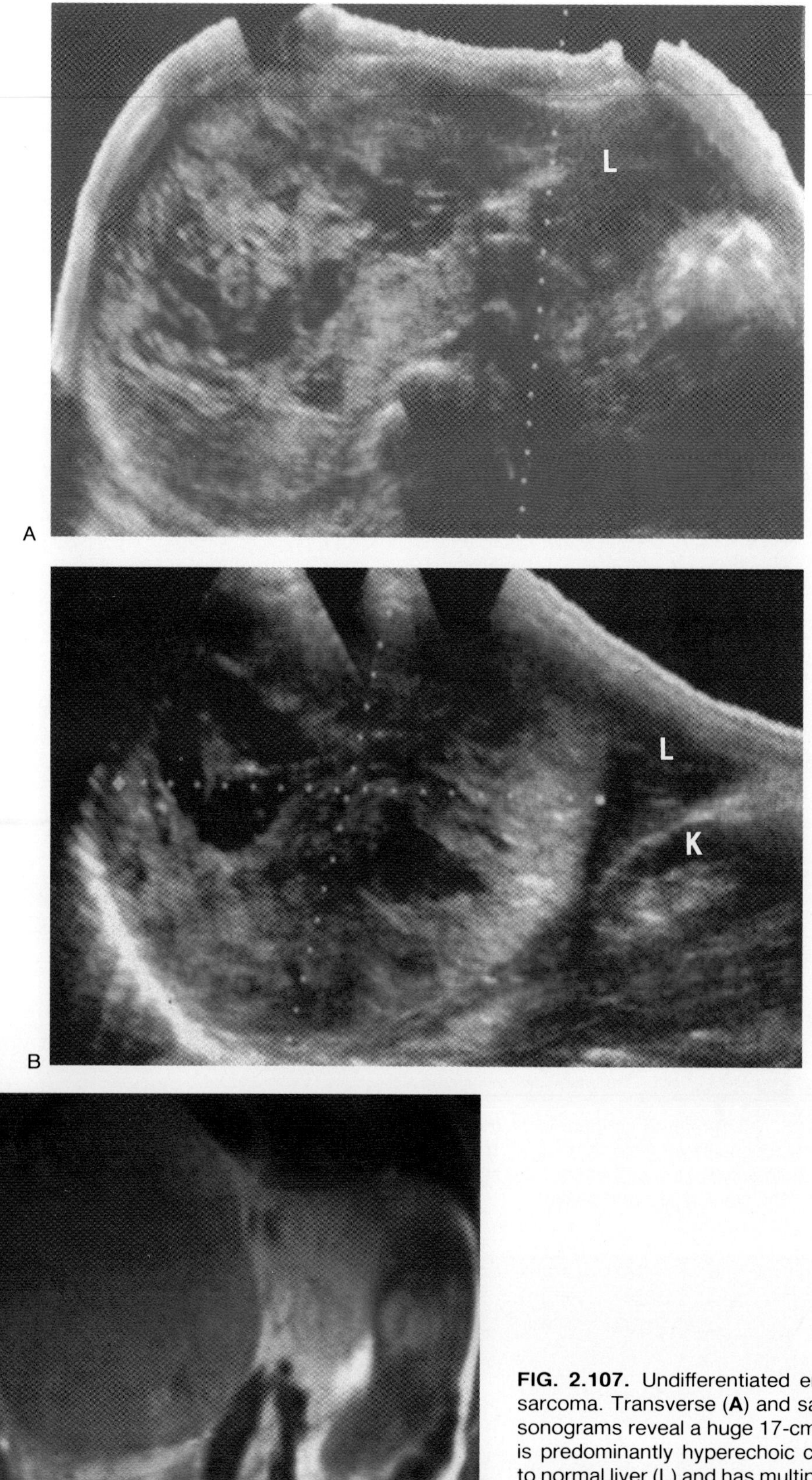

FIG. 2.107. Undifferentiated embryonal sarcoma. Transverse (**A**) and sagittal (**B**) sonograms reveal a huge 17-cm mass. It is predominantly hyperechoic compared to normal liver (L) and has multiple irregular areas that are anechoic, presumably representing necrosis. A coronal T1-weighted MRI (**C**) shows the huge mass replacing most of the right lobe of the liver. Hepatic sarcomas are rare neoplasms. K, right kidney.

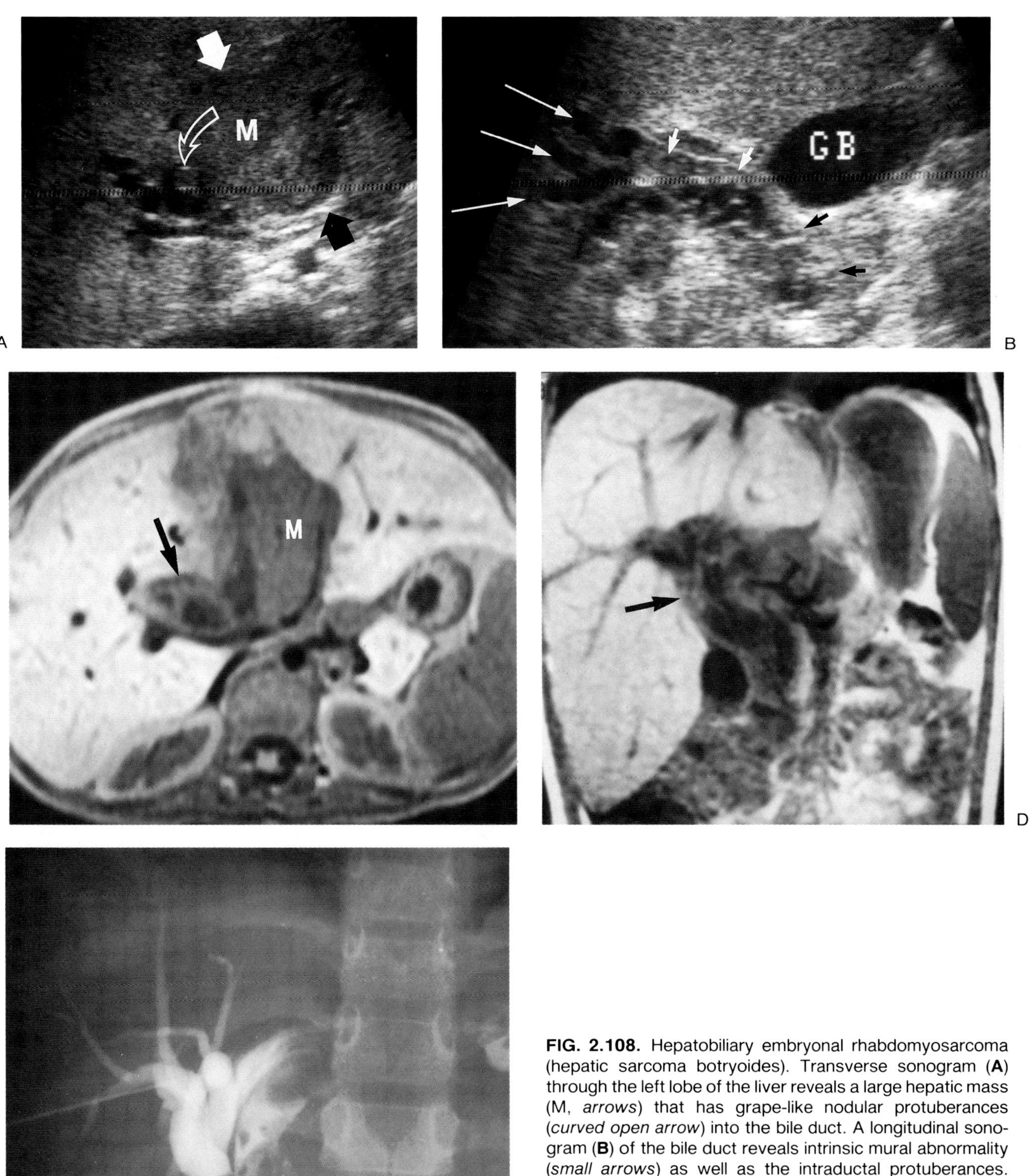

FIG. 2.108. Hepatobiliary embryonal rhabdomyosarcoma (hepatic sarcoma botryoides). Transverse sonogram (**A**) through the left lobe of the liver reveals a large hepatic mass (M, *arrows*) that has grape-like nodular protuberances (*curved open arrow*) into the bile duct. A longitudinal sonogram (**B**) of the bile duct reveals intrinsic mural abnormality (*small arrows*) as well as the intraductal protuberances. Proximal dilated ducts (*thin arrows*) are noted. Axial (**C**) and coronal (**D**) gadolinium-enhanced T1-weighted images reveal the hepatic mass (M) and the bile duct involvement (*arrow*). A transhepatic cholangiogram (**E**) reveals the medial imprint of the mass (M) and the rounded intraductal protuberances (*arrow*). The combination of the hepatic mass, bile duct involvement, and grape-like intraductal protuberances allowed a correct preoperative sonographic diagnosis.

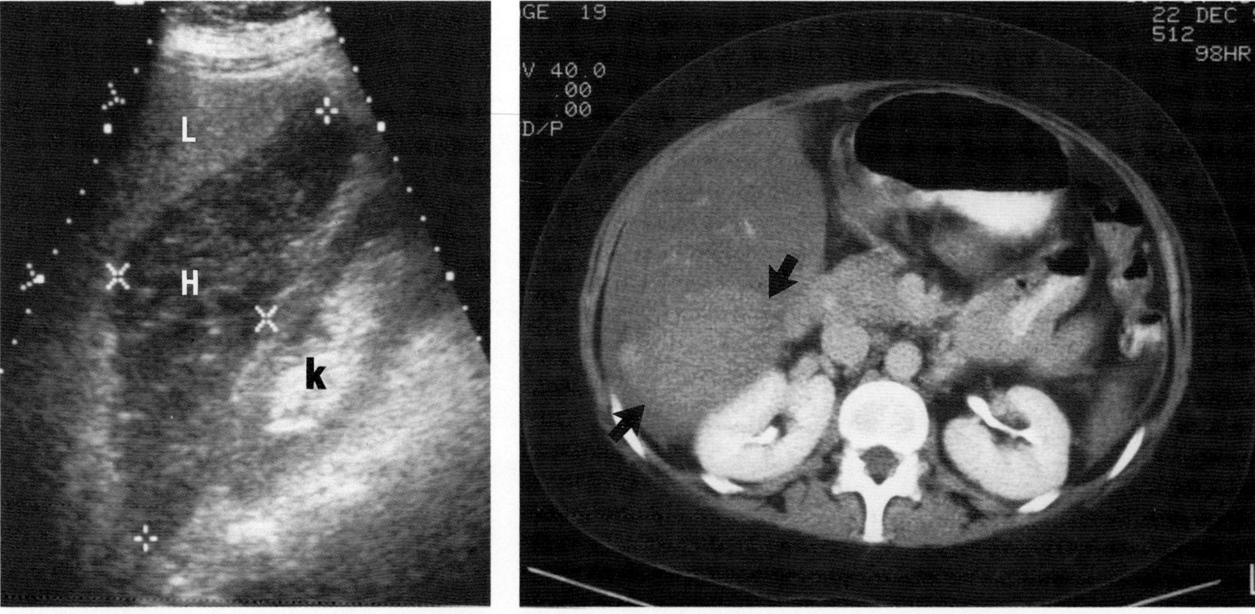

FIG. 2.109. Subcapsular hepatic hematoma. **A:** Longitudinal sonogram through the right lobe of the liver reveals a subcapsular hematoma (H, calipers) that is primarily hypoechoic compared to the liver parenchyma (L). Multiple internal echoes are indicative of relatively acute clot. **B:** The CT scan shows an area of higher attenuation (*arrows*), confirming the acute nature of the hematoma. k, right kidney.

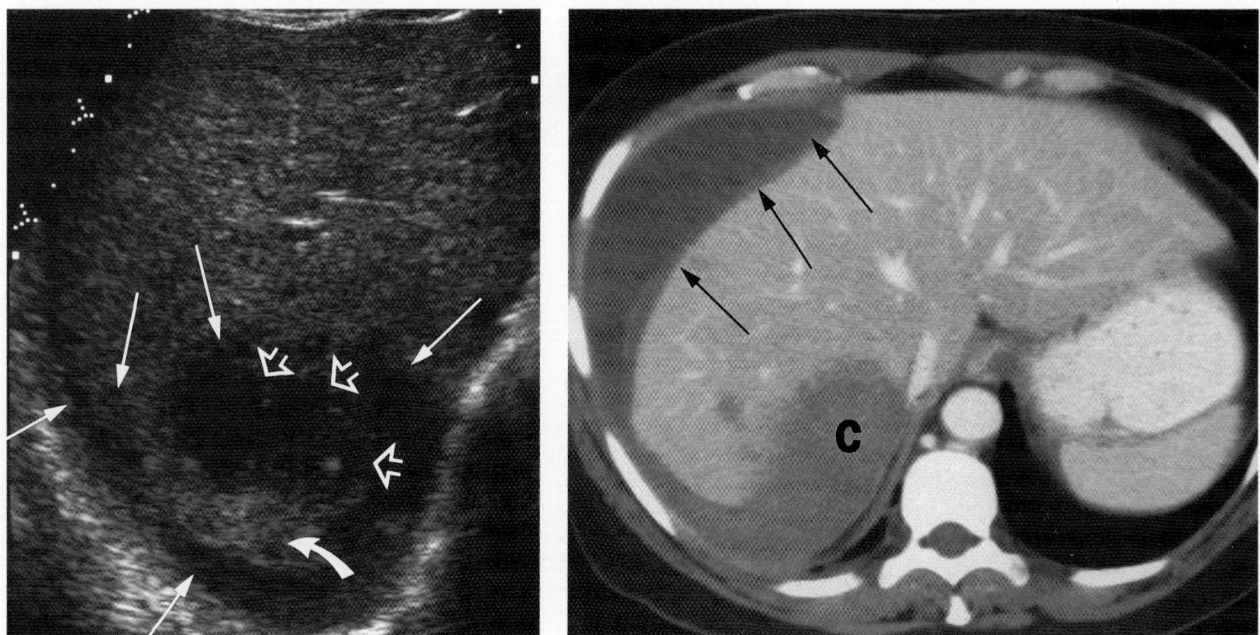

FIG. 2.110. Spontaneous subcapsular liver hematoma. **A:** Transverse sonogram through the right lobe of the liver reveals a mixed echogenicity, primarily hypoechoic, subcapsular hematoma (*thin arrows*), the largest part of which is near the dorsal right lobe of the liver. Some fibrin strands (*open arrows*) and an area of fresh clot (*curved arrow*) are noted. **B:** A CT scan shows fresh clot (C) of higher attenuation, while the more ventral older subcapsular hematoma (*thin arrows*) is of lower attenuation. This large subcapsular hematoma was unassociated with any neoplasm or other obvious predisposing condition.

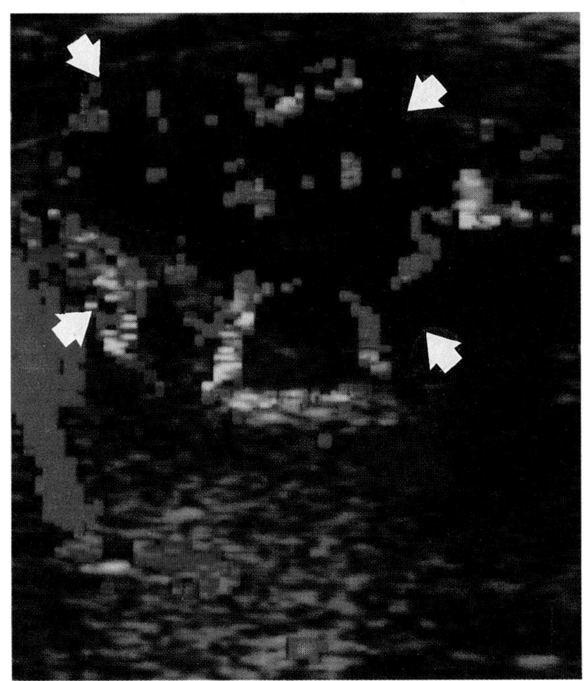

FIG. 2.111. AIDS-related lymphoma, increased color flow. This longitudinal color Doppler sonogram reveals prominent peripheral color flow. *Arrows* outline the mass. Many, but not all, AIDS-related lymphomas exhibit such increased flow peripherally.

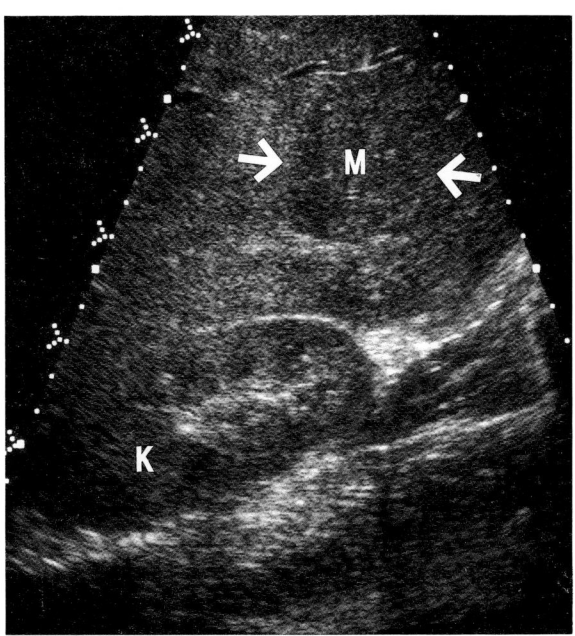

FIG. 2.113. Kaposi's sarcoma, focal mass. A subtle heterogeneous, mainly isoechoic, mass (M, *arrows*) is noted on this longitudinal sonogram through the right lobe of the liver. Hepatomegaly, probably related to diffuse infiltration of the liver by Kaposi's sarcoma, is present. K, right kidney.

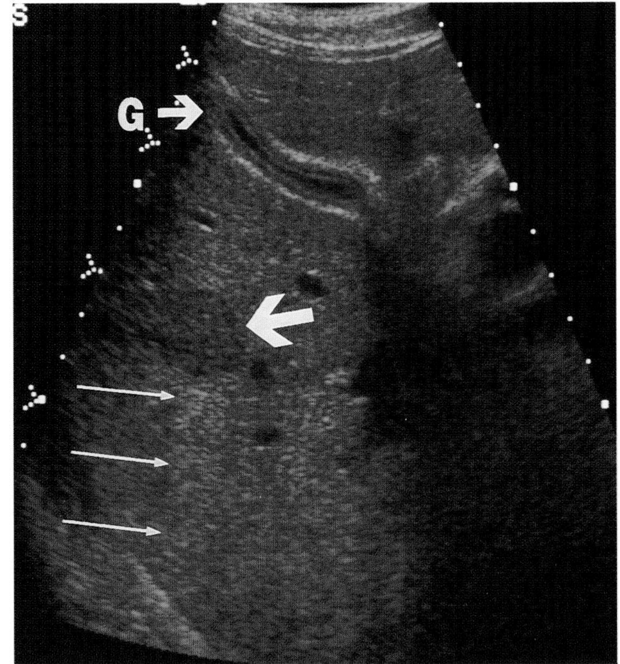

FIG. 2.112. Kaposi's sarcoma. A focal hypoechoic mass (*arrow*) is noted in this false color transverse sonogram through the liver. Note the subtle through transmission (*thin arrows*). Focal masses in Kaposi's sarcoma are unusual. G, gallbladder.

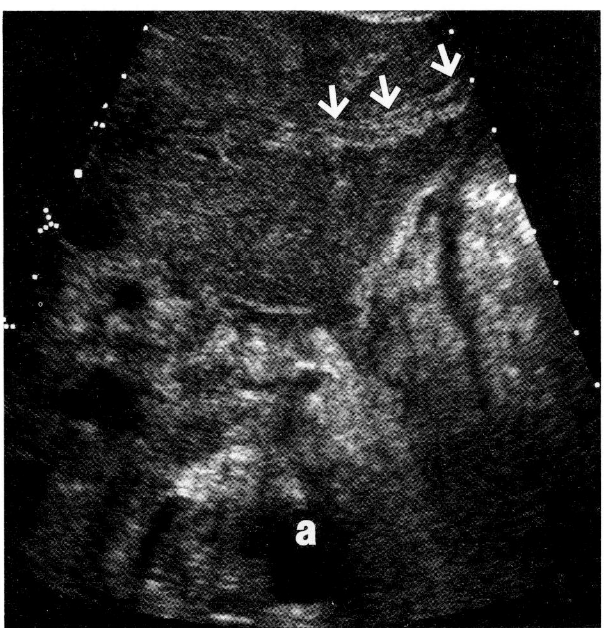

FIG. 2.114. Kaposi's sarcoma, increased periportal echogenicity. Transverse sonogram of the left lobe of the liver reveals marked increased echogenicity about the lateral segmental branch of the left portal vein (*arrows*). Periportal infiltration with Kaposi's sarcoma may cause this finding in some patients. a, aorta.

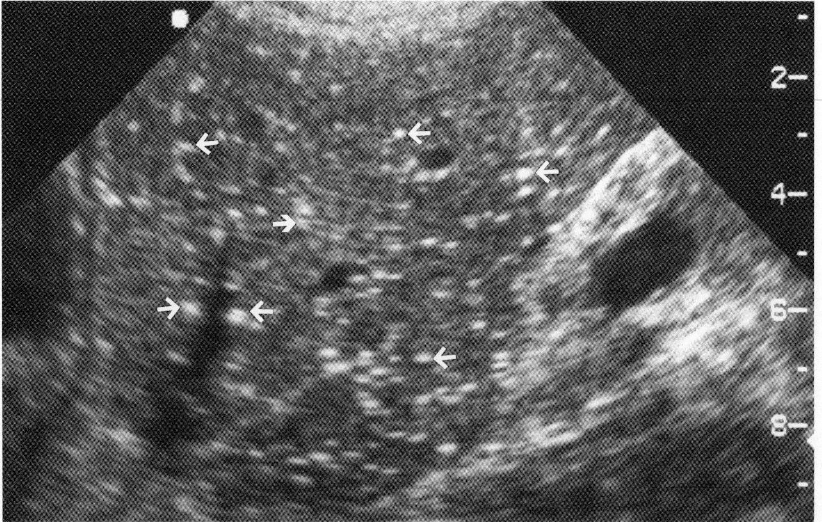

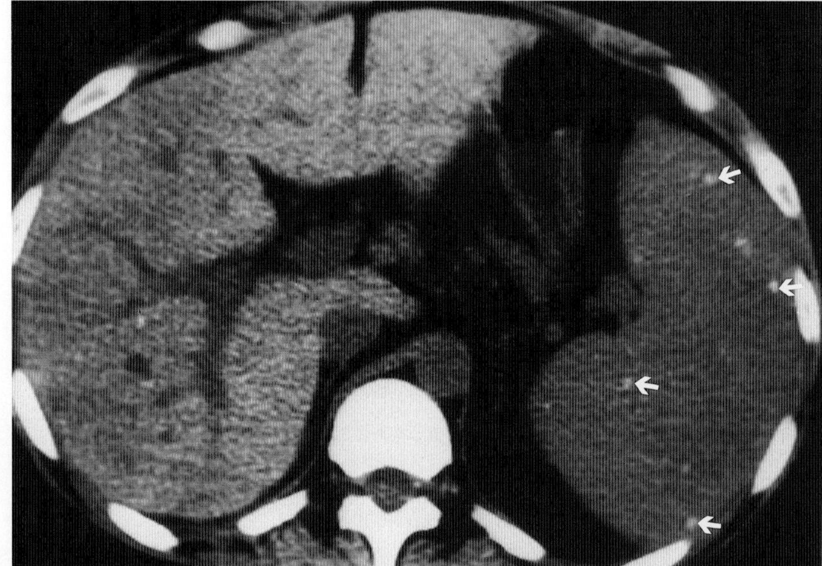

FIG. 2.115. Disseminated *Pneumocystis,* hepatic "starry sky" pattern. Longitudinal sonogram (**A**) of the left lobe of the liver reveals multiple tiny focal calcifications (some indicated by *arrows*) that are virtually invisible on the CT scan (**B**). This "starry sky" pattern is distinctive and should suggest the diagnosis of disseminated *Pneumocystis* in a patient with AIDS. The CT scan also shows some focal splenic calcifications (*arrows*). This pattern is highly suggestive, but not definitive, for disseminated *Pneumocystis* infection.

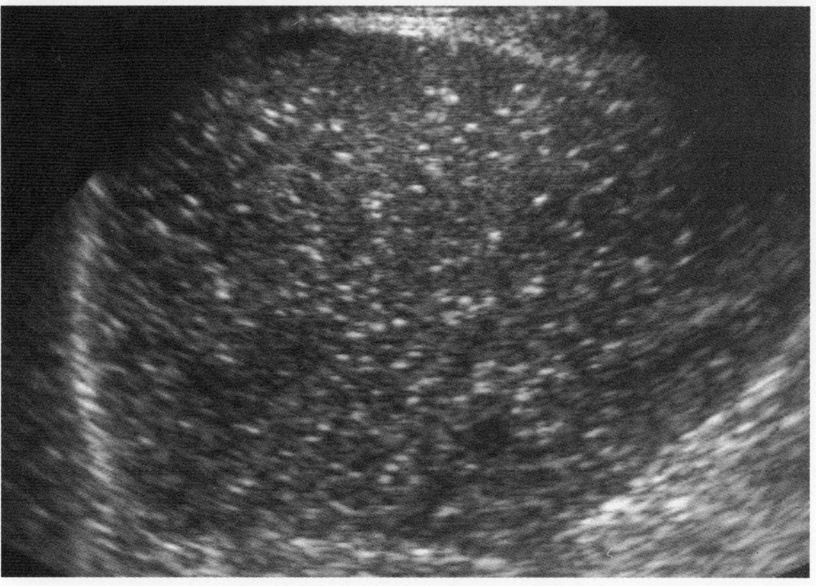

FIG. 2.116. Tuberculosis of the liver, "starry sky" pattern. An oblique longitudinal sonogram through the liver in this HIV-positive patient reveals myriad small focal calcifications, the "starry sky" pattern. Although this pattern is most frequently seen in patients with disseminated *Pneumocystis carinii* infection, other infectious processes in HIV patients may also produce this striking pattern. This patient had hepatic tuberculosis. Both mycobacterial and CMV infections occasionally produce findings similar to those illustrated here and in Fig. 2.115.

with central echogenic foci (the "wheel within a wheel" pattern, Fig. 2.91) (68). HIV infection is a risk factor for amebic liver abscess (see Liver Abscess section).

DIFFUSE DISEASE

Hepatomegaly, a feature of many diffuse liver diseases, is difficult to diagnose objectively with sonography. Accurate measurement is hampered by the limited field of view imaged by real-time instruments. The most reliable measurement is probably the sagittal dimension from the dome to the tip of the right lobe, measured at the midclavicular line. If this exceeds 15.5 cm, the liver is probably enlarged (98). Hepatomegaly can be confidently diagnosed when the liver extends caudal to the right kidney and the left lobe is of normal size or larger. Obviously, volumetric measurement would be superior, but obtaining appropriate measurements is tedious and inaccurate with conventional CT, MRI, or sonography. New techniques in all three modalities (three-dimensional MRI and sonography, spiral CT) promise to make volumetric measurements feasible soon.

Diffuse liver disease does not always cause distortion of liver anatomy or architecture, making sonographic detection difficult. Liver surface nodularity or atrophy of the right lobe, when present, can be useful signs of cirrhosis. Parenchymal echogenicity may be increased in diffuse disease but is difficult to evaluate as no absolute echo amplitude standard exists (analogous to CT attenuation numbers). The sonographer must appraise echogenicity by comparing the liver to adjacent organs such as the kidney or pancreas. The liver is normally of equal or lesser echogenicity than the pancreas. It is of equal or greater echogenicity than the renal cortex.

Sonographic findings in diffuse liver disease are often not specific. The findings depend on the type and severity of the disease: hepatitis of various etiologies, fatty infiltration, cirrhosis, and precirrhotic conditions.

Hepatitis

Hepatitis is a generic term for inflammation of the liver. Since many different diseases cause hepatic inflammation, sonographic findings are variable. Acute hepatitis is usually caused by viral infection. Other causes of acute inflammation include alcoholism, toxins, and drug reactions, among others.

Acute Viral Hepatitis

Viral hepatitis can be divided conveniently into types that cause chronic liver disease and types that do not. Most important of those causing chronic disease are hepatitis B and C, both transmitted parenterally. Hepatitis A and E, which have an enteric mode of transmission, do not cause chronic disease. Acute hepatitis is usually easily diagnosed by clinical, laboratory, and serologic data; imaging is unnecessary. Sonography may be requested when the diagnosis is unclear.

Some studies (99,100) have suggested that sonographic findings in acute hepatitis include increased periportal echogenicity coupled with decreased echogenicity. This pattern, however, is uncommon; the liver is generally normal in acute viral hepatitis. In a large series, only 19 of 791 patients with acute viral hepatitis demonstrated this pattern (101). In the same study, there was no difference in ultrasound findings between a normal control group and patients with acute viral hepatitis.

Striking irregular gallbladder wall thickening is sometimes present in patients with acute hepatitis, especially hepatitis A (102). This wall thickening, sometimes as much as 2 cm, is caused by direct inflammation and edema (see Chapter 3). This finding should not suggest intrinsic gallbladder disease.

Chronic Viral Hepatitis

Viral hepatitis B or C may lead to chronic inflammation with its attendant complications: chronic active hepatitis, cirrhosis, and hepatocellular carcinoma. Chronic active hepatitis is usually related to persistent viral-induced inflammation, although nonviral causes are known (103). Sonographic findings in chronic active hepatitis vary. Hepatomegaly and inhomogeneous patchy or diffuse increased echogenicity are common and are related to the amount of fatty infiltration and fibrosis present. The liver surface is smooth, unless cirrhosis is present. Enlarged arteries are noted on color flow sonography because of increased arterial flow. This may cause a "double channel" sign on grayscale images that can potentially be confused with biliary dilatation (Fig. 2.117). This occurs most often in the lateral segment of the left lobe, as the left hepatic artery is horizontally oriented, perpendicular to the ultrasound beam. Lymph nodes may be seen in the hepatoduodenal ligament (104).

Alcoholic Hepatitis

Alcoholic hepatitis results in focal or diffuse cell necrosis and inflammation. Patients with alcohol-related cirrhosis have usually had alcoholic hepatitis, but it is probably not a necessary precursor to cirrhosis. Symptoms vary and may be either mild (tender hepatomegaly, generalized malaise, mild jaundice) or severe (progressive jaundice, fever, leukocytosis, coagulopathy, renal failure, and encephalopathy). Cholestasis and reversible portal hypertension may occur.

Ultrasound findings depend on the amount of fibrosis

(text continues on page 145)

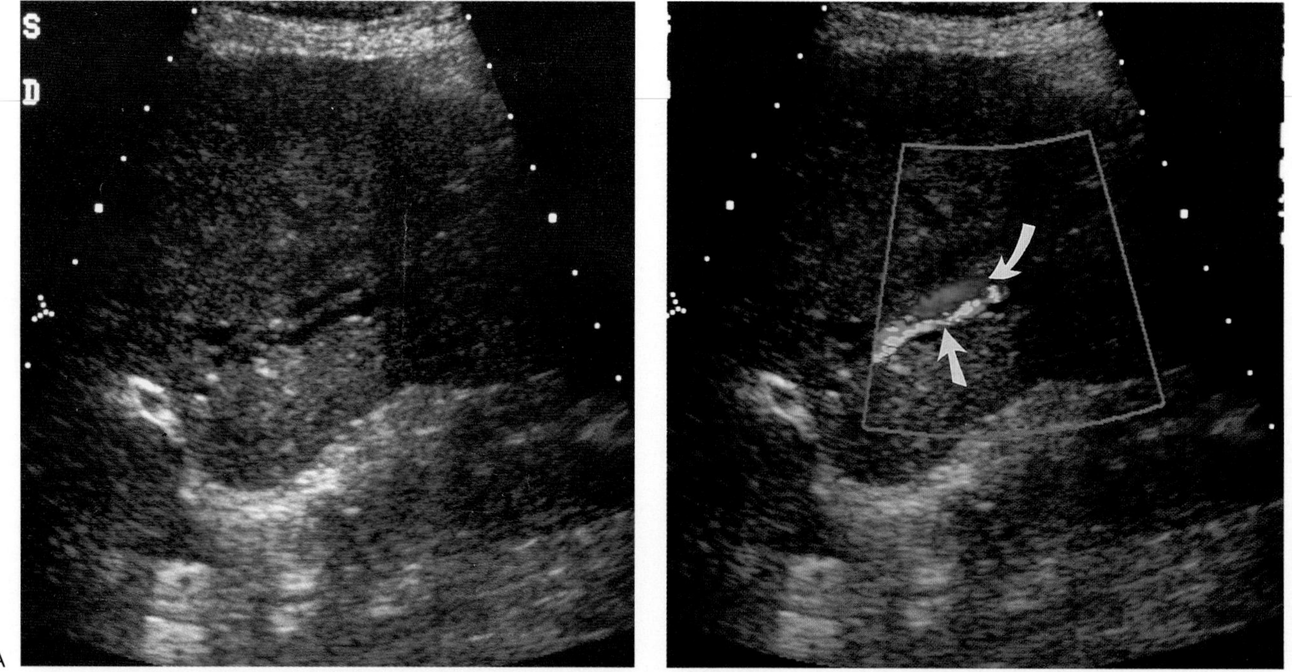

FIG. 2.117. Chronic active hepatitis, false-positive double-channel sign. **A:** Transverse grayscale sonogram of the left lobe in this jaundiced patient referred to rule out biliary dilatation revealed a "double-channel sign," a finding suspicious for biliary dilatation. **B:** The transverse color Doppler sonogram demonstrates that both channels are vascular structures. Flow reversal is noted in the ventral portal vein (*curved arrow*). An enlarged hepatic artery (*slant tailed arrow*) was responsible for the false-positive double-channel sign.

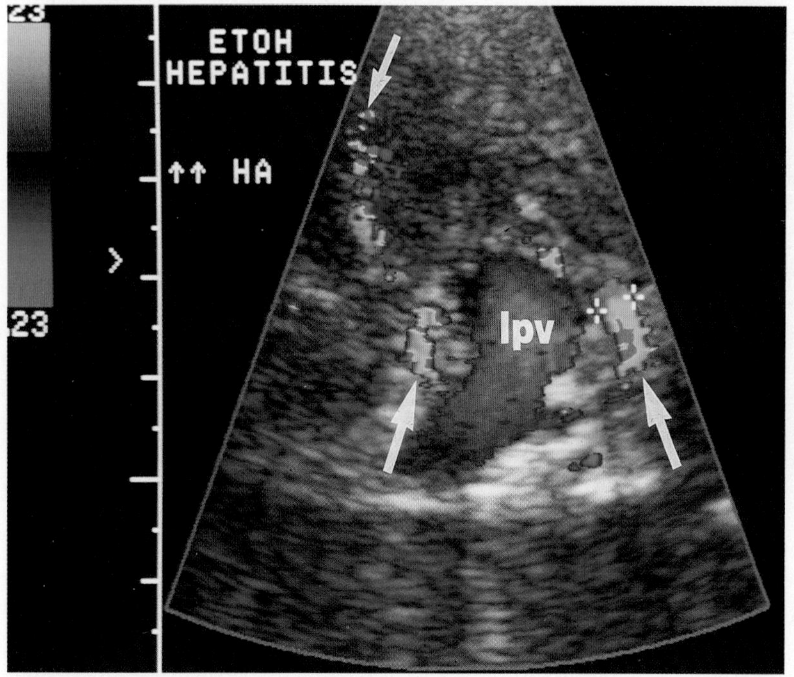

FIG. 2.118. Hepatic arterial enlargement, alcoholic hepatitis. Transverse color Doppler sonogram of the region of the left portal vein (lpv) reveals markedly enlarged hepatic arteries (*arrows*) that exhibit high-velocity aliased flow. Although the cause of the arterial enlargement is unknown in patients with alcoholic hepatitis, it may be related to increased flow from hepatic inflammation. Arterial enlargement occurs in many diffuse liver diseases.

or fat present. Parenchymal echogenicity is usually increased, with a patchy, irregular pattern. The liver is often enlarged, but the surface is usually smooth, in contrast to the nodularity sometimes detected in cirrhosis. Because arterial blood supply to the liver is increased, the arteries may be enlarged. Color flow sonography demonstrates enlarged arteries with aliased flow (Fig. 2.118).

Fatty Infiltration

Fatty infiltration is a nonspecific response to liver injury (e.g., alcoholic, toxins). It may occur in dysnutritional states including obesity, hyperalimentation, starvation, or diabetes mellitus. Sonographically, the liver is increased in echogenicity and may be enlarged. Cirrhosis may coexist with fatty infiltration. When fatty infiltration is diffuse, the liver is homogeneously increased in echogenicity (Fig. 2.119). Despite this, there is usually little difficulty obtaining adequate acoustic penetration. This is unlike patients with echogenic fibrotic livers, which significantly attenuate the sound beam. The liver surface is smooth.

Fatty infiltration is often patchy or focal. Geographic fatty infiltration typically has fairly well-defined margins between areas of greater and lesser involvement (Fig. 2.120). A less affected region of the liver (a "spared" area) may appear as a conspicuous hypoechoic mass that simulates a neoplasm (Fig. 2.118), standing out in stark contrast to the increased echogenicity of the surrounding fatty liver. Both focal fatty infiltration (Fig. 2.121) and focal sparing (Figs. 2.122 and 2.123) can simulate neoplasm (105–107). Both areas of focal fat and areas of sparing have a tendency to be pyramidal in configuration. Often, they have flame-shaped, tapered margins. Frequent locations include the region of the porta hepatis, near the falciform ligament, in the dorsal left lobe, and in the caudate lobe. An appreciation of the usual appearance and location of spared areas and focal fat generally suffices to avoid confusion with neoplasm or other masses. Color flow imaging reveals normal, undisplaced vessels in these areas (Fig. 2.124). Tumors are virtually always associated with displaced or abnormal vessels. Occasionally, noncontrast CT scanning, MRI, or biopsy may be required to clarify the diagnosis in a problematic case.

A recent study showed that the total amount of fat in relatively hypoechoic spared areas and more echogenic nonspared areas may be equivalent (108). Variations in echogenicity were related to the size of the fat globules. Smaller globules led to more interfaces and greater echogenicity, even though the total volume of fat in all areas was identical (108). These results are interesting, but do not explain the findings in other studies in which hypoechoic spared areas corresponded to areas with higher attenuation on CT scan (107) (Fig. 2.123).

An unusual form of fatty infiltration may occur with Langerhans' cell granulomatosis (formerly the group of diseases known as histiocytosis X, eosinophilic granuloma, and others). Large mass-like areas of fat may occur in unusual locations, simulating tumor on ultrasound (Fig. 2.125). CT reveals the low-attenuation, fatty nature of the lesion.

Cirrhosis

Hepatic cirrhosis results from fibrotic and reparative processes after a diffuse hepatic insult. Common causes include alcohol abuse, viral hepatitis, biliary obstruction, and toxic drugs. Sonographic findings of cirrhosis include increased parenchymal echogenicity, poor tissue penetration of sound, and parenchymal inhomogeneity (Fig. 2.126). Unfortunately, these signs are both insensitive and insufficiently specific to diagnose cirrhosis reliably.

For reasons not understood, but possibly related to differences in vascularity, the caudate and left lobes tend to be relatively less affected by cirrhotic scarring than the right lobe. The right lobe tends to shrink preferentially, especially in hepatitis B (109). This sometimes results in a small right lobe with left and caudate lobe hypertrophy. Because of this, it has been suggested that cirrhosis can be diagnosed by ratios comparing the size or volume of the caudate to the shrunken right lobe (110,111). Many observers have not found these ratios of practical use. A large series revealed a sensitivity of 43 percent and an accuracy of 79 percent for the caudate to right lobe ratio (109).

Another potentially valuable approach is to evaluate the smoothness or nodularity of the liver surface using a high-resolution near-field optimized linear array transducer (112,113). When using this technique, careful real-time evaluation is needed. The transducer must be held parallel to the liver surface, as angulation may simulate nodularity in normal patients. In DiLelio's series (113), nodularity of the liver surface was identified in 50 of 57 cirrhotics. Surface nodularity was a much more accurate parameter than echo inhomogeneity, increased echogenicity, and increased attenuation (Figs. 2.127 and 2.128). Other investigators have not confirmed the usefulness of evaluating surface nodularity. Ladenheim et al. (114) found that surface nodularity appraisal was not useful, leading to many false-positive and false-negative studies. The patients in this study probably had milder disease overall and there were fewer alcoholic cirrhotic patients. Clearly, further investigation is needed to determine the usefulness of sonographic liver surface nodularity evaluation. In our laboratory, we evaluate the liver surface routinely in all patients undergoing hepatic sonography. One potential pitfall is surface nodularity caused by subcapsular metastasis (see Fig. 2.41).

(text continues on page 151)

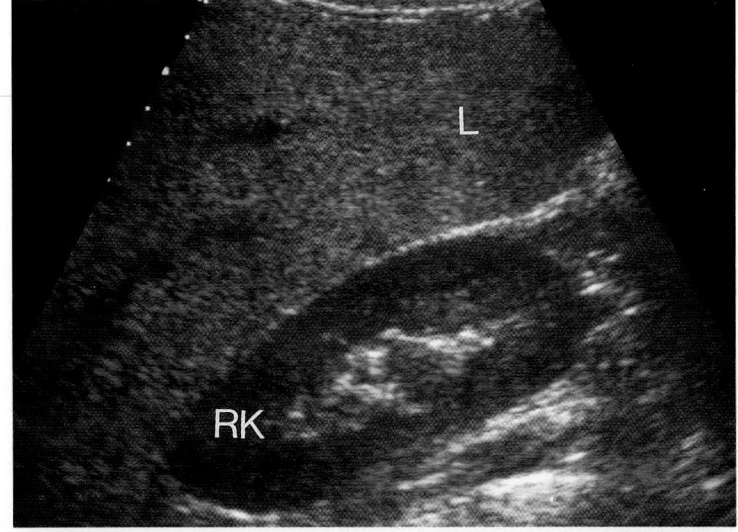

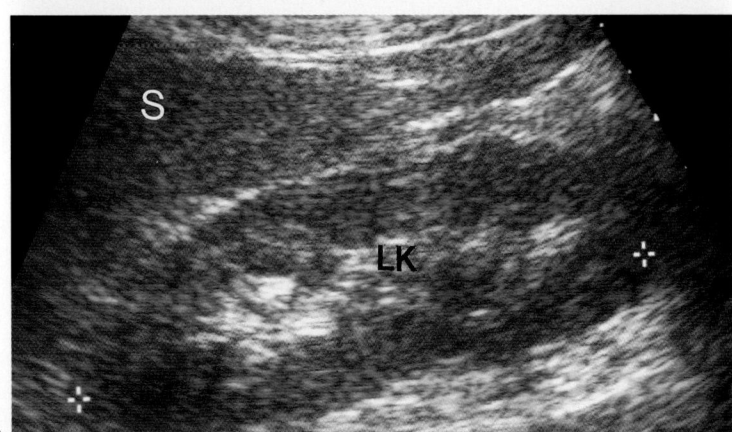

FIG. 2.119. Fatty infiltration of the liver. **A:** Longitudinal sonogram through the liver and right kidney reveals an enlarged, increased attenuation liver (L). Note the discrepancy in echogenicity between the right kidney (RK) and the liver. **B:** A longitudinal sonogram through the spleen and left kidney reveals that the left kidney (LK) is comparable in echogenicity to the spleen (S). The increased echogenicity of the liver suggests the presence of diffuse fatty infiltration. Since no absolute standards for hepatic echogenicity exist, accurate appraisal of hepatic echogenicity requires comparing the liver to the right kidney, as well as the spleen to the left kidney. The relative echogenicity of both the liver and spleen, when compared to the renal cortex, should be roughly the same. In this patient with fatty infiltration, the liver is much more echogenic than the spleen (using the kidneys as a standard). Its echogenicity is abnormally increased. Fatty infiltration usually causes increased echogenicity. Cirrhotic and precirrhotic conditions, which increase echogenicity because of fibrosis, can also result in a similar pattern.

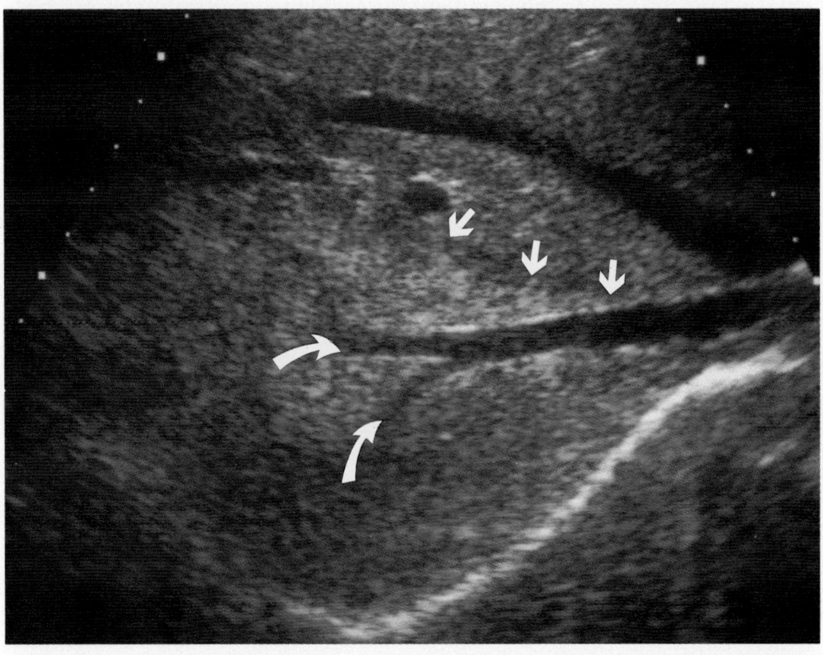

FIG. 2.120. Geographic fatty infiltration of the liver. Transverse sonogram of the right lobe of the liver reveals an area of increased echogenicity representing geographic fatty infiltration. Note the fairly well-defined margins between areas of greater and lesser involvement (*arrows*). One finding that facilitates the correct diagnosis is the fact that fatty liver does not displace the normal vessels that run through it (*curved arrows*).

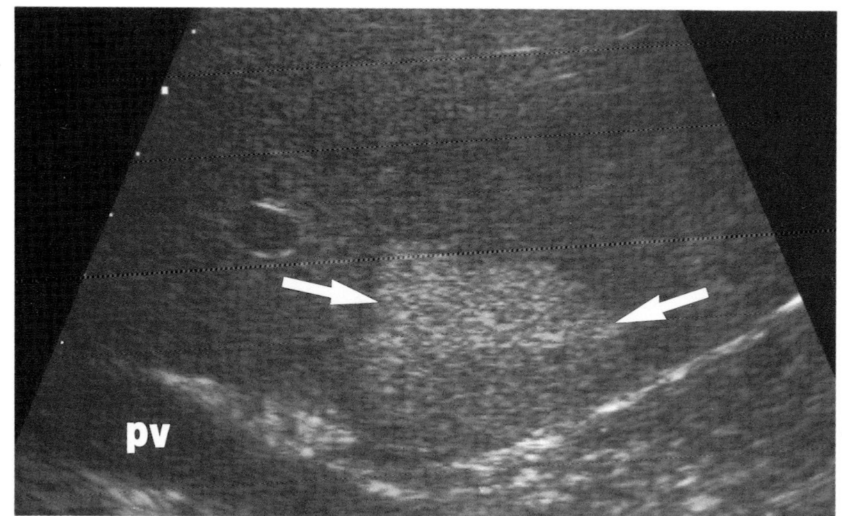

FIG. 2.121. Focal fatty infiltration simulates neoplasm. Longitudinal sonogram through the left lobe of the liver reveals a well-defined echogenic area of focal fatty infiltration (*arrows*). Well-defined echogenic areas of fatty infiltration such as this can raise the concern of neoplasm. A knowledge of the usual appearance and location (dorsal aspect of the left lobe in this instance) can often facilitate the correct diagnosis. pv, Main portal vein.

A

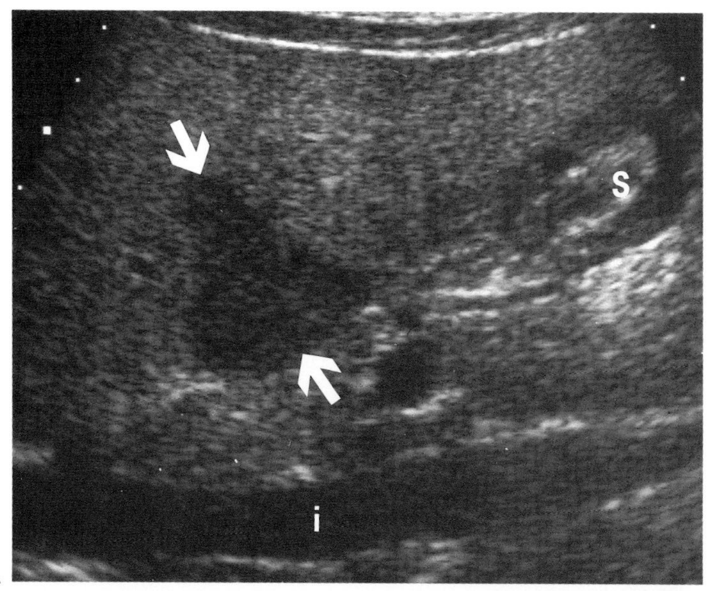

B

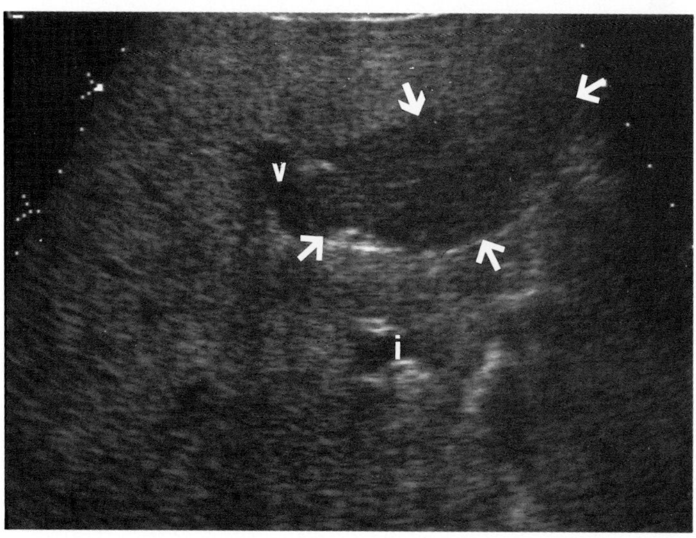

FIG. 2.122. Fatty liver, hypoechoic mass-like spared area. **A:** Longitudinal sonogram through the left lobe of the liver near the region of the inferior vena cava (i) reveals a pyramidal shaped, hypoechoic area (*arrows*) that represents a spared area within a fatty liver. **B:** The transverse sonogram through the left lobe reveals the same spared area (*arrows*) to the left of the left portal vein (v). Hypoechoic areas like this can simulate neoplasm. An appreciation of the usual appearance (pyramidal or flame-shaped) and an appreciation for the usual location (dorsal aspect of the lateral segment of the left lobe in this instance) can help make the diagnosis. Other common locations for areas of sparing in a fatty liver include around the falciform ligament, near the porta hepatis, and near the gallbladder. S, stomach.

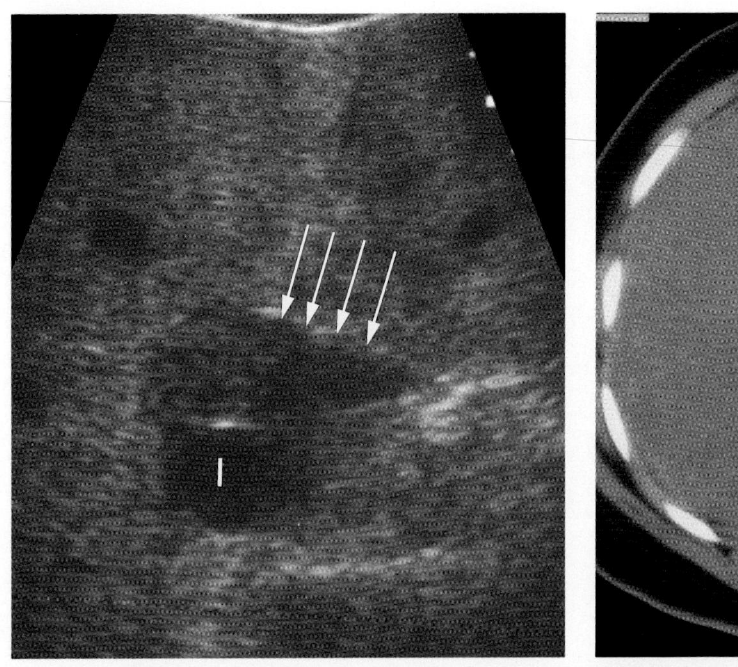

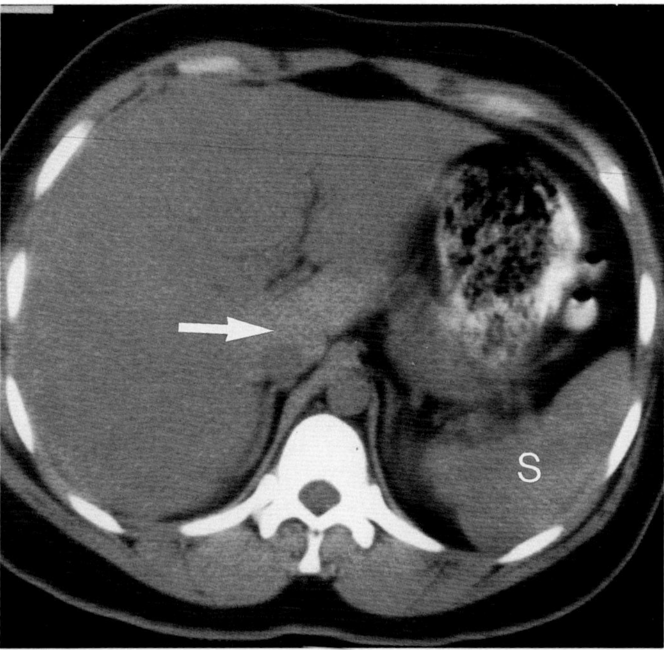

FIG. 2.123. Fatty liver, hypoechoic spared area. **A:** Transverse area through the region of the left and caudate lobes reveals a hypoechoic spared area between the IVC (I) and the fissure for ligamentum venosum (*thin arrows*). **B:** The CT scan reveals higher attenuation (*arrow*) within the caudate lobe, documenting this as a spared area within a fatty liver. Note that the liver is of lower attenuation than the spleen (S) on this noncontrast CT scan. The caudate lobe is another favored location for either focal sparing in a fatty liver or an area of focal fatty infiltration.

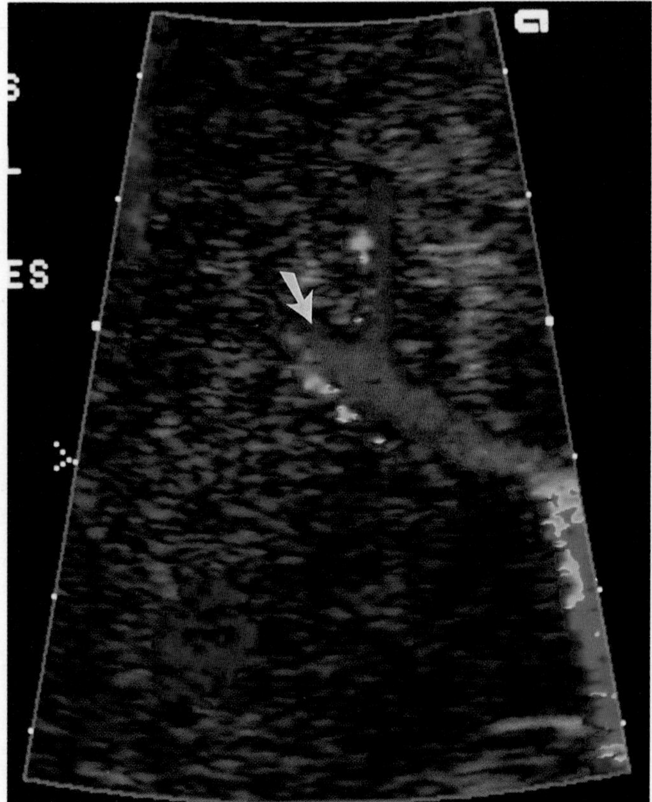

FIG. 2.124. Fatty liver, nondisplaced vessel. Transverse color Doppler sonogram of the right portal vein (*arrow*). The echogenic area of fatty infiltration surrounding the right portal vein does not displace or distort the vessel. Masses virtually always displace or distort vessels that run adjacent to or through them. Fatty infiltration causes no such distortion.

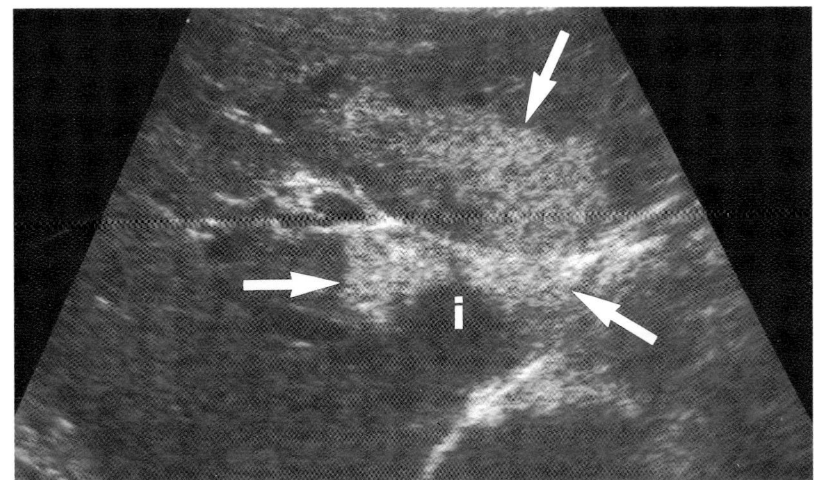

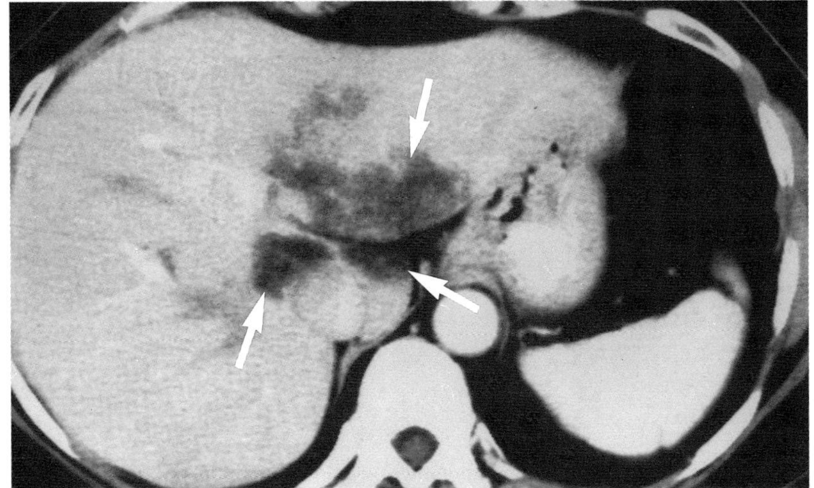

FIG. 2.125. Fatty masses, Langerhans' cell granulomatosis. **A:** Transverse sonogram through the liver reveals several fatty masses (*arrows*) in the left and caudate lobes. **B:** The CT scan also shows these findings and demonstrates low attenuation, compatible with fat. Unusual mass-like collections of intrahepatic fat may occur in Langerhans' cell granulomatosis (formerly the group of diseases known as histiocytosis X, Letterer–Siwe disease, and others). i, inferior vena cava. Although the fatty nature of the lesion can be suspected by the location and echogenicity sonographically, CT's ability to demonstrate fat attenuation allows a definitive diagnosis.

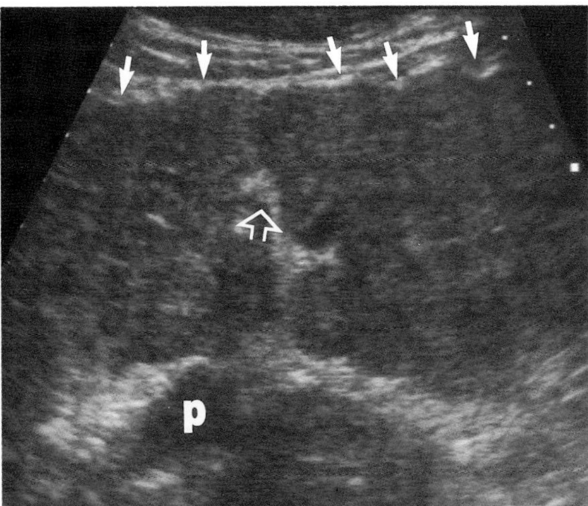

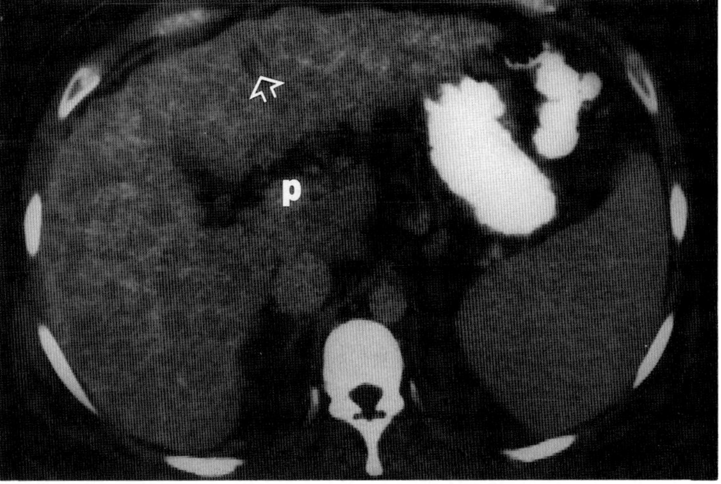

FIG. 2.126. Cirrhosis, unusual pattern. **A:** Transverse sonogram shows frank surface nodularity (*small arrows*) and textural inhomogeneity with fairly well-defined areas of increased and decreased echogenicity. **B:** A contrast-enhanced CT scan reveals an unusual pattern of enhancement and again confirms the nodular surface. The areas of higher and lower attenuation on the CT scan form a nodular pattern. Liver biopsy was compatible with the diagnosis of primary biliary cirrhosis. It is possible that the findings displayed may represent multiple adenomatous hyperplastic nodules (regenerating nodules). *Open arrow,* ligamentum teres; p, portal vein.

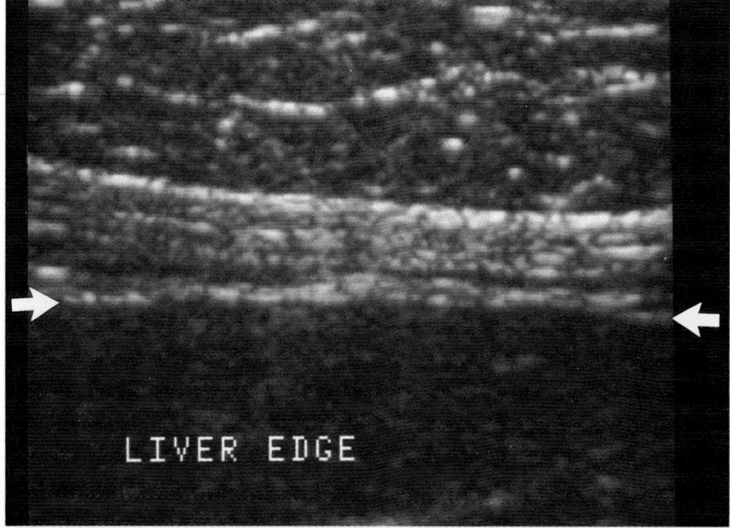

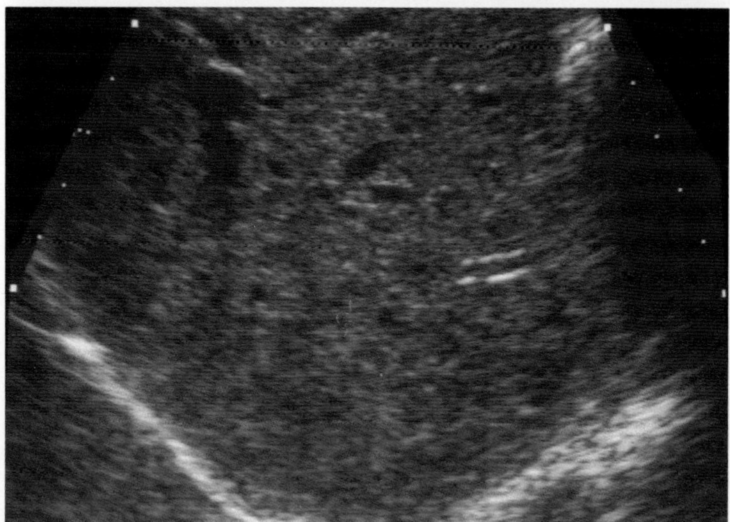

FIG. 2.127. Cirrhosis, subtle surface nodularity. **A:** Longitudinal high-resolution sonogram of the liver surface reveals very subtle nodularity/irregularity of the surface. The liver surface is indicated by the *arrows*. This degree of subtle nodularity is difficult to appreciate on frozen images and is better appreciated during real-time examination. Care must be taken to hold the transducer parallel to the liver surface during the examination, as angulation can simulate nodularity when none is present. **B:** A transverse sonogram through the right lobe reveals parenchymal inhomogeneity, a nonspecific indicator of diffuse liver disease. This patient had cirrhosis related to alcoholism.

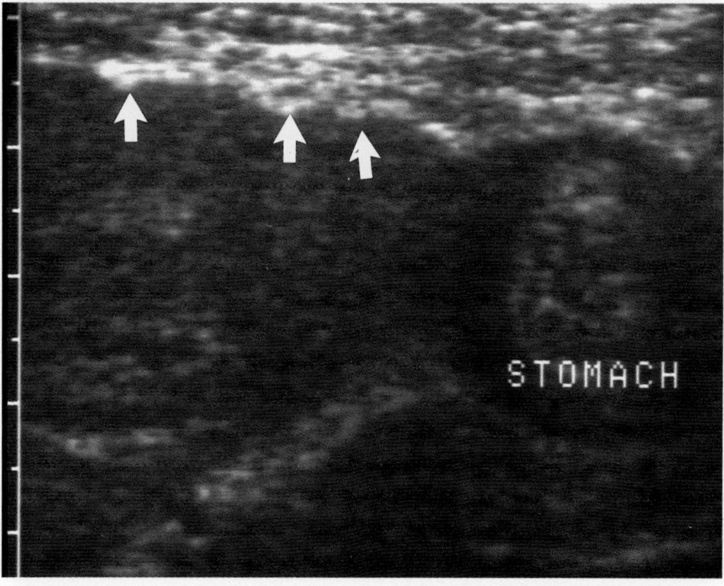

FIG. 2.128. Cirrhosis with gross surface nodularity. Longitudinal high-resolution sonogram in this patient reveals gross nodularity with surface indentations (*arrows*). There is little difficulty in diagnosing cirrhosis based on surface abnormalities in patients with gross changes like this.

Color flow sonography may detect portal vein flow reversal (Fig. 2.129) or portal collaterals (Fig. 2.130), prompting the diagnosis of portal hypertension. These may be the only findings indicating severe liver disease in a patient with an otherwise normal or nearly normal study. Enlarged tortuous arteries are sometimes imaged by color flow sonography in cirrhotic livers (Fig. 2.131). This finding, similar to "corkscrew" arteries seen angiographically, probably occurs because of truncation of arteries from liver atrophy related to cirrhosis, coupled with the increased arterial flow (115) that occurs when portal venous flow decreases.

Focal fatty infiltration, hepatocellular carcinoma, regenerating nodules (adenomatous hyperplastic nodule) (Fig. 2.63), or other focal lesions may occur in a cirrhotic liver. A liver mass in a cirrhotic patient strongly suggests the possibility of hepatocellular carcinoma; further evaluation should proceed (see Hepatocellular Carcinoma section).

HEPATIC VASCULAR DISEASES

Spectral Doppler and color flow imaging have revolutionized sonography's ability to detect and evaluate vascular abnormalities of the liver. Color flow sonography (CFS) passively and automatically displays blood flow in real-time. Flow in unsuspected vascular abnormalities (Fig. 2.132) or vessels invisible or inconspicuous on grayscale images is automatically displayed. Transient alterations in flow dynamics and pulsatility (Fig. 2.133) can be defined without affecting flow patterns (115), an ability other imaging modalities currently lack. Diagnoses that were previously possible only with angiography can now be made noninvasively with CFS. CFS allows some diagnoses impossible even with angiography. It can also evaluate the results and adequacy of vascular surgery and interventional angiographic procedures.

Spectral Doppler sonography is used when quantitative flow velocity or detailed waveform analysis is desired. CFS facilitates quick and accurate sample volume placement when spectral Doppler information is needed. CFS is used when flow detection or global anatomical information about blood flow is needed to make the diagnosis. CFS's ability to provide a global view of flow in real-time minimizes the chance of missing flow in an unexpected area and facilitates comparison of flow in different anatomic locations.

Despite their usefulness, spectral and color flow sonography have limitations. Acoustic access may be limited, obscuring vessels or collaterals, especially in the retroperitoneum. Flow in vessels deep in fibrotic livers is occasionally difficult to image even with low-frequency transducers. Static flow (very rare) or very slow flow in deep vessels can mimic an anechoic clot. Portal flow is often bidirectional in very low flow states.

Spectral Doppler sonography of normal portal veins reveals a uniform waveform with minor respiratory and cardiac variation. Hepatic veins have a triphasic waveform, reflecting the contractility of the right atrium (116). When a hepatic vein is "shielded" from cardiac-induced pressure waves, a uniform hepatic venous waveform results, devoid of the usual triphasic fluctuations (Fig. 2.134). This results in "portalization"—a waveform similar to that noted in normal portal veins. Hepatic vein shielding has many causes, including cirrhosis, any mass compressing a hepatic vein, partial hepatic vein thrombosis, hepatic vein valves, and obstruction of the inferior vena cava (IVC) above the level of the hepatic veins.

An interesting abnormality of the portal venous waveform occurs when there is tricuspid valve insufficiency. Portal flow becomes bidirectional, a phenomenon that can be seen with both spectral and color flow images (Fig. 2.133). This waveform sometimes occurs in patients with congestive heart failure and, rarely, cirrhosis. While the cause for this waveform is unknown, it is probably related to transient increased sinusoidal pressure.

Venous Thrombosis

CFS highlights a clot by displaying flow around the clot and in adjacent patent vessels. Portal venous thrombosis can be diagnosed when (a) no intravascular color-coded flow is detected, (b) an adequate Doppler scan angle and acoustic access are obtained, and (c) flow can readily be demonstrated in other vessels at a comparable depth and angle of insonation (115). On grayscale imaging, intraluminal echoes suggest the diagnosis of clot, but their presence is not diagnostic. Clot detection by grayscale imaging alone is difficult when the thrombus is hypoechoic or anechoic. Anechoic thrombus is rare in neoplastic invasion (see Figs. 2.66 to 2.70) but is fairly common with bland clot (Fig. 2.135).

Venous thrombosis can result from neoplastic invasion, septic portal thrombosis (pylephlebitis) (Fig. 2.135), pancreatitis (Fig. 2.136), portocaval shunts, trauma, portal hypertension, endoscopic esophageal sclerotherapy, and other causes. We feel thrombosis in portal hypertensive patients (115,117) is considerably more common than the 1 percent previously reported (118).

CFS is unrivaled in diagnosing partially occluded vessels (Fig. 2.137). Small residual flow channels are automatically displayed in color (Fig. 2.138). Clot resolution or progression can be documented on serial examinations.

Cavernous transformation of the portal vein, resulting from main portal vein clot, consists of prominent normal flow direction (hepatopetal) portal collaterals (Fig.

(text continues on page 157)

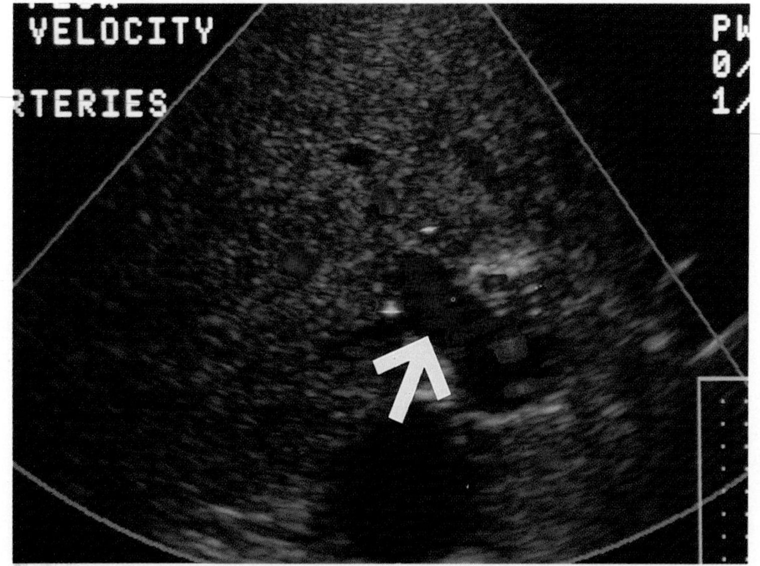

FIG. 2.129. Flow reversal in right portal vein. Transverse color Doppler sonogram of the right portal vein shows flow reversal (*arrow,* coded blue). This was the only abnormal finding in a patient with an otherwise normal grayscale examination. Detecting portal flow reversal (hepatofugal flow) allowed a diagnosis of severe portal hypertension in the face of a normal grayscale exam. Normally, blood in the right portal vein should be coded red, flowing out toward the periphery of the liver.

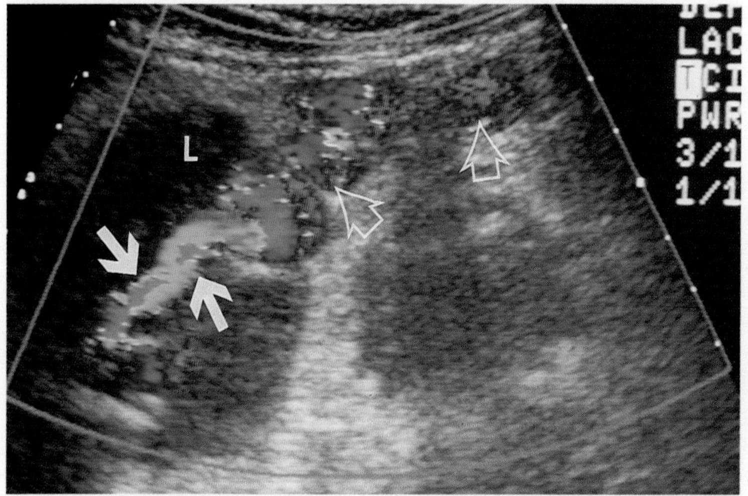

FIG. 2.130. Portal collateral, recanalized periumbilical vein. Longitudinal color Doppler sonogram of left lobe of the liver (L). The tortuous, twisting hepatofugal flow in the recanalized periumbilical vein (*arrows*) is the most common type of portosystemic collateral detected with color Doppler sonography. Coronary vein collaterals leading to esophageal varices are more frequent, but they are also more difficult to detect sonographically. The recanalized periumbilical vein feeds superficial peritoneal collaterals (*open arrows*).

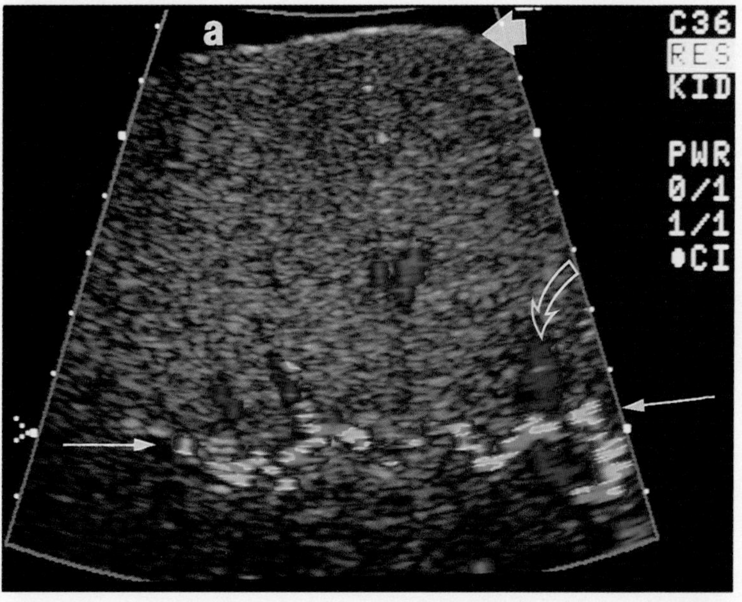

FIG. 2.131. "Corkscrew" artery, cirrhosis. Transverse sonogram through the right lobe of the liver reveals a tortuous, twisting, aliased corkscrew appearing artery (*thin arrows*). Note the flow reversal in the portal venous branch (*open curved arrow*) adjacent to the artery. This color flow sonography finding is similar to angiographic findings in cirrhosis. Note the nodular liver surface (*arrow*) and ascites (a).

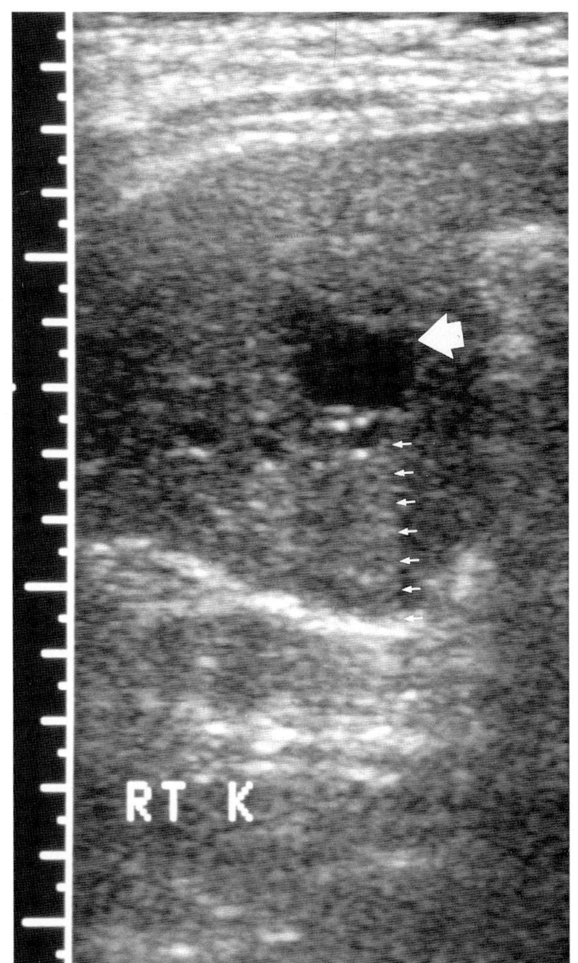

A

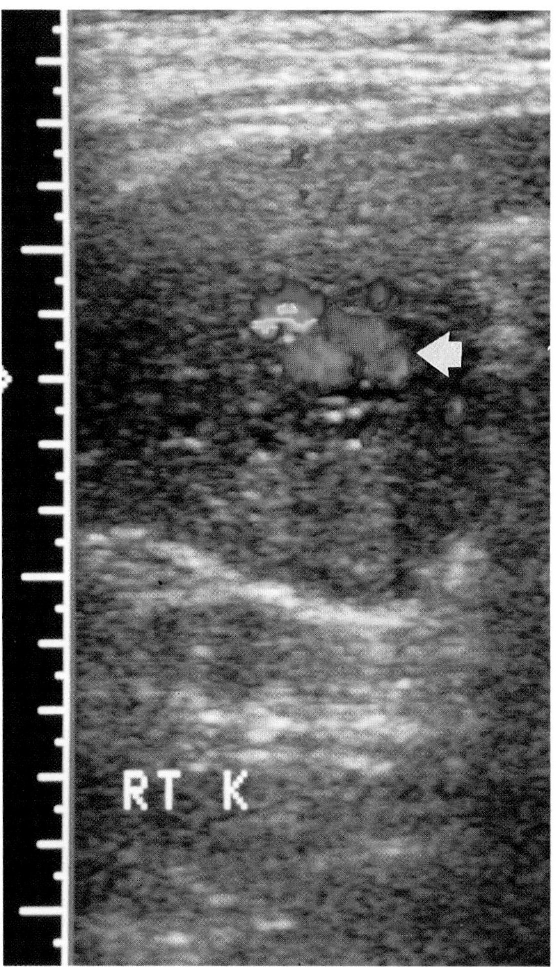

B

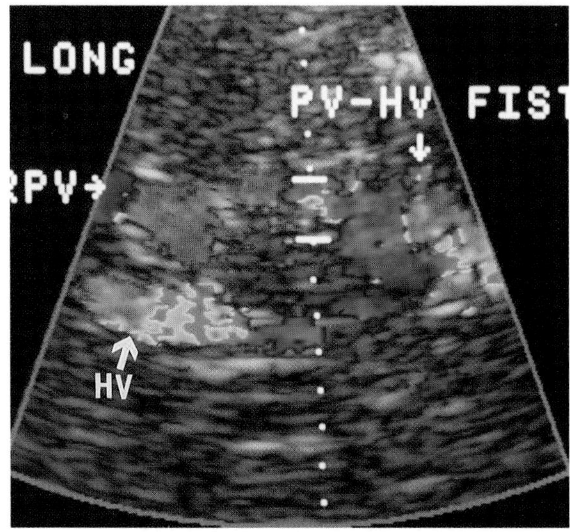

C

FIG. 2.132. Portal venous to hepatic venous malformation. **A:** Transverse sonogram through the right lobe of the liver reveals a hypoechoic lesion (*arrow*) that has through transmission deep to it (*tiny arrows*). This patient was referred for possible aspiration and drainage of an abscess. **B:** Color Doppler sonography of the same areas reveals that this is a vascular malformation. **C:** An oblique longitudinal color Doppler sonogram demonstrates a communication between the right portal vein (RPV) and the hepatic venous (HV) system—a portal venous to hepatic venous fistula. Color Doppler sonography should always be performed before hypoechoic lesions are aspirated. RT K, right kidney.

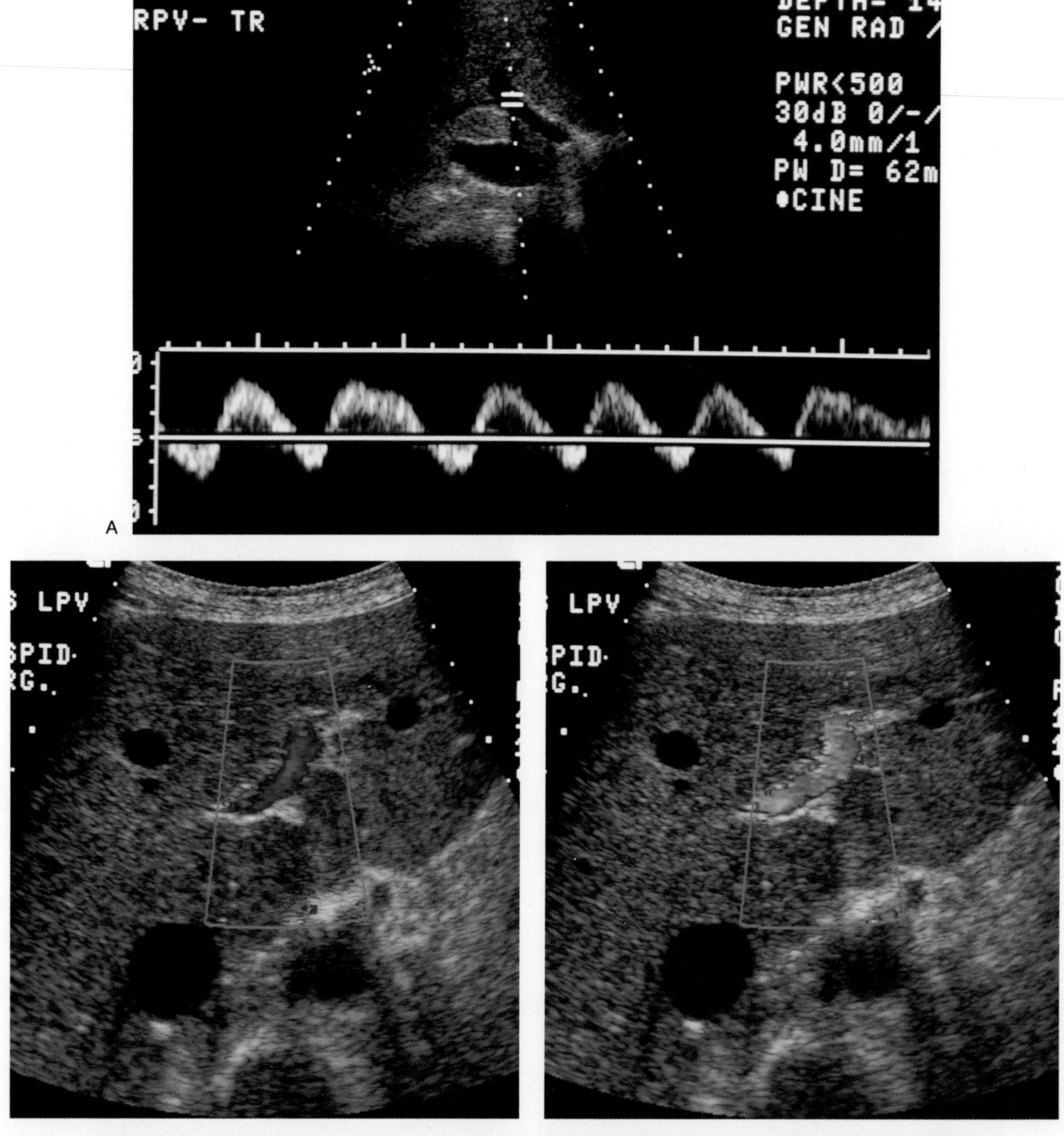

FIG. 2.133. Phasic portal vein flow, tricuspid regurgitation. Normally, the spectral Doppler flow profile of the portal venous system is uniform and rectangular with minor cardiac and respiratory variation. With tricuspid regurgitation, increased sinusoidal pressure is transmitted back to the portal vein and a striking biphasic spectral Doppler sonogram (**A**) may result. Transient alteration and flow dynamics can also be seen with color Doppler, where, on a color Doppler sonogram (**B**), flow in the left portal vein is reversed (coded blue) at one point of the cardiac cycle. During another phase of the cycle, flow is hepatopetal (coded red) on a color Doppler sonogram (**C**). Doppler sonography is the only imaging modality that can observe and record transient alterations in flow dynamics and pulsatility in real-time without affecting flow patterns.

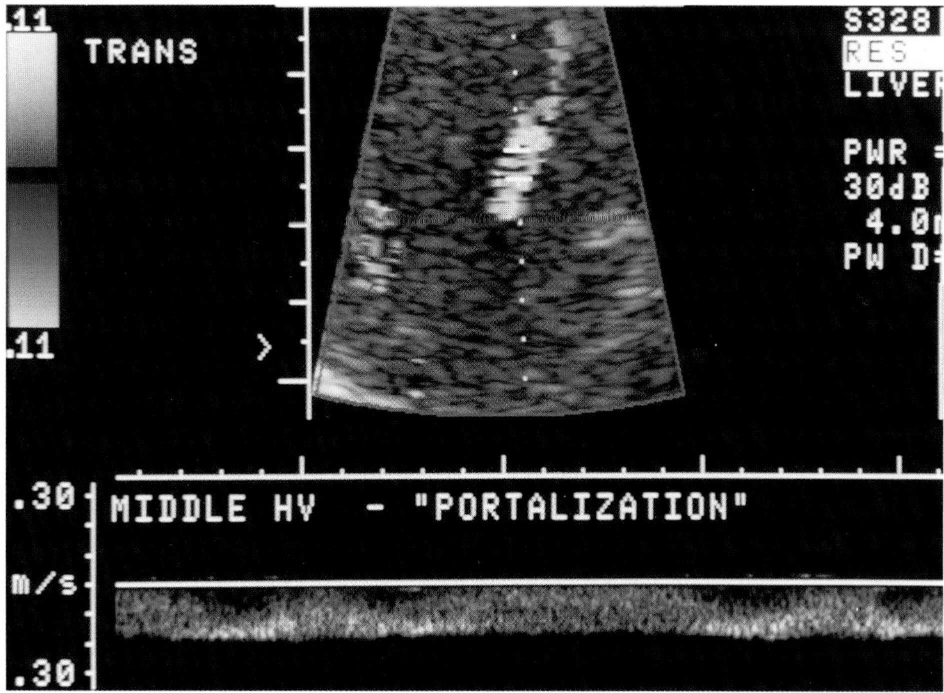

FIG. 2.134. Compressed hepatic vein, "portalized" waveform. Transverse color and spectral Doppler image of the middle hepatic vein reveals a monotonous, relatively aphasic waveform similar to that seen in normal portal veins. Normal hepatic veins reveal a triphasic "W-shaped" waveform. This "portalized" waveform, devoid of the usual triphasic fluctuation, occurs anytime that the hepatic venous flow is shielded from cardiac activity. Hepatic vein compression from mass, cirrhosis, partial thrombosis, hepatic vein valves, or obstruction or narrowing of the inferior vena cava above the level of the hepatic veins can cause this waveform pattern.

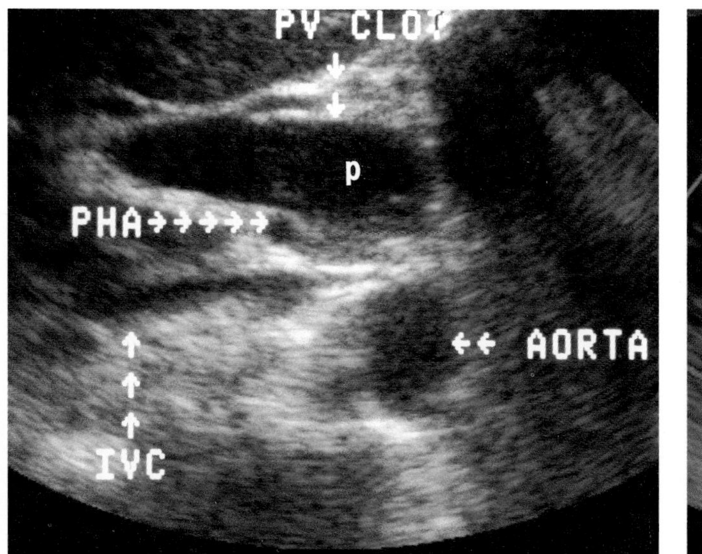

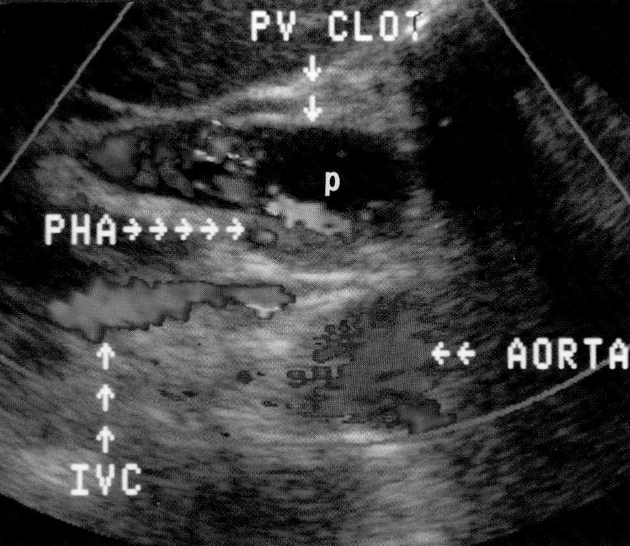

B

FIG. 2.135. Portal vein thrombosis associated with ascending cholangitis. **A**: Longitudinal oblique sonogram of the main portal vein (p) reveals no definite thrombus. **B:** The color Doppler sonogram reveals that there is partial thrombosis of the main portal vein (PV clot). Anechoic thrombus, as is present in this case, is very difficult to diagnose without color Doppler sonography, especially when there is partial thrombosis, as noted here. Anechoic thrombus such as this is fairly common in bland clot. It is rare with neoplastic invasion. PHA, proper hepatic artery; IVC, inferior vena cava; p, portal vein. (From ref. 115, with permission.)

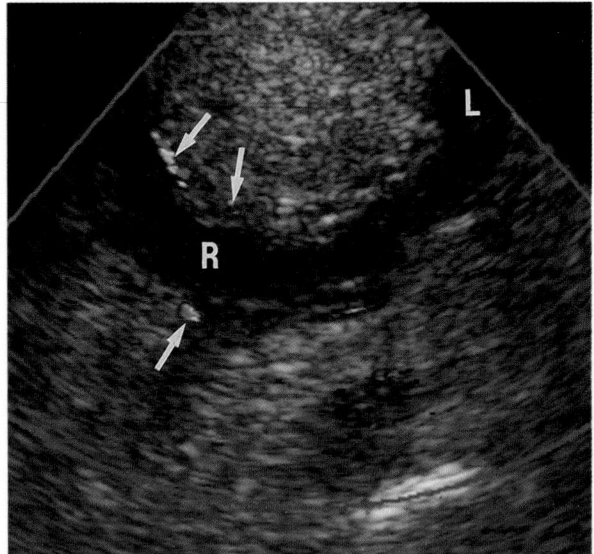

FIG. 2.136. Portal venous thrombosis from acute pancreatitis. Transverse oblique sonogram showing the left (L) and right (R) portal vein. There is complete thrombosis of the portal venous system in this patient with acute pancreatitis. Note the arterial flow adjacent to the right portal vein (*arrows*). Pancreatitis not infrequently causes thrombosis of portions of the portal system, most often by a splenic vein clot. Complete intrahepatic portal venous thrombosis from pancreatitis is rare.

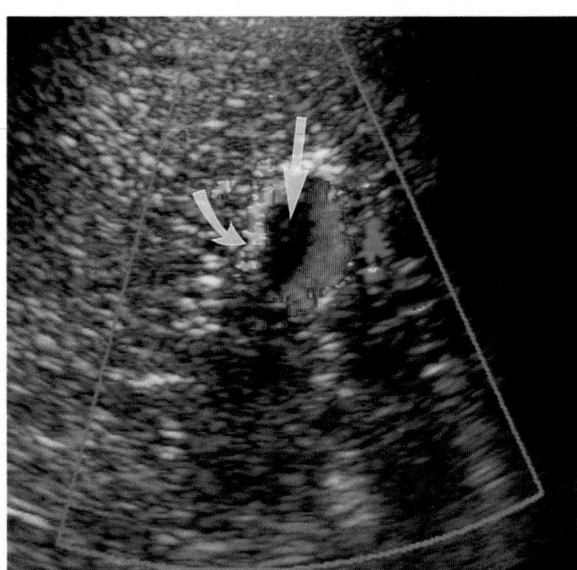

FIG. 2.137. Partial left portal vein clot. Transverse color Doppler sonogram at the level of the left portal vein reveals partial thrombosis (*arrow*) of the left portal vein. Hepatopetal flow is noted adjacent to the anechoic clot (flow coded red). An enlarged hepatic artery (*curved arrow*), presumably representing increased hepatic arterial flow, is noted adjacent to the portal vein. Partial thrombosis is difficult to diagnose without color Doppler sonography. Partial thrombosis is generally missed with spectral Doppler analysis.

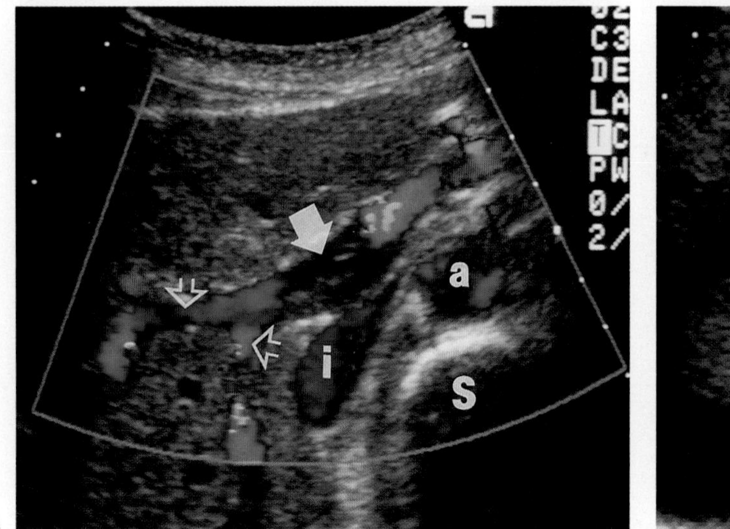

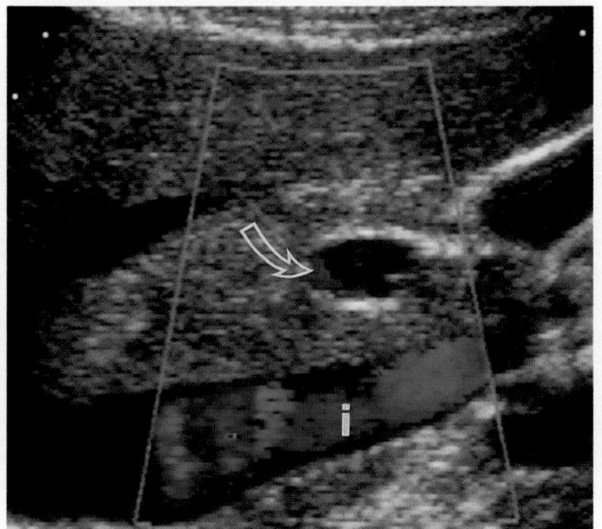

FIG. 2.138. Partial thrombosis, right portal vein. **A:** Transverse color Doppler sonogram at the level of the right portal vein reveals proximal right portal vein clot (*arrow*). Note the persistent portal vein flow (*open arrows*) peripheral to the region of thrombus. **B:** The longitudinal color Doppler sonogram through the region of the thrombus shows a small residual flow channel (*curved open arrow*). Color Doppler sonography is the only practical means to show small persistent flow channels such as the one present here. i, inferior vena cava; a, aorta; S, spine.

2.139). In acute portal vein thrombosis, CFS may reveal small acute hepatopetal portal collaterals, invisible on grayscale sonography. This may be a precursor to cavernous transformation of the portal vein. Gallbladder varices (Fig. 2.140) occur when portal vein thrombosis leads to hepatopetal collaterals involving the gallbladder.

Portal Hypertension

Portal hypertension results when venous obstruction occurs within the liver or in extrahepatic portal veins. Portal hypertension is most commonly caused by cirrhosis and portal vein clot. Other chronic causes include Budd–Chiari syndrome, veno-occlusive disease, schistosomiasis, peliosis hepatitis, chronic active hepatitis, nodular regenerative hyperplasia, and fibrotic noncirrhotic conditions. Idiopathic portal hypertension, often associated with noncirrhotic fibrotic conditions, may occur. Acute portal hypertension may occur with portal vein clot, severe acute hepatitis, alcoholic hepatitis, acute fatty liver of pregnancy, and acute veno-occlusive disease. Acute portal hypertension is often reversible (119).

Detection of portal collaterals may prompt diagnosis of unsuspected portal hypertension or reinforce it when suspected. Demonstration of collaterals is clinically useful in patients with unexplained jaundice, ascites, or upper gastrointestinal bleeding (120,121). Portal collaterals should be sought with CFS, since they may be invisible on grayscale images (Fig. 2.141). Some portosystemic collaterals, such as splenorenal shunts (122) and paraumbilical veins (123), may diminish the risk of hemorrhage from esophageal varices by diverting portal venous blood flow.

The most common collaterals are left gastric (coronary) and paraumbilical veins. Left gastric collaterals, though by far the most prevalent, are often difficult to image because of their deep location. Left gastric (coronary) vein collaterals are best detected by seeking their origin from the splenic (or portal) vein, then following their path cephalad within the lesser omentum (Figs. 2.142 and 2.143) as they run toward the esophagus. Paraumbilical veins are easier to image, as they are superficial. They arise from the ventral tip of the left portal vein and usually flow caudally through the ligamentum teres (Figs. 2.144 and 2.145), where they communicate with superficial peritoneal collaterals (Figs. 2.146 and 2.147). Other types of portal collaterals include retroperitoneal (Fig. 2.148), splenorenal (Fig. 2.149), splenoretroperitoneal (Fig. 2.150), short gastric, omental (Fig. 2.141), and many others (Fig. 2.151).

Normally, blood flows toward the liver (hepatopetal) in portal veins. Reversed (hepatofugal) flow, although often associated with collaterals (115), may be the sole indication of portal hypertension (Fig. 2.129). Other portal flow abnormalities include bidirectional flow and, rarely, nearly static blood flow. Very slow (nearly static) flow cannot be displayed with Doppler techniques. Differentiation from clot may be difficult in this rare situation. Bidirectional phasic flow represents a near equilibrium between hepatopetal and reversed flow. Eating causes increased portal venous flow. Thus reversed flow may become hepatopetal postprandially. Various drugs that increase portal flow may also convert reversed to antegrade flow. Local variations in portal flow can be displayed using CFS (Fig. 2.152).

Therapeutic Portosystemic Shunts

Surgically or transvenously created portosystemic shunts are created to prevent fatal gastrointestinal hemorrhage from bleeding esophageal varices or, occasionally, to decompress varices in other locations. Common surgical shunts include end-to-side portocaval (Fig. 2.153), side-to-side portocaval (Fig. 2.154), and distal splenorenal shunts (Fig. 2.155). CFS often displays surgical shunts (124), even when they are inapparent on preliminary grayscale images. Transjugular intrahepatic portosystemic shunt (TIPS) stents are also easily evaluated by CFS (Fig. 2.156). TIPS stents are performed via a transjugular approach. An expandable wire mesh stent is placed between an hepatic and portal vein, decompressing the hypertensive portal venous system. TIPSs are increasing in popularity because they interfere much less with subsequent liver transplantation than do surgical shunts. CFS is useful in TIPS patients before, after, and sometimes during the procedure.

Shunt thrombosis can be diagnosed reliably only when no anastomotic flow is seen with CFS. Only direct CFS evaluation of the shunt itself should be used to determine patency or thrombosis. Some suggested secondary signs of shunt thrombosis, such as hepatopetal intrahepatic portal flow (120), may be misleading (125). Color flow criteria for clot are described in the Venous Thrombosis section. Rarely, technical problems may result in nonvisualization of flow, even when the shunt is patent.

Arterial and venous abnormalities may result after shunt surgery. With end-to-side portocaval shunts, the intrahepatic portal veins may be patent or clotted. With side-to-side portocaval shunts, pronounced flow reversal in the native left, right, and main portal veins is usual (Fig. 2.154). Since portal blood supply is either nonexistent or net hepatofugal with both of these shunts, enlargement of the hepatic arteries from increased arterial flow is usual. This increased flow can be imaged by CFS (see the Arterialization section) (Fig. 2.157). Side-to-side shunts often result in intrahepatic portal blood flow that varies with respiration: it may be hepatopetal, static, or hepatofugal. Distal splenorenal shunts usually cause less

(text continues on page 168)

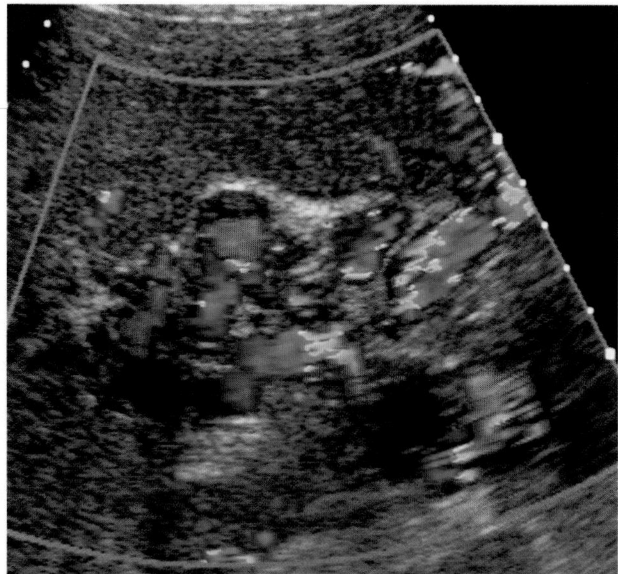

FIG. 2.139. Cavernous transformation of the portal vein. Longitudinal oblique color Doppler sonogram through the region of the hepatoduodenal ligament. No normal portal vein is identified in this patient. Instead, multiple dilated tortuous collateral veins are present, representing cavernous transformation of the portal vein. Cavernous transformation (cavernoma) results when the native portal vein is occluded and blood must find its way to the liver via collaterals. With time, the initially small collaterals become much larger, resulting in a chaotic, tangled mass, as noted here.

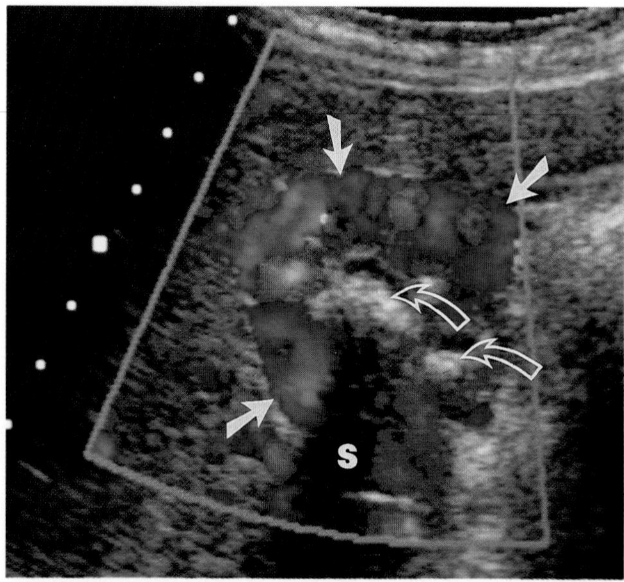

FIG. 2.140. Gallbladder varices. Transverse sonogram through the region of the gallbladder fossa. The entire wall of the gallbladder is replaced by dilated variceal vessels (*slant tailed arrows*). Note the gallstones (*open curved arrows*) within the gallbladder lumen. Shadowing (s) is noted deep to one of the stones. Gallbladder varices result when portal vein thrombosis occurs and hepatopetal collaterals that pass through the wall of the gallbladder are recruited. One wonders if this is a suitable candidate for laparoscopic cholecystectomy!

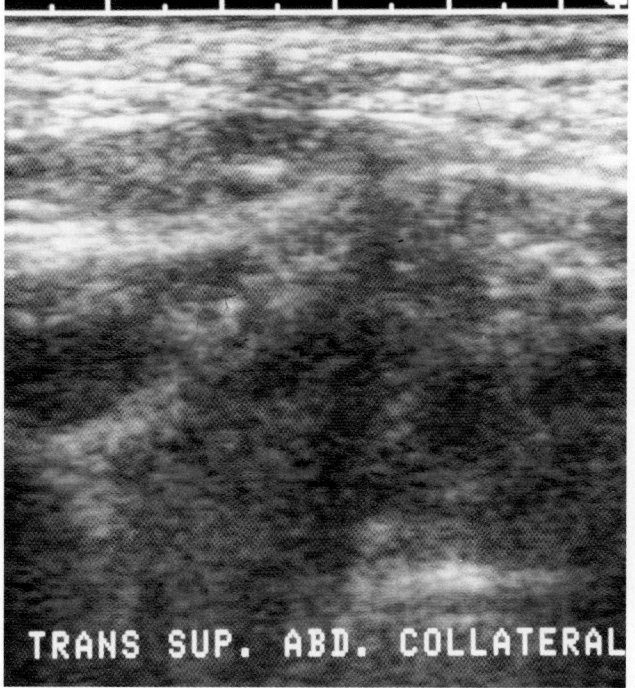

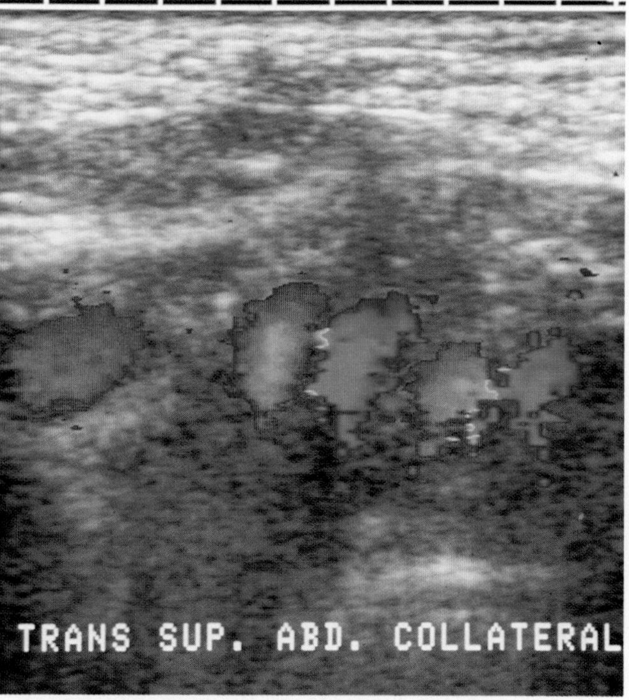

FIG. 2.141. Omental collaterals invisible on grayscale. Transverse high-resolution color and grayscale image pair (**A, B**). These superficial omental collaterals in the right upper abdomen are essentially invisible on the grayscale image (A). When seeking portosystemic collaterals related to portal hypertension, color Doppler should be employed at all times, because occult collaterals such as this would otherwise be missed.

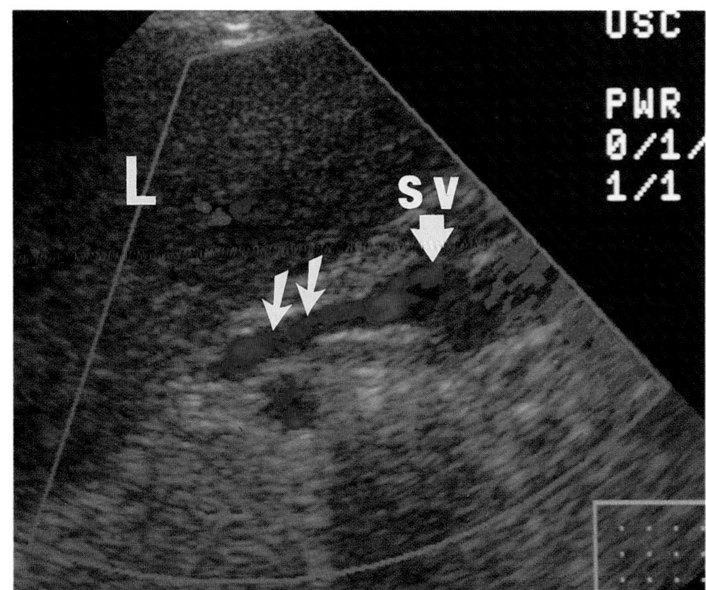

FIG. 2.142. Small coronary vein collateral. Longitudinal color Doppler sonogram in the region of the lesser omentum reveals flow reversal (hepatofugal flow) in a small coronary (left gastric) vein (*twin arrows*). Blood flow is coded blue, flowing away from the splenic vein (SV) toward the gastroesophageal junction (not visualized). If blood were flowing in the usual hepatopetal direction, it would be color coded red (toward the splenic vein) on this image. Virtually all patients with left gastric (coronary) vein flow reversal will have esophageal varices on endoscopy.

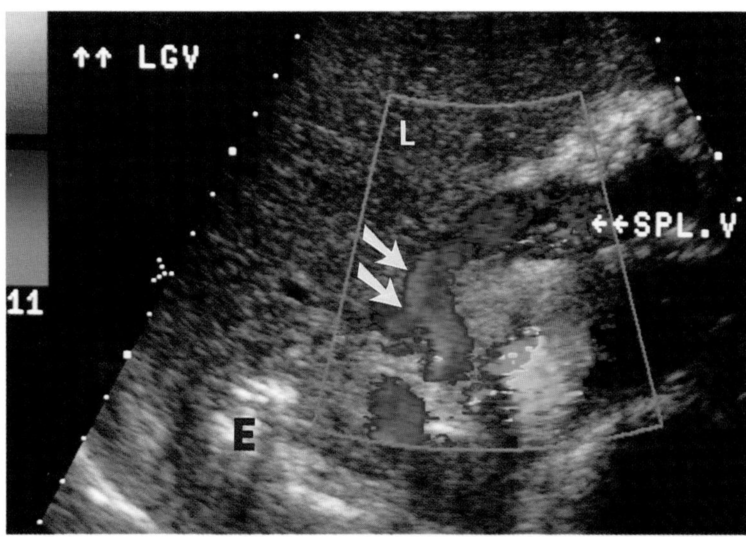

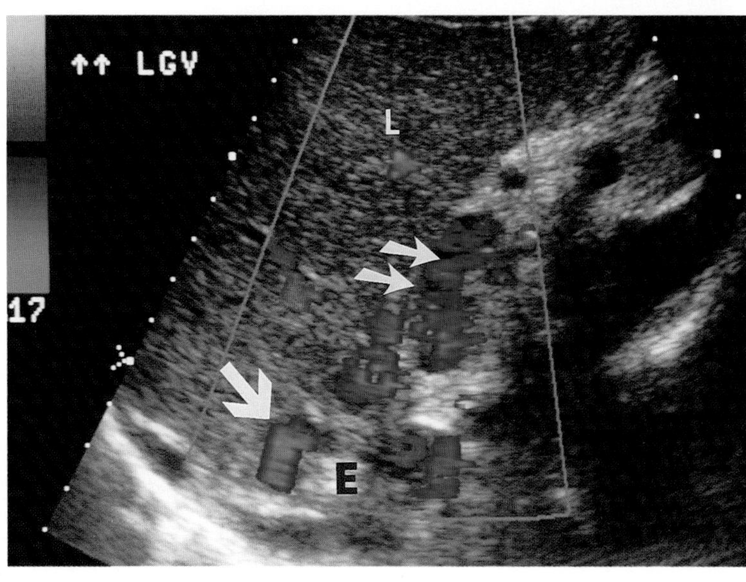

FIG. 2.143. Large coronary vein collateral, esophageal varix. Two longitudinal oblique color Doppler sonograms (**A, B**) in the region of the lesser omentum. A very large tortuous coronary vein collateral (*twin arrows*) is noted. Blood is flowing in a reversed, hepatofugal direction toward the gastroesophageal junction (esophagus, *black E*). An esophageal varix (*block arrow*) in the wall of the esophagus (*black E*) is demonstrated on the second image. It is very unusual to image mural esophageal varices with color flow sonography. Usually, all that can be shown is flow reversal in the coronary vein, not the esophageal varices themselves. Flow reversal in left gastric (coronary) vein is the commonest collateral in portal hypertension. Demonstration of this type of collateral is somewhat technically demanding. LGV, left gastric vein; SPL.V, splenic vein.

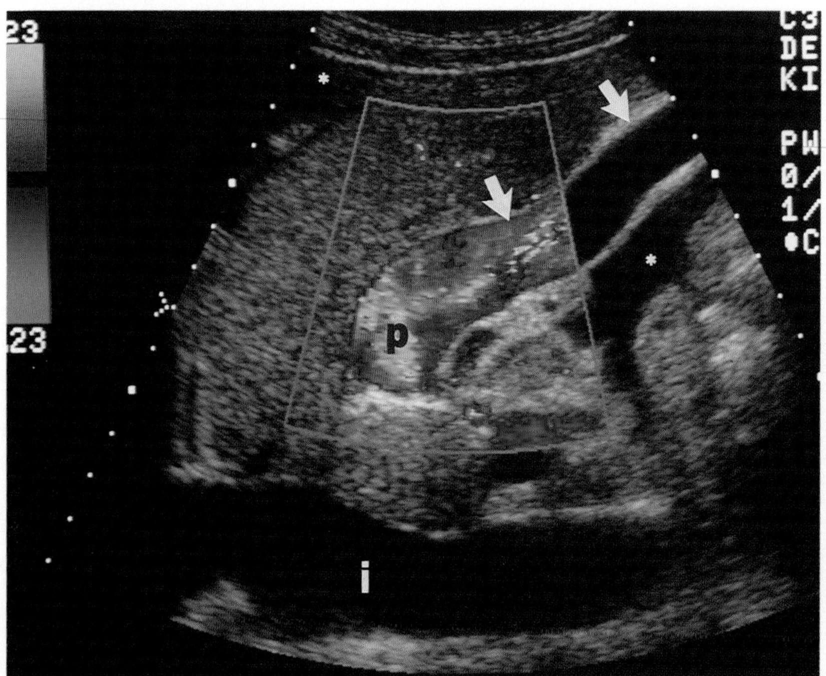

FIG. 2.144. Large paraumbilical vein. Longitudinal color Doppler sonogram at the level of the left portal vein (p) reveals a huge hepatofugal paraumbilical venous collateral (*arrows*). Flow in the vessel is away from the liver and directed caudally to superficial peritoneal collaterals. Paraumbilical veins are easy to image because they arise dorsally from the distal left portal vein, carrying blood away from the liver, usually into superficial peritoneal collaterals that flow caudally toward the umbilicus. Note the exuberant hepatofugal flow within the color flow box. The enlarged vessel is seen extending caudally (*arrows*). Ascites (*) is present. i, inferior vena cava.

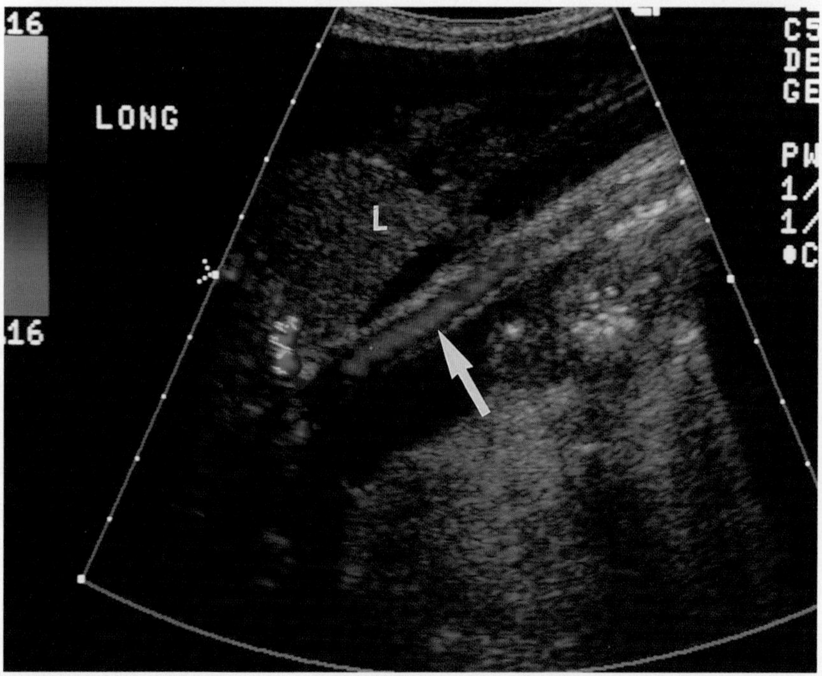

FIG. 2.145. Small paraumbilical vein. A longitudinal color Doppler sonogram reveals a small (3 mm) paraumbilical vein (*arrow*) just dorsal to the irregular left lobe of the liver (L) in this patient with cirrhosis. A large amount of ascites is present.

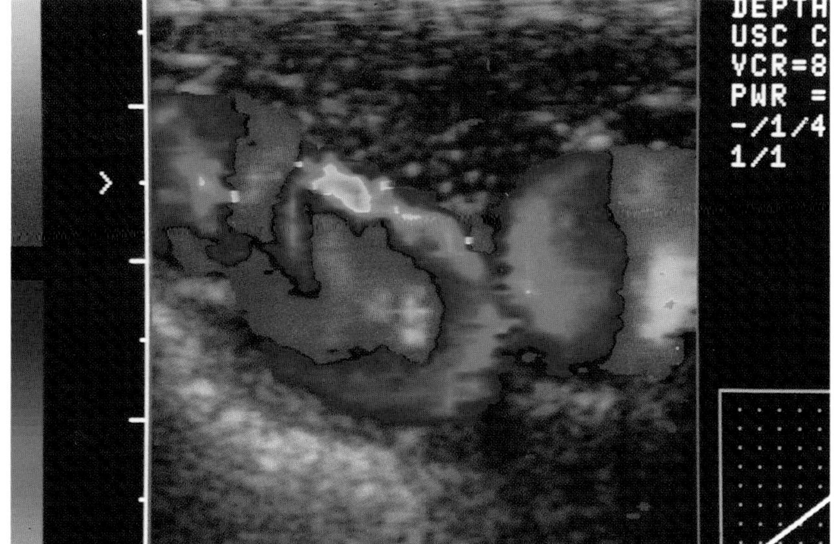

FIG. 2.146. Superficial abdominal collateral. Longitudinal high-resolution sonogram in the upper abdomen reveals a superficial abdominal collateral in a patient with hepatofugal flow via a recanalized paraumbilical vein. Note the swirling flow within this twisted, tortuous collateral. In patients with paraumbilical veins, flow typically communicates with superficial peritoneal collaterals such as this. Collateral flow then proceeds caudally, where ramifying collaterals are often found around the umbilicus. Subsequently, blood flows in superficial lower abdominal collaterals to the inferior epigastric vein or into pelvic collaterals. Other pathways of collateralization occur, but more rarely (see Fig. 2.147).

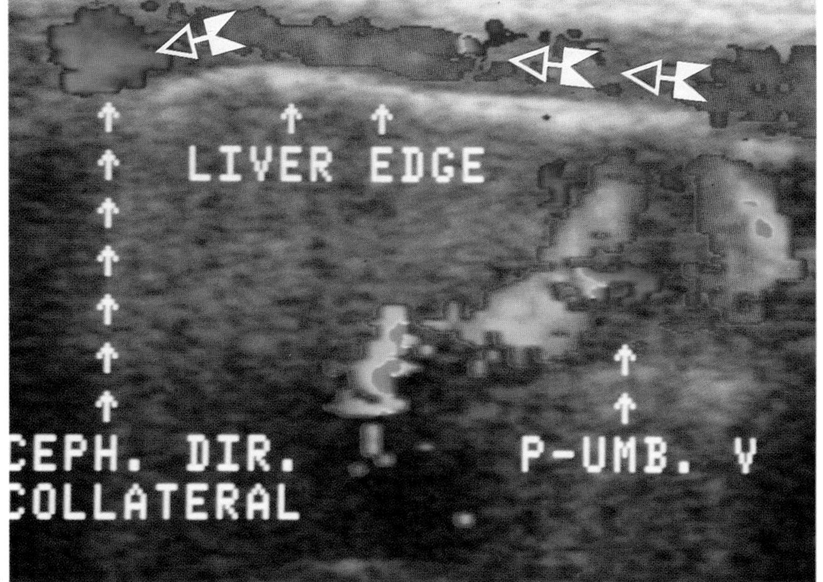

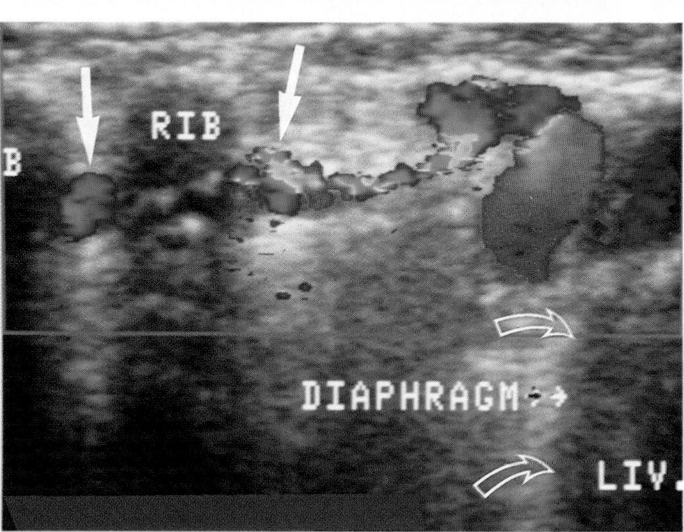

FIG. 2.147. Paraumbilical vein with collaterals to internal mammary veins. An unusual collateral pathway from an enlarged paraumbilical vein is demonstrated in this patient. **A:** The longitudinal color Doppler sonogram in the region of the left lobe of the liver demonstrates hepatofugal flow via a paraumbilical vein (P-UMB.V). Slightly caudal to this image, the collateral turned back on itself and blood flowing cephalad in a collateral anterior (ventral) to the liver edge was detected (Ceph. dir. collateral). The direction of blood flow in this collateral is indicated by the *tailed arrows*. **B:** A longitudinal color Doppler sonogram, cephalad to (A), in the region of the lower thorax allows us to follow this collateral cephalad. Note that the diaphragm (*curved open arrows*) and liver (LIV) are at the caudal (right) edge of this image. The collateral communicated with internal mammary vessels that can be seen adjacent to the ribs (*arrows*). Hepatofugal flow via paraumbilical veins is generally directed caudally. Cephalad directed collaterals from paraumbilical veins are occasionally present, as in this case.

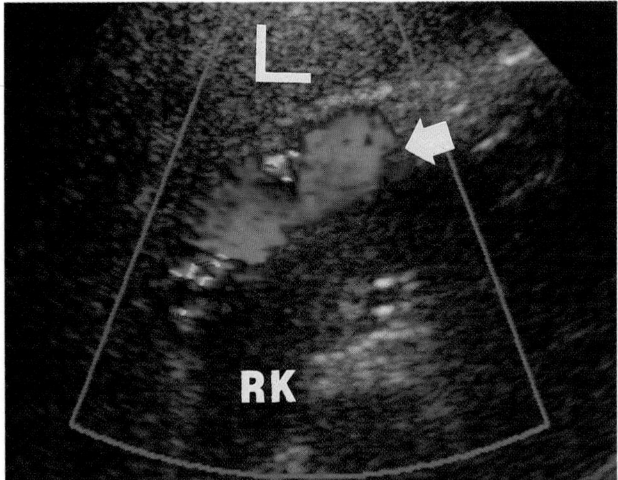

FIG. 2.148. Retroperitoneal collateral, Morison's pouch. Longitudinal color Doppler sonogram in the right upper abdomen reveals a prominent retroperitoneal collateral (*arrow*) in the region of Morison's pouch. This collateral was thought to represent a fluid collection in the subhepatic space on the grayscale real-time image, before color Doppler was performed. Aspiration and drainage of a suspected abscess had been requested in this patient. It is prudent to perform color Doppler in all anechoic "fluid collections" prior to aspiration. Retroperitoneal collaterals such as this one are often hard to identify when more centrally located, as they tend to be obscured by gas. L, liver; RK, right kidney.

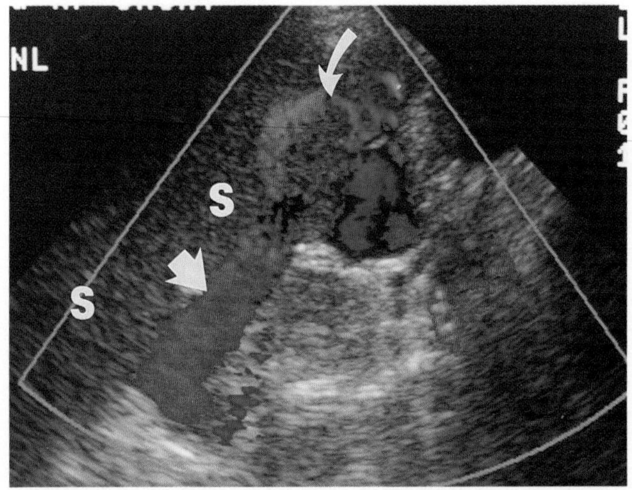

FIG. 2.149. Splenorenal shunt, splenic vein flow reversal. Longitudinal coronal color Doppler sonogram performed through the left flank reveals a splenorenal shunt. The patient's left flank is at the top of the image and the bottom of the image is medial. Blood flow is reversed in the splenic vein (*arrow*) coded red. Normal splenic vein flow direction would be toward the midline (coded blue). A splenorenal shunt (*curved arrow*) is present. Enlargement of the left renal vein (not shown) and some associated retroperitoneal collaterals (also not shown) were noted. Splenorenal and splenoretroperitoneal shunts are not unusual. Most splenorenal and splenoretroperitoneal collaterals are not associated with flow reversal in the splenic vein. S, spleen. (From ref. 115, with permission.)

A

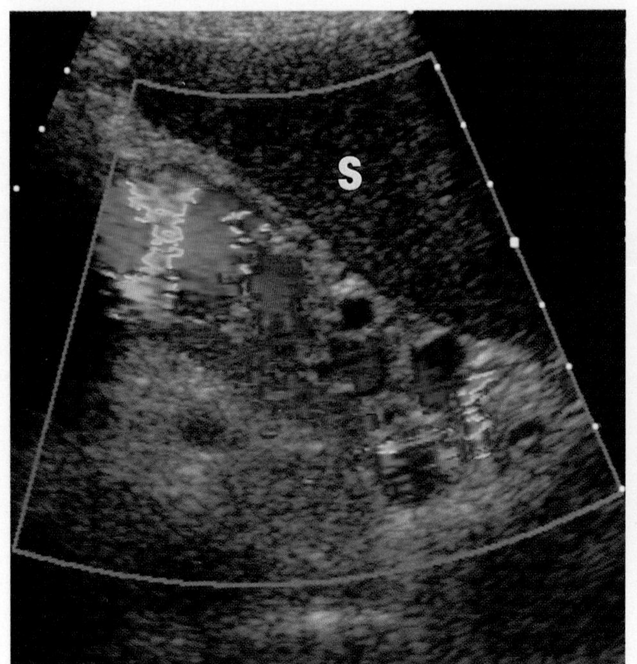

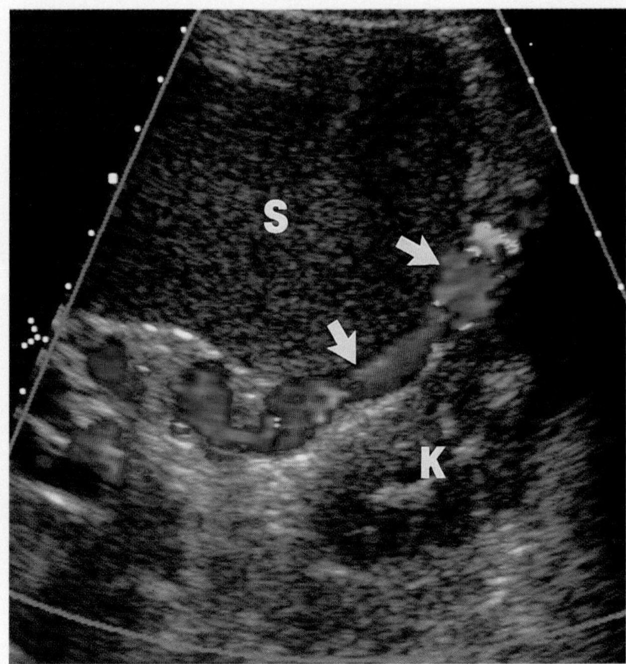

B

FIG. 2.150. Splenoretroperitoneal and flank collaterals. Transverse color Doppler sonogram (**A**) reveals tangled splenoretroperitoneal collaterals medial to the spleen (S). This patient also had collaterals extending to the flank lateral to the spleen (not shown). These collaterals were fed by the vessels shown on the longitudinal coronal color Doppler sonogram (**B**). This collateral (*arrows*) flows between the spleen (S) and left kidney (K).

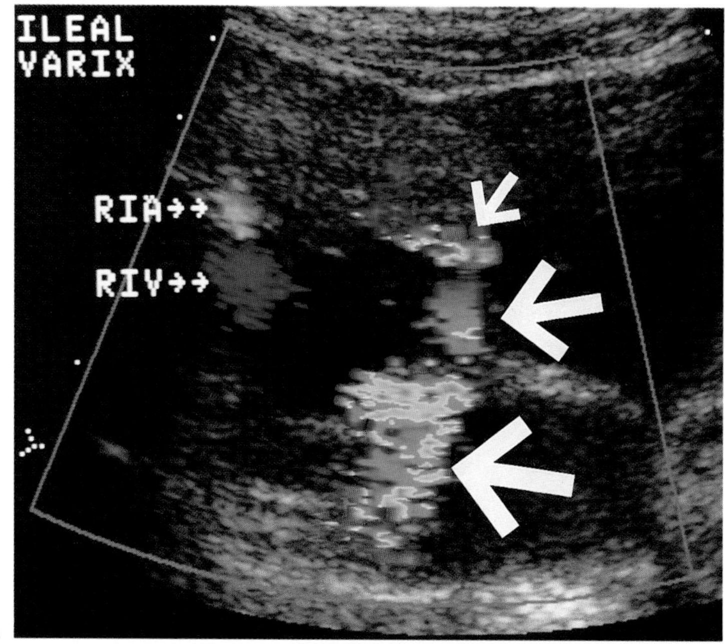

A

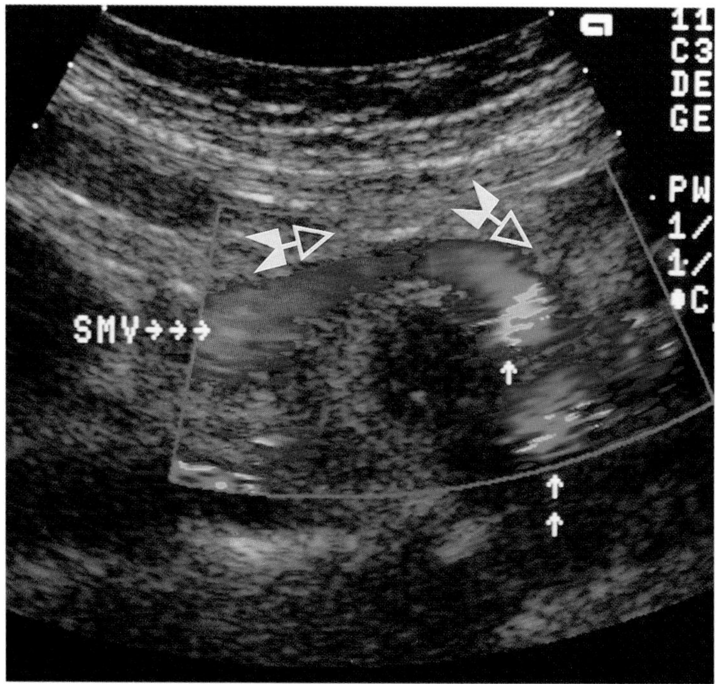

B

FIG. 2.151. Varices of the ileum, causing gastrointestinal (GI) hemorrhage. This patient had GI bleeding, the source of which could not be detected with upper or lower endoscopy or contrast GI studies. **A:** A transverse right lower quadrant color Doppler sonogram revealed enlarged abnormal variceal masses (*arrows*) associated with the ileum. Note the internal iliac artery (RIA) and vein (RIV) lateral to the variceal collaterals. **B:** Longitudinal color Doppler sonogram demonstrated flow reversal in the superior mesenteric vein (SMV), feeding the right lower quadrant varices (*small arrows*). The reverse flow direction in the SMV is indicated by the *tailed arrows*. While GI bleeding caused by portal hypertension and portosystemic collaterals generally originates from esophageal varices, varices in other locations occasionally cause bleeding. This patient was successfully treated with a TIPS procedure and direct embolization of the varices. Follow-up color Doppler sonogram showed diminished, but not completely obliterated, varices (not shown).

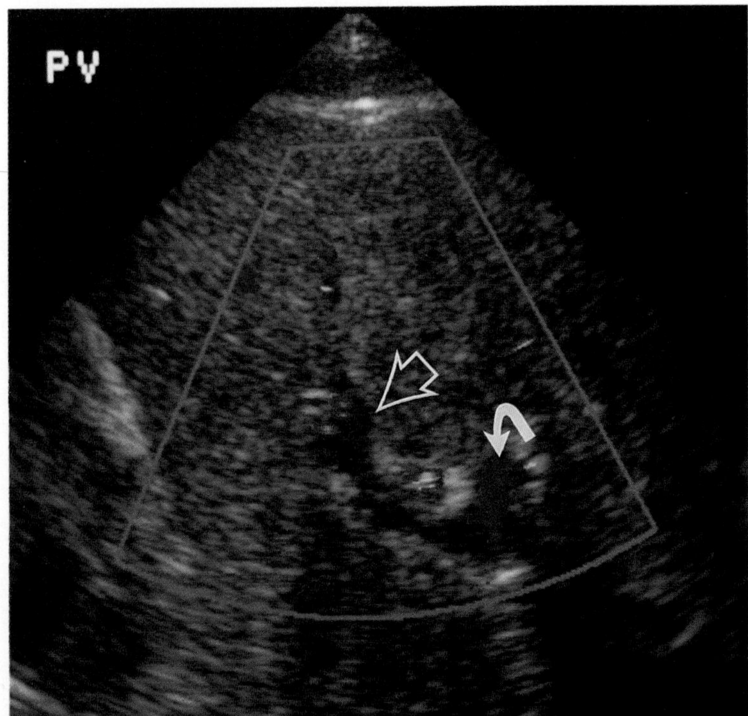

FIG. 2.152. Local portal venous flow variations. Transverse color Doppler sonogram of the right portal vein reveals different direction flow in two right portal venous branches. In one area, flow is hepatopetal (correct direction) (coded red, *curved arrow*). In a nearby area, flow direction is reversed (coded blue, *open arrow*). Color flow sonography is the only imaging modality capable of showing local flow conditions in such fine detail. Another unique ability is color flow sonography's ability to depict flow in real-time.

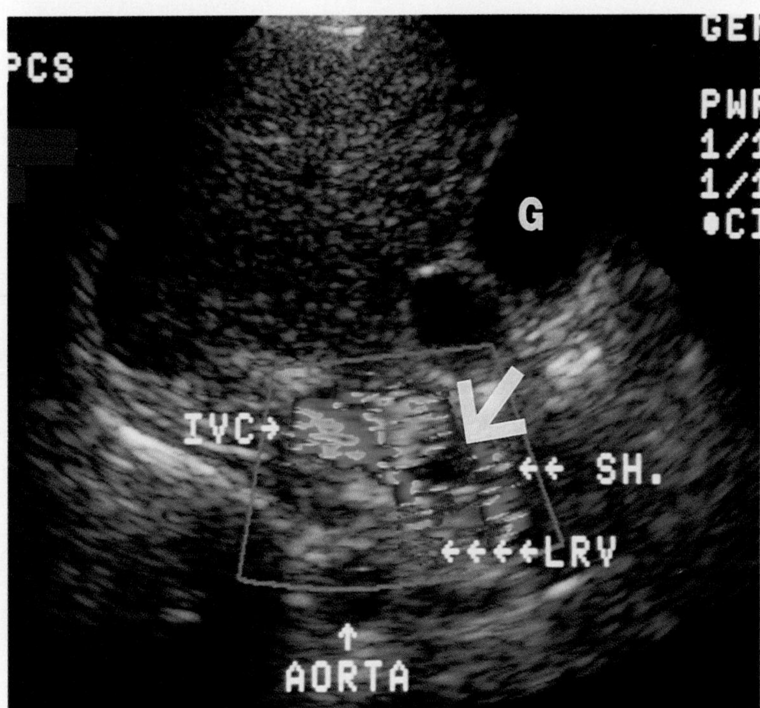

FIG. 2.153. Patient end-to-side portocaval shunt. Transverse upper abdominal color Doppler sonogram with the patient in a right anterior oblique (RAO) position reveals a patent end-to-side portocaval shunt (SH). The anastomosis with the inferior vena cava (IVC) is indicated (*arrow*). End-to-side portocaval shunts, performed to prevent fatal hemorrhage from esophageal varices, are formed by transecting the portal vein and sewing its end directly into the inferior vena cava. As the anastomosis is often close to the level of the left renal vein (LRV), it is important to identify the left renal vein separate from the portal vein. Only direct visualization of the anastomosis should be considered adequate to evaluate whether the shunt is patent or not. Indirect signs, such as flow in the vessels near the shunt, may be misleading.

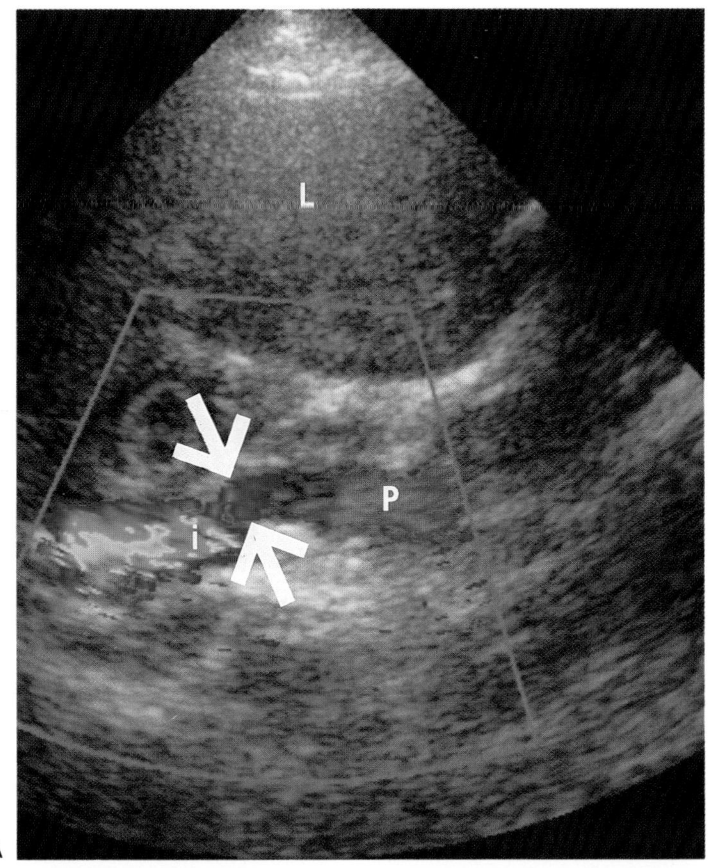

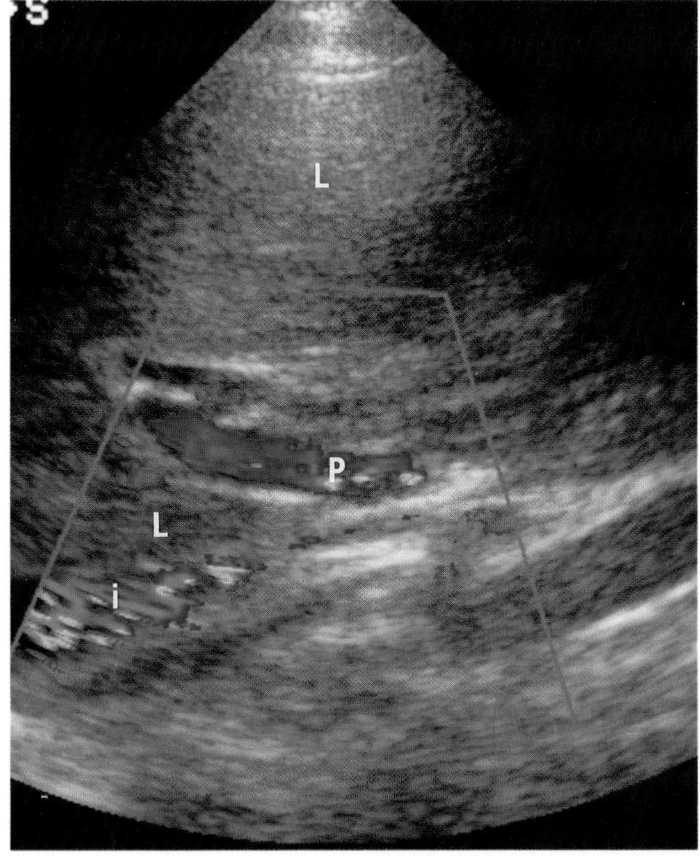

FIG. 2.154. Side-to-side portocaval shunt. In side-to-side portocaval shunts, decompression of portal hypertension is achieved by opening a window of communication between the portal vein and inferior vena cava (side-to-side anastomosis). **A:** A transverse oblique color Doppler sonogram reveals the location of the side-to-side anastomosis (*arrows*) between the portal vein (P) and the inferior vena cava (i). **B:** A longitudinal oblique color Doppler sonogram reveals flow reversal (coded blue) within the main portal vein (P). Typically, after side-to-side shunt, the main portal vein becomes an outflow tract through which portal venous blood drains from the liver into the inferior vena cava (i). L, liver.

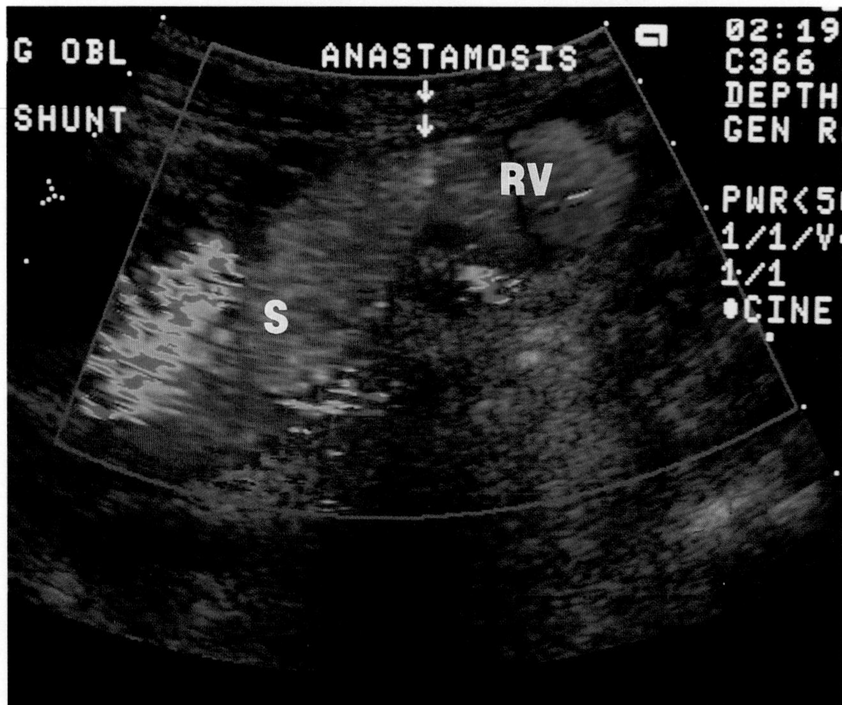

FIG. 2.155. Patent distal splenorenal shunt. Longitudinal oblique color Doppler sonogram in the left upper abdomen reveals a patent splenorenal shunt. The anastomosis is indicated by the small arrows. In this type of shunt, the splenic vein (S) is connected with the left renal vein (RV). This is the most difficult shunt to visualize with color flow sonography as GI gas sometimes intervenes. Persistence and the use of multiple scan planes generally allow visualization of the anastomosis.

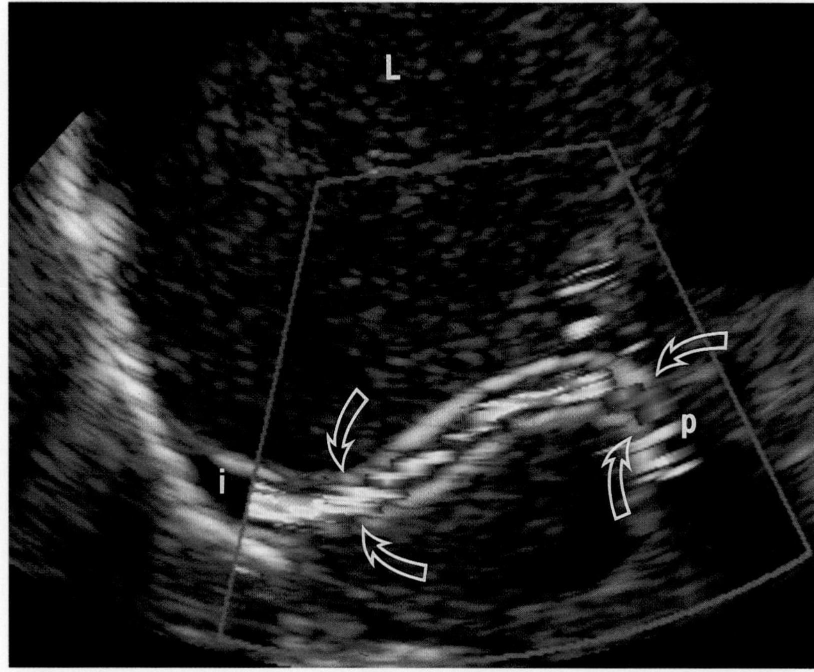

FIG. 2.156. Patent TIPS stent. Transverse oblique color Doppler sonogram reveals color-coded flow through a patent stent. The ends of the echogenic wire mesh stent are shown by the *curved open arrows*. Blood is flowing from the portal venous system (p) through a hepatic vein into the inferior vena cava (i). Visualization of flow within the wire mesh often requires low-frequency transducers and meticulous attention to scanning at a low angle. Color flow sonography can be useful in evaluating patients with TIPS stents before, after, and even during the procedure. L, liver.

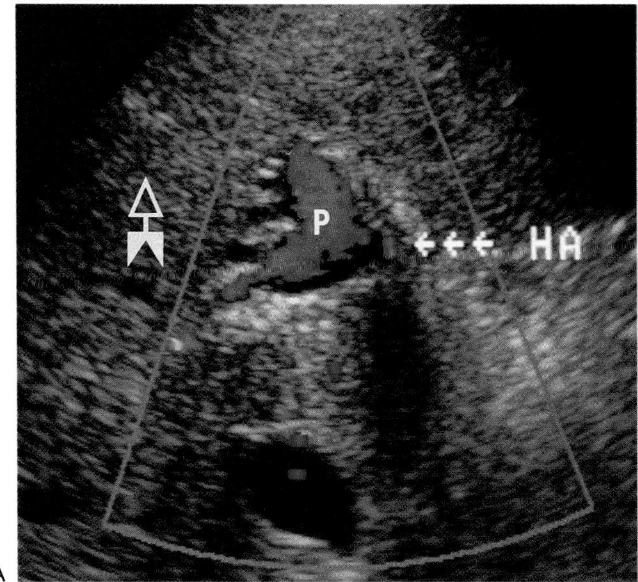

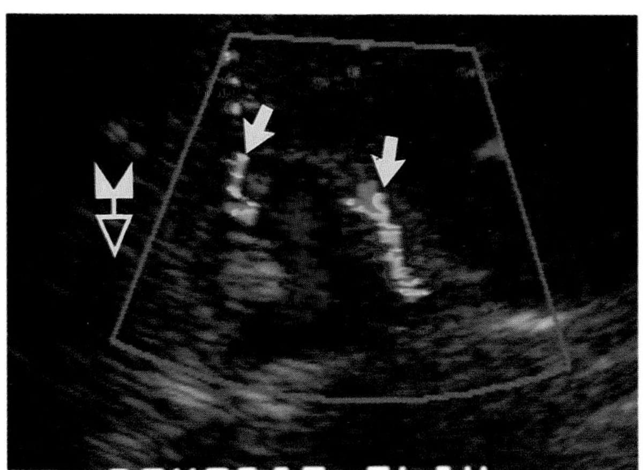

A B

FIG. 2.157. Enlarged hepatic arteries after portocaval shunt. **A**: Transverse sonogram of the left portal vein performed 1 day before an end-to-side portocaval shunt reveals normal direction flow in the left portal vein (p). Flow direction is indicated by the *tailed arrow*. Several normal sized hepatic arteries (HA) are present. **B:** Three days later, after the end-to-side portocaval shunt had been performed, flow direction is now reversed (coded blue). Flow direction is indicated by the *tailed arrow*. Note the prominent enlargement and aliased flow now present in the hepatic arteries (*arrows*). Enlargement of the hepatic arteries (arterialization) occurs when portal blood flow is interrupted, as occurred here when the end-to-side portocaval shunt was performed. Increased flow with enlarged arteries may also occur when portal blood flow is net hepatofugal because of portosystemic collaterals.

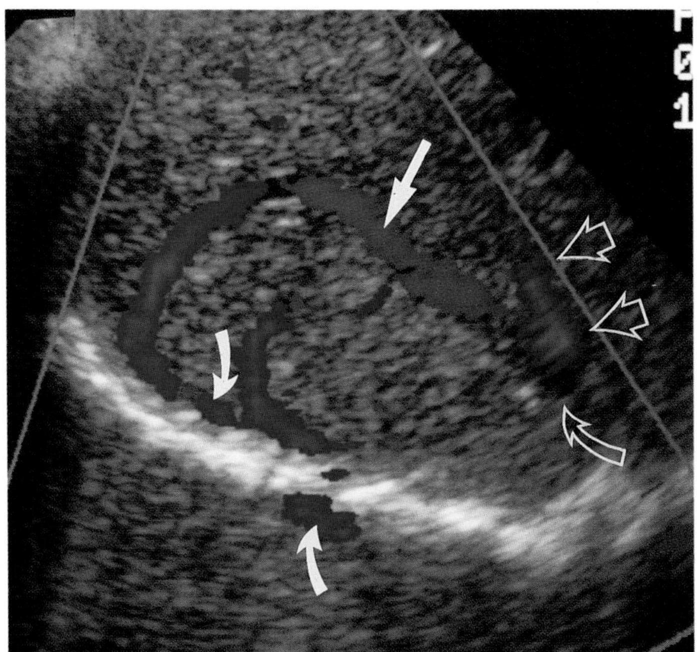

FIG. 2.158. Budd–Chiari syndrome, capsular systemic collaterals. This transverse oblique sonogram reveals normal direction flow in a hepatic vein (*open arrows*) that is interrupted (*curved open arrow*) before it reaches the inferior vena cava. Flow in this vein is coded blue. A hepatic venous collateral (*arrow*) leads to systemic capsular veins (*curved arrows*), through which this patient's hepatic venous blood is exiting the liver. The red and blue coded V-shaped hepatic vein configuration, representing the normal flow direction of the hepatic vein and reverse flow direction of the hepatic venous collateral, is a typical finding in Budd–Chiari syndrome. (From ref. 128, with permission.)

pronounced portal venous and arterial changes. Native portal thrombosis and increased arterial flow occur less frequently with this type of shunt.

Increased Hepatic Artery Flow: Arterialization

As portal venous flow to the liver decreases, hepatic arterial flow increases (122,123,126), presumably as a homeostatic mechanism to maintain hepatic perfusion. Increased arterial flow may be very pronounced when there is (a) clot or surgical interruption of the main portal vein (Fig. 2.157) or (b) more blood exiting the liver via portal veins than entering (net hepatofugal portal flow). In some cirrhotics, this may result in a "corkscrew" artery pattern (Fig. 2.131). Net hepatofugal portal flow is usually caused by large collaterals or large portosystemic shunts.

In this setting, color flow imaging reveals a striking arterial pattern: conspicuously enlarged hepatic arteries with a high-velocity, aliased (chaotic, mixed colors flow) appearance, referred to as "arterialization" of the hepatic blood supply. Arterialization is only observed occasionally in cirrhosis, since portal blood flow remains nearly normal until cirrhosis is advanced (123,127).

Other conditions may result in arterial enlargement. Inflammation related to chronic active hepatitis (Fig. 2.117) or alcoholic hepatitis (Fig. 2.118), or intrahepatic AV shunting (e.g., neoplasms, hereditary hemorrhagic telangiectasia) may result in hepatic arterial enlargement. Color flow findings in these conditions are usually less striking than the increased arterial flow caused by portal flow abnormalities.

Budd–Chiari Syndrome

The Budd–Chiari syndrome (BCS) is a rare condition that is characterized by obstruction or stenosis of the hepatic veins, sometimes accompanied by stenosis or obstruction of the inferior vena cava. Obstruction may be primary—caused by webs or membranes (more common in Asia)—or secondary—caused by hypercoagulable conditions (polycythemia rubra vera, sickle cell disease, etc.), trauma, neoplasm, medications, pregnancy, and other conditions. The cause cannot be determined in the majority (as many as 70 percent) of patients. Clinical features of BCS are quite variable and most often include ascites (93 percent), hepatomegaly (70 percent), and pain, edema, and superficial abdominal collateral veins (about 55 percent each) (128).

Since blood entering the liver cannot exit via the hepatic veins, collateral pathways are recruited: portal vein collaterals via enlarged paraumbilical veins, reversed hepatic venous flow to systemic veins (via capsular veins) (Fig. 2.158), and intrahepatic hepatic venous (HV) to hepatic venous collaterals ("spider web" collaterals) (Fig. 2.159) (128).

Grayscale findings in BCS include hepatic venous abnormalities: absence, stenosis, dilatation, irregularity, and abnormal or absent junction with the IVC (Fig. 2.159). The IVC may itself be occluded or stenosed. Less specific changes include parenchymal inhomogeneity (Fig. 2.160) or caudate hypertrophy and atrophy/enlargement of the other lobes and segments. Absent or reversed hepatic venous flow and intrahepatic HV to HV "spider web" collaterals (Fig. 2.159) are diagnostic of BCS. A flat HV waveform, lacking the normal phasic fluctuation, indicates HV compression—a finding that, though nonspecific, supports the diagnosis of BCS. Color Doppler Sonography (CDS) allows reliable and confident identification of irregular or compressed hepatic veins (Fig. 2.161), demonstrates flow reversal, and clearly displays collaterals (128). All these findings are easy to miss with conventional Doppler sonography and other imaging modalities.

Hepatic Veno-occlusive Disease

Hepatic veno-occlusive disease most often occurs in patients after bone marrow transplantation and, rarely, other conditions. It results in fibrous obliteration of microscopic central hepatic lobular venules (terminal hepatic venules). Sonographic findings are nonspecific secondary changes related to the microscopic venular occlusion. These findings, not universally present, include thickened gallbladder wall, abnormal or reversed portal venous flow (129), and increased hepatic artery peripheral resistance (as measured by resistive index, RI) (130).

Hereditary Hemorrhagic Telangiectasia

Hereditary hemorrhagic telangiectasia (HHT), also known as Osler–Weber–Rendu disease, is a rare autosomal dominant condition characterized by telangiectases, arteriovenous fistulas, and aneurysms involving the skin and mucosa, as well as blood vessels of the lung, liver, and central nervous system. The most common clinical manifestations are epistaxis (78 percent) and gastrointestinal bleeding (44 percent). AV shunting leads to hepatic congestion. Congestive heart failure may occur (131,132).

Grayscale findings in HHT include enlarged hepatic arteries and increased echogenicity from fatty infiltration (133) or cirrhosis. CFS (134) reveals enlarged, tortuous, arteries with high-velocity, aliased flow (Fig. 2.162). CFS clarifies the potentially confusing grayscale appearance that may mimic biliary dilatation. Visualization of the actual hepatic AV fistulas probably depends on their size

(*text continues on page 171*)

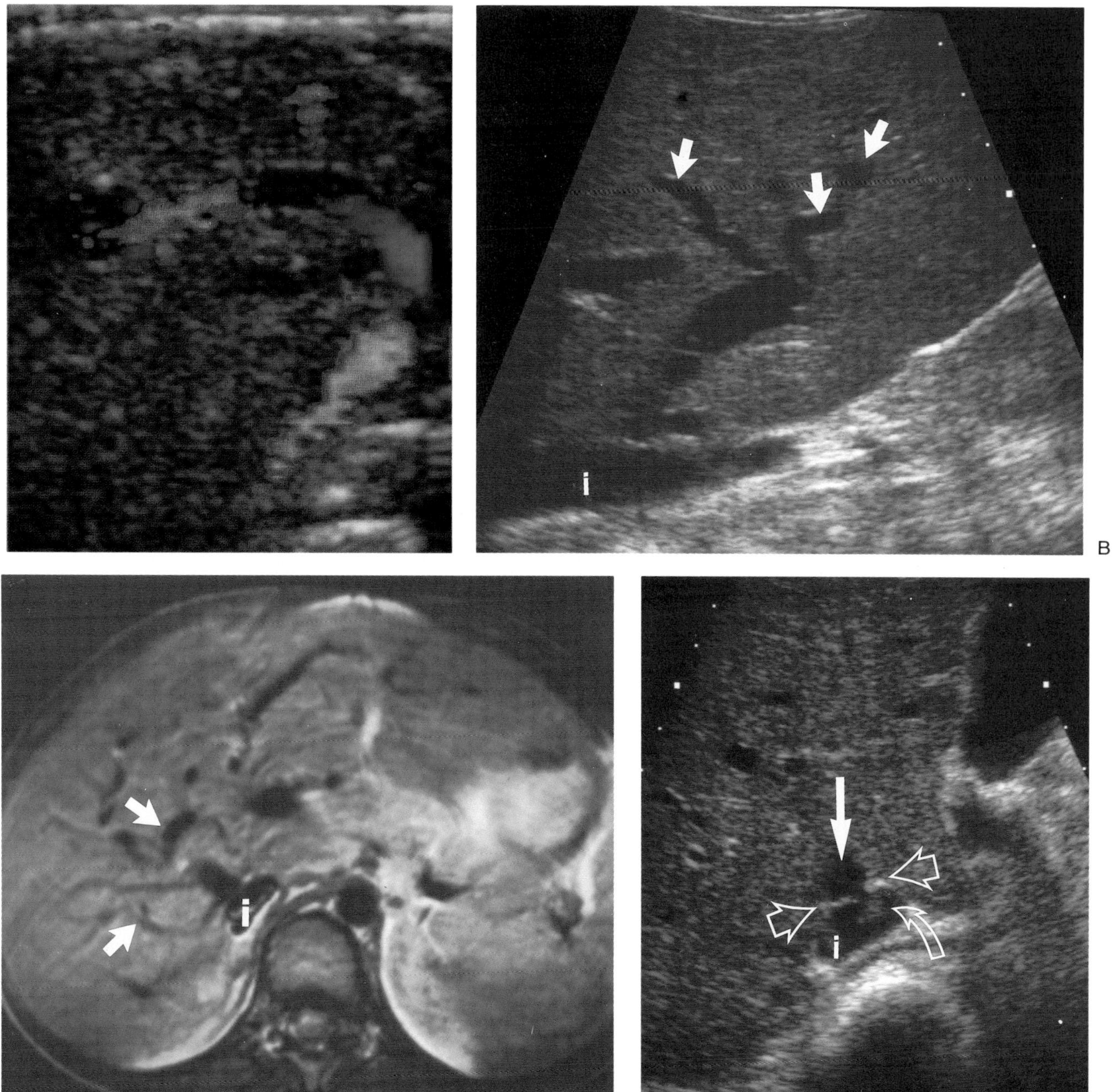

FIG. 2.159. Spider web collaterals, Budd–Chiari syndrome. **A:** Oblique color Doppler sonogram through the liver reveals communicating color-coded hepatic venous to hepatic venous collaterals. This type of collateral results when hepatic venous intercommunication occurs, related to obstruction of outflow into the inferior vena cava. Because of the interconnecting mesh of veins, they are called ''spider web'' collaterals. ''Spider web'' collaterals are much easier to appreciate on real-time scanning than on a single frozen image. With real-time, one can rapidly scan through the liver and easily appreciate the hepatic venous intercommunications. **B:** An oblique longitudinal grayscale sonogram also reveals spider web collaterals (*arrows*). **C:** An MR examination of the liver revealed the same collaterals (*arrows*). **D:** The only hepatic vein seen entering the inferior vena cava was noted caudally in the right lobe on this transverse grayscale sonogram. A band-like stenosis was present (*open arrow*) at the IVC orifice. A small clot (*curved open arrow*) was demonstrated within the inferior vena cava (i). A spectral Doppler sonogram (not shown) of the hepatic vein (HV) revealed a flat waveform, lacking the normal phasic fluctuation, an indicator of impaired hepatic venous flow and presumed stenosis. (From ref. 128, with permission.)

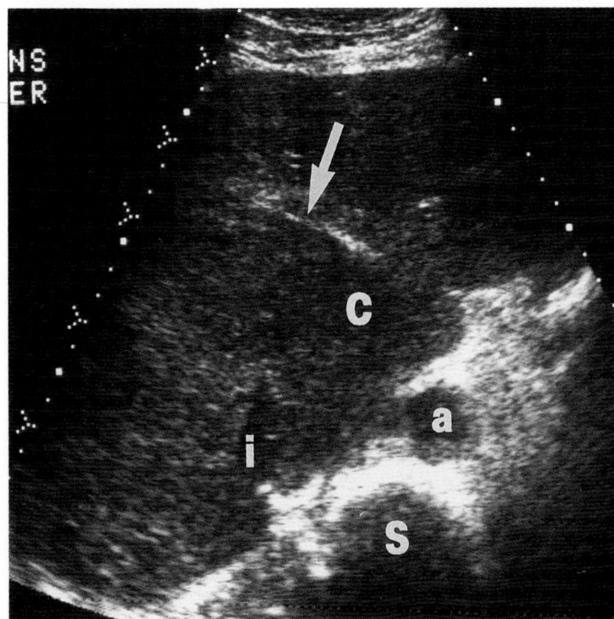

FIG. 2.160. Budd–Chiari syndrome, caudate hypertrophy. Transverse sonogram reveals enlargement of the caudate lobe (C). Note the ventral displacement of the fissure for the ligamentum venosum (*arrow*). Parenchymal inhomogeneity, a nonspecific finding that often occurs in Budd–Chiari syndrome, is also present. S, spine; a, aorta; i, inferior vena cava.

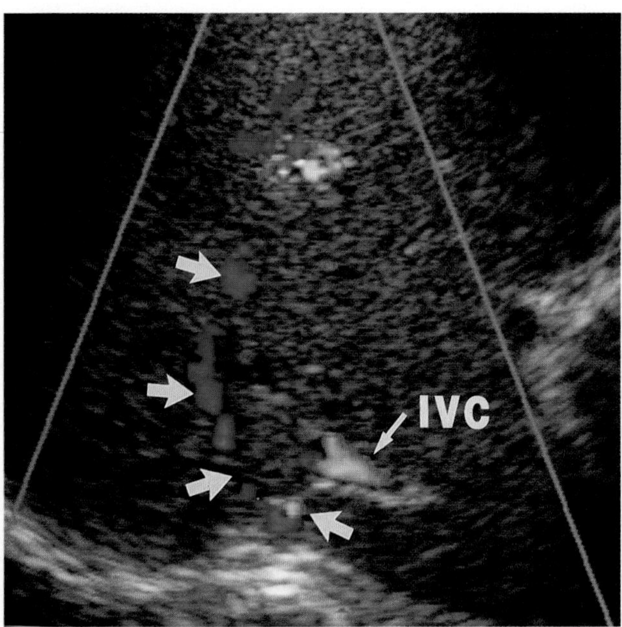

FIG. 2.161. Budd–Chiari syndrome, aberrant hepatic vein. Transverse color Doppler sonogram through the region of the middle hepatic vein reveals a narrowed irregular hepatic venous collateral (*arrows*) that enters the inferior vena cava (IVC) dorsally, rather than from the ventral/anterior direction. Hepatic venous abnormalities such as this, as well as absent or otherwise abnormal hepatic veins (see Fig. 2.159), are typical of Budd–Chiari syndrome.

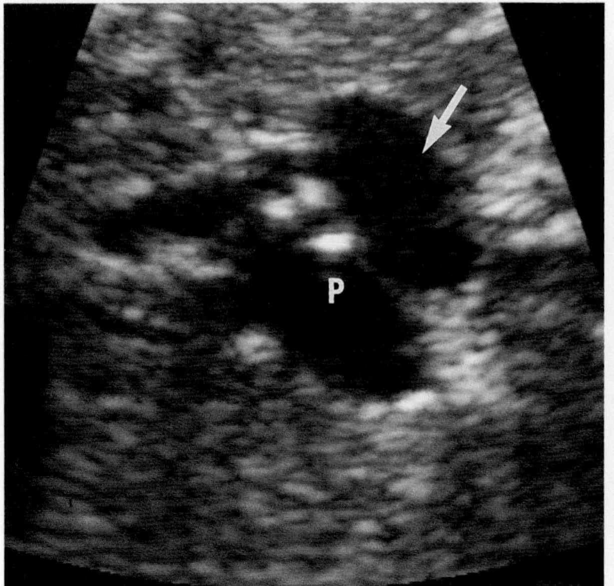

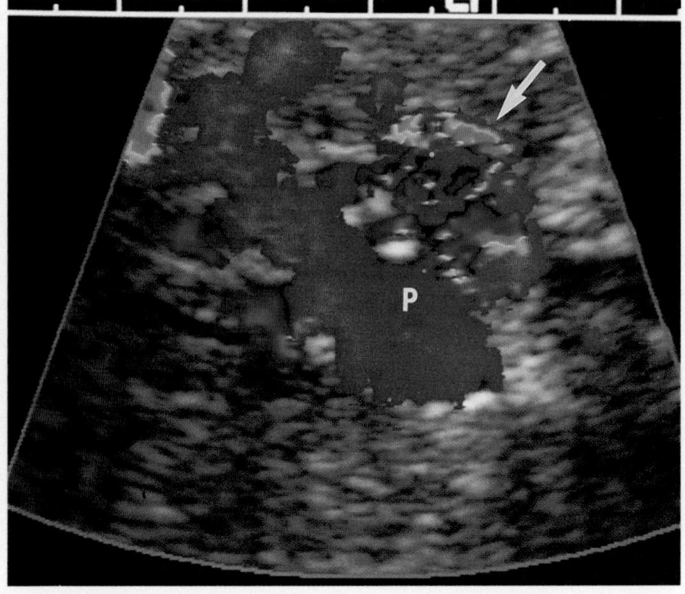

FIG. 2.162. Hereditary hemorrhagic telangiectasia, enlarged arteries. A transverse grayscale (**A**) and color Doppler (**B**) image pair in the region of the right portal vein (P) reveal a tangled mass of enlarged arteries (*arrow*). In hereditary hemorrhagic telangiectasia (Osler–Weber–Rendu disease), arteries enlarge because of markedly increased flow related to multiple intrahepatic AV fistulas. In this patient, an earlier outside ultrasound had incorrectly diagnosed biliary dilatation related to Caroli's disease. Color Doppler sonography demonstrated the arterial nature of the mass and made the diagnosis clear. (From ref. 134, with permission.)

(Fig. 2.163). Tangled arterial masses resulting from the enlarged arteries may be difficult to differentiate from AV fistulas.

Vascular Malformations

Hepatic pseudoaneurysms (Figs. 2.164 and 2.165) and AV fistulas (Fig. 2.166) can be diagnosed and followed noninvasively by CFS. CFS can also assess the results and adequacy of vascular interventional procedures without recourse to angiography. Portal vein and hepatic vein malformations (Fig. 2.132) may be demonstrated by CFS.

LIVER TRANSPLANTATION

Sonography, especially color flow imaging, is important in evaluating liver transplant candidates and in assessing complications after transplantation (135,136). Detecting and defining portal hypertension-related collaterals in the recipient may impact surgical planning. Portal vein clot, although not a contraindication, often means that donor venous grafts must be used. Spontaneous or surgical portosystemic shunts must be detected and delineated so that post-transplant vascular steals can be avoided. Detection of HCC in the native liver is not a contraindication but may alter planning.

After transplantation, sonography's most important function is screening for hepatic arterial occlusion (137). Portal vein complications are less frequent. Hepatic artery occlusion should be suspected when there is acute deterioration in the first few weeks after transplant; rejection is the other major potential problem at this time. Hypoechoic infarcts or intrahepatic fluid collections may result when arterial occlusion occurs. Bile duct complications, often ischemic, should also prompt evaluation of the hepatic artery. Color flow imaging serves a screening function. When abnormalities are noted, arteriographic evaluation and intervention are often indicated (138).

Other post-transplant complications include portal venous and inferior vena caval clot, venous stenosis (Fig. 2.167), biliary complications, and intra- and perihepatic fluid collections. Biliary leaks may cause bilomas; ductal obstruction may cause biliary dilatation. Cholangiography is generally needed, as sonography may miss as many as 50 percent of bile duct complications (135,139). Fluid collections must often be diagnostically aspirated and therapeutically drained. Ultrasound, with CT, is useful in these situations. Post-transplant fluid collections include abscess, biloma, seroma, lymphocele, and hematoma.

No specific sonographic findings occur with rejection. In this setting, color Doppler sonography is useful to ensure that hepatic artery occlusion is not the cause of the symptoms.

REFERENCES

1. Kudo M, Hirasa M, Takakuwa H, et al. Small hepatocellular carcinomas in chronic liver disease: detection with SPECT. *Radiology* 1986;159:697–703.
2. Heiken JP, Weyman PJ, Lee JKT, et al. Detection of focal hepatic masses: prospective evaluation with CT, delayed CT, CT during arterial portography, and MR imaging. *Radiology* 1989;171:47–51.
3. Nelson RC, Chezmar JL, Sugarbaker PH, et al. Hepatic tumors: comparison of CT during arterial portography, delayed CT, and MR imaging for preoperative evaluation. *Radiology* 1989;172:27–34.
4. Wernecke K, Rummeny E, Bongartz G, et al. Detection of hepatic masses in patients with carcinoma: comparative sensitivities of sonography, CT, and MR imaging. *AJR* 1991;157:731–739.
5. Takayasu K, Moriyama N, Muramatsu Y, et al. The diagnosis of small hepatocellular carcinomas: efficacy of various imaging procedures in 100 patients. *AJR* 1990;155:49–54.
6. Barnes PF, DeCock KM, Reynolds TN, et al. A comparison of amebic and pyogenic abscesses of the liver. *Medicine (Baltimore)* 1987;66(6):472–483.
7. Holm J, Jacobson B. Accuracy of dynamic ultrasonography in the diagnosis of malignant liver lesions. *J Ultrasound Med* 1986;5:1–4.
8. Parker GA, Lawrence W Jr, Horsley JS III, et al. Intraoperative ultrasound of the liver affects operative decision making. *Ann Surg* 1989;209(5):569–577.
9. Clarke MP, Kane RA, Steele G Jr, et al. Prospective comparison of preoperative imaging and intraoperative ultrasonography in the detection of liver tumors. *Surgery* 1989;106(5):849–855.
10. Tanaka S, Kitamura T, Fujita M, et al. Color Doppler imaging of liver tumors. *AJR* 1990;154:509–514.
11. Ralls PW, Johnson MB, Lee KP, et al. Color Doppler sonography in hepatocellular carcinoma. *Am J Physiol Imaging* 1991;6:57–61.
12. Nino-Murcia M, Ralls PW, Jeffrey RB Jr, et al. Color Doppler characterization of focal hepatic lesions. *AJR* 1992;159:1195–1197.
13. Taylor KJW, Ramos I, Morse SS, et al. Focal liver masses: differential diagnosis with pulsed Doppler US. *Radiology* 1987;164:643–647.
14. Ohnishi K, Nomura F. Ultrasonic Doppler studies of hepatocellular carcinoma and comparison with other hepatic focal lesions. *Gastroenterology* 1989;97:1489–1497.
15. Sherlock S, Dick R. The impact of radiology on hepatology. *AJR* 1986;147:116–122.
16. Gaines PA, Sampson MA. The prevalence and characterization of simple hepatic cysts by ultrasound examination. *Br J Radiol* 1988;62:335–337.
17. Edmondson HA, Peters RL. Tumors of the liver: pathologic features. *Semin Roentgenol* 1983;18(2):75–82.
18. DeBakey ME, Jorgan GL. Surgery of the liver. In: Schiff L, Schiff ER, eds. *Diseases of the liver,* 6th ed. Philadelphia: Lippincott; 1987:1216.
19. Witzleban CL. Cystic diseases of the liver. In: Zakim D, Boyer TD, eds. *Hepatology: a textbook of liver diseases.* Philadelphia: Saunders; 1990:1395–1411. Vol 2.
20. Ralls PW, Eto R, Quinn MF, et al. Gray-scale ultrasonography of a traumatic biliary cyst. *J Trauma* 1981;21:176–177.
21. Ralls PW, Quinn MF, Boswell WD, et al. Patterns of resolution in successfully treated hepatic amebic abscess: sonographic evaluation. *Radiology* 1983;149:541–543.
22. Korobkin M, Stephens DH, Lee JKT. Biliary cystadenoma and cystadenocarcinoma: CT and sonographic findings. *AJR* 1989;153:507–511.
23. Craig JR, Peters RL, Edmondson HA. In: Hartmann WH, Sobin

(*text continues on page 175*)

A

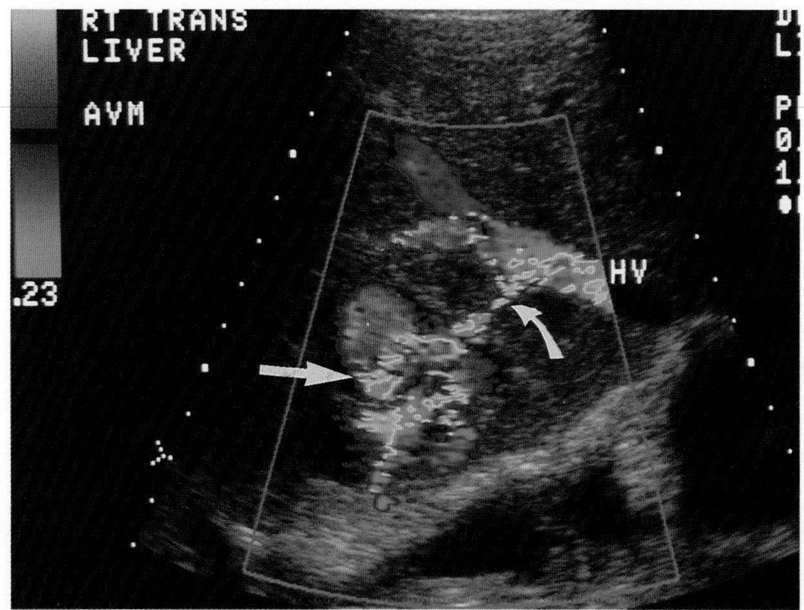

B

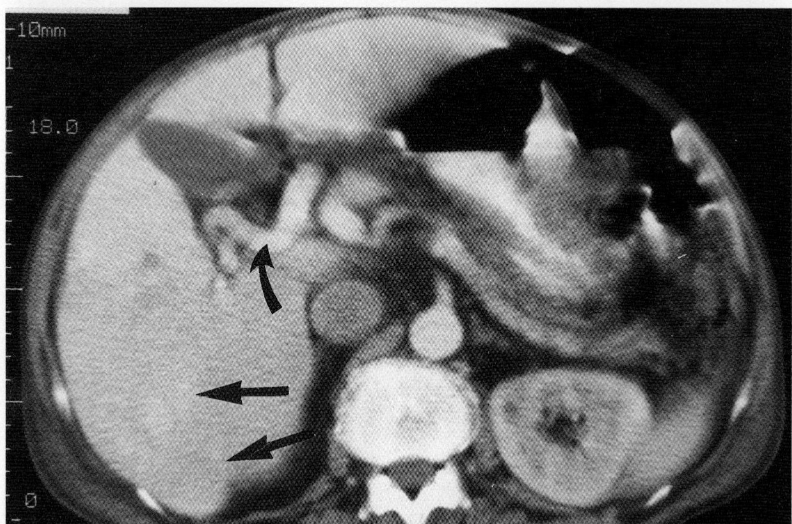

FIG. 2.163. Hereditary hemorrhagic telangiectasia, large arteriovenous fistula. **A:** Transverse color Doppler sonogram reveals a large AV fistula (*arrow*) in this patient with hereditary hemorrhagic telangiectasia (Osler–Weber–Rendu disease). Communication with the hepatic vein (HV) is shown (*curved arrow*). **B:** A dynamic contrast-enhanced CT scan shows the hepatic arterial enlargement (*curved arrow*) associated with the AV fistula. It shows the AV fistula much less well (*arrows*) than does the color Doppler sonogram. (From ref. 134, with permission.)

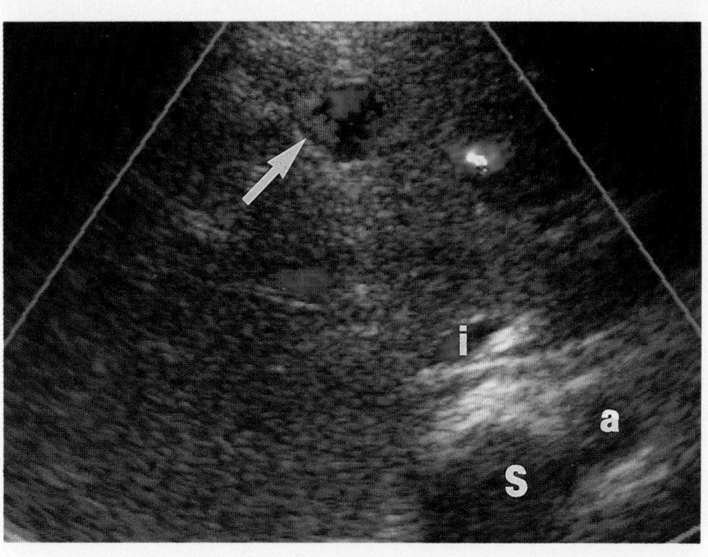

FIG. 2.164. Traumatic hepatic artery pseudoaneurysm. Transverse color Doppler sonogram reveals swirling alternately red and blue coded flow within a post-traumatic hepatic artery pseudoaneurysm (*arrow*). Color Doppler sonography can probably detect most clinically significant pseudoaneurysms, although its actual sensitivity has not yet been determined. S, spine; a, aorta; i, inferior vena cava.

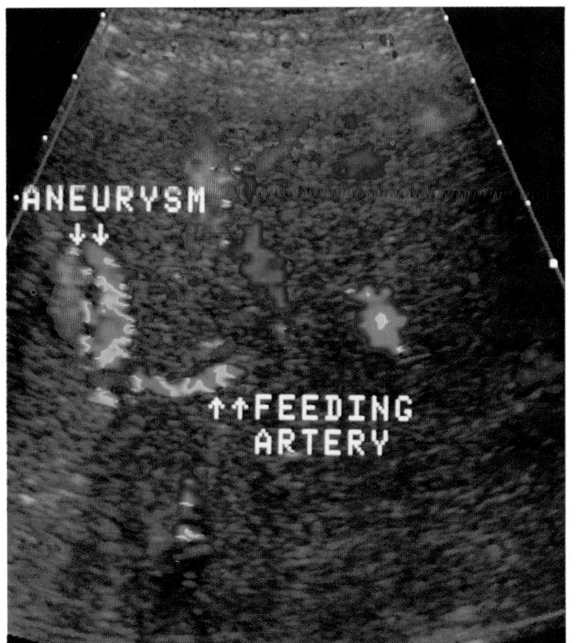

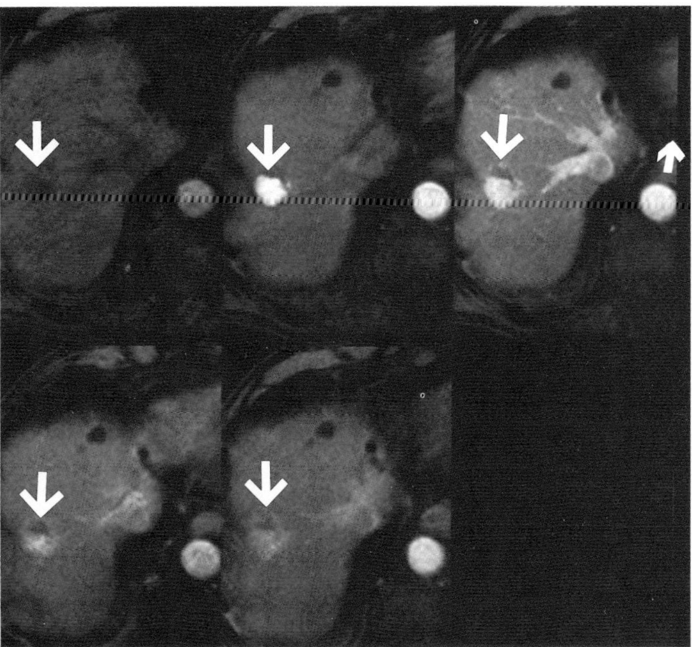

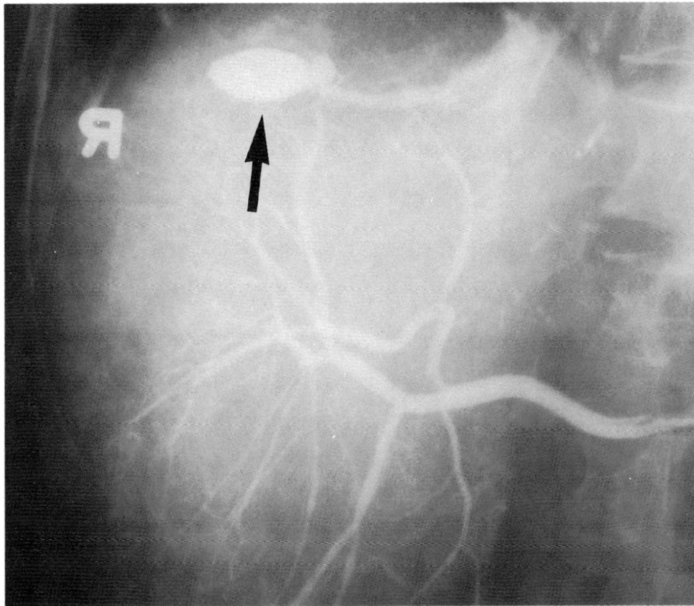

FIG. 2.165. Hepatic artery pseudoaneurysm, polyarteritis nodosa. **A:** Transverse color Doppler sonogram reveals the swirling alternately red and blue coded flow within a pseudoaneurysm (aneurysm) related to polyarteritis nodosa. In this instance, the feeding artery (*arrows*) is detected. **B:** MR angiography with gadolinium enhancement also reveals the pseudoaneurysm (*arrow*) on multiple sequential images. **C:** The angiogram delineates the lesion (*arrow*) prior to transluminal embolization for therapy.

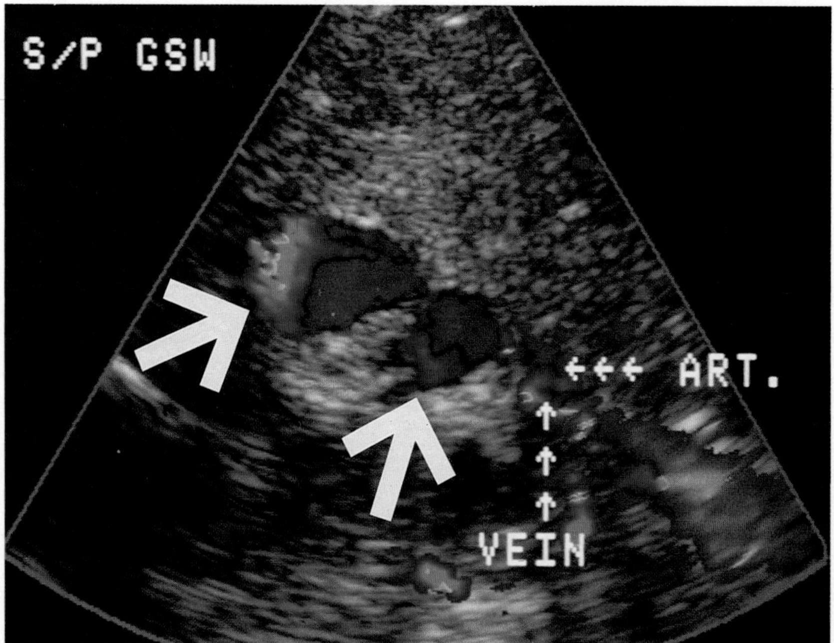

FIG. 2.166. Traumatic bilobed AV fistula. Transverse sonogram in the region of the right lobe of the liver reveals two AV fistulas (*arrows*) that exhibit swirling internal flow, alternately coded blue and red. This bilobed AV fistula resulted from a gunshot wound injury. The feeding hepatic artery (ART) and draining vein are indicated.

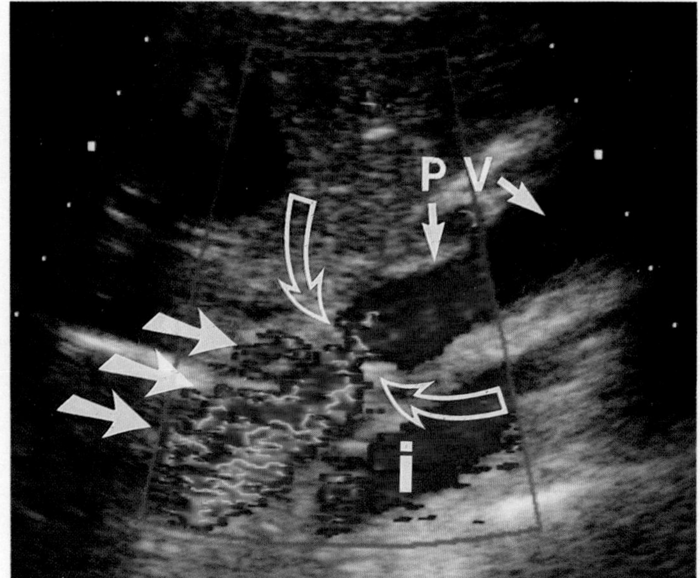

FIG. 2.167. Portal vein stenosis. Longitudinal oblique sonogram through the portal vein (PV) reveals a high-grade stenosis at the level of the portal venous post-transplant anastomosis (*curved arrows*). Marked increased velocity, manifested as aliasing (*slanted arrows*), is noted in the poststenotic portal vein. Portal vein stenosis, when mild, may be an incidental finding. On occasion, transplant patients with portal vein stenosis may present with variceal bleeding. i, inferior vena cava.

LH, eds. *Tumors of the liver and intrahepatic bile ducts,* 2nd series, Fascicle 26. Washington, DC: Armed Forces Institute of Pathology; 1989:45–51.
24. Frick MP, Feinberg SB. Biliary cystadenoma. *AJR* 1982;139:393–395.
25. Esfahani F, Rooholamini SA, Vessal K. Ultrasonography of hepatic hydatid cysts: new diagnostic signs. *J Ultrasound Med* 1988;7(8):443–450.
26. Didier D, Weiler S, Rohmer P, et al. Hepatic alveolar echinococcosis: correlative US and CT study. *Radiology* 1985;154:179–186.
27. Lewall DB, McCorkell SJ. Hepatic echinococcal cysts: sonographic appearance and classification. *Radiology* 1985;155:773–775.
28. Gharbi HA, Hassine W, Brauner MW. Ultrasound examination of the hydatid liver. *Radiology* 1981;139:459–463.
29. Niron EA, Ozer H. Ultrasound appearances of liver hydatid disease. *Br J Radiol* 1981;54:335–338.
30. Bret PM, Fond A, Bretagnolle M, et al. Percutaneous aspration and drainage of hydatid cysts in the liver. *Radiology* 1988;168:617–620.
31. Khuroo MS, Zargar SA, Mahajan R. *Echinococcus granulosus* cysts in the liver: management with percutaneous drainage. *Radiology* 1991;180:141–145.
32. Edmonson HA, Craig JR. Neoplasms of the liver. In: Shiff L, Shiff ER, eds. *Diseases of the liver,* 6th ed. Philadelphia: Lippincott; 1987:1147.
33. Cronan JJ, Esparza AR, Dorfman GS, et al. Cavernous hemangioma of the liver: role of percutaneous biopsy. *Radiology* 1988;166:135–138.
34. Taboury J, Porcel A, Tubiana JM, et al. Cavernous hemangiomas of the liver studied by ultrasound. *Radiology* 1983;149:781–785.
35. Choji K, Shinohara M, Nojima T, et al. Significant reduction of the echogenicity of the compressed cavernous hemangioma. *Acta Radiol* 1988;29:317–320.
36. Gibney RG, Hendin AP, Cooperberg PL. Sonographically detected hepatic hemangiomas: absence of change over time. *AJR* 1987;149:953–957.
37. Solbiati L, Livraghi T, DePa L, et al. Fine needle biopsy of hepatic hemangioma with sonographic guidance. *AJR* 1985;144:471–474.
38. Marchal GJ, Pylyser K, Tshibwabwa-Tumba, EA, et al. Anechoic halo in solid liver tumors: sonographic, microangiographic, and histologic correlation. *Radiology* 1985;156:479–483.
39. Wernecke K, Henke L, Vassallo P, et al. Sonographic halo sign in liver tumors: histopathologic correlation. Presented at RSNA 77th Scientific Assembly and Annual Meeting, Chicago, 1991. Paper 372, p 153.
40. Araki T, Suda K, Sekikawa T, et al. Portal venous tumor thrombosis associated with gastric adenocarcinoma. *Radiology* 1990;174:811–814.
41. Atri M, deStempel J, Bret PM, et al. Incidence of portal vein thrombosis complicating liver metastasis as detected by duplex ultrasound. *J Ultrasound Med* 1990;9(5):285–289.
42. Takayasu K, Moriyama N, Muramatsu Y, et al. The diagnosis of small hepatocellular carcinomas: efficacy of various imaging procedures in 100 patients. *AJR* 1990;155:49–54.
43. Sheu JC, Sung JL, Chen DS, et al. Ultrasonography of small hepatic tumors using high-resolution linear-array real-time instruments. *Radiology* 1984;150:797–802.
44. Ebara M, Ohto M, Shinagawa T, et al. Natural history of minute hepatocellular carcinoma smaller than three centimeters complicating cirrhosis. *Gastroenterology* 1986;90:289–298.
45. Tanaka S, Kitamura T, Imaoka S, et al. Hepatocellular carcinoma: sonographic and histologic correlation. *AJR* 1983;140:701–707.
46. Yoshikawa J, Matsui O, Takashima T, et al. Fatty metamorphosis in hepatocellular carcinoma: radiologic features in 10 cases. *AJR* 1988;151:717–720.
47. Brandt DJ, Johnson CD, Stephens DH, et al. Imaging of fibrolamellar hepatocellular carcinoma. *AJR* 1988;151:295–299.
48. Titelbaum DS, Burke DR, Meranze SG, et al. Fibrolamellar hepatocellular carcinoma: pitfalls in nonoperative diagnosis. *Radiology* 1988;167:25–30.
49. Rummeny E, Weissleder R, Sironi S, et al. Central scars in primary liver tumors: MR features, specificity, and pathologic correlation. *Radiology* 1989;171:323–326.
50. Okazaki M, Higashihara H, Koganemaru F, et al. Intraperitoneal hemorrhage from hepatocellular carcinoma: emergency chemoembolization or embolization. *Radiology* 1991;180:647–651.
51. Livraghi T, Salmi A, Bolondi L, et al. Small hepatocellular carcinoma: percutaneous alcohol injection—results in 23 patients. *Radiology* 1988;168:313–317.
52. Shiina S, Tagawa K, Unuma T, et al. Percutaneous ethanol injection therapy of hepatocellular carcinoma: analysis of 77 patients. *AJR* 1990;155:1221–1226.
53. Savader SJ, Benenati JF, Venbrux AC, et al. Choledochal cysts: classification and cholangiographic appearance. *AJR* 1991;156:327–331.
54. Lack EE, Khettry U, Legg MA. The pancreas and extrahepatic biliary system. In: Silverberg SG, ed. *Principles and practice of surgical pathology,* 2nd ed. New York: Churchill Livingstone; 1990:1379.
55. Klatskin G. Adenocarcinoma of the hepatic duct at its bifurcation within the porta hepatis. *Am J Med* 1965;38:241–256.
56. Nesbit GM, Johnson CD, James EM, et al. Cholangiocarcinoma: diagnosis and evaluation of resectability by CT and sonography as procedures complementary to cholangiography. *AJR* 1988;151:933–938.
57. Ros PR, Buck JL, Goodman ZD, et al. Intrahepatic cholangiocarcinoma: radiologic–pathologic correlation. *Radiology* 1988;167:689–693.
58. Choi BI, Lee JH, Han MC, et al. Hilar cholangiocarcinoma: comparative study with sonography and CT. *Radiology* 1989;172:689–692.
59. Machan L, Muller NL, Cooperberg PL. Sonographic diagnosis of Klatskin tumors. *AJR* 1986;147:509–512.
60. Jeffrey RB Jr. *CT and sonography of the acute abdomen.* New York: Raven Press; 1989:41.
61. Ralls PW. Hepatic section. In: Sarti DA, ed. *Diagnostic ultrasound: text and cases,* 2nd ed. Chicago: Year Book Publishers; 1987:70–85.
62. Jeffrey RB, Tolentino CS, Chang FC, et al. CT of small pyogenic hepatic abscesses: the cluster sign. *AJR* 1988;151:487–489.
63. Plemmons M, Sones PJ Jr, Price RB, et al. Percutaneous drainage of multiseptated hepatic abscess. *J Comput Assist Tomogr* 1984;8:38–41.
64. Ralls PW, Barnes PF, Radin DR, et al. Sonographic features of amebic and pyogenic liver abscesses: a blinded comparison. *AJR* 1987;149:499–501.
65. Ralls PW, Barnes PF, Johnson MB, et al. Medical treatment of hepatic amebic abscess: rare need for percutaneous drainage. *Radiology* 1987;165:805–807.
66. Van Allan RJ, Katz M, Johnson MB, et al. Uncomplicated amebic liver abscess: prospective evaluation of percutaneous therapeutic aspiration. *Radiology* 1992;183:827–830.
67. Callen PW, Filly RA, Marcus FS. Ultrasonography and computed tomography in the evaluation of hepatic microabscesses in the immunosuppressed patient. *Radiology* 1980;136:433–434.
68. Pastakia B, Shawker TH, Thaler M, et al. Hepatosplenic candidiasis: wheels within wheels. *Radiology* 1988;166:417–421.
69. Andrew WK, Thomas RG, Gollach BL. Miliary tuberculosis of the liver—another cause of the "bright liver" on ultrasound examination. *S Afr Med J* 1982;62:808–809.
70. Blangy S, Cornud F, Silbert A, et al. Hepatitis tuberculosis presenting as tumoral disease on ultrasonography. *Gastrointest Radiol* 1988;13:52–54.
71. Brauner M, Buffard MD, Jeantils V, et al. Sonography and computed tomography of macroscopic tuberculosis of the liver. *J Clin Ultrasound* 1989;17:563–568.
72. Alvarez SZ, Carpio R. Hepatobiliary tuberculosis. *Dig Dis Sci* 1983;28:193–200.
73. Welch TJ, Sheedy PF II, Johnson CM, et al. Focal nodular hyperplasia and hepatic adenoma: comparison of angiography, CT, US, and scintigraphy. *Radiology* 1985;156:593–595.
74. Sandler MA, Petrocelli RD, Marks DS, et al. Ultrasonic features and radionuclide correlation in liver cell adenoma and focal nodular hyperplasia. *Radiology* 1980;135:393–397.

75. Rogers JV, Mack LA, Freeny PC, et al. Hepatic focal nodular hyperplasia: angiography, CT, sonography, and scintigraphy. *AJR* 1981;137:983–990.
76. Scatarige JC, Fishman EK, Sanders RC. The sonographic "scar sign" in focal nodular hyperplasia of the liver. *J Ultrasound Med* 1982;1:275–278.
77. Ginaldi S, Bernardino ME, Jing BS, et al. Ultrasonographic patterns of hepatic lymphoma. *Radiology* 1980;136:427–431.
78. Wernecke K, Peters PE, Kruger KG. Ultrasonographic patterns of focal hepatic and splenic lesions in Hodgkin's and non-Hodgkin's lymphoma. *Br J Radiol* 1987;60:655–660.
79. Jackson FI, Lalani Z. Ultrasound in the diagnosis of lymphoma: a review. *J Clin Ultrasound* 1989;17:145–171.
80. Lepke R, Pagani JJ. Sonography of hepatic chloromas. *AJR* 1982;138:1176–1177.
81. Livraghi T, Sangalli G, Vettori C. Adenomatous hyperplastic nodules in the cirrhotic liver: a therapeutic approach. *Radiology* 1989;170:155–157.
82. Freeman MP, Vick GW, Taylor KJW, et al. Regenerating nodules in cirrhosis: sonographic appearance with anatomic correlation. *AJR* 1986;146:533–536.
83. Laing FC, Jeffrey RB, Federle MP, et al. Noninvasive imaging of unusual regenerating nodules in the cirrhotic liver. *Gastrointest Radiol* 1992;7:245–249.
84. Ros PR, Olmsted WW, Dachman AH, et al. Undifferentiated (embryonal) sarcoma of the liver: radiologic–pathologic correlation. *Radiology* 1986;160:141–145.
85. Radin DR, Craig JR, Colletti PM, et al. Hepatic epithelioid hemangioendothelioma. *Radiology* 1988;169:145–148.
86. Furui S, Itai Y, Ohtomo K, et al. Hepatic epithelioid hemangioendothelioma: report of five cases. *Radiology* 1989;171:63–68.
87. Dachman AH, Pakter RL, Ros PR, et al. Hepatoblastoma: radiologic–pathologic correlation in 50 cases. *Radiology* 1987; 164:15–19.
88. Wiener MD, Halvorsen RA Jr, Vollmer RT, et al. Focal intrahepatic hematopoiesis mimicking neoplasm. *AJR* 1987;149:1171–1172.
89. Park JH. Sonography of extramedullary hematopoiesis of the liver. *AJR* 1990;154:900–901.
90. Stanley P, Hall TR, Woolley MM, et al. Mesenchymal hamartomas of the liver in childhood. *AJR* 1986;147:1035–1039.
91. Ros PR, Goodman ZD, Ishak KG, et al. Mesenchymal hamartoma of the liver: radiologic–pathologic correlation. *Radiology* 1986;158:619–624.
92. Klein MA, Slovia TL, Chang CH, et al. Sonographic and Doppler features of infantile hepatic hemangiomas with pathologic correlation. *J Ultrasound Med* 1990;9:619–624.
93. Nyberg DA, Federle MP. AIDS-related Kaposi sarcoma and lymphomas. *Semin Roentgenol* 1987;22:54–65.
94. Luburich P, Bru C, Ayuso MC, et al. Hepatic Karposi sarcoma in AIDS: US and CT findings. *Radiology* 1990;175:172–174.
95. Radin DR, Baker EL, Klatt EC, et al. Visceral and nodal calcification in patients with AIDS-related *Pneumocystis carinii* infection. *AJR* 1990;154:27–31.
96. Spouge AR, Wilson SR, Gopinath N, et al. Extrapulmonary *Pneumocystis carinii* in a patient with AIDS: sonographic findings. *AJR* 1990;155:76–78.
97. Towers MJ, Withers CE, Hamilton PA, et al. Visceral calcification in patients with AIDS may not always be due to *Pneumocystis carinii*. *AJR* 1991;156:745–747.
98. Grant EG. Parenchymal disease of the liver. Presented at RSNA 77th Scientific Assembly and Annual Meeting, Chicago, 1991, pp 281–292. In: Rifkin MD, Charboneau JW, Laing FC, eds. *Ultrasound 1991 syllabus: special course.*
99. Kurtz AB, Rubin CS, Cooper HC. Ultrasound findings in hepatitis. *Radiology* 1980;136:717–723.
100. Needleman L, Kurtz AB, Rifkin MD, et al. Sonography of diffuse benign liver disease: accuracy of pattern recognition and grading. *AJR* 1986;146:1011–1015.
101. Giorgio A, Ambroso P, Fico P, et al. Ultrasound evaluation of uncomplicated and complicated acute viral hepatitis. *J Clin Ultrasound* 1986;14:675–679.
102. Juttner HU, Ralls PW, Quinn MF, et al. Thickening of the gallbladder wall in acute hepatitis: ultrasound demonstration. *Radiology* 1982;142:465–466.
103. Koff RS, Golombas JT. Viral hepatitis. In: Schiff L, Schiff ER, eds. *Diseases of the liver.* Philadelphia: Lippincott; 1987:527.
104. Forsberg L, Floren CH, Hederstrom E, et al. Ultrasound examination in diffuse liver disease. Clinical significance of enlarged lymph nodes in the hepato-duodenal ligament. *Acta Radiol* 1987;28:281–284.
105. White EM, Simeone JF, Mueller PR, et al. Focal periportal sparing in hepatic fatty infiltration: a cause of hepatic pseudomass on US. *Radiology* 1987;162:57–59.
106. Quinn SF, Gosink BB. Characteristic sonographic signs of hepatic fatty infiltration. *AJR* 1985;145:753–755.
107. Sauerbrei EE, Lopez M. Pseudotumors of the quadrate lobe in hepatic sonography: a sign of generalized fatty infiltration. *AJR* 1986;147:923–927.
108. Caturelli E, Costarelli L, Giordano M, et al. Hypoechoic lesions in fatty liver. *Gastroenterology* 1991;100:1678–1682.
109. Giorgio A, Ambroso P, Lettieri G, et al. Cirrhosis: value of caudate to right lobe ratio in diagnosis with ultrasound. *Radiology* 1986;161:443–445.
110. Harbin WP, Robert NJ, Ferrucci JT Jr. Diagnosis of cirrhosis based on regional changes in hepatic morphology. *Radiology* 1980;135:273–283.
111. Hess CF, Schmiedl U, Koelbel G, et al. Diagnosis of liver cirrhosis with US; receiver-operating characteristic analysis of multidimensional caudate lobe indexes. *Radiology* 1989;171:349–351.
112. Ralls PW. Hepatic section. In: Sarti DA, ed. *Diagnostic ultrasound: text and cases,* 2nd ed. Chicago: Year Book Publishers; 1987:70–85.
113. DiLelio A, Cestari C, Lomazzi A, et al. Cirrhosis: diagnosis with sonographic study of the liver surface. *Radiology* 1989;172:389–392.
114. Ladenheim JA, Luba DG, Yao F, et al. Limitations of liver surface US in the diagnosis of cirrhosis. *Radiology* 1992;185:21–24.
115. Ralls PW. Color Doppler sonography of the hepatic artery and portal venous system. *AJR* 1990;155:517–525.
116. Taylor KJW, Burns PN, Woodcock JP, et al. Blood flow in deep abdominal and pelvic vessels: ultrasonic pulsed-Doppler analysis. *Radiology* 1985;154:487–493.
117. Leach SD, Meier GH, Gusberg RJ. Endoscopic sclerotherapy: a risk factor for splanchnic venous thrombosis. *J Vasc Surg* 1989;10:9–13.
118. Okuda K, Ohnishi K, Kimura K, et al. Incidence of portal vein thrombosis in liver cirrhosis. *Gastroenterology* 1985;89:279–286.
119. Lebrec D, Benhamou JP. Noncirrhotic intrahepatic portal hypertension. *Semin Liver Dis* 1986;6:332–340.
120. Lafortune M, Patriquin H, Pomier G, et al. Hemodynamic changes in portal circulation after portosystemic shunts: use of duplex carotid sonography in 43 patients. *AJR* 1987;149:701–706.
121. Hanson KM, Johnson PC. Local control of hepatic arterial and portal venous flow in the dog. *Am J Physiol* 1966;211:712–720.
122. Bookstein J, Boijsen E, Olin T, et al. Angiography after end-to-side portacaval shunt. *Invest Radiol* 1971;6:101–109.
123. Moriyasu F, Nishida O, Ban N, et al. "Congestion index" of the portal vein. *AJR* 1986;146:735–739.
124. Ralls PW, Lee KP, Mayekawa DS, et al. Color Doppler sonography of portocaval shunts. *J Clin Ultrasound* 1990;18:379–381.
125. Rice S, Lee KP, Johnson MB, et al. Portal venous system after portosystemic shunts or endoscopic sclerotherapy: evaluation with Doppler sonography. *AJR* 1991;156:85–89.
126. Reuter SR, Berk RN, Orloff MJ. An angiographic study of the pre- and postoperative hemodynamics in patients with side-to-side portacaval shunts. *Radiology* 1975;116:33–39.
127. Reynolds TB. The role of hemodynamic measurements in portosystemic shunt surgery. *Arch Surg* 1974;108:276–281.
128. Ralls PW, Johnson MB, Radin DR, et al. Budd–Chiari syndrome: detection with color Doppler sonography. *AJR* 1992;159:113–116.
129. Kriegshauser JS, Charboneau JW, Letendre L. Hepatic venocclusive disease after bone-marrow transplantation: diagnosis with duplex sonography. *AJR* 1988;150:289–290.

130. Herbetko J, Grigg AP, Bucklev AR, et al. Veno-occlusive liver disease after bone marrow transplantation: findings at duplex sonography. *AJR* 1992;158:1001–1005.

131. Peery WH. Clinical spectrum of hereditary hemorrhagic telangiectasia (Osler–Weber–Rendu disease). *Am J Med* 1987;82:989–997.

132. Reilly PJ, Nostrant TT. Clinical manifestations of hereditary hemorrhagic telangiectasis. *Am J Gastroenterol* 1984;79:363–367.

133. Cloogman HM, DiCapo RD. Hereditary hemorrhagic telangiectasia: sonographic findings in the liver. *Radiology* 1984;150:521–522.

134. Ralls PW, Johnson MB, Radin DR, et al. Hereditary hemorrhagic telangiectasia: findings in the liver with color Doppler sonography. *AJR* 1992;159:59–61.

135. Davis PL, VanThiel DH, Zajko AB, et al. Imaging in hepatic transplantation. *Semin Liver Dis* 1989;9:90–101.

136. Oliver JH, Federle MP, Campbell WL, et al. Imaging the hepatic transplant. *Radiol Clin North Am* 1991;29:1285–1298.

137. Segel MC, Zajko AB, Bowen A, et al. Hepatic artery thrombosis after liver transplantation: radiologic evaluation. *AJR* 1986;146:137–141.

138. Dalen K, Day DL, Ascher NL, et al. Imaging of vascular complications after hepatic transplantation. *AJR* 1988;150:1285–1290.

139. Zemel G, Zajko AB, Skolnick ML, et al. The role of sonography and transhepatic cholangiography in the diagnosis of biliary complications after liver transplantation. *AJR* 1988;151:943–946.

CHAPTER 3

Gallbladder and Bile Ducts

GALLBLADDER

Technique

Sonography of the gallbladder is best performed with a 5-MHz curved array transducer. A 5-MHz linear array transducer may be helpful in patients with very superficial gallbladders. In obese patients or in patients with difficult sonographic access, a 3.5-MHz sector or curved linear transducer is necessary. The gallbladder is generally imaged with patients in both supine and left posterior oblique (LPO) positions. Upright and, on occasion, prone scans may be helpful to visualize very small gallstones. When stones are not immediately apparent, the region of the cystic duct and neck of the gallbladder should carefully be scrutinized for stones in both transverse and sagittal views. When a gallstone is identified in the neck of the gallbladder, it is important to scan the patient in multiple positions to determine if the stone is impacted. All patients with acute right upper quadrant pain should be evaluated for secondary signs of acute cholecystitis (sonographic Murphy's sign, wall thickening, pericholecystic fluids, etc.)

Acute Calculous Cholecystitis

In the United States alone there are over 20 million individuals with gallstones (1). Acute calculous cholecystitis is, not surprisingly, one of the most common causes of right upper quadrant pain. A stone obstructing the cystic duct is the cause of acute cholecystitis in 90 to 95 percent of the cases (1). Cystic duct obstruction leads to gallbladder distention and stimulation of afferent nerve fibers, resulting in "biliary colic." The pain of acute cholecystitis, however, is typically constant rather than colicky. Prolonged cystic duct obstruction and gallbladder distention cause secondary venous and lymphatic obstruction and subserosal edema. Infiltration of the gallbladder wall with inflammatory cells then leads to acute cholecystitis. If not treated promptly, gangrenous cholecystitis may develop, resulting in gallbladder perforation, pericholecystic abscess formation, and sepsis.

Patients with acute calculous cholecystitis typically present with right upper quadrant or midepigastric pain, nausea, vomiting, and fever (2). Twenty-five percent of the patients demonstrate localized right upper quadrant peritoneal signs with rebound tenderness (2). The clinical Murphy's sign, one of the classic physical findings in acute cholecystitis, refers to abrupt inspiratory arrest during palpation of the right upper quadrant (2). It is not present in all patients. Indeed, the clinical diagnosis of acute cholecystitis is often imprecise; only 13 to 35 percent of patients with suspected acute cholecystitis ultimately have that diagnosis verified at surgery (3). Thus imaging with either sonography or scintigraphy is essential to confirm the clinical diagnosis of cholecystitis and avoid unnecessary surgery.

Sonography and biliary scintigraphy are equally accurate techniques for diagnosing acute calculous cholecystitis (4–9). Whether sonography or cholescintigraphy is the initial imaging study is often a matter of institutional preference. The choice is often influenced by availability, cost, imaging expertise, and, most importantly, the acceptance of a positive study by surgeons and referring clinicians.

Sonography has several clear advantages in the evaluation of patients with possible acute cholecystitis. It is less expensive than biliary scintigraphy and often can be performed and interpreted more quickly. Sonography provides considerably more anatomic information and can definitively diagnose gallstones. In addition, sonography can be used to elicit the sonographic Murphy's sign and other important secondary findings such as gallbladder wall edema, pericholecystic fluid, or abscesses. Unlike scintigraphy, sonography is independent of hepatic function and biliary obstruction. It may be performed at the bedside in critically ill patients. In patients with gangrenous cholecystitis, sonography may guide percutaneous cholecystostomy when clinically appropriate. Finally, sonography can survey the entire abdomen if the gallbladder is normal, an important capability as only a minority of patients referred for imaging with right upper quadrant pain prove to have cholecystitis.

Despite these advantages, sonography has a number of significant limitations in the diagnosis of acute cholecystitis. Cystic duct stones may be missed due to the small lumen of the cystic duct and lack of surrounding bile (Fig. 3.1) (10). While cystic duct obstruction can generally be inferred when a stone is identified impacted in the neck of the gallbladder, sonography cannot directly diagnose cystic duct obstruction (Fig. 3.2).

The sonographic diagnosis of acute cholecystitis is based on a combination of primary and secondary signs taken in the clinical context of a patient with fever, leukocytosis, and right upper quadrant pain (4,9). Gallstones are the single most important finding. In the absence of stones, other observations, such as wall thickening or focal tenderness over the gallbladder (sonographic Murphy's sign), indicate the need for cholescintigraphy.

The sonographic Murphy's sign is an important finding in suspected acute cholecystitis. It differs significantly from the clinical sign and refers to focal tenderness directly over the gallbladder when pressure is applied by the ultrasound transducer. In order for the sonographic Murphy's sign to be positive, it must be obvious and unequivocal. Thus it does not require a great deal of expertise to determine a positive sign. Gangrenous cholecystitis may cause necrosis and denervation of afferent nerve fibers from the gallbladder and result in a negative sonographic Murphy's sign (11). However, there are generally other significant sonographic abnormalities such as gallstones, wall thickening, or pericholecystic fluid to suggest the diagnosis of cholecystitis. Scintigraphy should be performed in all equivocal cases.

Thickening of the gallbladder wall is an important sonographic observation in acute cholecystitis (Fig. 3.3). The normal gallbladder wall measures 3 mm or less (3). Measurements are most accurate when obtained from the anterior subhepatic gallbladder wall using a long axis image. This avoids side-lobe artifacts from adjacent bowel gas and difficulties encountered by dependent intraluminal sludge. Measurements of the gallbladder wall are not reliable in postprandial patients with a contracted gallbladder.

Symmetric thickening of the gallbladder wall is often not related to intrinsic biliary disease. In the absence of gallstones, this finding must be interpreted with caution in patients with possible cholecystitis (12–15). Generalized gallbladder wall thickening may occur in a broad spectrum of other disorders including hepatitis, acquired immunodeficiency syndrome (AIDS), congestive heart failure, hypoalbuminemia, ascites, hyperplastic cholecystosis, and chronic cholecystitis (Fig. 3.4) (3,12–15). Asymmetric thickening of the gallbladder wall may be due to carcinoma, metastases, adenomyomatosis, or gangrenous cholecystitis.

Four distinct patterns of gallbladder wall thickening have been identified with sonography (16). These include (a) a striated pattern of multiple hypoechoic layers separated by echogenic zones (Fig. 3.5) (17), (b) asymmetric thickening of the gallbladder wall with echogenic tissue projecting into the gallbladder lumen (Fig. 3.6), (c) a single central hypoechoic zone separated by two echogenic layers (Fig. 3.7), and (d) a uniformly echogenic appearance (Fig. 3.8) (16). Unfortunately, no one pattern of wall thickening as an isolated finding is specific for acute cholecystitis. Furthermore, there is considerable overlap with many other causes of gallbladder wall thickening. Teefey et al. (16) have noted that in patients with compelling clinical features of acute cholecystitis, a striated pattern or asymmetric pattern is suggestive of gangrenous cholecystitis (Fig. 3.9).

Color Doppler sonography may prove to be a valuable adjunct in evaluating patients with possible cholecystitis. In our experience, the cystic artery can be visualized with 5-MHz color Doppler transducers optimized for low-flow sensitivity in approximately 40 percent of normal patients. The anterior branch of the cystic artery can be demonstrated with color Doppler sonography on sagittal scans of the anterior subhepatic portion of the gallbladder wall. The normal cystic artery is generally only visible in the neck and proximal portion of the gallbladder. It is rarely visible in the distal half of the gallbladder. In some, but not all, patients with cholecystitis, the cystic artery may enlarge. It may be visualized over 50 percent of the length of the gallbladder wall (Fig. 3.10). Prominent cystic artery flow in the distal half of the gallbladder is suggestive of acute cholecystitis. Increased blood flow within echogenic areas of inflamed pericholecystic fat and omentum is another secondary finding of acute cholecystitis (Fig. 3.11). Potential false-positive color Doppler diagnoses for acute cholecystitis may occur in patients with gallbladder varices or enlargement of the cystic artery secondary to portal hypertension (Fig. 3.12). Spectral Doppler sonography can confirm venous flow in gallbladder varices. Whether color Doppler sonography of the gallbladder wall will prove helpful in acute cholecystitis is unclear at the present time. It certainly warrants further investigation, particularly in patients with acalculous cholecystitis.

Biliary scintigraphy remains an extremely useful modality in suspected cholecystitis. It should be performed routinely if there is any question about the sonographic diagnosis. Scintigraphy is performed with an intravenous injection of ^{99m}Tc-labeled derivatives of iminodiacetic acid (6–9). In normal patients there is prompt hepatic uptake and excretion of isotope into the biliary system. Visualization of the gallbladder, bile duct, and gastrointestinal tract generally occurs within 1 hr. Failure to visualize the gallbladder at 4 hr is reliable evidence

(*text continues on page 188*)

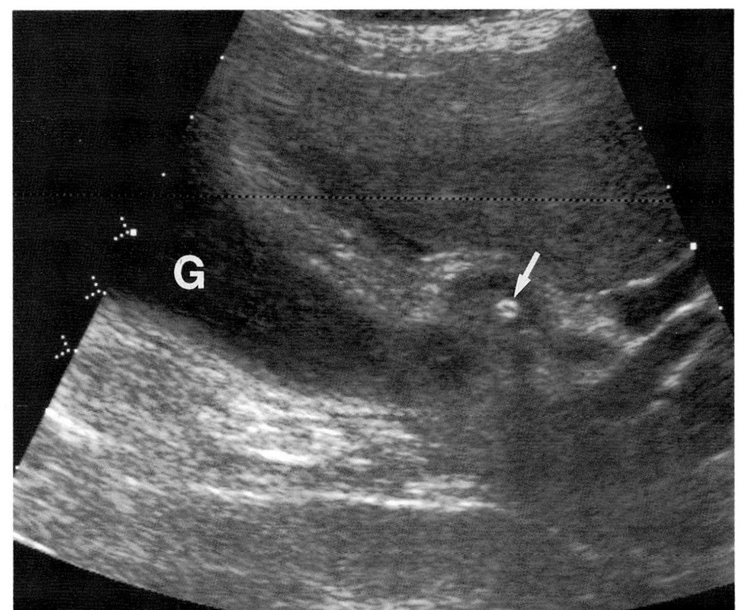

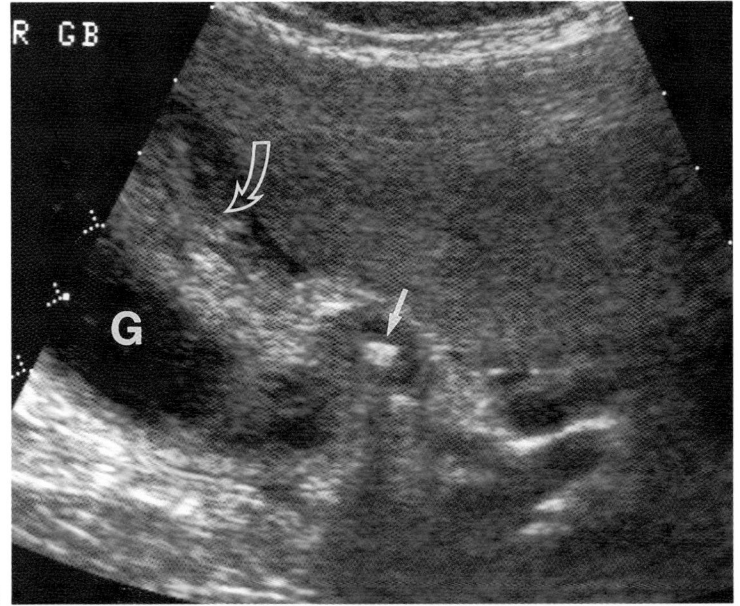

FIG. 3.1. Acute cholecystitis with small cystic duct stones. **A:** Transverse scan of a gallbladder demonstrates a small cystic duct stone (*arrow*). The stone is difficult to visualize due to lack of surrounding bile (G, gallbladder). **B:** Note additional cystic duct (*arrow*) as well as marked gallbladder wall thickening and edema (*curved arrow*). G, gallbladder.

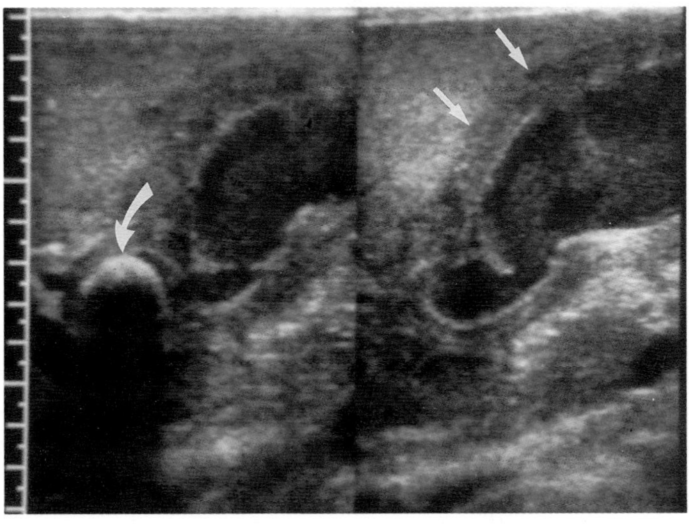

FIG. 3.2. Acute cholecystitis with impacted stone in the neck of the gallbladder. Sagittal sonogram demonstrates impacted stone (*curved arrow*) and marked thickening of gallbladder wall (*arrows*).

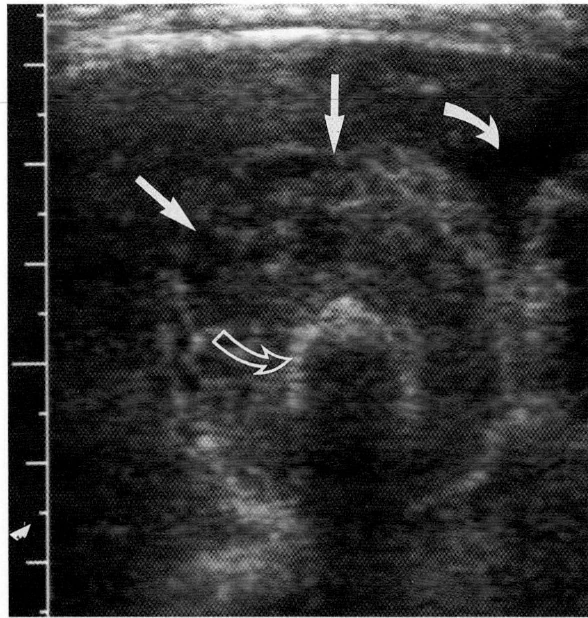

FIG. 3.3. Thickened gallbladder wall in acute cholecystitis. Transverse sonogram of the gallbladder demonstrates marked mural thickening (*arrows*) and gallstone (*curved open arrow*). Note adjacent pericholecystic fluid (*curved arrow*).

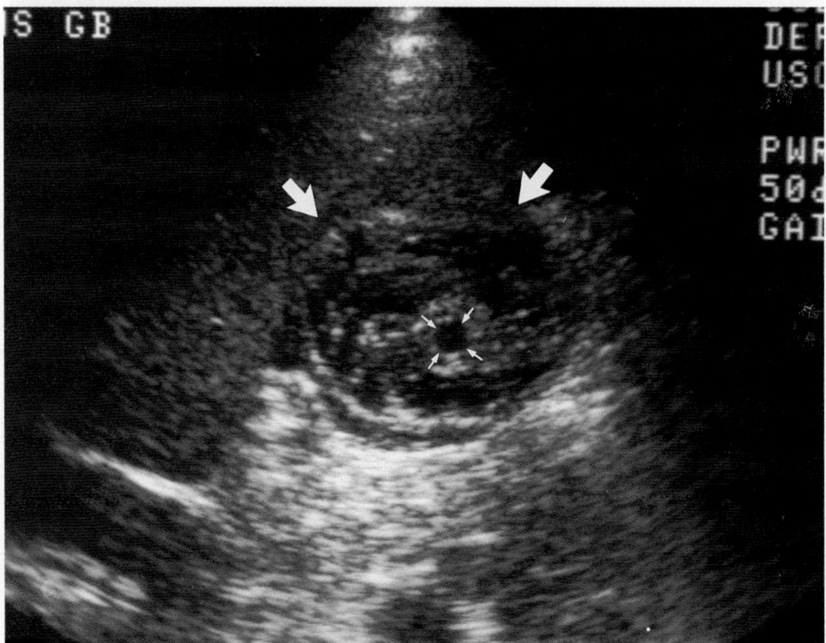

FIG. 3.4. Symmetric thickening of the gallbladder wall due to hepatitis. Transverse sonogram of the gallbladder demonstrates marked mural edema almost obliterating the gallbladder lumen (*small arrows*). Outer wall is indicated by *large arrows.* Patient had viral hepatitis.

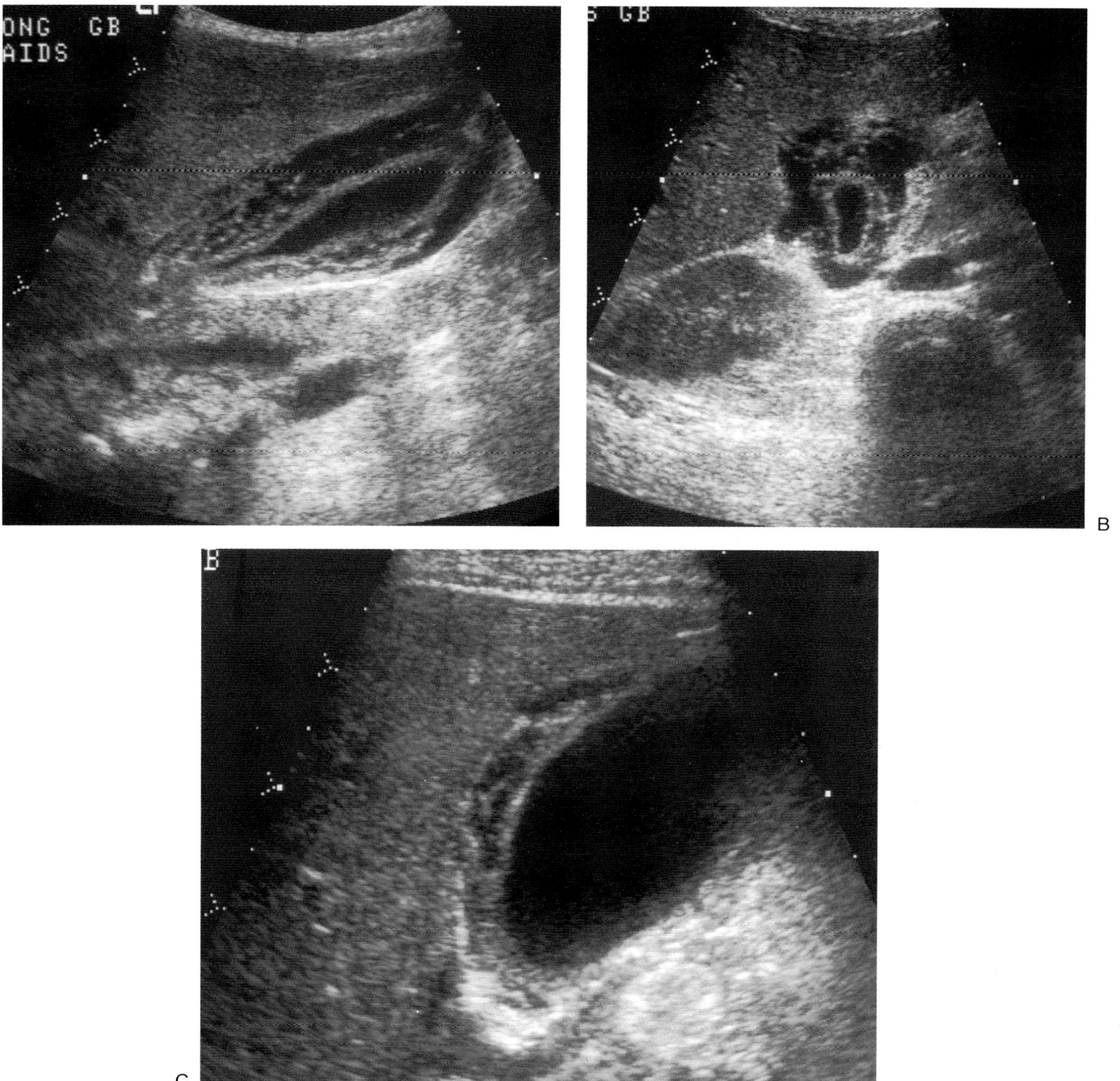

FIG. 3.5. Striated gallbladder wall in two patients without cholecystitis. Sagittal (**A**) and transverse (**B**) views of edematous gallbladder wall with striated pattern in a patient with AIDS. **C:** Striated gallbladder wall in patient with acute pancreatitis.

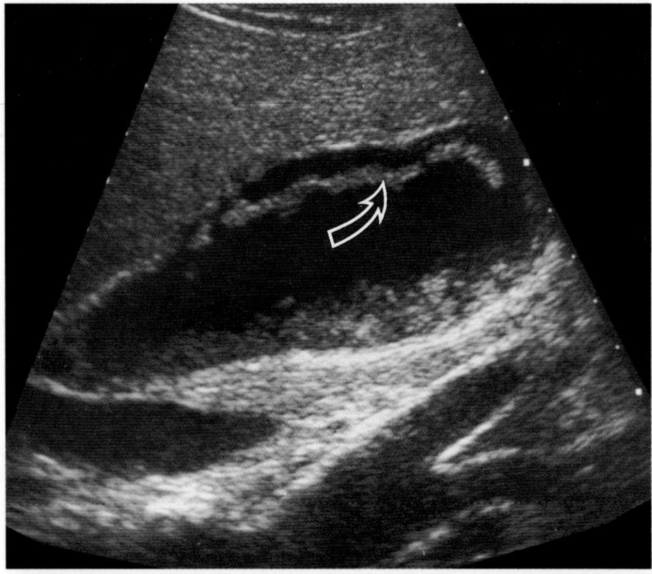

FIG. 3.6. Mucosal sloughing in acute cholecystitis. Note irregular membrane floating within lumen of gallbladder (*arrow*) on sagittal sonogram. (Case courtesy of Lincoln Berland, MD, Birmingham, AL.)

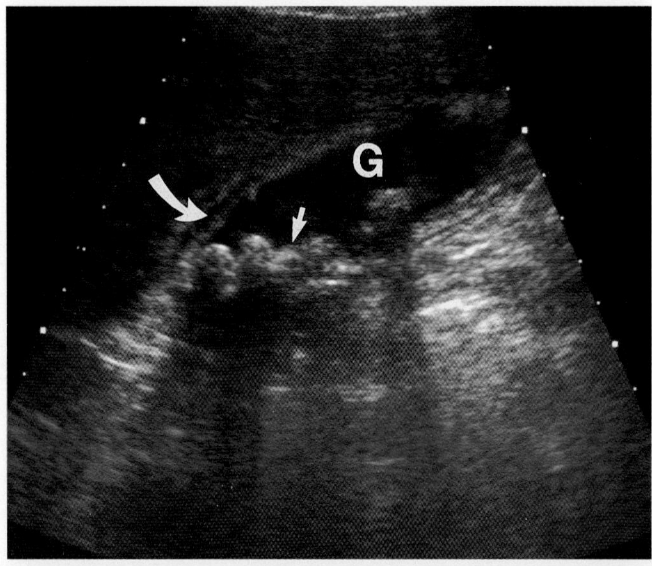

FIG. 3.7. Acute cholecystitis with subserosal gallbladder wall edema. Sagittal scan of gallbladder (G) demonstrates gallstones (*arrow*) and hypoechoic area of subserosal edema of gallbladder wall (*curved arrow*).

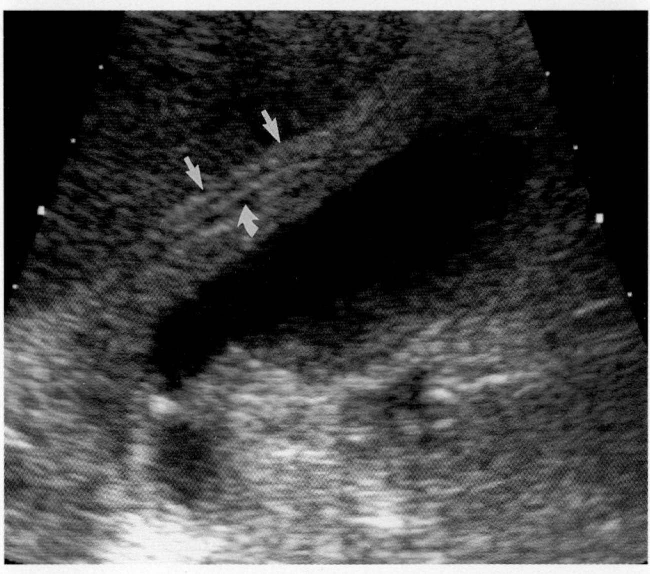

FIG. 3.8. Diffusely echogenic gallbladder wall in congestive heart failure. Sagittal sonogram demonstrates markedly thickened and echogenic gallbladder wall (*arrows*) with areas of striation (*curved arrows*).

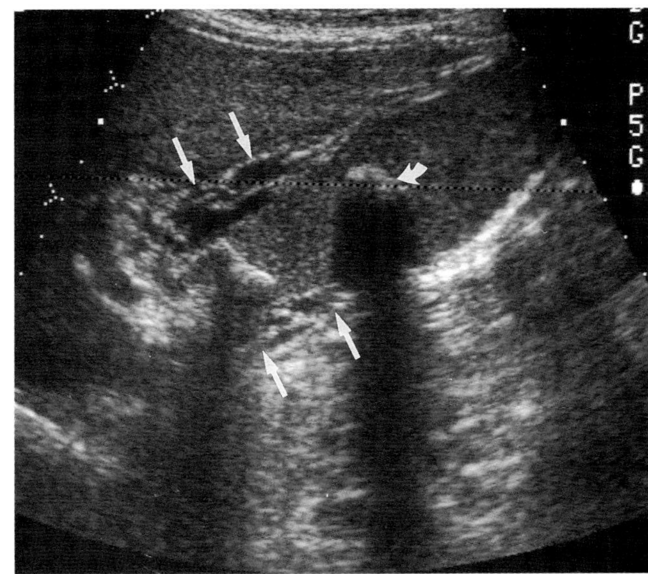

FIG. 3.9. Striated gallbladder wall in gangrenous cholecystitis. Sagittal sonogram demonstrates floating gallstone (*curved arrow*) within sludge-filled gallbladder. Note striations within gallbladder wall (*arrows*).

A

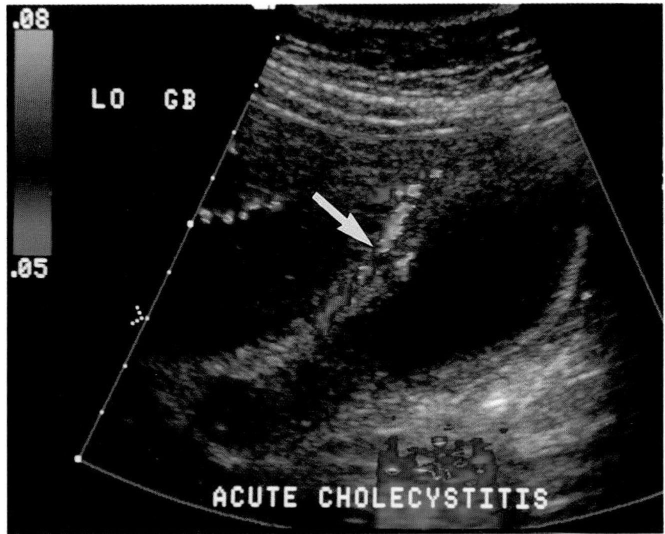

B

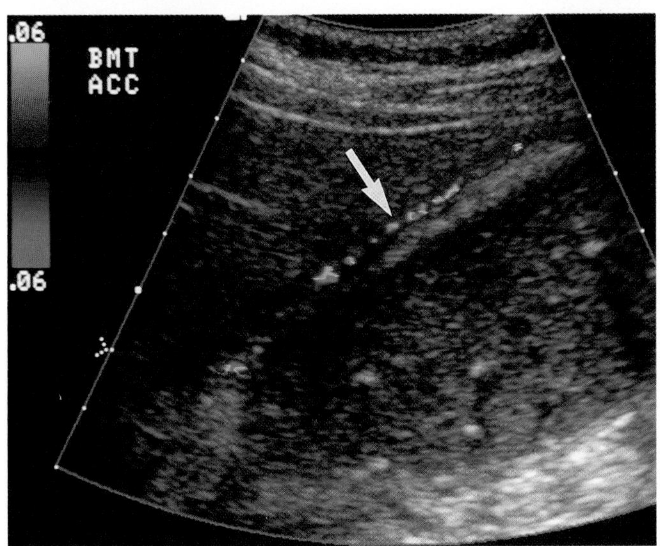

FIG. 3.10. Color Doppler sonography of acute cholecystitis in two patients. Note prominent cystic artery (*arrows,* **A** and **B**) seen extending over 50 percent of the length of gallbladder wall. Both patients had cholecystitis confirmed surgically.

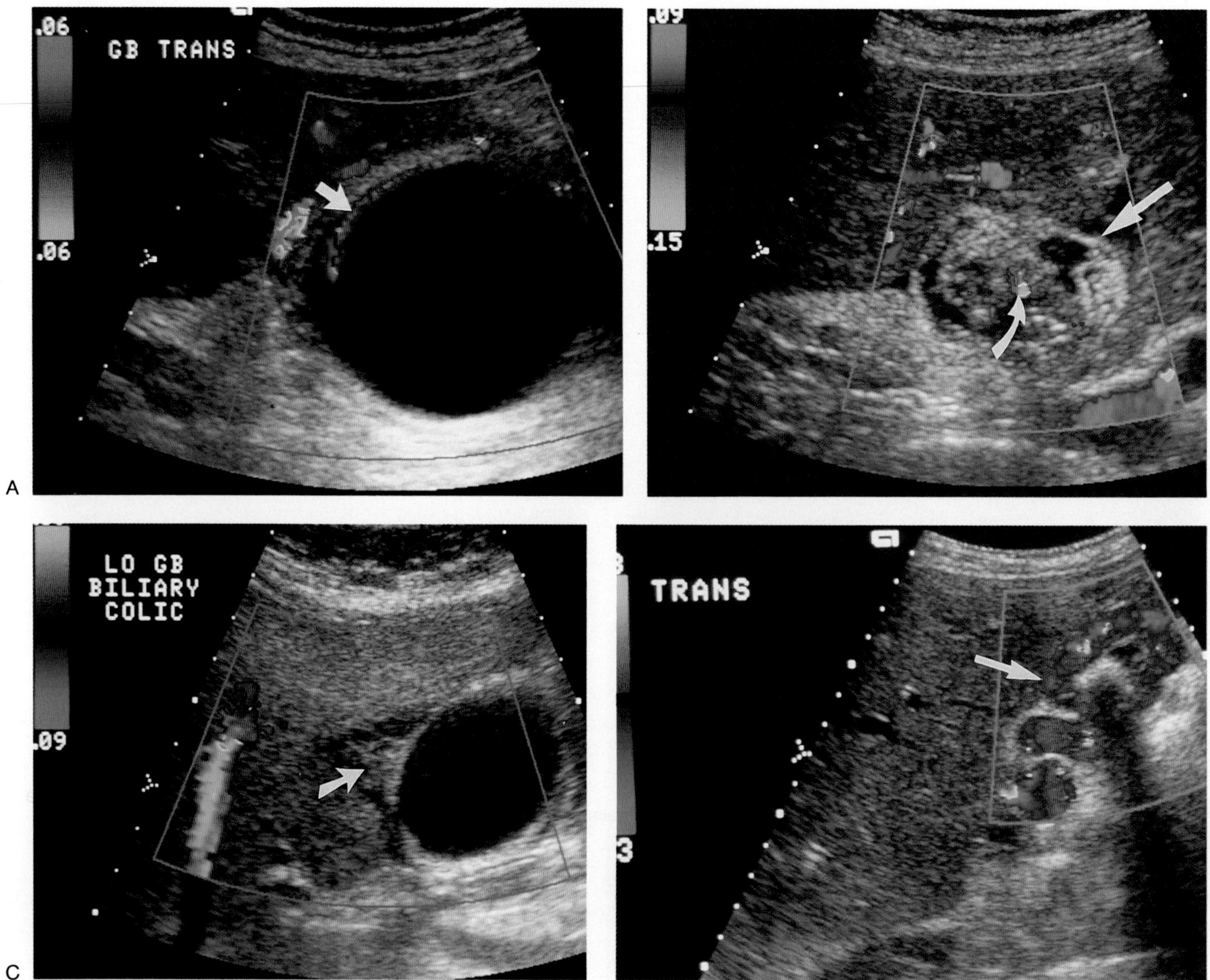

FIG. 3.11. Pericholecystic fat in acute cholecystitis and biliary colic. **A:** Demonstration of increased vascularity within gallbladder wall (*arrow*). **B:** Note increased vascularity within echogenic inflamed pericholecystic fat (*arrow*). **C** and **D:** Another patient had biliary colic and no evidence of acute inflammation. Note echogenic edematous pericholecystic fat (*arrow, C and D*) without increased vascularity on color Doppler sonogram, indicating lack of acute inflammation.

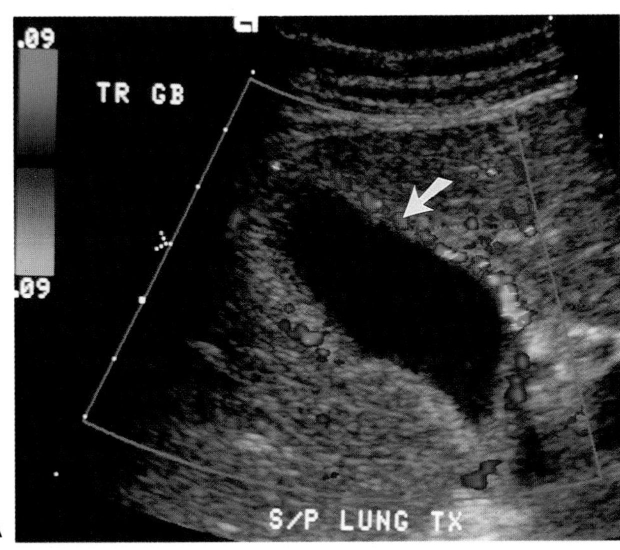

A

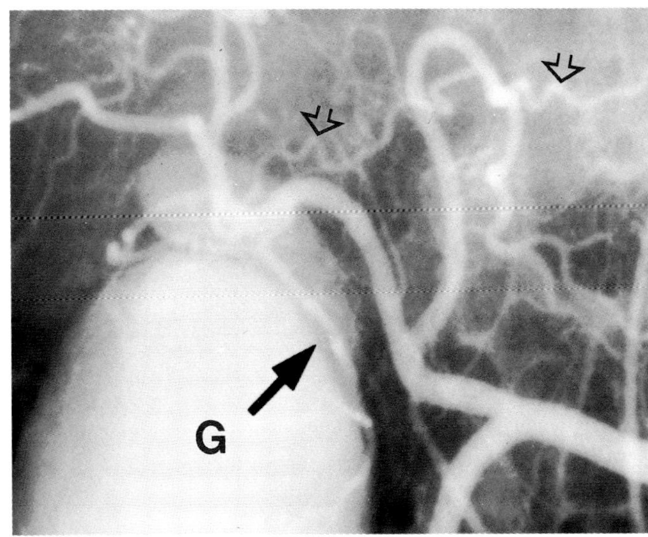

B

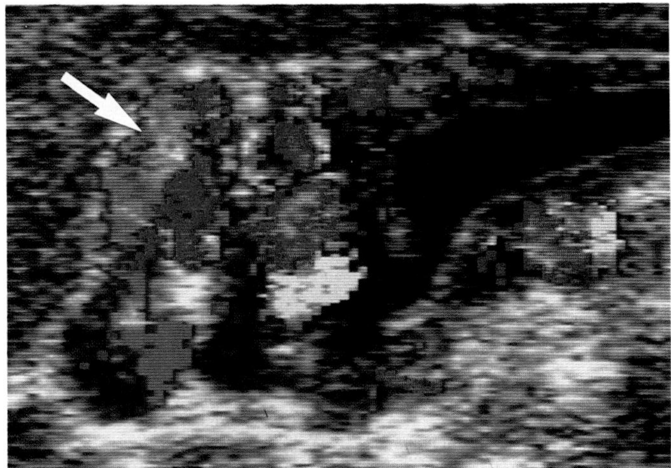

C

FIG. 3.12. Potential false-positive color Doppler sonograms for acute cholecystitis. **A:** Color Doppler sonogram reveals prominent cystic artery (*arrow*) from cirrhosis. **B:** Celiac arteriogram demonstrates tortuous pattern of intrahepatic arterial branches typical of cirrhosis (*open arrow*). Note enlarged cystic artery (*arrow*). Gallbladder (G) had been opacified by retrograde cholangiogram. **C:** In another patient prominent gallbladder varices (*arrow*) are noted that could be misdiagnosed as increased arterial flow in cholecystitis. The patient had portal hypertension.

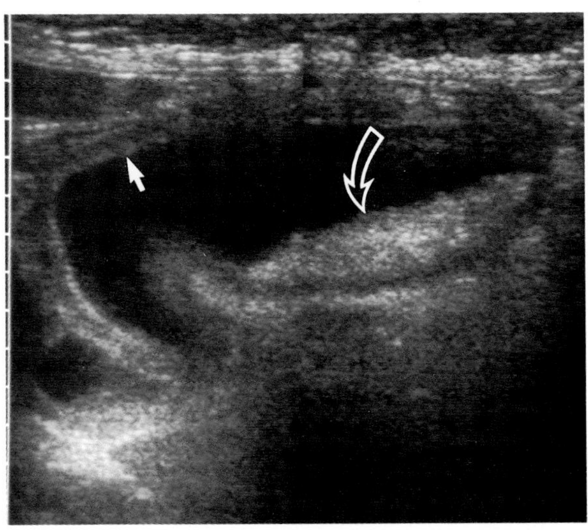

FIG. 3.13. Nonspecific sonographic findings in early acalculous cholecystitis. A sagittal sonogram demonstrated mild gallbladder wall thickening (*arrow*) and sludge (*curved arrow*). Acalculous cholecystitis proved at surgery.

of cystic duct obstruction and acute cholecystitis (6–10). Rarely, patients with acute cholecystitis will demonstrate delayed visualization of the gallbladder, a finding much more frequent in chronic cholecystitis. False-positive cholescintigrams may occur in patients with gallbladder sludge due to hyperalimentation or alcoholic liver disease (18).

Both sonography and scintigraphy have diagnostic accuracies exceeding 90 percent for suspected acute calculous cholecystitis (10,11). In general, sonography is most reliable if multiple signs are present such as gallstones, a thickened gallbladder wall, and a positive sonographic Murphy's sign (9). In patients with a sonographically normal gallbladder, acute cholecystitis can be excluded with a high degree of confidence. Scintigraphy is most reliable when there is intestinal uptake of isotope by 4 hr without visualization of the gallbladder, thus indicating cystic duct obstruction (6,8).

Acute Acalculous Cholecystitis

Acalculous cholecystitis is relatively uncommon and accounts for only 5 to 10 percent of all patients with acute cholecystitis (18). Numerous conditions have been associated with acalculous cholecystitis including trauma, major surgical procedures, hyperalimentation, burns, sepsis, diabetes, and other severe intercurrent illnesses (19–22). Acalculous cholecystitis, however, is not confined to hospitalized patients with critical illnesses. Savoca et al. (20) noted that acalculous cholecystitis may occur in elderly men with atherosclerosis who are otherwise healthy outpatients.

Early clinical diagnosis of acalculous cholecystitis is often exceedingly difficult (19). Delay in diagnosis has resulted in a much higher morbidity and mortality than for calculous cholecystitis. Morbidity approximates 10 percent in some clinical series (19). Unexplained fever may, in fact, be the first sign of acute acalculous cholecystitis (19). This is particularly true in patients who are either unresponsive, ventilatory dependent, or unable to relate symptoms of right upper quadrant pain.

The pathophysiology of acalculous cholecystitis is unknown but likely to be multifactorial. A number of diverse etiologies have been proposed for acalculous cholecystitis, including gallbladder ischemia, cholestasis, and factor XII (Hageman factor), which secondarily activates specific mediators of gallbladder wall inflammation (14,19–22).

Diagnostic imaging also has significant limitations in the early diagnosis of acute acalculous cholecystitis (19–24). Cystic duct obstruction may not be present in early acalculous cholecystitis, resulting in a false-negative scintigraphic examination (22). Another potential cause of falsely positive scintigram is viscous sludge, which may prevent or delay gallbladder filling. As with calculous cholecystitis, the scintigraphic diagnosis is based on nonvisualization of the gallbladder at 4 hr. Because of the potential for false-positive and false-negative diagnoses, the reported sensitivities of isotope studies range from 68 to 93 percent (22).

The sonographic findings in early acalculous cholecystitis may be subtle or nonspecific (Fig. 3.13) (24). The gallbladder may, in fact, appear normal (Fig. 3.14). As previously emphasized, symmetric thickening of the gallbladder wall is often not due to cholecystitis and must be interpreted with caution. Sludge within the gallbladder is similarly nonspecific. Sonographic abnormalities in acalculous cholecystitis include gallbladder wall thickening, pericholecystic fluid, intraluminal membranes, echogenic debris (i.e., hemorrhage or pus), and a positive sonographic Murphy's sign (24,25). Because initial studies of the gallbladder may be normal, a follow-up examination in 24 to 48 hr may be quite valuable in demonstrating interval gallbladder wall edema or pericholecystic fluid. In the appropriate clinical setting, progressive mural thickening is highly suggestive of acalculous cholecystitis (Fig. 3.14).

Computed tomography (CT) may be a valuable adjunct to sonography or scintigraphy in patients with possible acalculous cholecystitis (24,25). One of the main advantages of CT is the ability to clearly demonstrate focal inflammatory changes (edema and soft tissue infiltration) within adjacent pericholecystic fat (24,25).

Some authors have advocated sonographically guided needle aspiration or percutaneous drainage of the gallbladder to diagnose and treat acalculous cholecystitis (Fig. 3.15) (26–28). However, immediate gram stain of the bile aspirate has shown only a 48 percent sensitivity for infected bile due to prior intravenous antibiotic administration (26). Clearing of sepsis has been used as the criterion for success of percutaneous cholecystostomy in critically ill patients with unexplained fever and leukocytosis. Because of the somewhat ambiguous criteria for diagnosis and cure, it is difficult to judge the current efficacy of percutaneous cholecystostomy for acalculous cholecystitis. Reported success rates range from only 36 to 58 percent (27,28). Even though percutaneous cholecystostomy has a relatively low morbidity, further clinical studies are needed to establish more specific indications.

COMPLICATIONS OF CHOLECYSTITIS

Gangrenous Cholecystitis

Two to 38 percent of all patients with acute cholecystitis develop gangrenous changes characterized pathologically by intramural hemorrhage, necrosis, and microabscess formation (29–33). Sonography is generally not very reliable in differentiating uncomplicated cholecysti-

(*text continues on page 191*)

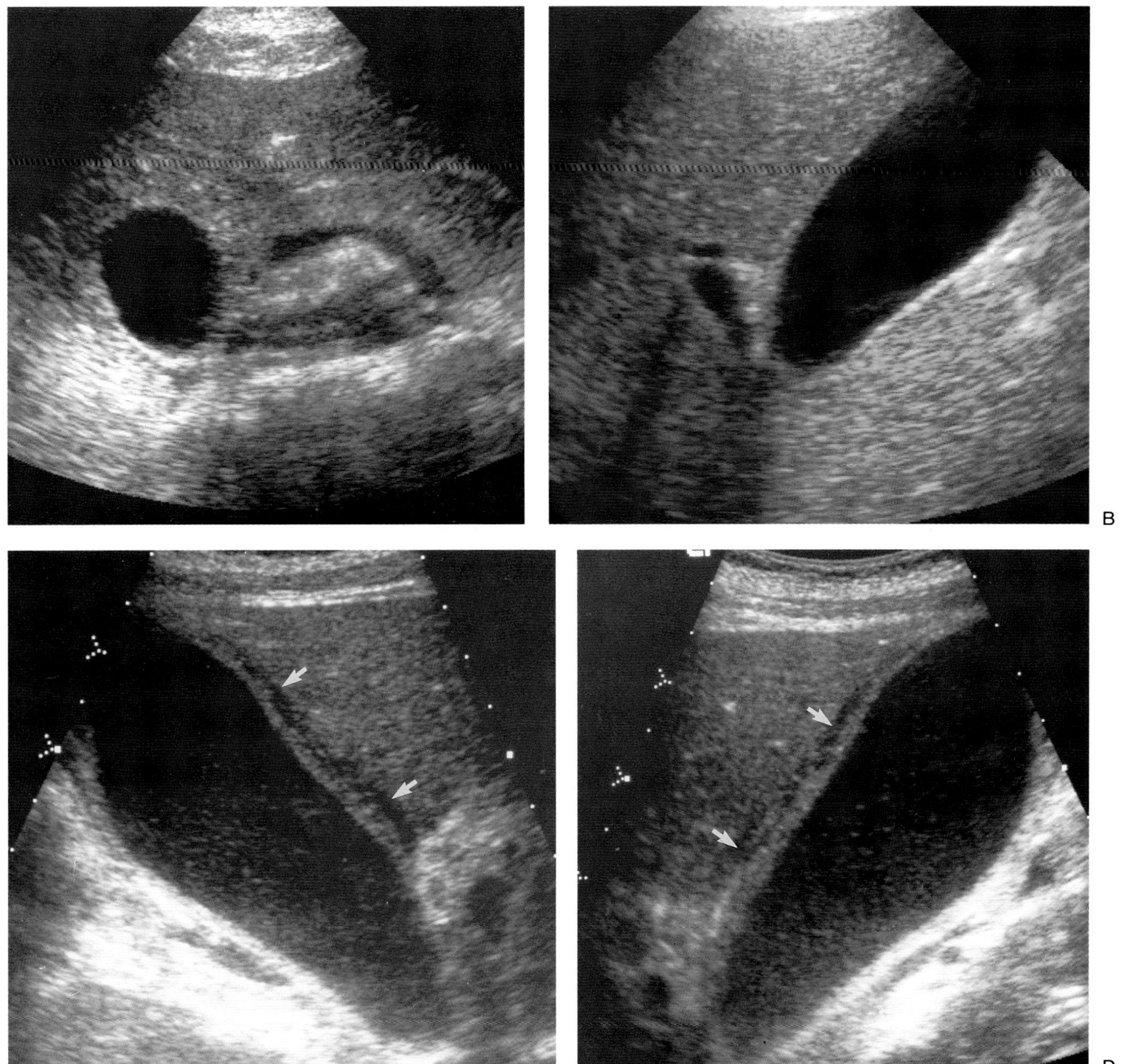

FIG. 3.14. Progressive edema of gallbladder wall in acalculous cholecystitis. Initial transverse (**A**) and sagittal (**B**) sonograms demonstrate no definite abnormalities. Follow-up transverse (**C**) and sagittal (**D**) sonograms 12 hr later reveal interval edema of gallbladder wall (*arrows,* **C** and **D**). Acalculous cholecystitis proved at surgery.

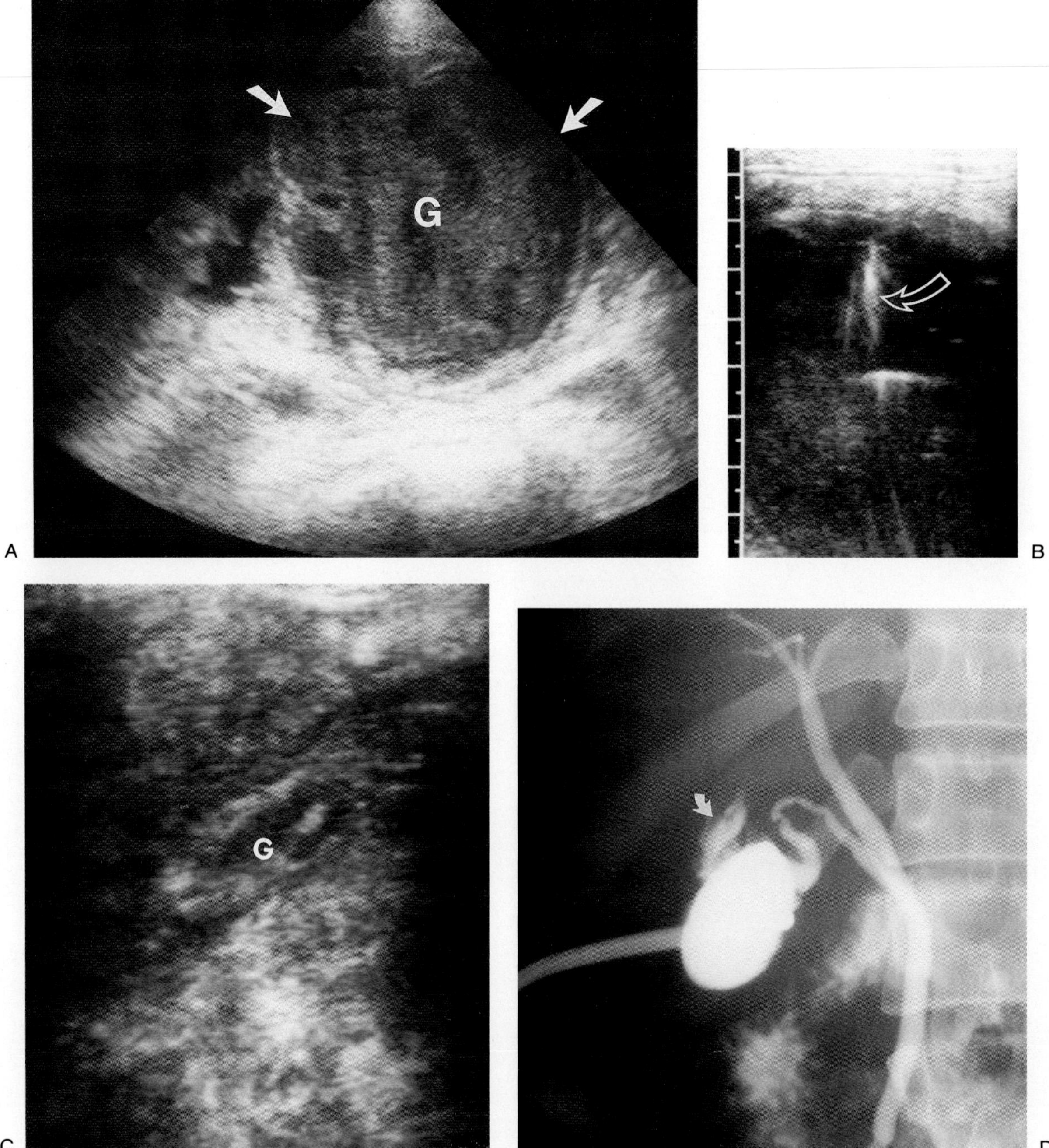

FIG. 3.15. Successful percutaneous cholecystostomy in acalculous cholecystitis and staphylococcal empyema. **A:** Transverse sonogram demonstrating a distended gallbladder (G) filled with echogenic pus (*arrows*). **B:** Following insertion of 18 gauge needle, a guide wire (*arrows*) was coiled in the gallbladder under sonographic guidance. **C:** Immediately after evacuation of pus, the gallbladder (G) is now decompressed. **D:** Tube cholecystogram 5 days later reveals patent cystic duct and focal area (*curved arrow*) of gallbladder perforation. Cultures grew staphylococcus.

tis from gangrenous cholecystitis (32,33). Because the treatment is generally the same (i.e., urgent cholecystectomy), this distinction is not of critical clinical importance. There are, however, several sonographic findings that suggest the diagnosis of gangrenous cholecystitis. These include pericholecystic fluid, intraluminal membranes (sloughed mucosa or fibrinous debris), and asymmetric thickening of the gallbladder wall (microabscess formation or hemorrhage) (Fig. 3.16) (16,32,33). In a prospective study in patients with acute cholecystitis, pericholecystic fluid was the single most common finding in gangrenous cholecystitis (33). However, fluid in the subhepatic space or pericholecystic spaces is not specific for gangrenous cholecystitis. It may occur in patients with ascites, pancreatitis, duodenitis, and severe peptic ulcer disease. Despite extensive mucosal ischemia in gangrenous cholecystitis, some patients demonstrate an enlarged cystic artery with color Doppler sonography (Fig. 3.17). Increased blood flow to the omentum and inflamed pericholecystic fat may also be demonstrated with color Doppler sonography. Areas of necrosis of the gallbladder fundus result in focal loss of the normal echogenicity of the gallbladder wall (Fig. 3.18).

Hemorrhagic Cholecystitis

In some patients, submucosal or intraluminal hemorrhage may be a prominent feature of gangrenous cholecystitis (34). Intraluminal membranes, coarse intraluminal echoes, and asymmetric wall thickening may occur in both gangrenous and hemorrhagic cholecystitis (Fig. 3.19). Echogenic clot may be visible within the gallbladder lumen (Fig. 3.16). At times it may be difficult to distinguish clot from viscous or tumefactive sludge within the gallbladder (Fig. 3.20). Noncontrast CT scans are valuable in confirming the diagnosis of hemorrhage due to its characteristic high attenuation values (greater than 30 HU).

Gallbladder Perforation and Pericholecystic Abscess Formation

Gallbladder perforation and pericholecystic abscess formation are the primary causes of sepsis in acute cholecystitis (35,36). Due to delay in diagnosis, gallbladder perforation is more common in diabetics and patients with acalculous cholecystitis. Advanced age, poor vascular profusion of the gallbladder from atherosclerosis, steroid administration, and associated malignancy also predispose to perforation (36). The gallbladder fundus is the most common anatomic site of perforation due to its relatively limited blood supply.

Sonographically, pericholecystic abscesses are quite variable in appearance. Some abscesses are complex fluid collections adjacent to the gallbladder (Figs. 3.21 and 3.22) (37,38). Due to attenuation of sound by proteinaceous debris, the sonographic appearance in some patients may mimic a "solid" hypoechoic mass (Fig. 3.23). In other patients, prominent echogenic areas are noted due to inflamed omental and pericholecystic fat (Fig. 3.24). The site of perforation of the gallbladder wall may be visualized as a focal interruption of the gallbladder wall (Figs. 3.18 and 3.24). However, this is an inconsistent finding that may be better demonstrated by contrast CT. Pericholecystic abscesses are classified as either intramural, intraperitoneal, or within the pericholecystic space. There may be direct extension of the abscess into the liver (38). Intraperitoneal pericholecystic abscesses are often associated with significant septic complications and early surgery or percutaneous drainage is indicated (37). CT is superior to sonography in delineating gas-forming pericholecystic abscesses (24). In selected patients, CT may also be quite valuable in guiding percutaneous catheter drainage.

Pericholecystic abscesses are often "walled off" from the remainder of the peritoneal cavity by thickened and inflamed omentum (Fig. 3.23). This appears sonographically as a focal echogenic mass adjacent to the abscess. Increased blood flow to the inflamed omentum can be demonstrated with color Doppler sonography.

Emphysematous Cholecystitis

Emphysematous cholecystitis is a rare infection caused by gas-forming organisms within either the wall or lumen of the gallbladder (39,40). Surgical or percutaneous intervention is usually required as antibiotic therapy alone is rarely successful. Emphysematous cholecystitis is significantly more common in diabetic and elderly patients and has a slight male predominance. It has also been reported following endoscopic retrograde cholangiopancreatography (40). *Escherichia coli* is the most common associated organism, although other gram-negative organisms may cause emphysematous cholecystitis.

Plain abdominal radiographs in patients with emphysematous cholecystitis may demonstrate gas within the wall of the gallbladder or an air–fluid level in the lumen of the gallbladder. In patients with small amounts of gas, plain radiographs may be normal. Sonographically, gas bubbles within the gallbladder cause echogenic foci with reverberation or comet tail artifacts. Extensive gas may result in diffuse acoustic shadowing from the gallbladder (Figs. 3.25 and 3.26). Rarely, rising gas bubbles have been noted on real-time examination of the gallbladder and termed the "effervescent gallbladder" (40). In some patients it may be difficult to distinguish intramural gas from mural calcification (i.e., a porcelain gallbladder). Either plain abdominal radiographs or CT scans can readily confirm the diagnosis (39).

(text continues on page 199)

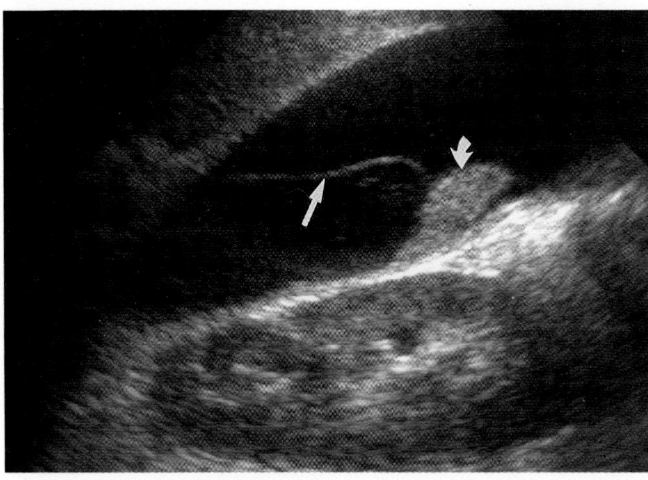

FIG. 3.16. Intraluminal membrane in gangrenous cholecystitis. This sagittal scan of gallbladder demonstrates prominent intraluminal membrane (*arrow*) and echogenic area of hemorrhage (*curved arrow*).

A

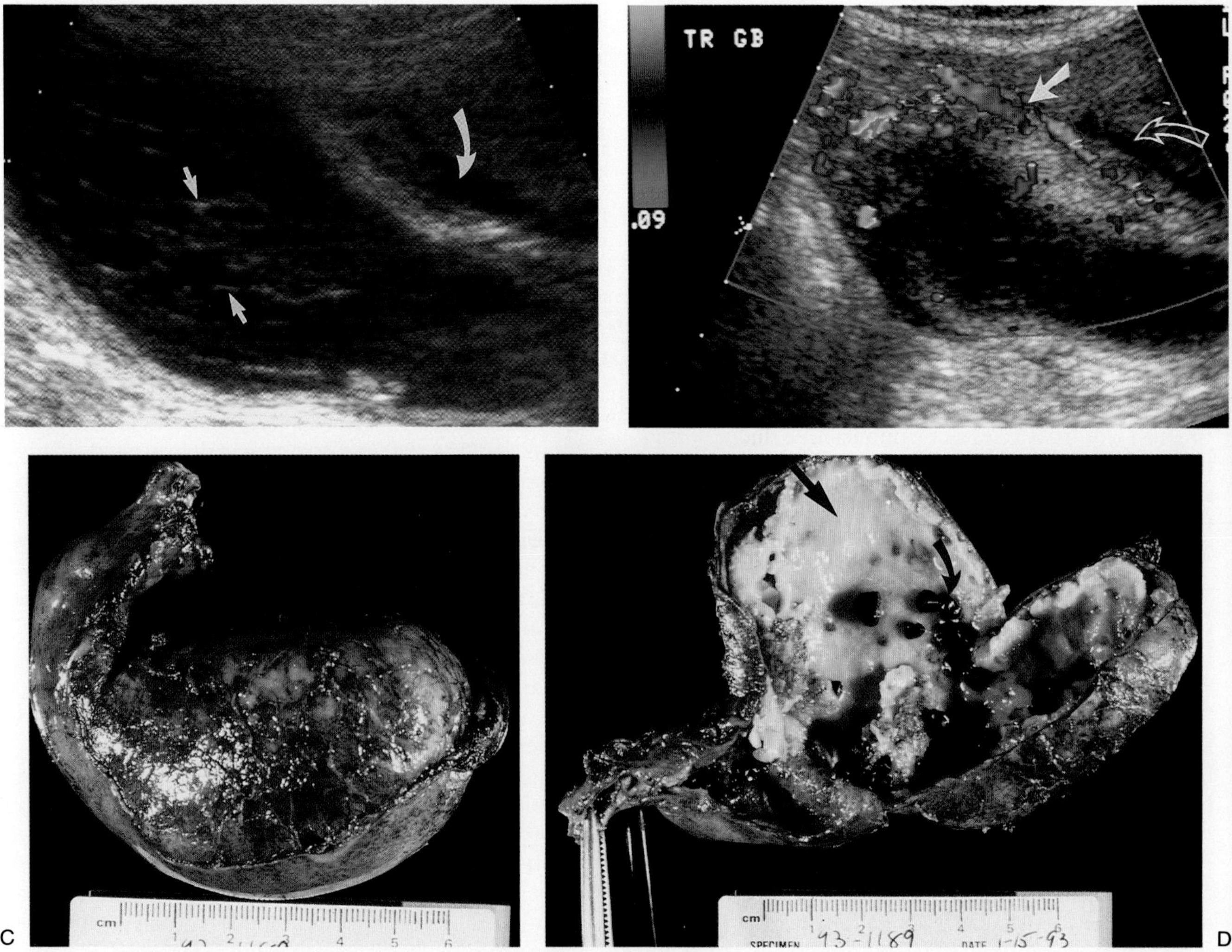

C

D

FIG. 3.17. Gangrenous gallbladder with intraluminal membranes and marked increased mural vascularity. **A:** Note intraluminal membranes (*arrows*) and pericholecystic fluid (*curved arrows*). **B:** Note prominent cystic artery on color Doppler scan within thickened gallbladder wall (*arrow*). Pericholecystic fluid is evident (*curved arrows*). **C:** Gross pathologic specimen demonstrates marked serosal inflammation. **D:** Cut specimen demonstrates necrotic gallbladder mucosa (*arrow*) and stones (*curved arrow*).

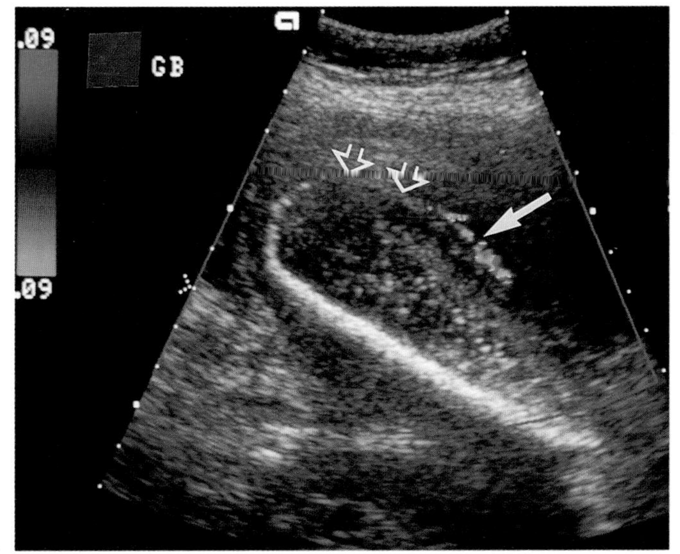

A

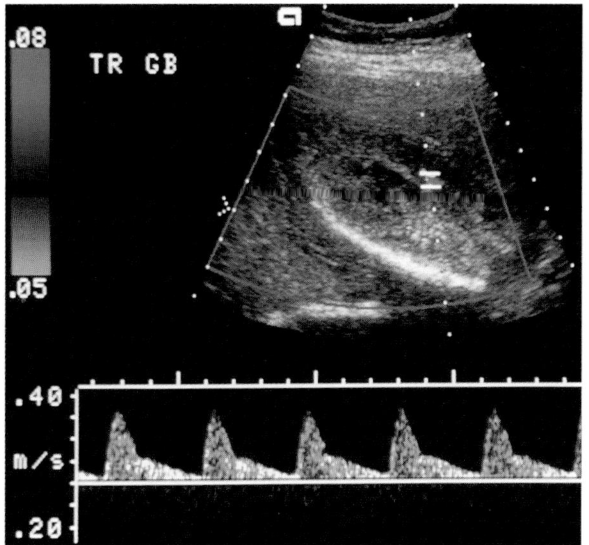

B

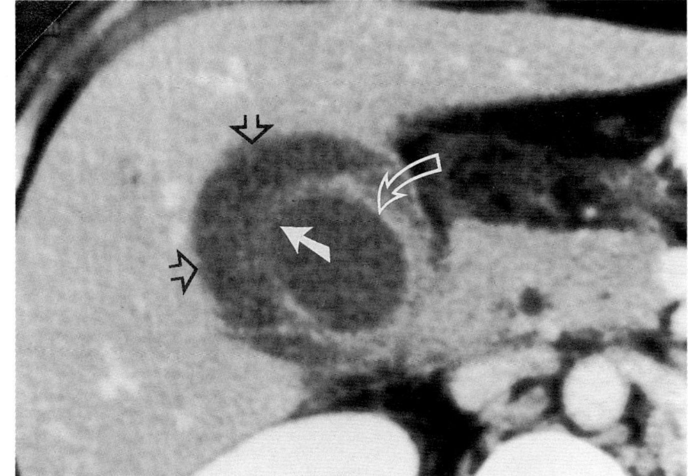

C

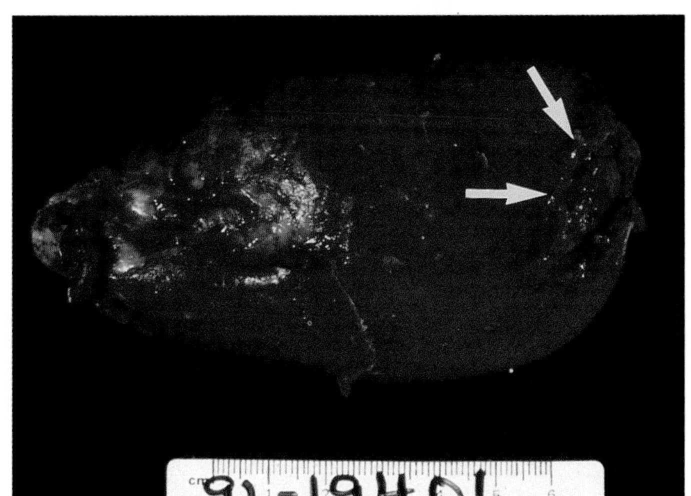

D

FIG. 3.18. Gangrenous gallbladder with focal necrosis of fundus. **A:** Prominent cystic artery (*arrow*) within distal half of gallbladder wall is demonstrated. Note abrupt termination of cystic artery and lack of normal reflectivity of necrotic area in fundus (*open arrow*). **B:** Spectral tracing confirms arterial waveform of cystic artery. **C:** Contrast CT scan demonstrates marked edema of gallbladder wall (*open arrows*) and lack of mucosal enhancement in focal area of necrosis (*white arrow*). Note normal enhancement of gallbladder mucosa (*curved arrow*). **D:** Gross pathology specimen reveals transmural necrosis of fundus (*arrows*).

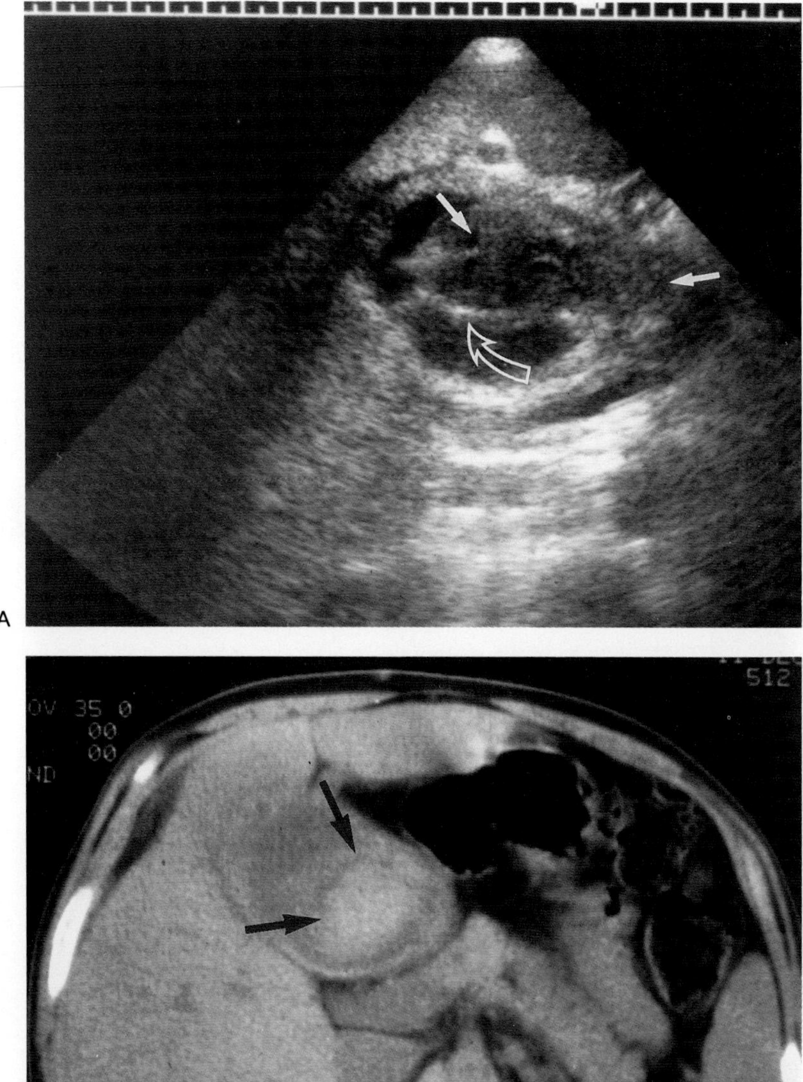

FIG. 3.19. Hemorrhagic cholecystitis. **A:** Transverse sonogram demonstrates echogenic fluid (*arrows*) and membranes (*curved arrow*) representing hemorrhage. **B:** Noncontrast CT confirms high-attenuation clot within gallbladder (*arrows*).

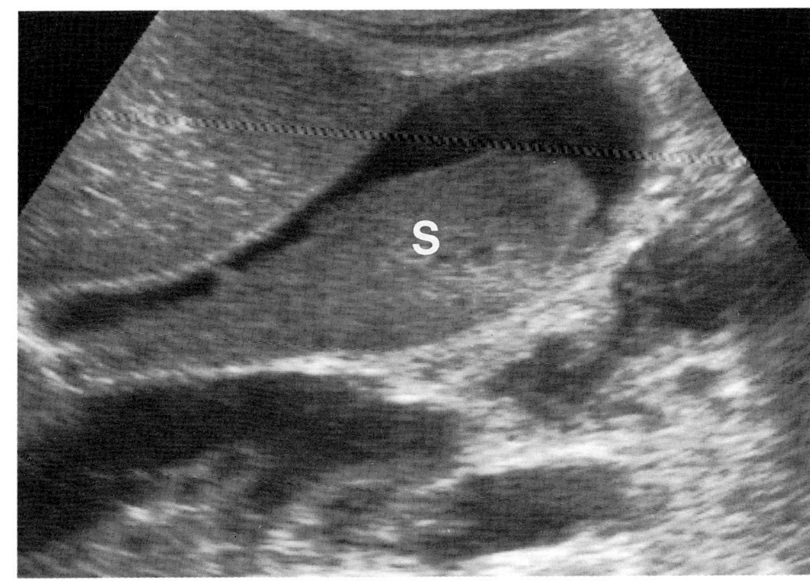

FIG. 3.20. Tumefactive sludge mimicking intraluminal clot. Note echogenic mass within gallbladder representing tumefactive sludge (S).

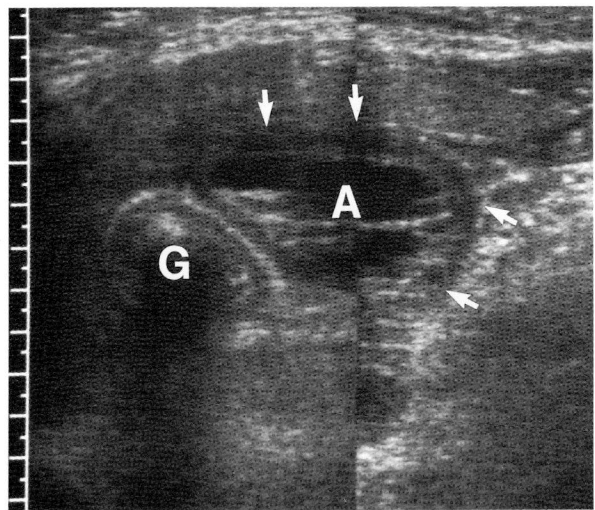

FIG. 3.21. Pericholecystic abscess. Septated pericholecystic abscess (A) is noted adjacent to stone-filled gallbladder (G). *Arrows* indicate margins of abscess.

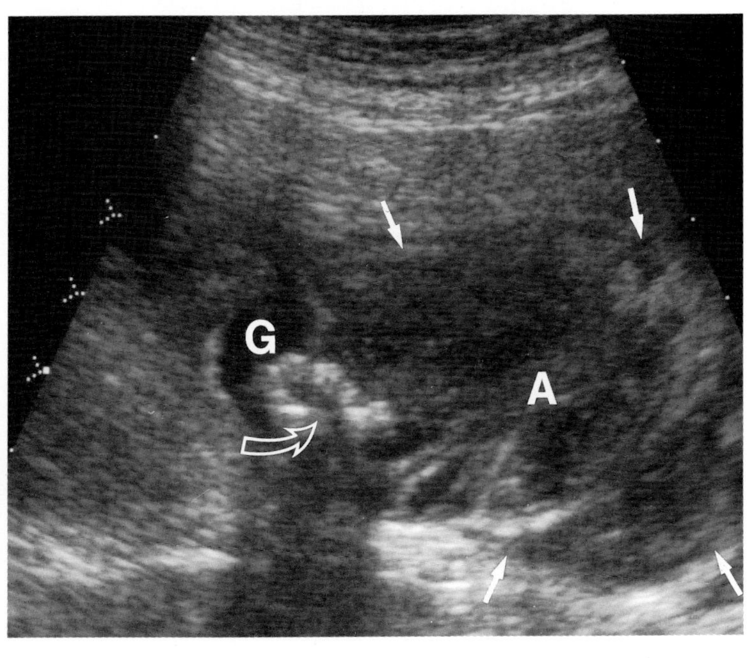

FIG. 3.22. Solid appearing pericholecystic abscess. Transverse scan of gallbladder (G) demonstrates stones (*curved arrows*) and large pericholecystic abscess (A). *Arrows* denote limit of abscess. Note lack of enhanced through sound transmission. Abscess mimics a solid mass.

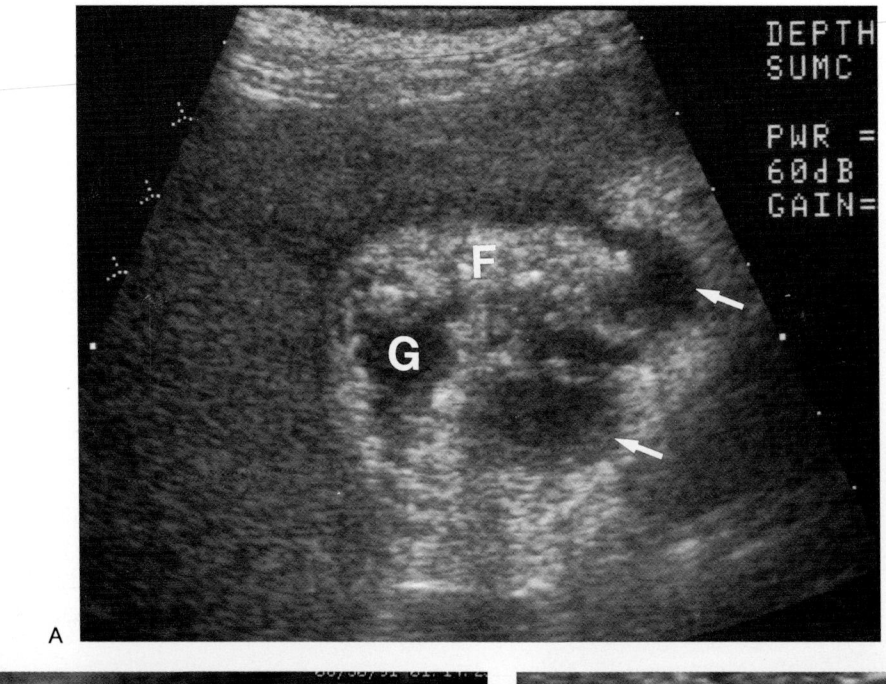

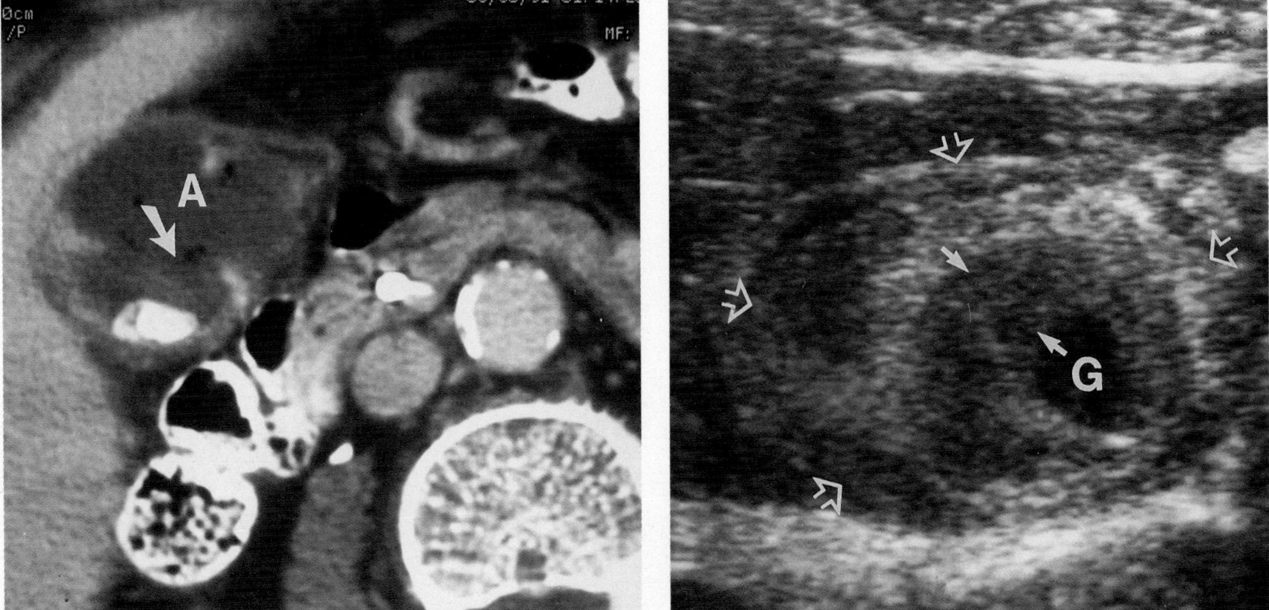

FIG. 3.23. Pericholecystic abscess with surrounding echogenic fat in two patients. **A:** Transverse scan of gallbladder (G) demonstrates echogenic inflamed omental fat (F) adjacent to gallbladder. Hypoechoic areas (*arrows*) correspond to liquefied pus. **B:** CT scan in same patient identifies area of mural necrosis (*arrow*) and surrounding abscess (A). **C:** In another patient, note the marked mural thickening of gangrenous gallbladder (*arrows*). Also note extensive echogenic pericholecystic fat (*open arrows*). G, gallbladder.

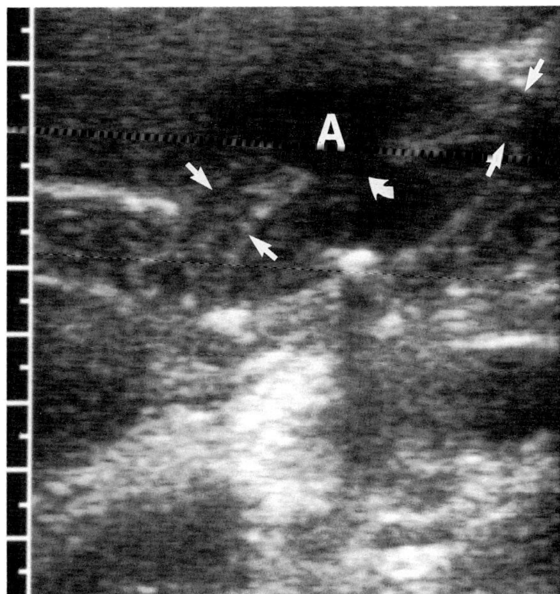

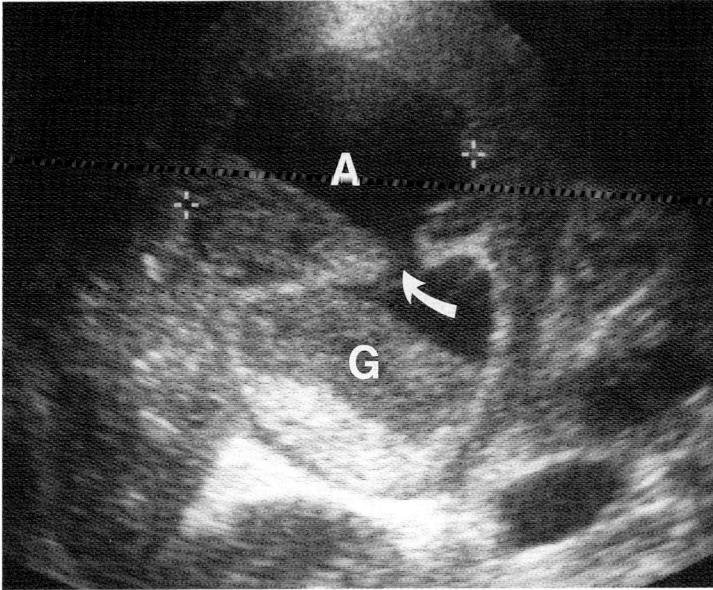

B

FIG. 3.24. Site of gallbladder perforation identified by sonography in two patients. **A:** Sagittal scan of gallbladder demonstrates marked mural thickening (*arrows*), pericholecystic abscess (A), and focal site of mural necrosis (*curved arrow*). **B:** In another patient, pericholecystic abscess (A) is noted anterior to sludge-filled gallbladder (G). *Curved arrow* indicates site of gallbladder perforation.

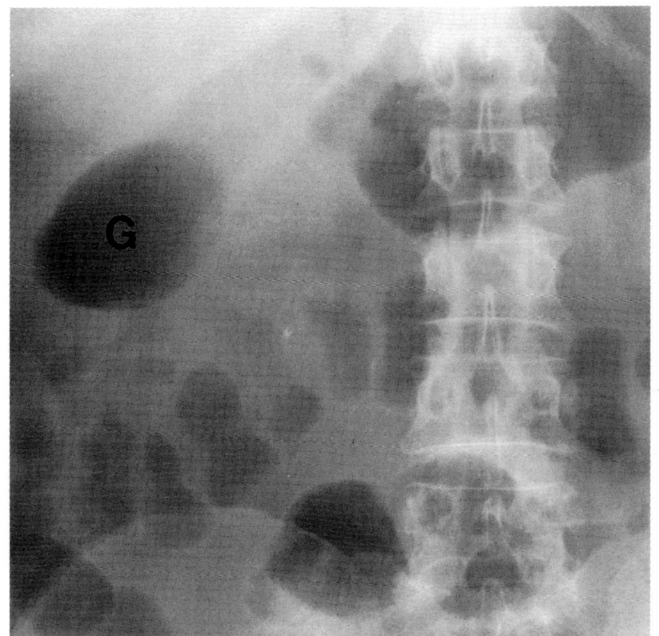

A

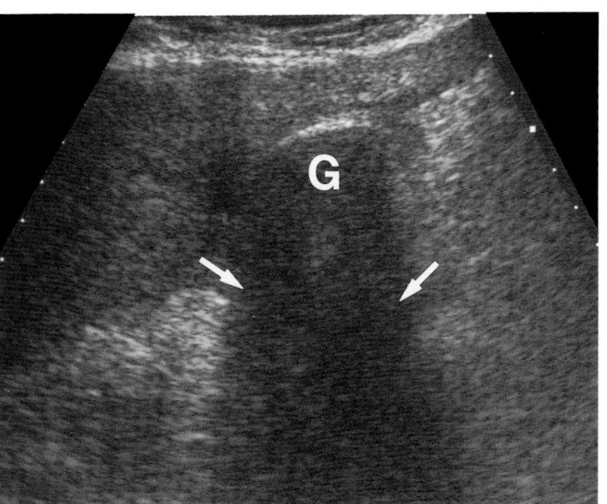

B

FIG. 3.25. Emphysematous cholecystitis with intraluminal gas. **A:** Plain abdominal radiography demonstrates gas in the lumen of the gallbladder (G). **B:** Transverse sonogram of the gallbladder (G) reveals extensive shadowing from gas with acoustic shadowing (*arrow*).

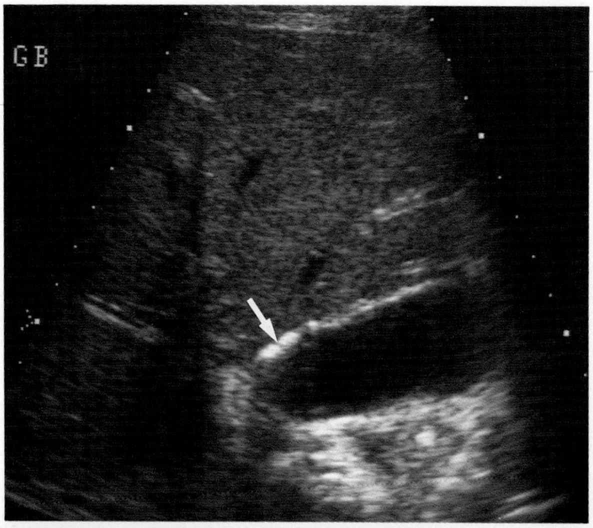

A 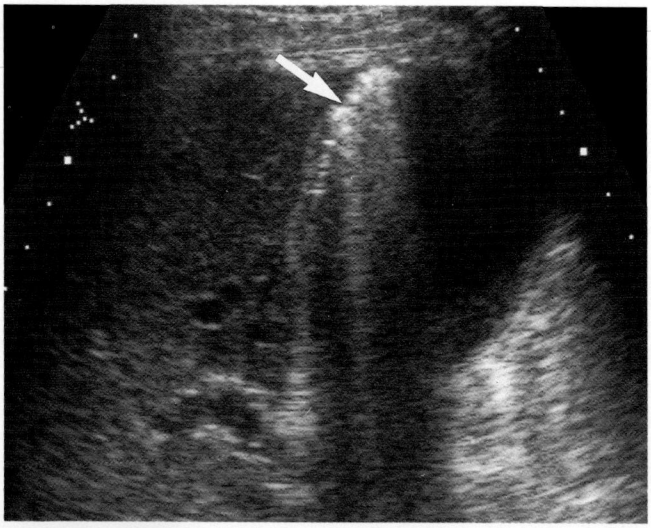 B 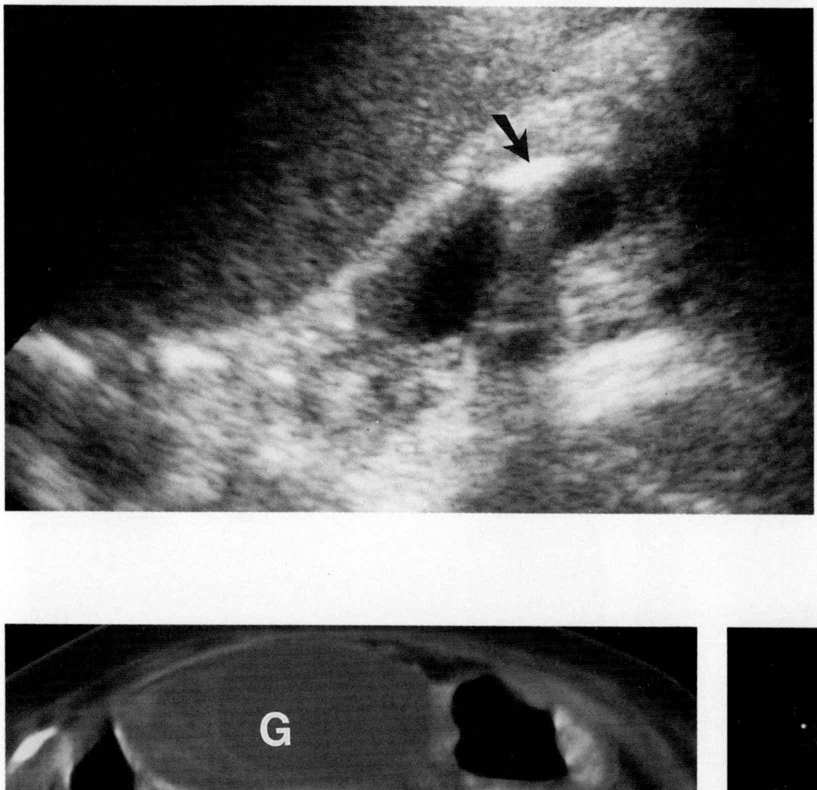 C

FIG. 3.26. Intramural gas in three patients with emphysematous cholecystitis. *Arrows* (**A, B,** and **C**) demonstrate focal gas accumulations in the gallbladder wall in three patients with emphysematous cholecystitis.

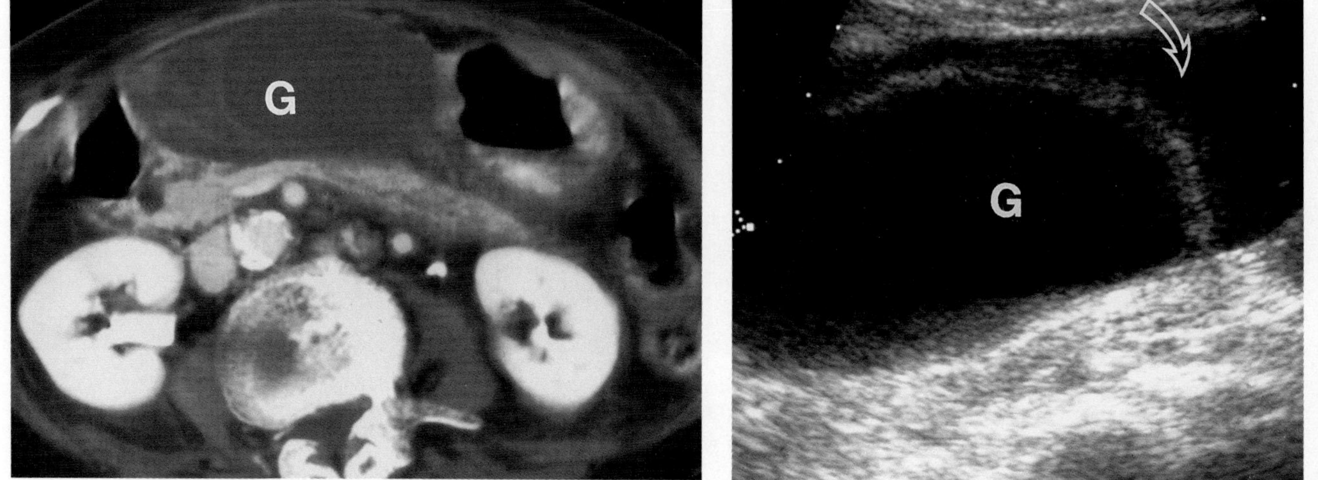

FIG. 3.27. Gallbladder infarction from torsion. **A:** Contrast-enhanced CT scan demonstrates a distended gallbladder with an unusually horizontal axis. **B:** Transverse sonogram of the gallbladder 2 days later demonstrates horizontal axis of the gallbladder as well as new pericholecystic fluid (*arrow*). Gallbladder torsion with infarction was noted at surgery.

Gallbladder Torsion

In approximately 5 percent of patients the gallbladder and cystic duct have a true mesentery (41). The gallbladder may rarely undergo torsion along the axis of its mesentery, causing acute right upper quadrant pain. Torsion of the gallbladder results in vascular compromise with secondary intramural hemorrhage, edema, and ultimately transmural infarction. Depending on the degree of rotation of the gallbladder, the gallbladder may demonstrate an unusually horizontal axis on either sonography or CT (Fig. 3.27).

Empyema of the Gallbladder

An empyema, or pus-filled gallbladder, accounts for biliary sepsis in a small percentage of patients with cholecystitis. These patients often cannot be identified clinically as their symptoms mimic acute cholecystitis. Sonographically, the gallbladder is distended and filled with echogenic pus (Fig. 3.15). Pus within the gallbladder lumen may mimic either sludge or hemorrhage. Diagnostic needle aspiration or percutaneous cholecystostomy must be performed in some patients to confirm the diagnosis.

Xanthogranulomatous Cholecystitis

Xanthogranulomatous cholecystitis is a rare form of chronic inflammation caused by infiltration of the gallbladder wall by lipid-laden histiocytes and multinucleated giant cells (42). The gallbladder wall is replaced by xanthoma cells, resulting in marked mural thickening. Often there are dense adhesions in the right upper quadrant involving the transverse colon, liver, and duodenum. Sonographically, the findings may mimic gangrenous cholecystitis or gallbladder carcinoma due to the extensive mural thickening (Fig. 3.28) (42).

Hyperplastic Cholecystosis

Adenomyomatosis and cholesterolosis are the two pathologic forms of hyperplastic cholecystoses. Adenomyomatosis is characterized by mucosal outpouchings extending through the muscularis layer of the gallbladder wall known as Rokitansky–Aschoff sinuses. Oral cholecystography has historically been the primary method of diagnosis of adenomyomatosis by demonstrating contrast accumulation within the Rokitansky–Aschoff sinuses (43). Involvement of the gallbladder with adenomyomatosis may be circumferential, localized, or diffuse. In patients without gallstones, the need for surgery in adenomyomatosis is controversial.

Sonographic characteristics of adenomyomatosis include intramural calculi (trapped within Rokitansky–Aschoff sinuses) and focal mural thickening of the fundus of the gallbladder (Fig. 3.29) (43). Stones may become isolated within a thickened segmented portion of the fundus (Fig. 3.30). Diffuse forms of adenomyomatosis may be difficult to distinguish from chronic cholecystitis or other causes of gallbladder wall thickening. Intramural calculi or crystal deposition within the gallbladder wall may result in ringdown artifacts (comet tails) (Figs. 3.31 and 3.32). When circumferential this results in a "diamond ring" appearance described by Fowler and Reid (44). Rarely, a double lumen may be demonstrated due to the eccentric extension of the sinuses and creation of a false lumen.

Cholesterolosis is due to deposition of esters within lipid-laden macrophages in the lamina propria of the gallbladder. On gross inspection the mucosal surface of the gallbladder has numerous yellow excrescences superimposed on a hyperemic gallbladder mucosa (Fig. 3.33). Sonographically, cholesterolosis is characterized by echogenic polypoid lesions that are immobile and nonshadowing (45). As with adenomyomatosis, the absence of gallstones makes clinical management of this entity somewhat controversial.

Not infrequently, solitary gallbladder polyps are identified sonographically (Fig. 3.34). Polyps are echogenic mucosal lesions without shadowing. Polyps less than 1 cm are almost always benign and can be followed sonographically. When 1 cm or larger, surgery is indicated to exclude a polypoid carcinoma (Fig. 3.35).

Gallbladder Carcinoma

Gallbladder carcinoma is the fifth most common gastrointestinal malignancy in the United States (46). It is three times more common in women than in men (46). Primary carcinoma of the gallbladder is most often identified in elderly patients with a mean age of approximately 72 years (46). In 1 percent of patients carcinoma may be discovered incidentally at the time of cholecystectomy for acute cholecystitis (46). Gallstones and chronic cholecystitis are typically present. Gallbladder carcinoma is also associated with mural calcification (porcelain gallbladder), colonic polyposis, and inflammatory bowel disease (46). In patients with porcelain gallbladder, approximately 25 percent have associated carcinoma (46). The clinical features of gallbladder carcinoma are often nonspecific. Many patients present with right upper quadrant pain indistinguishable from cholecystitis or biliary colic. There are three gross pathologic forms of gallbladder carcinoma: (a) a polypoid intraluminal mass, (b) focal or diffused circumferential thickening of the gallbladder wall, and (c) a mass replacing the entire gallbladder.

The most common sonographic abnormality in pa-

(*text continues on page 204*)

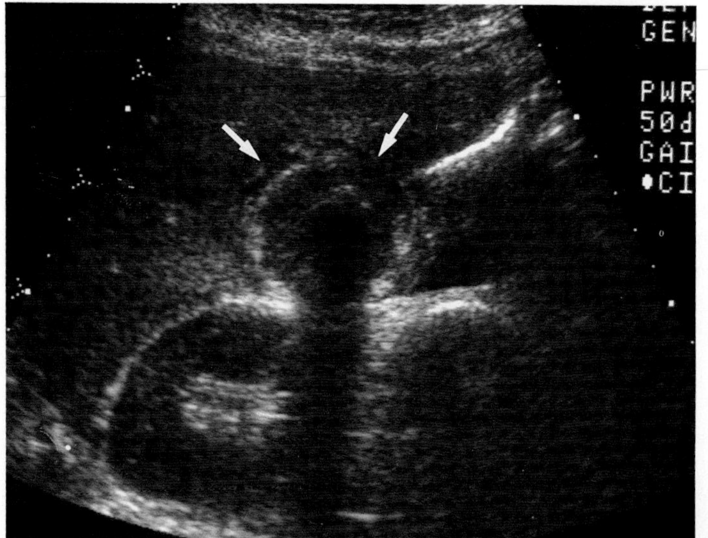

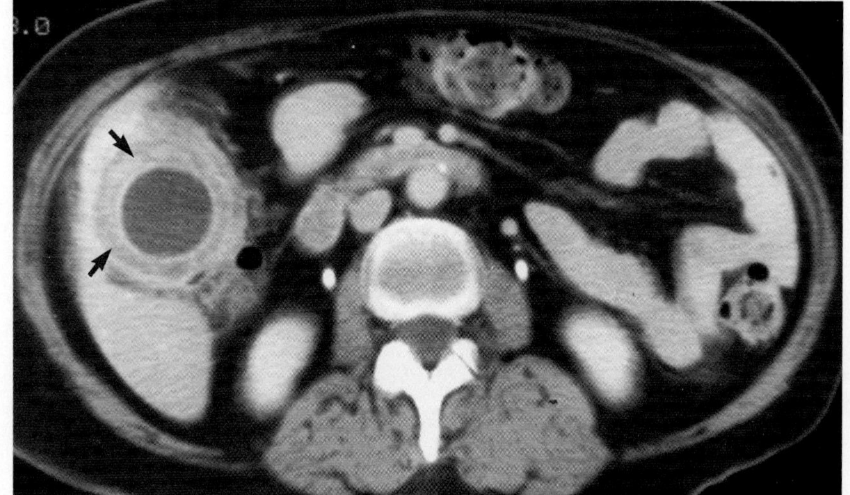

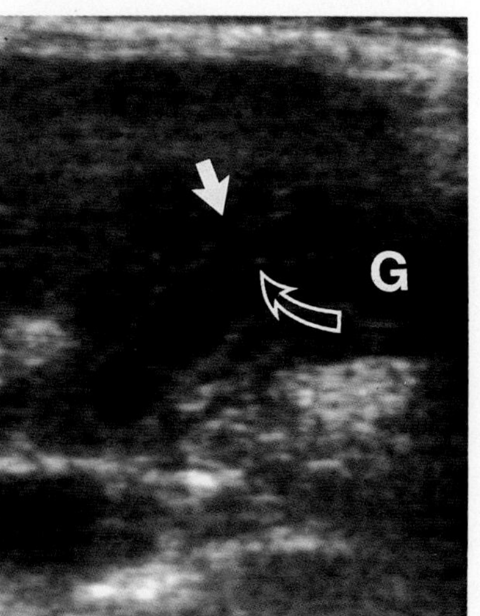

FIG. 3.28. Nonspecific appearance of xanthogranulomatous cholecystitis in two patients. **A:** Transverse sonogram shows gallbladder with a markedly thickened wall (*arrows*). **B:** Note extensive low-attenuation areas demonstrated within the gallbladder on contrast CT scan (*arrows*). **C:** In another patient, note marked mural thickening of the gallbladder wall (*arrow*) and intraluminal membranes (*curved arrow*). G, gallbladder. Findings mimic gangrenous cholecystitis.

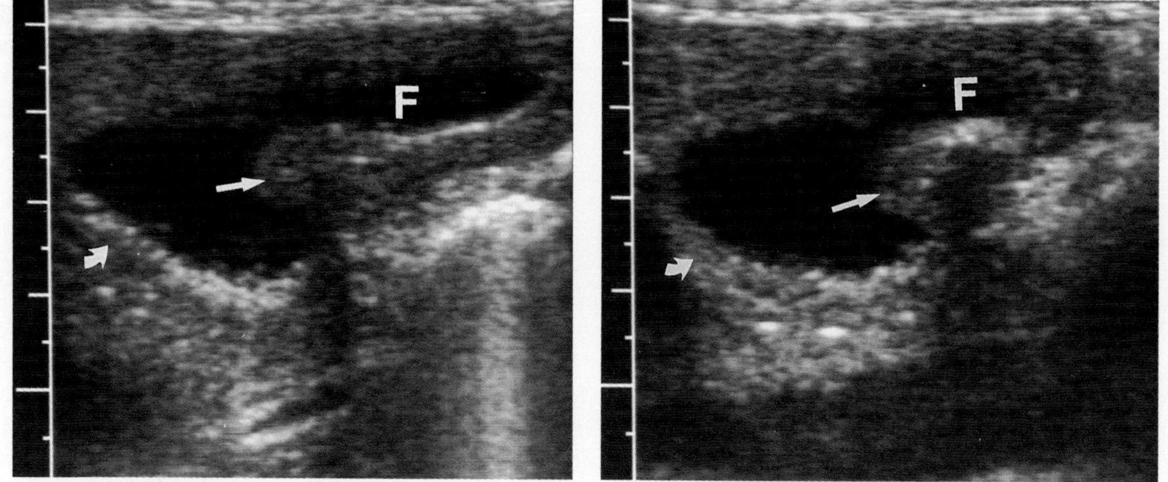

FIG. 3.29. Adenomyomatosis of the gallbladder with mural thickening of the fundus. Oblique views (**A, B**) of the gallbladder demonstrate mural thickening confined to the gallbladder fundus (*arrow*). F, lumen of gallbladder fundus. *Curved arrow* denotes relatively normal gallbladder wall thickness in proximal portion of gallbladder.

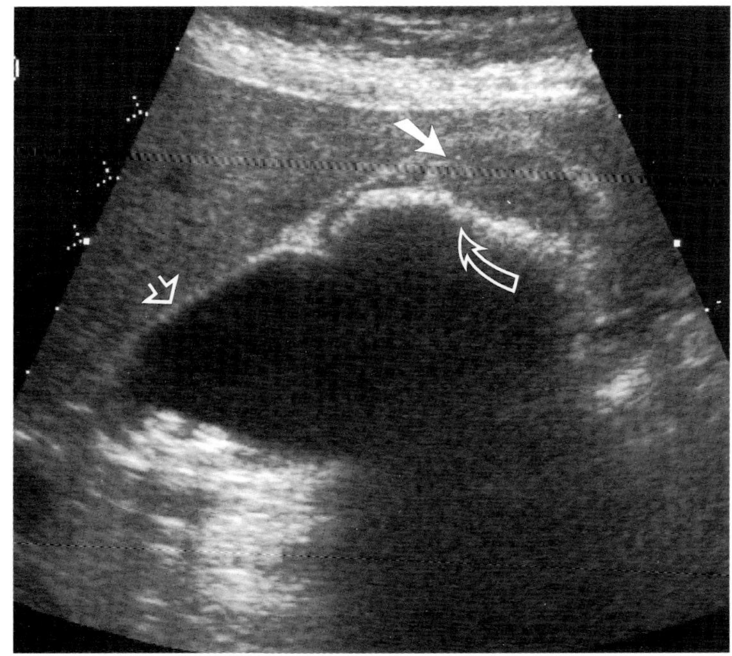

FIG. 3.30. Stones trapped in segmented fundus in adenomyomatosis. Note fundal wall thickening (*arrow*) and shadowing from multiple fundal calculi (*curved arrow*). Note normal wall thickness (*open arrow*) of proximal gallbladder.

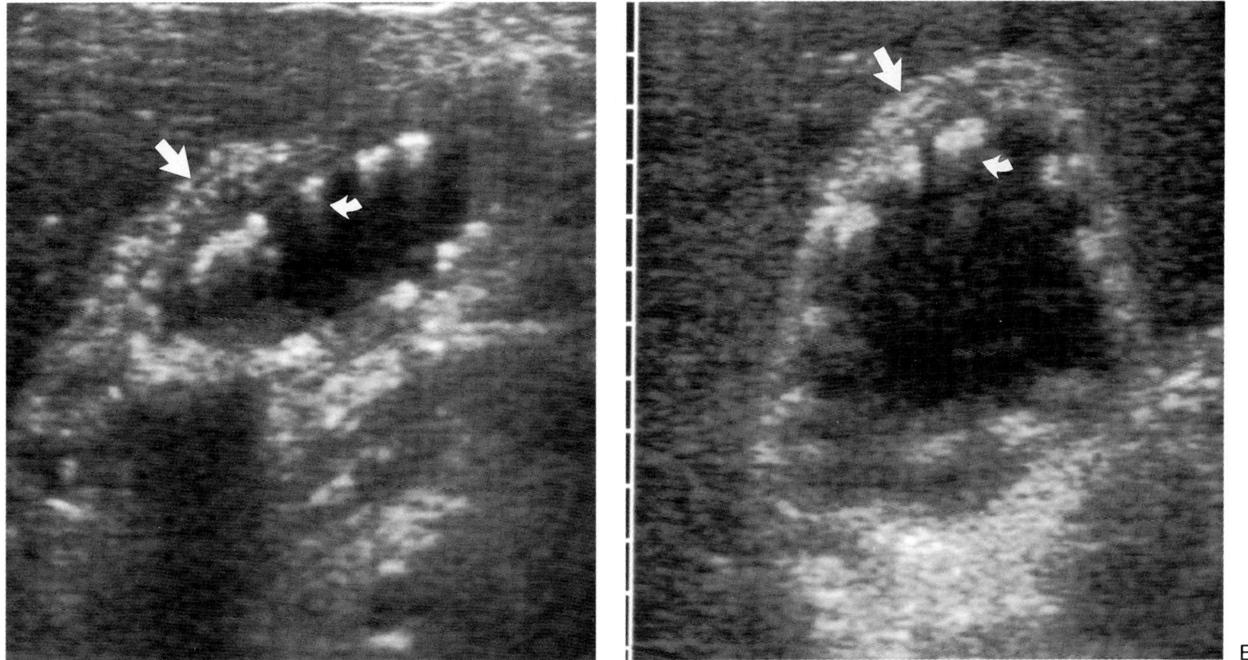

FIG. 3.31. Ringdown artifacts from intramural calculi in adenomyomatosis. Note diffuse mural thickening (*arrows* in **A** and **B**) and reverberation artifacts (comet tails) from intramural calculi (*curved arrows*, **A** and **B**).

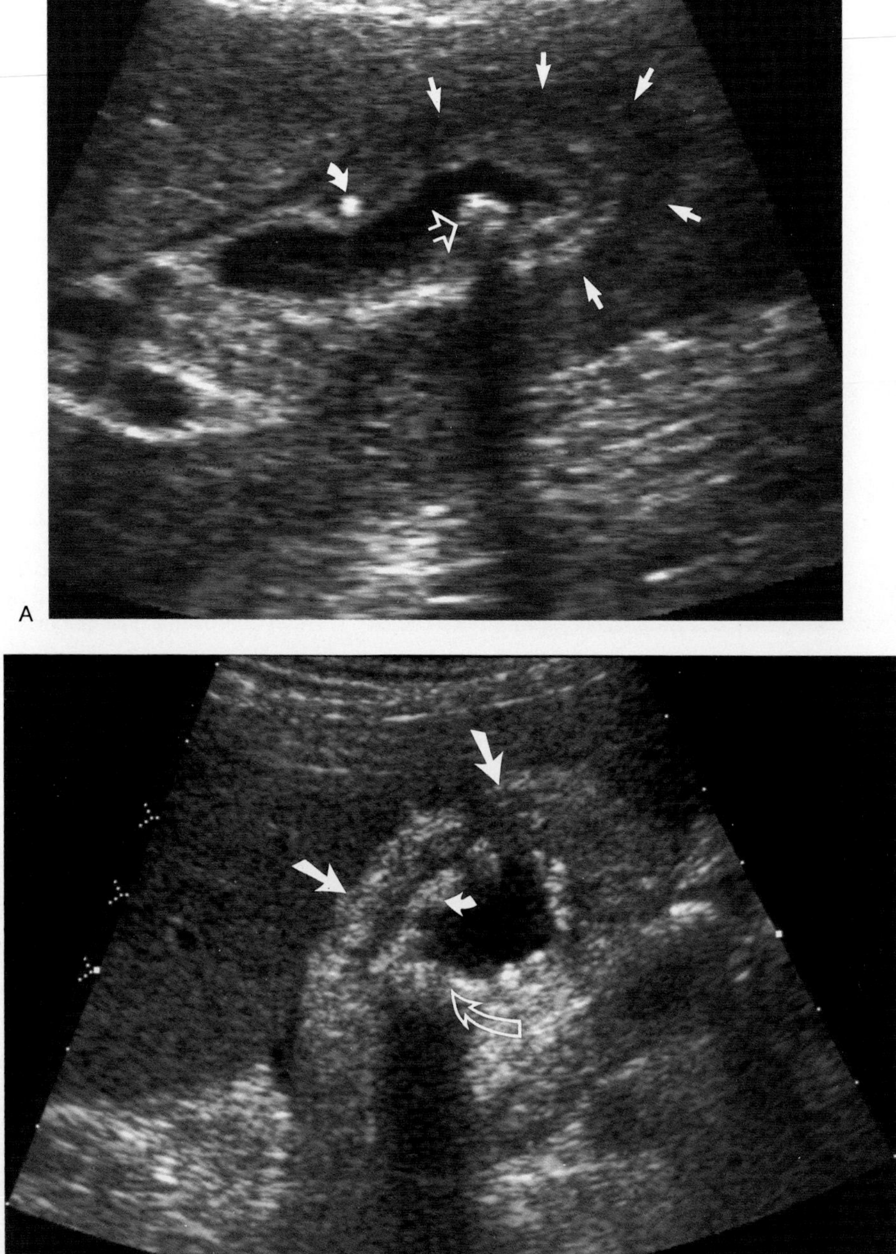

FIG. 3.32. Diffuse form of adenomyomatosis in two patients. **A:** Oblique sonogram of gallbladder demonstrates diffuse mural thickening (*arrows*), intramural stone (*curved arrow*), and intraluminal stone (*open arrow*). **B:** In another patient, note the diffuse wall thickening (*arrows*), intramural calculi (*curved arrow*), and intraluminal calculi (*curved open arrow*).

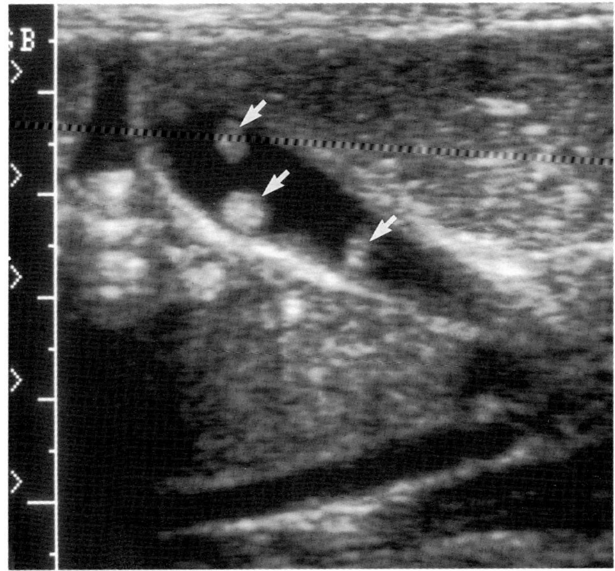

FIG. 3.33. Cholesterolosis with multiple polyps. Multiple polyps are identified on transverse view of gallbladder (*arrows*).

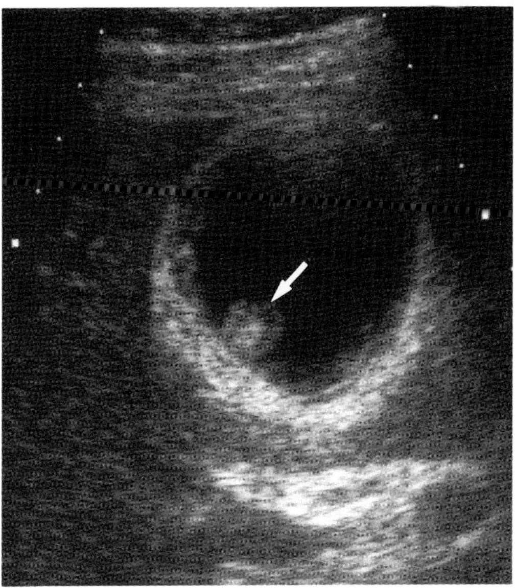

FIG. 3.34. Gallbladder polyp. Echogenic polyp (*arrow*) is identified on transverse sonogram. Note lack of distal acoustic shadowing.

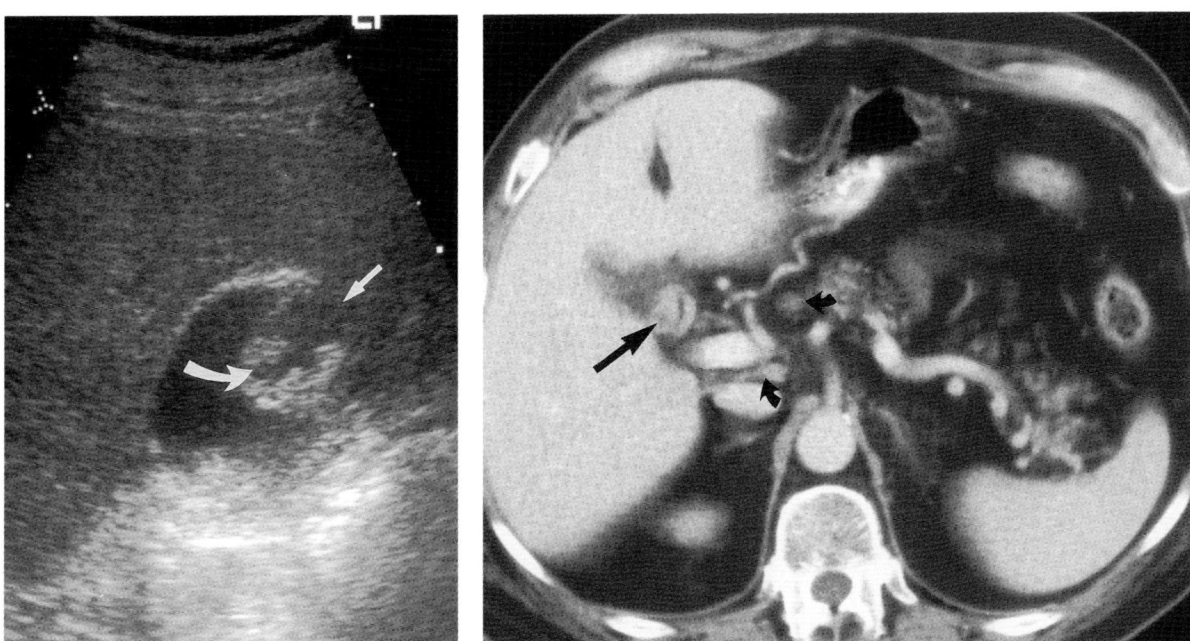

FIG. 3.35. Polypoid gallbladder carcinoma. **A:** Small polypoid carcinoma (*curved arrow*) is identified on transverse sonogram. Mural invasion at the base of the carcinoma is evident by loss of mucosal echogenicity (*arrow*). **B:** Corresponding CT scan demonstrates enhancing mass in gallbladder (*arrow*). Note small adjacent nodes (*curved arrows*). Metastatic gallbladder carcinoma was found at surgery.

tients with gallbladder carcinoma is a mass replacing the entire gallbladder (Fig. 3.36) (47). The second most common finding on both sonography and CT is evidence of hepatic invasion from a gallbladder mass (Fig. 3.37) (47). This typically appears as a hypoechoic hepatic lesion immediately adjacent to a thickened gallbladder wall. Gallbladder carcinoma has a poor clinical prognosis. The majority of patients will have advanced disease at the time of diagnosis and approximately 84 percent have hepatic or lymph node metastases (47).

There are a number of sonographic pitfalls in the diagnosis of gallbladder carcinoma. Small polypoid carcinomas may mimic benign polyps (Fig. 3.38). Thus in patients with polyps larger than 1 cm either surgery or close-interval follow-up is indicated to document stability and exclude carcinoma. Intraluminal masses may appear similar to tumefactive sludge on grayscale images (Fig. 3.39). Color Doppler sonography or contrast CT may be extremely helpful to distinguish sludge from carcinoma (Figs. 3.40 and 3.41). Most gallbladder carcinomas will demonstrate both intrinsic vascularity with color Doppler sonography and contrast enhancement with dynamic bolus CT. Diffuse infiltration of the gallbladder wall, however, may be impossible to distinguish from other forms of chronic cholecystitis.

There are several characteristic patterns of spread of gallbladder carcinoma that may be diagnosed with sonography and CT (47). The most common abnormality is contiguous spread of the tumor into the liver. Nodal metastases are also common to the porta hepatis. Hematogenous metastases to the liver may also be identified by sonography (Fig. 3.42) but are often better identified with contrast CT.

Gallbladder Metastases

Hematogenous metastases to the gallbladder are rare but may occur in melanoma, carcinoma of the lung, breast, or other widespread malignancies. A solitary metastasis may be indistinguishable from a primary carcinoma (Fig. 3.43) or a large benign polyp.

Gallbladder Duplication

Complete gallbladder duplication is a rare anomaly. Its importance lies in not mistaking the duplication for pericholecystic fluid (Fig. 3.44).

BILE DUCTS

Technique

Real-time sonography with color Doppler is an ideal method to visualize early biliary ductal dilatation. Bile ducts stand out in stark contrast to the color-coded vessels. It is now possible to routinely image normal intrahepatic bile ducts (Fig. 3.45). The use of color Doppler sonography is essential to distinguish small hepatic vessels from bile ducts. This is particularly true in the lateral segment of the left lobe as parallel branching structures representing the hepatic artery and portal vein may mimic dilated left intrahepatic bile ducts.

In general, biliary tract imaging is best performed with a 5-MHz curved array transducer. Color Doppler sonography should be employed routinely in all patients with possible biliary tract dilatation on grayscale images. The anatomic relationship between the biliary tree and the portal venous system is variable and inconstant. Bret et al. (48) have demonstrated that the widely held view that the bile ducts are always anterior to the portal venous system is incorrect. Bile ducts may be located posterior to the portal veins or intertwined between portal venous segments (48). These anatomic relationships can be clearly depicted with color Doppler sonography.

The intra- and extrahepatic ductal systems should be examined with patients in different positions. The common hepatic duct and proximal right and left ducts are best imaged with the patient in a supine LPO position, scanning in sagittal and transverse planes. The intrapancreatic portion of the distal extrahepatic bile duct is best visualized with the patient in a semi-erect slight right posterior oblique (RPO) position. Transverse scans of the head of the pancreas are essential to visualize the distal common bile duct free from overlying duodenal bowel gas.

Sonographic Diagnosis of Biliary Ductal Dilatation

The right and left main bile ducts are extrahepatic in their course and lie in close proximity to the right portal vein or anterior segment of the left portal vein. Based on endoscopic cholangiograms, Davies et al. (49) have demonstrated that the "extrahepatic common bile duct" measured anterior to the right portal vein, in fact, represents the right hepatic duct. Thus what has been loosely termed the extrahepatic bile duct or common hepatic bile duct in the prior sonographic literature may, in fact, be the right hepatic duct. In general, intrahepatic bile ducts should be 2 mm or less in normal patients. The internal diameter of the extrahepatic bile duct is generally 5 mm or less. An extrahepatic duct measuring 6 to 9 mm is equivocal for biliary dilatation and the patient's age must be taken into account. Aging causes elastic fiber degeneration within the bile duct wall, and therefore the internal diameter of the extrahepatic duct dilates with age (50). A reasonable rule to follow is to allow 1 mm of internal diameter of the bile duct for each decade after 50. A 7-mm bile duct is considered normal in a 70-year-old patient (51).

(text continues on page 213)

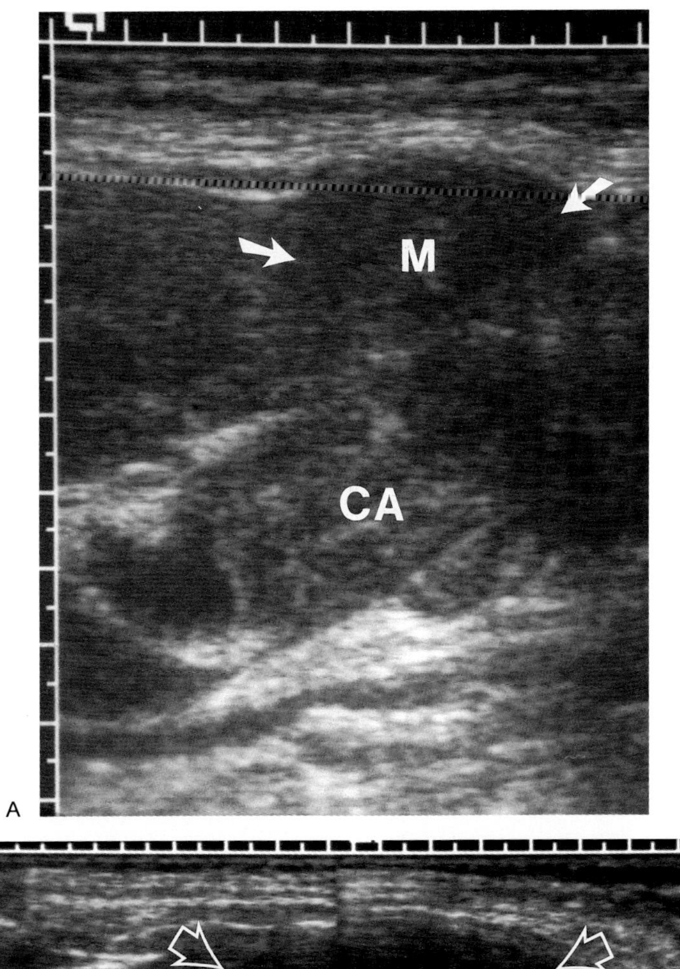

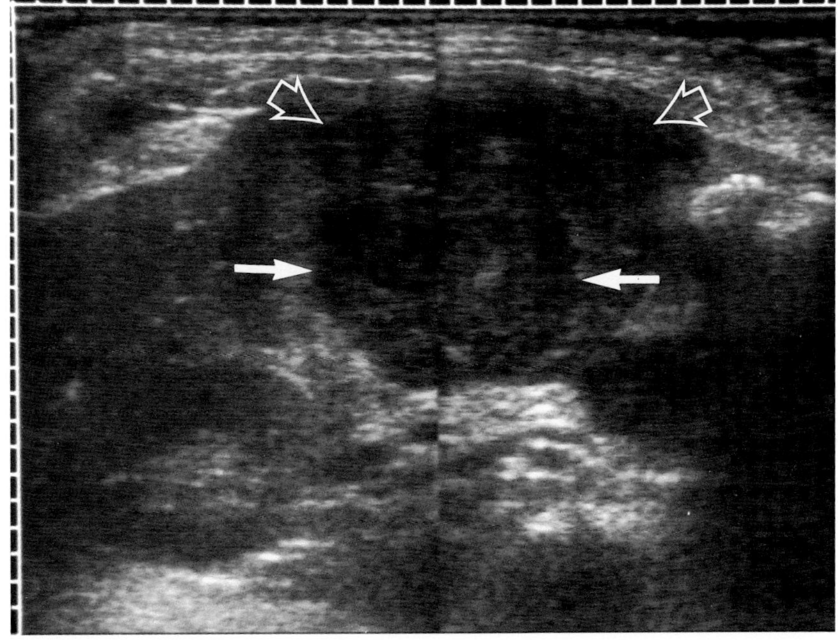

FIG. 3.36. Gallbladder carcinoma with direct hepatic invasion. **A:** Sagittal sonogram of gallbladder demonstrates large hypoechoic carcinoma (CA) with direct metastasis (M) to liver. *Arrows* denote edges of metastasis. **B:** Transverse scan of gallbladder demonstrates extensive carcinoma (*arrows*) replacing the gallbladder. Direct invasion of liver is evident (*open arrows*).

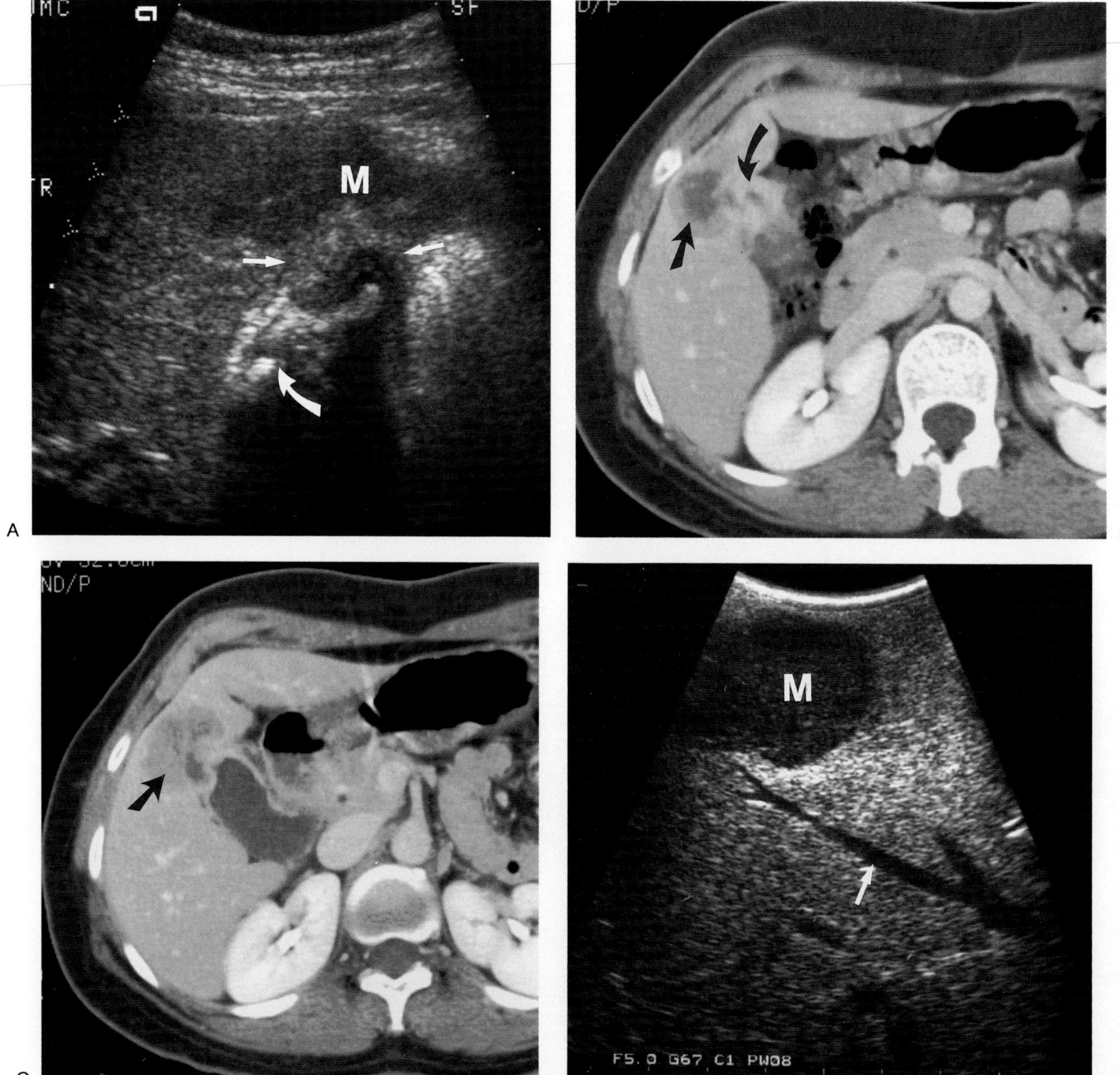

FIG. 3.37. Fundal carcinoma directly invading liver. **A:** Transverse scan of the gallbladder fundus demonstrates a hypoechoic carcinoma (*arrows*) with direct liver metastasis (M). Note gallstones (*curved arrow*). **B, C:** Contrast CT scans demonstrate similar findings of fundal mass (*curved arrow,* **B**) with liver metastasis (*arrows,* **B** and **C**). **D:** Intraoperative sonogram shows liver metastasis (M) during successful surgical resection. Note relationship of metastasis to middle hepatic vein (*arrow*).

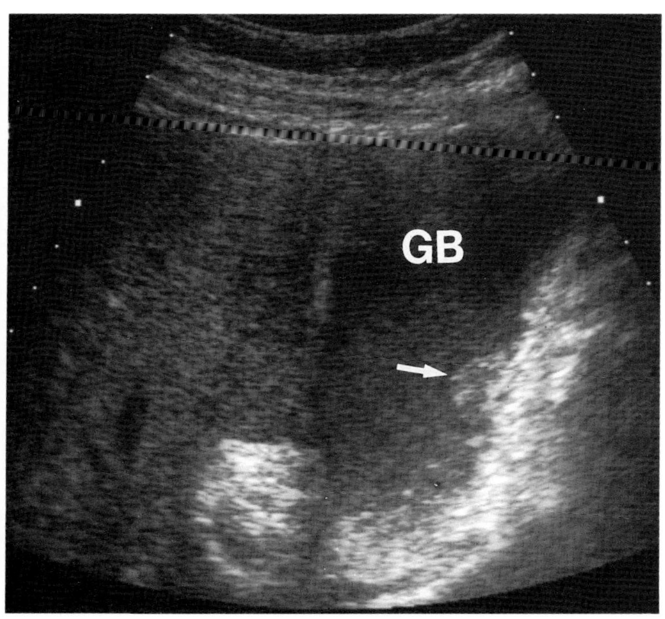

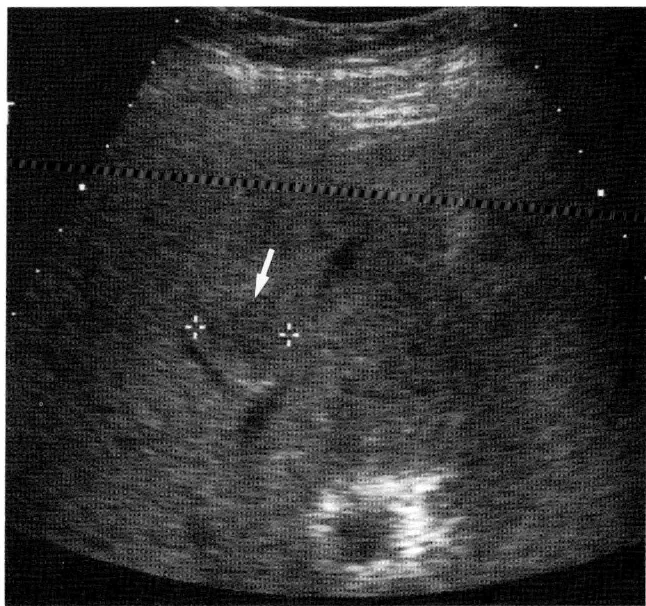

B

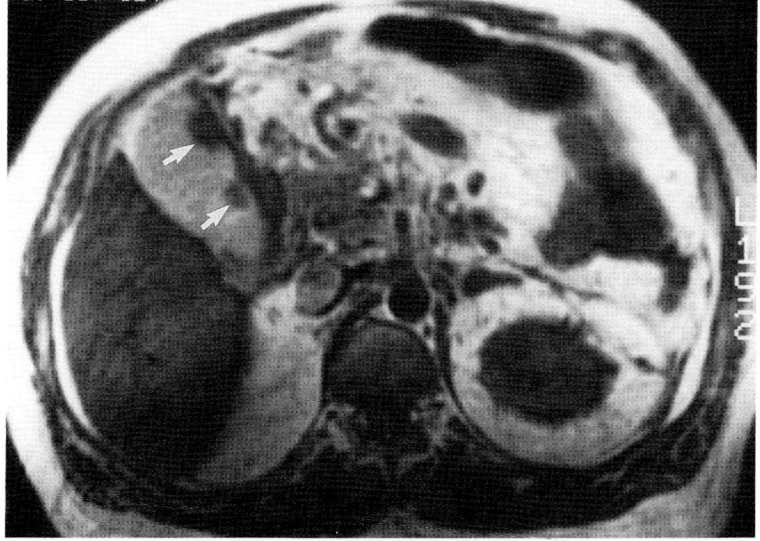

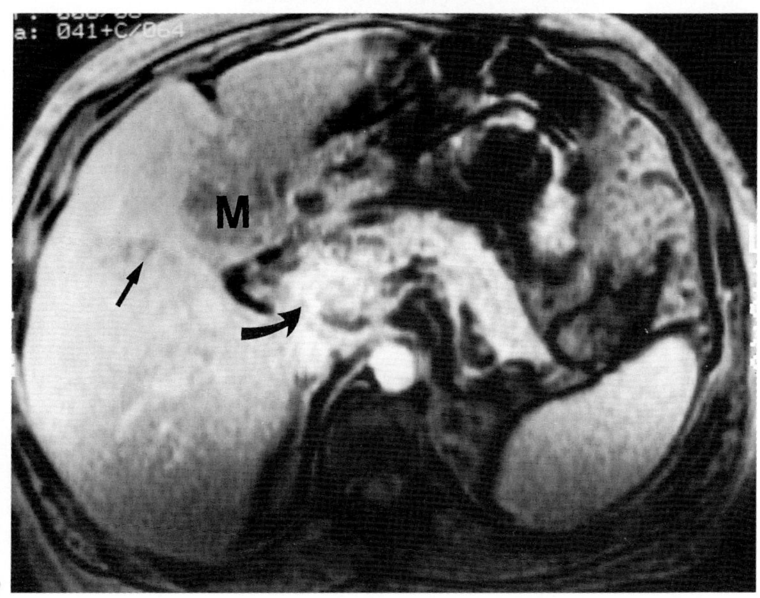

FIG. 3.38. Small polypoid carcinoma. **A:** Oblique scan of the gallbladder (GB) demonstrates small polypoid carcinoma (*arrow*). **B:** Subtle liver metastasis is identified (*arrow*). **C:** T1-weighted MR scan demonstrates two gallbladder polyps. The larger polyp was malignant. **D:** Extent of metastases are better demonstrated by gadolinium-enhanced MRI sequence. Note large liver metastasis (M) not appreciated by sonography. Note enhancing nodal metastasis (*curved arrow*) in porta hepatis and smaller intrahepatic metastasis (*arrow*).

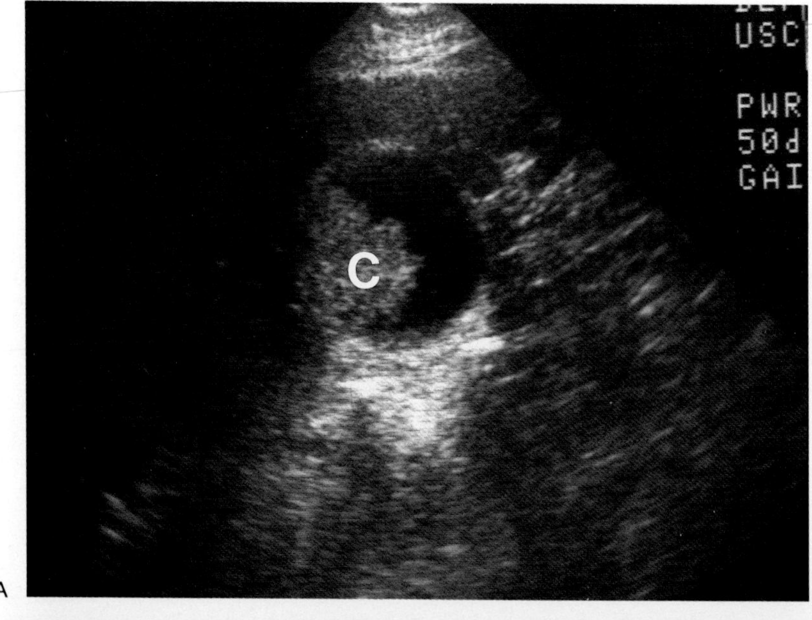

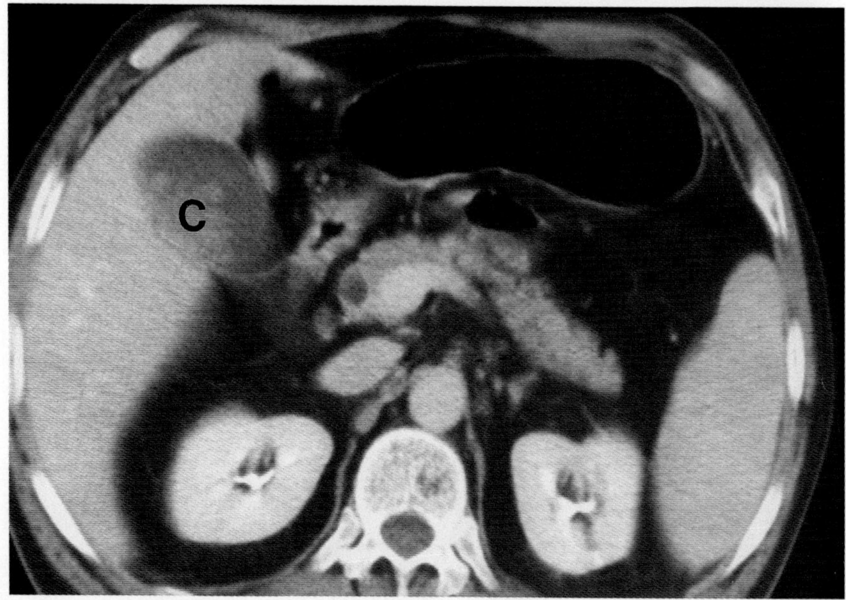

FIG. 3.39. Polypoid carcinoma mimicking tumefactive sludge. **A:** Transverse scan of gallbladder demonstrates lobulated villous carcinoma (C). The appearance mimics tumefactive sludge. **B:** Contrast CT scan demonstrates enhancement of carcinoma (C) and no evidence of liver metastases.

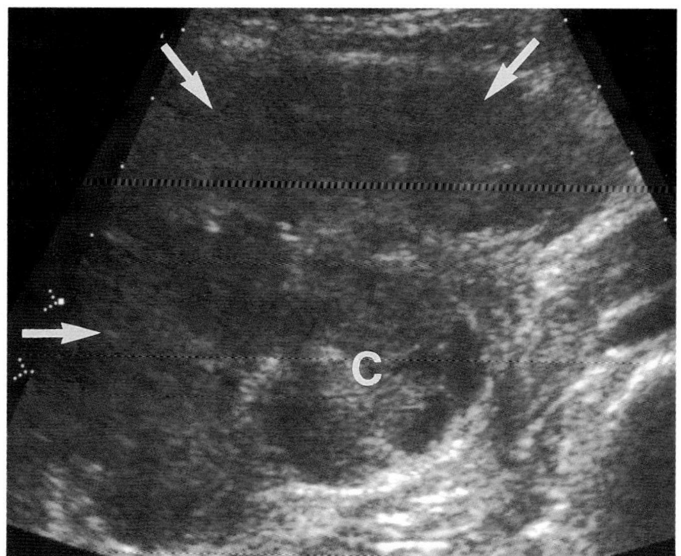

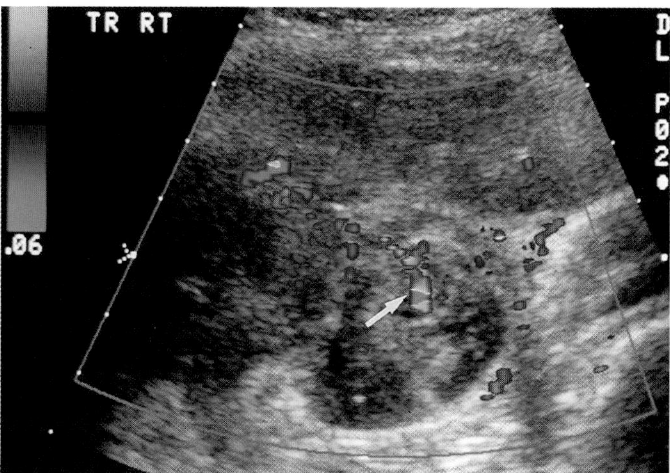

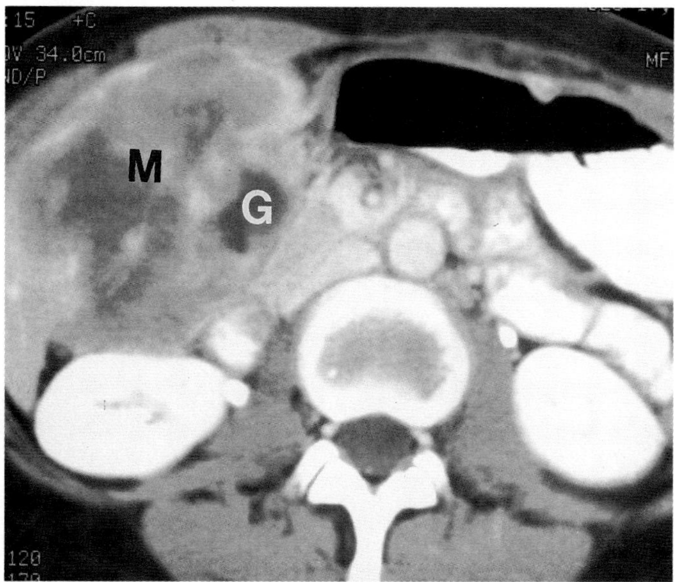

FIG. 3.40. Color Doppler sonography of gallbladder carcinoma. **A:** Transverse grayscale image of gallbladder demonstrates echogenic carcinoma (C) replacing most of gallbladder. Note vague hypoechoic mass within adjacent liver (*arrows*). **B:** Color Doppler sonogram demonstrates intrinsic vascularity consistent with carcinoma (*arrow*). **C:** Contrast CT scan better depicts extensive liver metastases (M) and small residual gallbladder lumen (G).

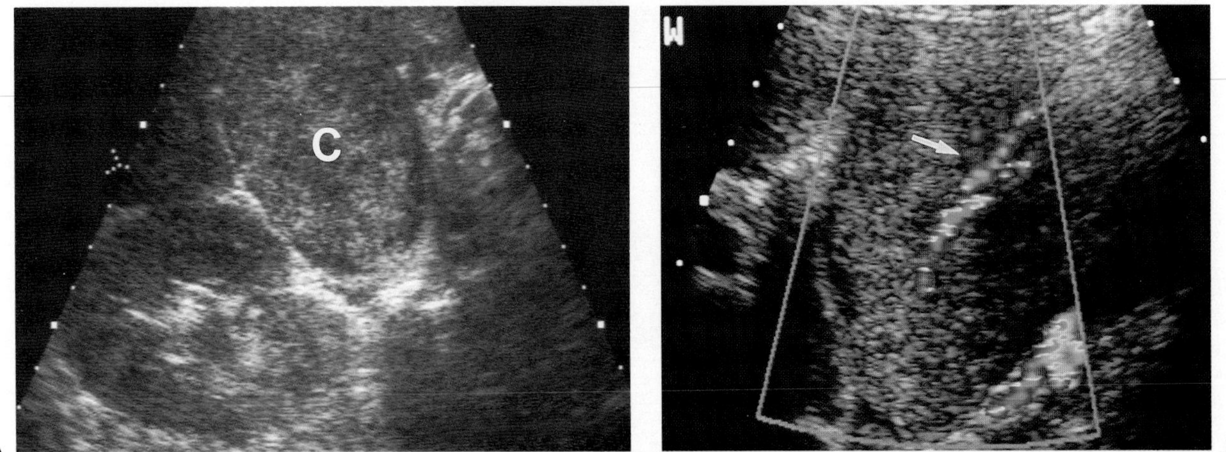

FIG. 3.41. Value of color Doppler sonography in distinguishing intraluminal carcinoma from sludge. **A:** Transverse scan of gallbladder demonstrates echogenic carcinoma (C) filling the entire lumen. The appearance is indistinguishable from sludge. **B:** Color Doppler sonogram demonstrates internal vascularity (*arrow*) within the mass, diagnostic of tumor.

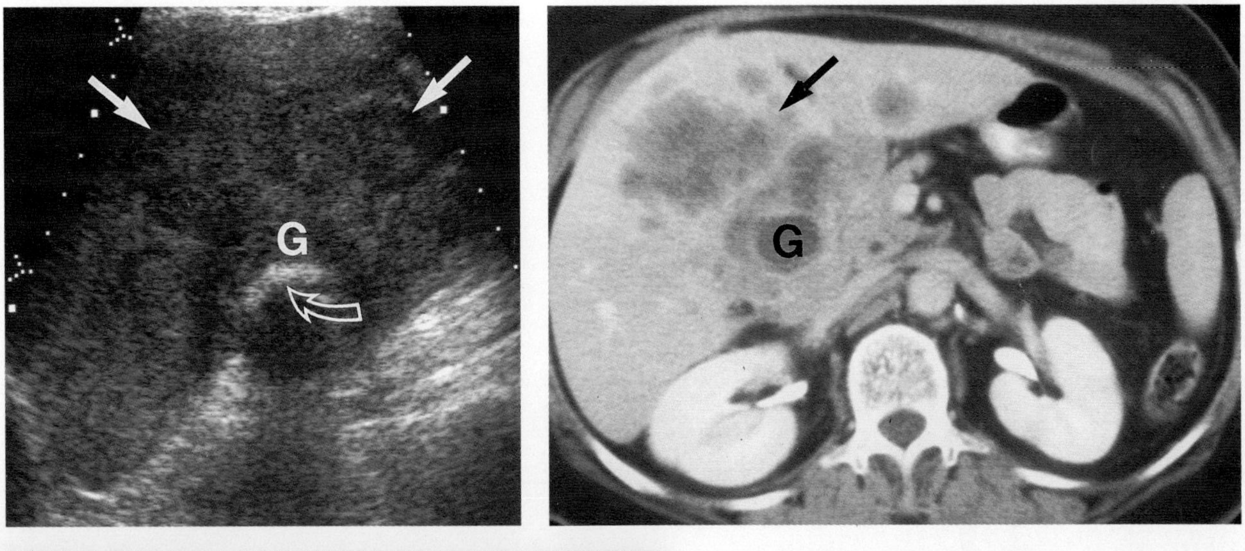

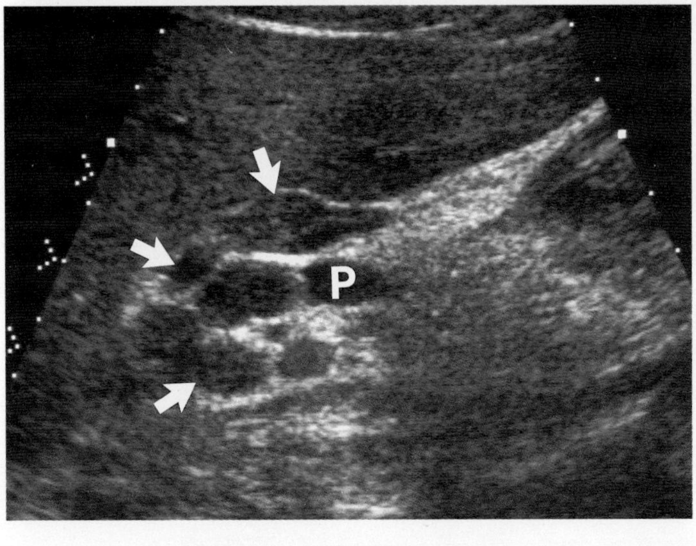

A B C

FIG. 3.42. Nodal metastases from gallbladder carcinoma. **A:** Demonstration of a direct hepatic invasion from gallbladder carcinoma (*arrows*). G, gallbladder. **B:** CT scan demonstrates hepatic metastases (*arrow*). G, gallbladder; *curved arrow,* stones. **C:** Nodal metastases to porta hepatis are noted (*arrows*). P, portal vein.

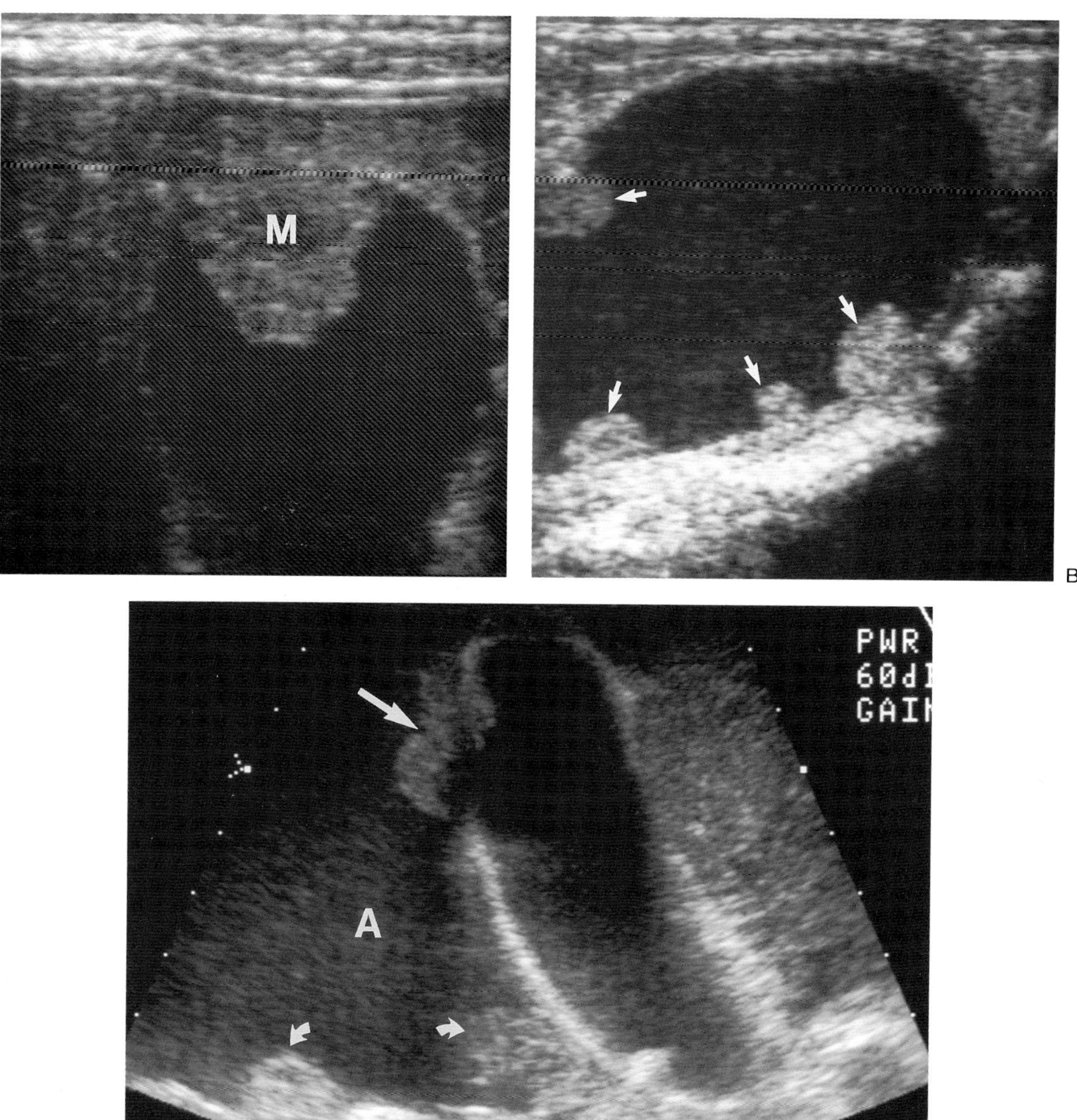

FIG. 3.43. Sonographic spectrum of gallbladder metastases in three patients. **A:** Solitary gallbladder metastasis (M) from lung carcinoma is shown. **B:** In another patient, multiple polypoid metastases (*arrows*) from adenocarcinoma are noted. **C:** In a third patient, serosal metastasis (*arrow*) to gallbladder is noted. Patient had carcinomatosis from pancreatic cancer. Note echogenic ascites (A) and peritoneal implants (*curved arrows*).

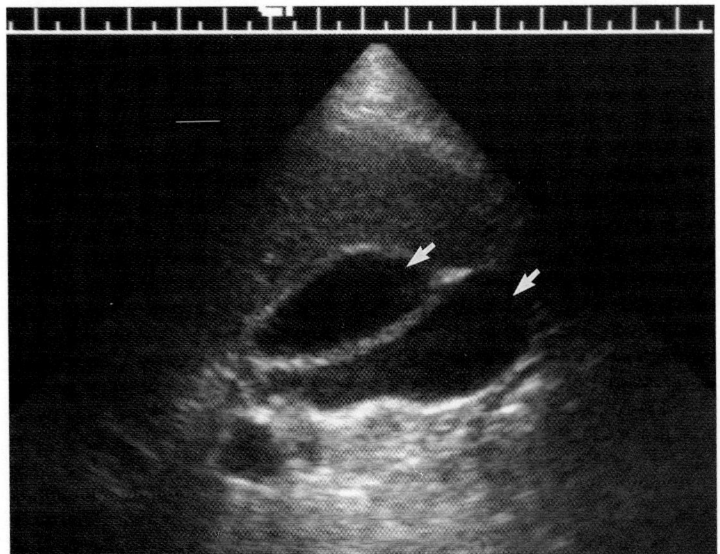

FIG. 3.44. Complete gallbladder duplication. Two separate gallbladders (*arrows*) are visualized in this sagittal sonogram.

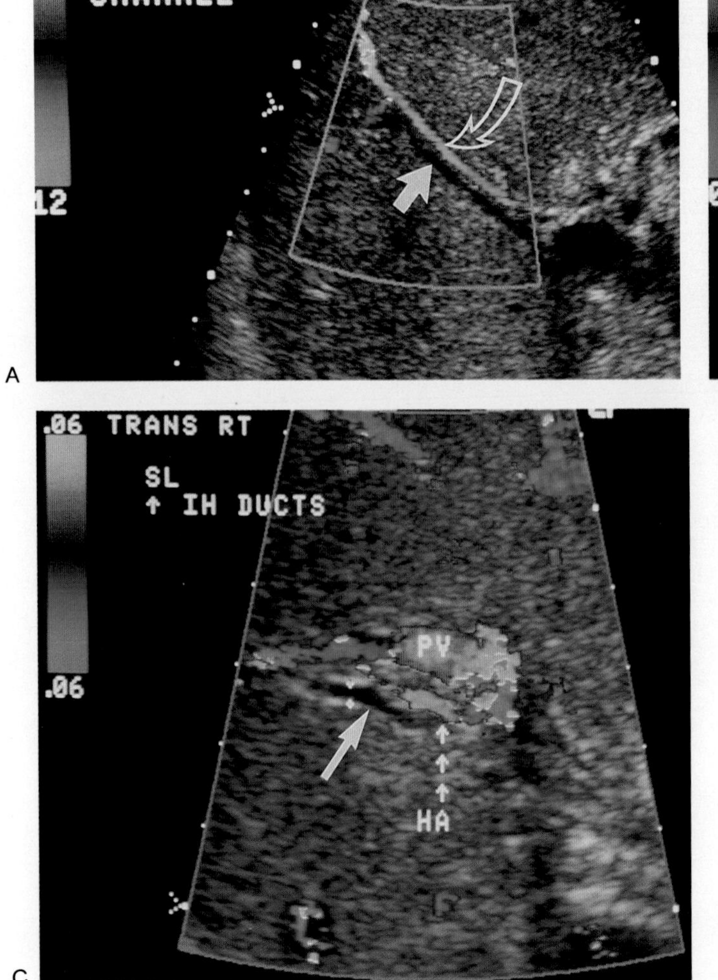

FIG. 3.45. Value of color Doppler sonography in demonstrating normal and minimally dilated intrahepatic bile ducts in three patients. **A:** Note normal peripheral bile duct (*arrow*) adjacent to color-coded portal vein (*curved arrow*). **B:** In another patient, note minimally dilated bile ducts (*arrows*). **C:** In a third patient, note minimally dilated intrahepatic bile ducts (*arrow*). PV, portal vein; HA, hepatic artery.

Bile ducts greater than 10 mm in internal diameter are generally due to obstruction (52,53). Rarely, this degree of dilatation may be noted in elderly patients with dilated but nonobstructed ducts due to elastic fiber breakdown. Direct cholangiography is often required to further evaluate these patients. Whether bile duct dilatation occurs after cholecystectomy is a subject of considerable controversy (51). It is our view that in most instances dilatation is due to precholecystectomy stone passage with intermittent obstruction and subsequent elastic fiber breakdown in the bile duct wall.

Administration of a fatty meal may be of value in selected patients with equivocally enlarged bile ducts (54–56). Thirty minutes after a fatty meal, the unobstructed bile duct usually decreases 2 mm in diameter (Fig. 3.46). Enlargement of the duct by 2 mm indicates a positive study suggestive of partial obstruction by a stone. Lack of change in size of the duct is equivocal and requires further evaluation with direct cholangiography.

Dilated intrahepatic ducts demonstrate a number of relatively constant sonographic findings with real-time imaging and color Doppler sonography. One typical feature is a stellate branching pattern of bile ducts extending from the porta hepatis. Unlike portal or hepatic veins, dilated intrahepatic ducts have irregular walls and may demonstrate distal acoustic enhancement (49). As previously emphasized, color Doppler imaging has greatly enhanced the ability to visualize both anatomic variation in the position of bile ducts and subtle biliary tract dilatation. On occasion, two parallel structures can be identified in the left lobe that mimic the "shotgun" sign of dilated intrahepatic bile duct adjacent to the left portal vein. Color Doppler sonography readily identifies both structures as vessels. The left hepatic artery is noted adjacent to the left portal vein (Fig. 3.47). Similarly, dilated intrahepatic vascular structures may mimic the grayscale appearance of obstructed bile ducts (Fig. 3.48). This may occur in patients with Osler–Weber–Rendu syndrome with intrahepatic arteriovenous malformations.

The main role of sonography in patients with jaundice and possible biliary tract obstruction is to exclude intra- or extrahepatic ductal dilatation. The level of obstruction may be identified correctly in 90 percent of cases with high-resolution real-time sonography (52). However, direct cholangiography and/or CT is often required to fully assess the cause and extent of biliary tract obstruction (52). In all patients with extrahepatic obstruction, a specific attempt should be made to determine its anatomic level. The level of obstruction is often critical in determining the etiology.

In the vast majority of patients with elevated liver function tests and hyperbilirubinemia, sonography can reliably determine the presence or absence of biliary tract obstruction. However, in a small percentage of cases, both false-negative and false-positive sonographic examinations may result (53). In some patients with biliary tract obstruction the intra- or extrahepatic bile ducts are of normal caliber minimally dilated (53). This occurs in selected forms of cholangitis such as sclerosing cholangitis or AIDS-related cholangitis (53,57). Similarly, partial or intermittent extrahepatic obstruction from a small common bile duct stone may produce little or no biliary dilatation (Fig. 3.49). Peripheral intrahepatic biliary obstruction from either an intrahepatic neoplasm, stricture, or stone may also not be detected on a screening sonogram unless the focal area of biliary tract dilatation is identified. Hemobilia may cause medium level homogeneous echoes within the bile duct that may make visualization of the extrahepatic bile duct difficult. Hemobilia may also be indistinguishable from sludge or infected bile and may create difficulties in differential diagnosis.

BILIARY TRACT PATHOLOGY

Cholangitis

Bacterial Cholangitis

Patients with bacterial cholangitis typically present with fever, right upper quadrant pain, and jaundice. The clinical manifestations may be indistinguishable from acute cholecystitis. On occasion, however, patients may present with hypotension and shock due to gram-negative septicemia. In approximately two-thirds of patients the etiology of cholangitis is due to benign disease either from common bile duct stones or postoperative biliary strictures. Neoplastic obstruction, choledochal cysts, parasitic infection, and iatrogenic causes are less common etiologies (58).

Sonography is an excellent screening method to evaluate patients with suspected bacterial cholangitis (Fig. 3.50). In the vast majority of patients, significant biliary ductal dilatation will be readily apparent. Contrast-enhanced CT, however, may provide important additional information in patients with cholangitis. Cholangitic abscesses from biliary tract obstruction may be better demonstrated by contrast CT if they are small or gas-containing. Percutaneous biliary drainage is often performed on an emergent basis in patients with bacterial cholangitis. Sonography may be particularly valuable in guiding percutaneous access to the biliary tree and avoiding bacteremia from direct contrast injection into an infected biliary tree.

Recurrent Pyogenic Cholangitis

Recurrent pyogenic cholangitis (also known as Oriental cholangitis or Oriental cholangiohepatitis) is endemic in areas of Asia although non-Asians may also suffer from this condition. This entity is being encountered with increasing frequency in Western countries due to

(*text continues on page 217*)

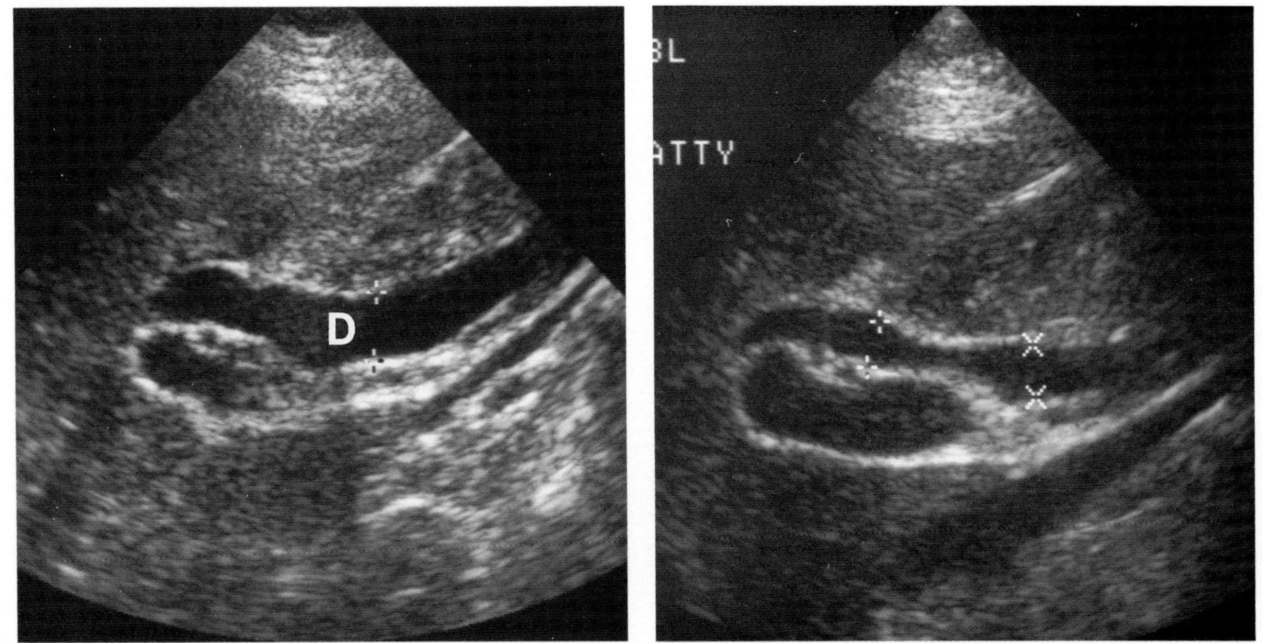

FIG. 3.46. Value of fatty meal in the evaluation of a dilated common duct. **A:** Initial scan demonstrates an 8-mm duct (D). **B:** Repeat scan 30 min after fatty meal reveals normal response with diminution of duct size to 6 mm.

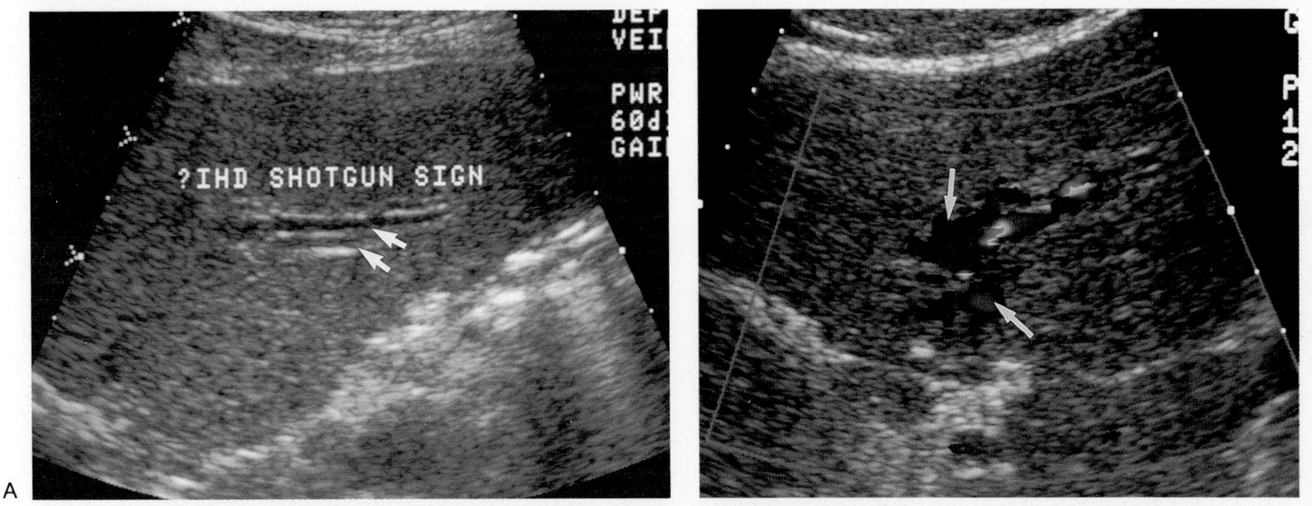

FIG. 3.47. Hepatic artery mimicking dilated intrahepatic bile duct. **A:** Initial grayscale images of left lobe demonstrate two parallel tubular structures (*arrows*). **B:** Color Doppler sonogram demonstrates that these structures (*arrows*) are both vessels (portal vein and hepatic artery) and not dilated intrahepatic ducts.

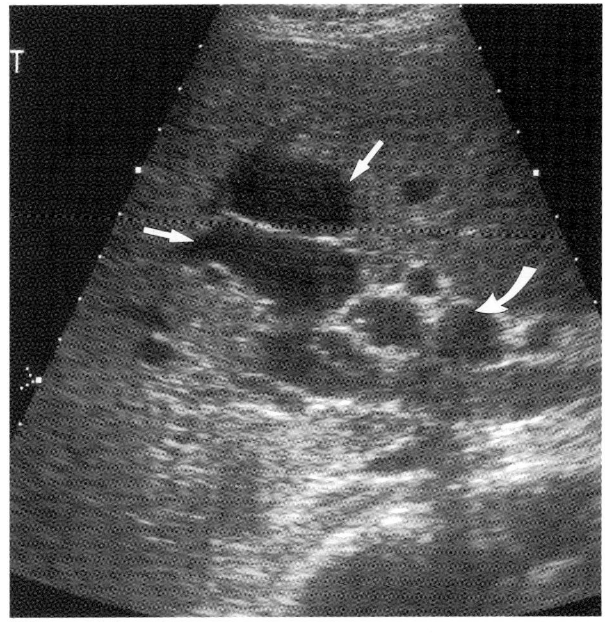

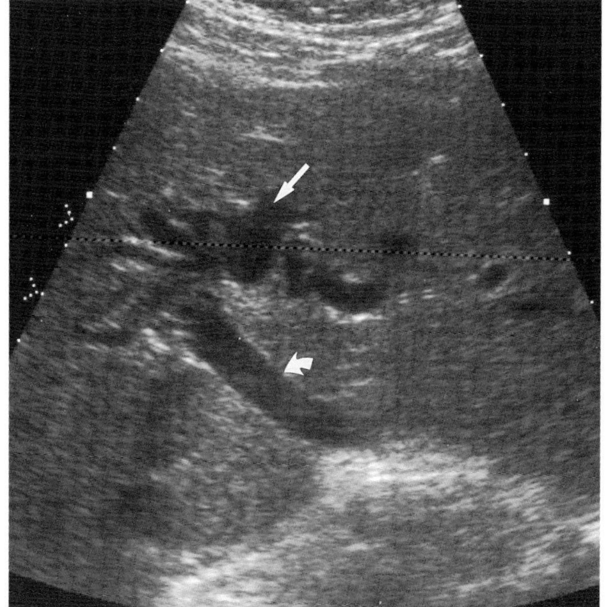

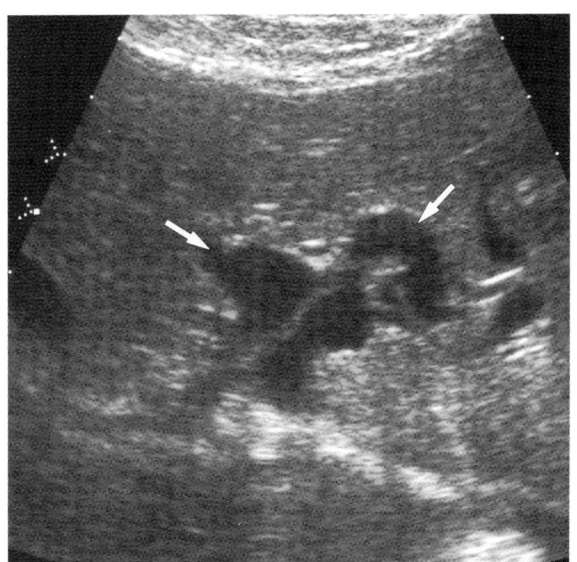

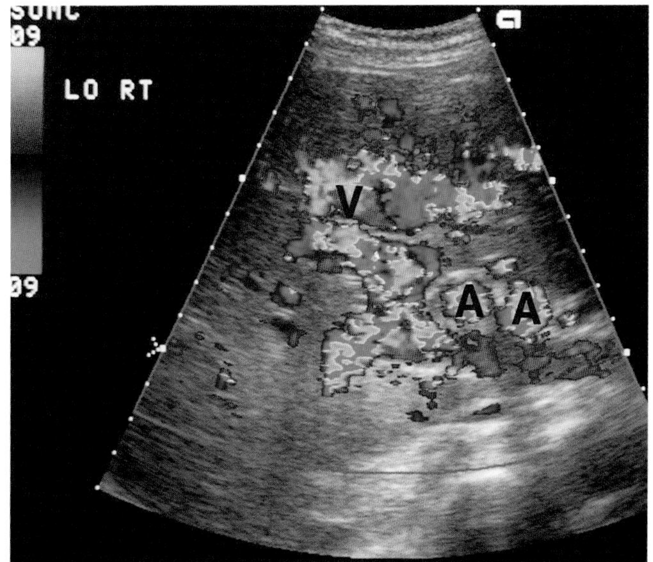

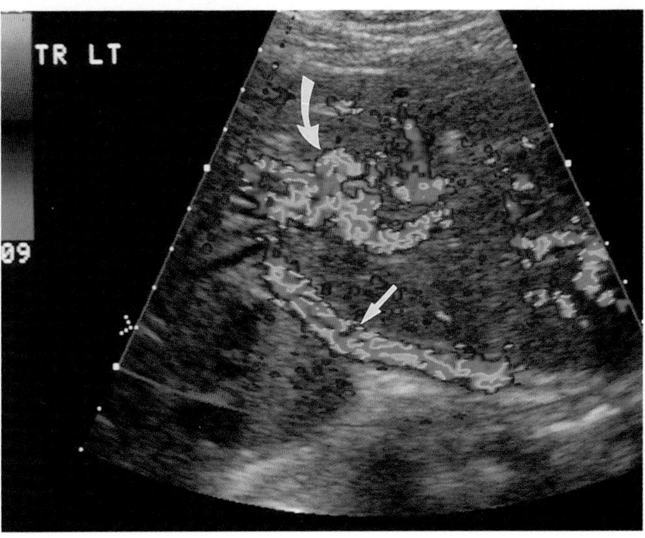

FIG. 3.48. Dilated intrahepatic vessels mimicking biliary obstruction. Patient has Osler–Weber–Rendu syndrome and hepatic arteriovenous malformations. An oblique grayscale scan (**A**) of the right lobe of liver demonstrates multiple dilated tubular structures (*arrows*) possibly representing dilated bile ducts. Note enlarged hepatic artery in porta hepatis (*curved arrow*). A similar configuration of dilated tubular structures is noted on transverse scans of left lobe (*arrows* in **B** and **C**). Note in (**B**) the enlarged replaced left hepatic artery traversing fissure ligamentum (*curved arrow*). Color Doppler images of right lobe (**C**) and left lobe (**D** and **E**) demonstrate arteriovenous malformations as the cause of dilated intrahepatic tubular structures. Enlarged hepatic arterial branches (A) are noted in porta hepatis in (**C**). Dilated portal veins (V) are also noted intrahepatically in (**C**). Scan (**D**) demonstrates enlarged left hepatic artery (*arrow*) replaced to the left gastric artery. Note dilated intrahepatic left portal veins (*curved arrow*) in (**E**).

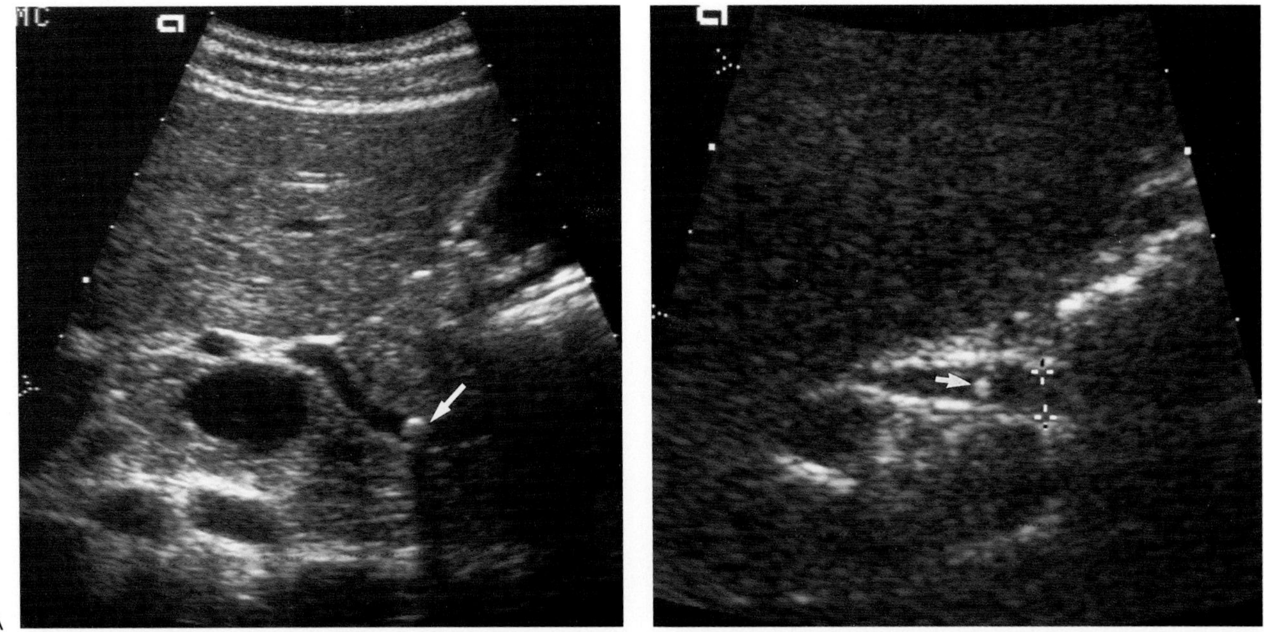

FIG. 3.49. Tiny nonobstructing common duct stones in two patients. Small stones (*arrows*) are identified (**A, B**). Note lack of proximal biliary dilatation.

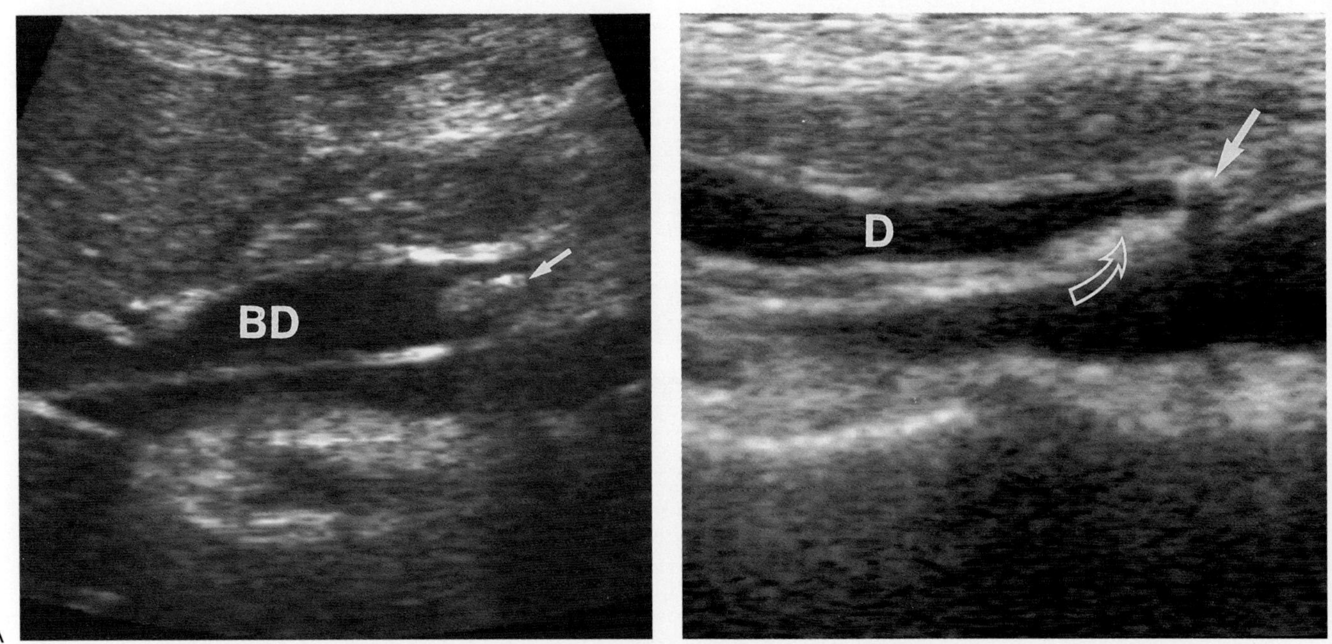

FIG. 3.50. Bacterial cholangitis due to obstructing common duct stone in two patients. **A:** Sagittal scan of common duct demonstrates stone (*arrow*) lodged in distal portion with secondary dilatation of proximal duct. **B:** In another patient, sagittal scan demonstrates stone obstructing distal duct (*arrow*) and echogenic pus (*curved arrow*) within duct. D, common duct.

recent Asian immigration (59,60). Although the exact etiology is unknown, recurrent pyogenic cholangitis is characterized pathologically by the development of pigment stones within the intra- and extrahepatic biliary ducts. Stones do not generally develop within the gallbladder. The pigment stones in recurrent pyogenic cholangitis often are of mud-like consistency and may completely fill segments of the biliary tree (60). Clinically, patients develop symptoms of cholangitis from secondary bacterial infection with fever, chills, and right upper quadrant pain.

Lim et al. (60) reviewed the sonographic features of recurrent pyogenic cholangitis in 48 patients. They noted a characteristic finding in 56 percent of patients of pigment stones in the left intrahepatic biliary system (Figs. 3.51 and 3.52). Although the majority of stones were echogenic and had distal acoustic shadowing, a small percentage lack acoustic shadowing and appeared as echogenic debris. Often the bile ducts are distended and the stones form a cast of the bile duct. Atrophy of a lobe or segment may occur after multiple episodes of cholangitis. Contrast CT is often of additional value in patients with persistent fever as it may more clearly demonstrate associated intrahepatic abscesses. On CT scan, intrahepatic pigment stones may have either soft tissue attenuation values (25 HU) or higher density due the presence of calcium bilirubinate (>150 HU). In patients with surgically created biliary–enteric anastomoses, CT is the imaging method of choice. Pneumobilia may preclude adequate evaluation with sonography (Fig. 3.53).

AIDS Cholangitis

In patients with acquired immunodeficiency syndrome (AIDS), opportunistic infection may involve the biliary tract or the gallbladder. The most common associated organisms are cytomegalovirus and cryptosporidium (57,61). A spectrum of biliary abnormalities may occur including acalculous cholecystitis (Fig. 3.54) and diffuse intrahepatic biliary strictures. These strictures may be difficult to distinguish from sclerosing cholangitis. Isolated involvement of the common bile duct may occur, characterized by either concentric mural thickening or distal stricture formulation (Figs. 3.55 and 3.56). Early involvement of the biliary tree with AIDS cholangitis may not be evident sonographically or may demonstrate only minimal mural thickening of the extrahepatic bile duct. In these patients direct cholangiography is the most specific method to detect the subtle mural irregularities, focal stricturing, and beading of the intrahepatic ducts.

Choledocholithiasis

Improvements in real-time sonographic equipment and scanning techniques have greatly facilitated the diagnosis of common bile duct stones. However, even with these technical refinements, only 50 to 70 percent of common bile duct stones can be detected sonographically (62). As previously noted, the majority of common duct stones lodge within the distal intrapancreatic portion of the common bile duct. This segment of the extrahepatic biliary tree should be examined in great detail in patients suspected of harboring common duct stones. Transverse semi-erect views of the intrapancreatic portion of the bile duct are essential to demonstrate small distal common duct stones (Fig. 3.57). Sagittal scans of the distal duct are often obscured by duodenal gas but may be of value in selected patients (Fig. 3.58). In 30 percent of patients with common duct stones there is no evidence of extrahepatic biliary dilatation. Sonography may be of only limited value in patients with a nondilated biliary tree (49).

In addition to calculi, sonography may demonstrate gas within the bile duct following sphincterotomy or biliary–enteric bypass surgery (Fig. 3.59). Parasitic infestation with *Ascaris* results in characteristic tubular filling defect within the duct (Fig. 3.60). Mucus strands within the biliary tree may, on occasion, simulate ascariasis (Fig. 3.61).

Malignant Biliary Obstruction

Malignant neoplasms of the bile ducts typically cause significant biliary dilatation. The differential diagnosis is related to the anatomic level of biliary obstruction. Distal obstructing lesions involving the intrapancreatic portions of the bile duct are most often caused by pancreatic carcinoma, ampullary carcinoma, or a distal cholangiocarcinoma. Suprapancreatic obstructions are characteristic of gallbladder carcinoma, periportal lymph nodes, or cholangiocarcinoma. Obstruction at the hilar confluence is typical of cholangiocarcinoma, gallbladder carcinoma, or metastases to periportal lymph nodes.

Accurate staging of biliary tract neoplasms often requires multiple diagnostic modalities such as CT, magnetic resonance imaging (MRI), and direct cholangiography. Although sonography is useful as a screening technique to detect the presence of biliary tract obstruction, contrast-enhanced CT is often required to define the intra- and extrahepatic extent of a malignant lesion. Contrast CT can more reliably identify associated hepatic metastases or regional lymphadenopathy. MRI is helpful in patients who cannot receive intravenous contrast for CT.

It is often not possible with imaging to determine the etiology of an obstructing biliary lesion. A combination of CT and sonography can often determine whether the lesion appears intrinsic or extrinsic to the biliary tract. Extrinsic lesions such as periportal lymph nodes may be suggested on the basis of typical imaging findings. How-

(*text continues on page 225*)

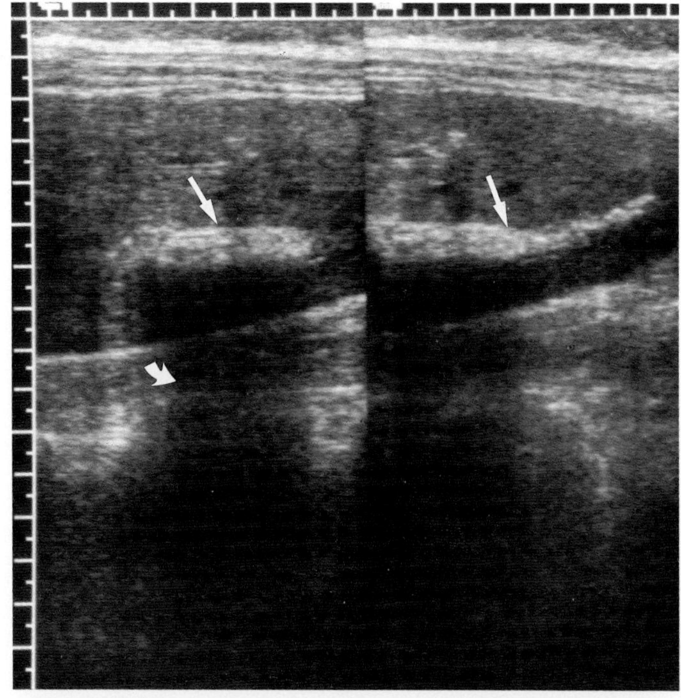

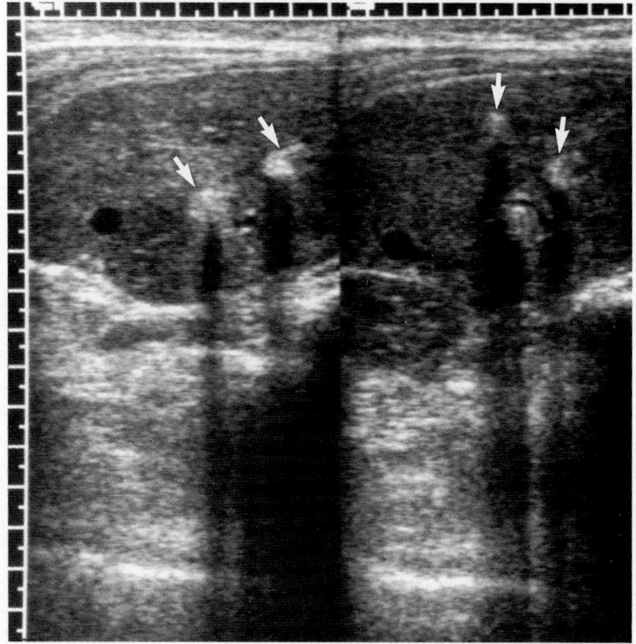

FIG. 3.51. Left hepatic ductal calculi in recurrent pyogenic cholangitis. **A:** Transverse scan of left hepatic lobe demonstrates left ductal system packed with echogenic debris and calculi (*arrows*). Note distal acoustic shadowing (*curved arrow*). **B:** Sagittal scan of left lobe demonstrates echogenic stones and debris (*arrows*).

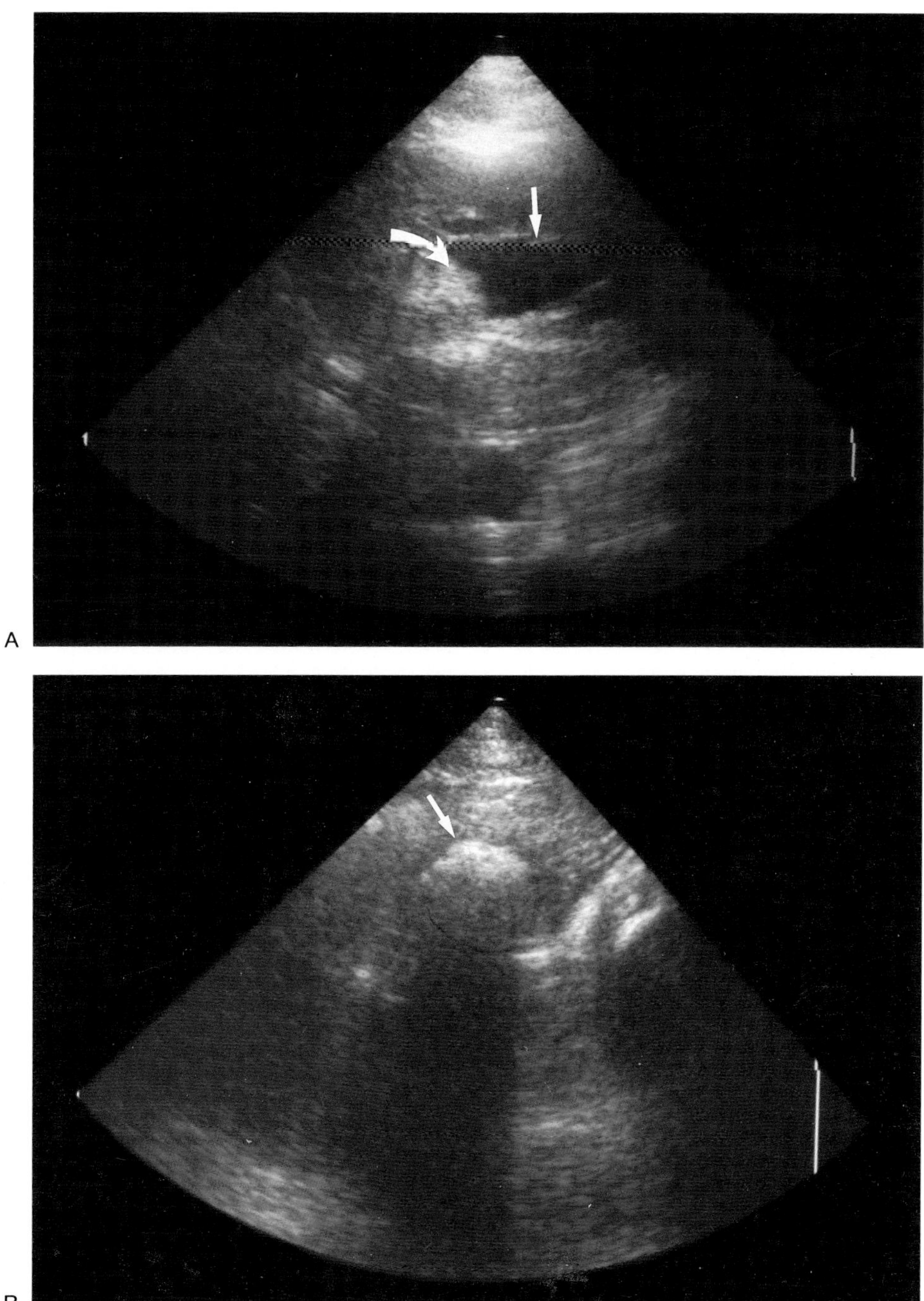

FIG. 3.52. Left hepatic duct and common duct stones in recurrent pyogenic cholangitis. **A:** Transverse scan shows left duct (*arrow*) obstructed by echogenic debris (*curved arrow*) casting little distal acoustic shadow. **B:** Transverse scan of common duct demonstrates large calculus (*arrow*). There were no stones in the gallbladder.

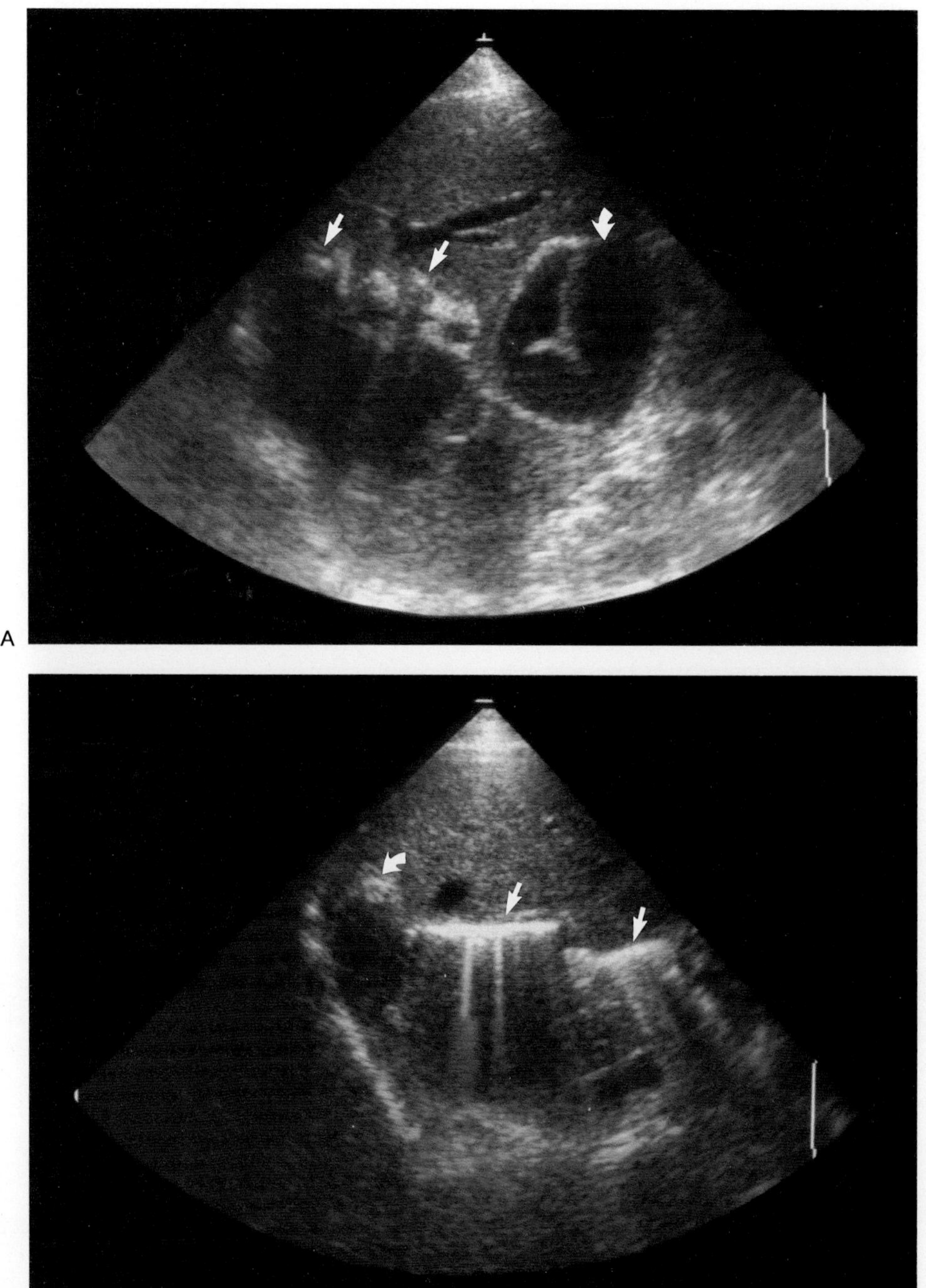

FIG. 3.53. Pneumobilia following biliary–enteric anastomosis for recurrent pyogenic cholangitis. **A:** Sagittal sonogram of right lobe of liver demonstrates normal gallbladder (*curved arrow*) and multiple intrahepatic stones (*arrows*). **B:** Following surgery, extensive pneumobilia is demonstrated in the right lobe (*arrows*). Note residual stones (*curved arrow*).

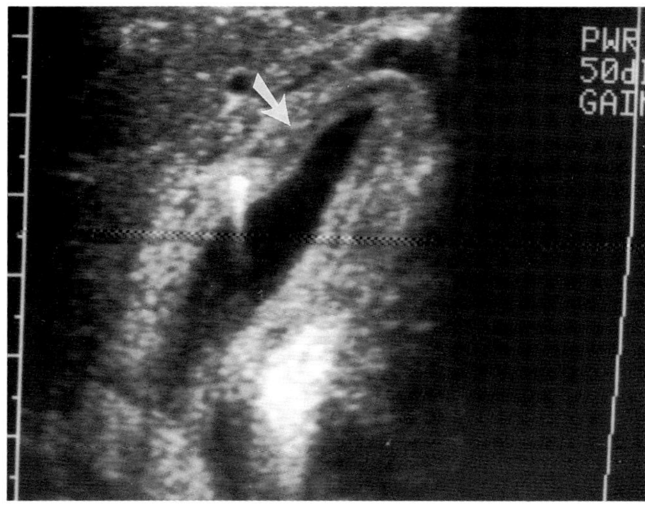

FIG. 3.54. Cryptosporidial cholecystitis in AIDS. Sagittal scan of gallbladder demonstrates thickened gallbladder wall with striations (*arrow*).

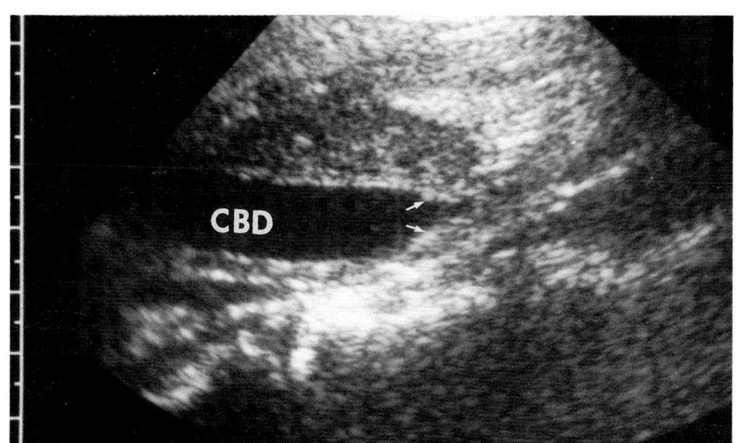

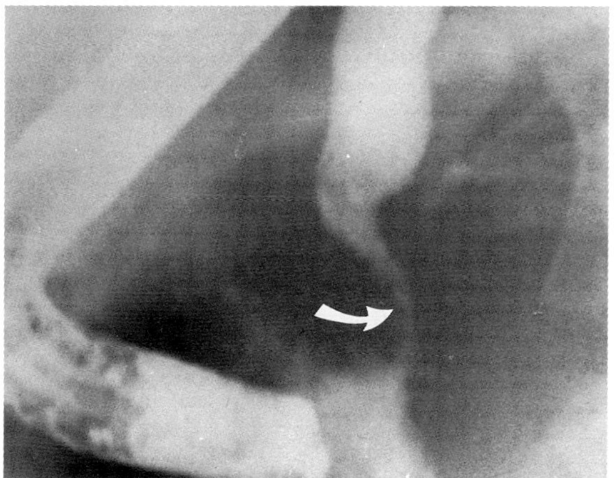

B

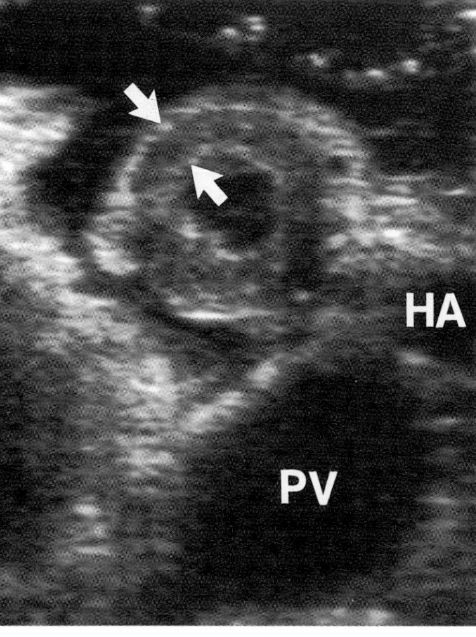

C

FIG. 3.55. Extrahepatic bile duct wall thickening in AIDS cholangitis in two patients. **A:** Note focal thickening of distal bile duct (*arrows*). CBD, common bile duct. **B:** Endoscopic retrograde cholangiopancreatography (ERCP) in same patient demonstrates distal bile duct stricture (*arrow*). **C:** In another patient, an intraoperative scan of porta hepatis demonstrates marked thickening of the wall of the bile duct (*arrows*). PV, portal vein; HA, hepatic artery.

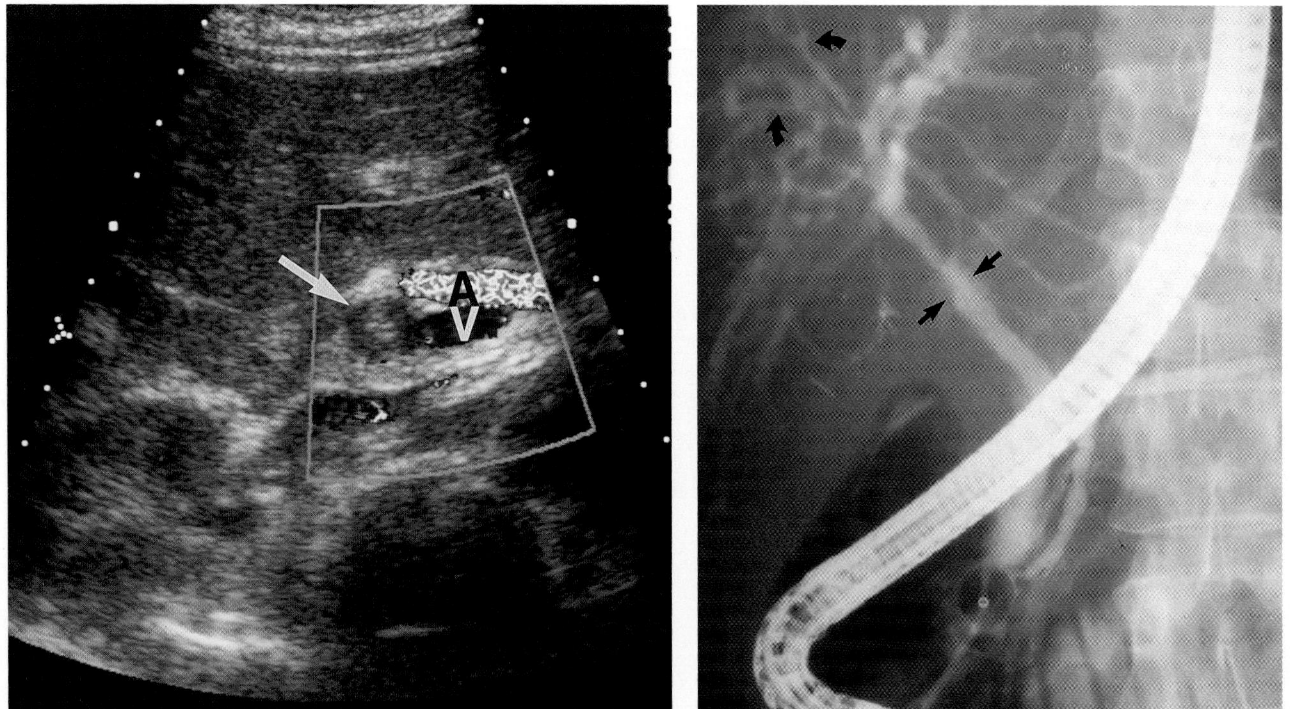

FIG. 3.56. AIDS cholangitis with extensive mural thickening and edema of bile duct. **A:** Transverse color Doppler sonogram demonstrates concentric thickening of bile duct in porta hepatis (*arrow*). A, hepatic artery; V, portal vein. **B:** ERCP demonstrates shaggy contour of extrahepatic (*arrows*) and intrahepatic ducts (*curved arrows*).

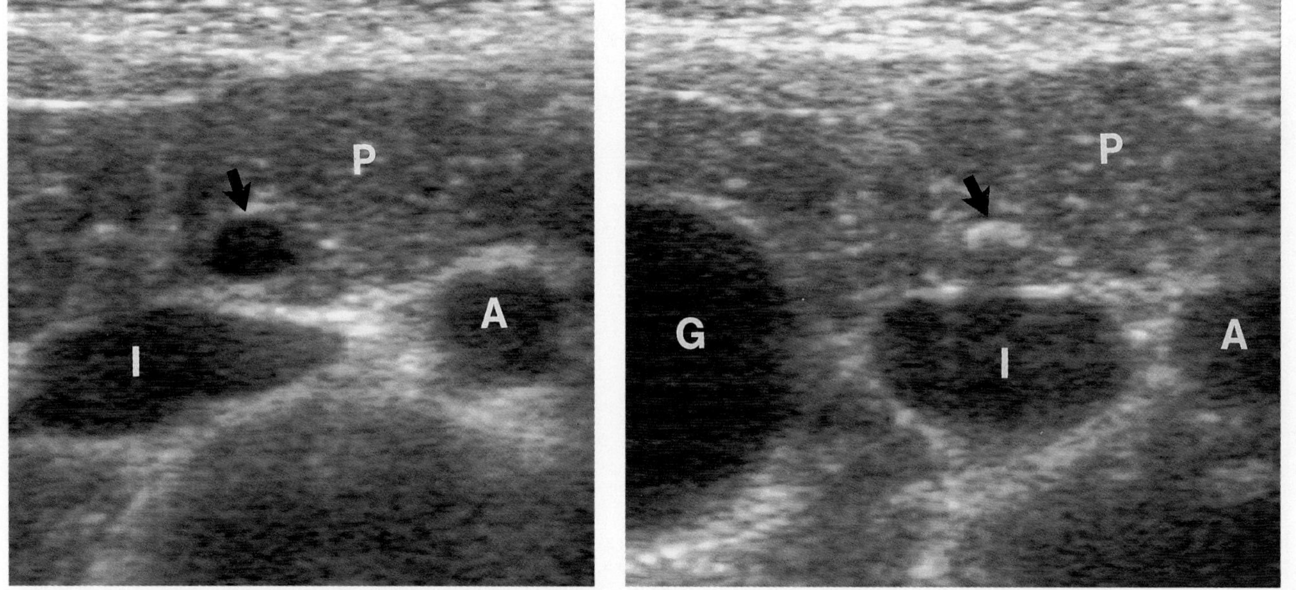

FIG. 3.57. Identification of distal common duct stone with transverse scans. **A:** Transverse scan of the distal duct (*arrow*) at the level of the head of the pancreas (P). A, aorta; I, inferior vena cava. **B:** By angling scan plane caudally, distal stone (*arrow*) is visualized. P, pancreas; A, aorta; I, inferior vena cava.

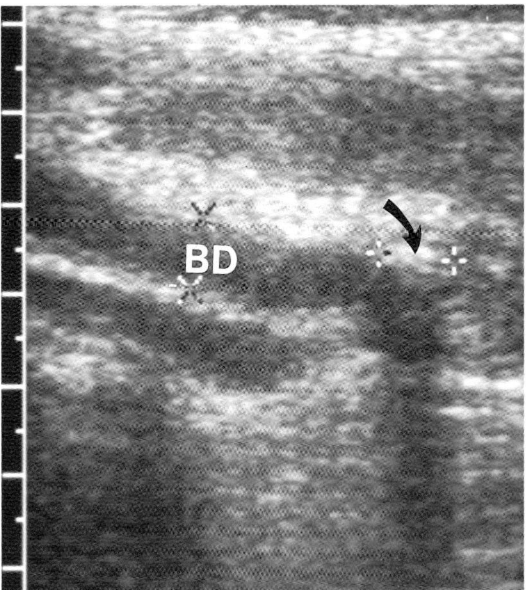

FIG. 3.58. Obstructing distal common duct stone. Sagittal scan of distal duct (BD) demonstrates impacted stone (*curved arrow*) with proximal biliary dilatation.

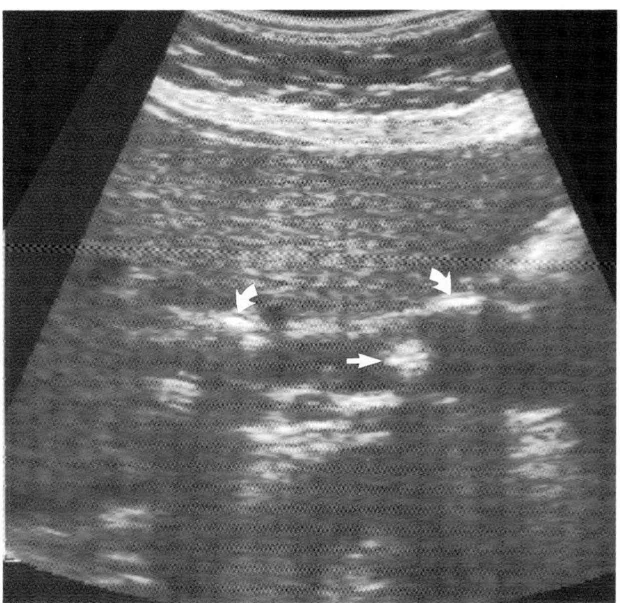

FIG. 3.59. Common duct stone and gas in extrahepatic duct. Sagittal scan of bile duct reveals rounded stone (*arrow*) and linear echoes caused by pneumobilia (*curved arrows*). Note that stone is surrounded by bile but gas rises to most nondependent portion of duct.

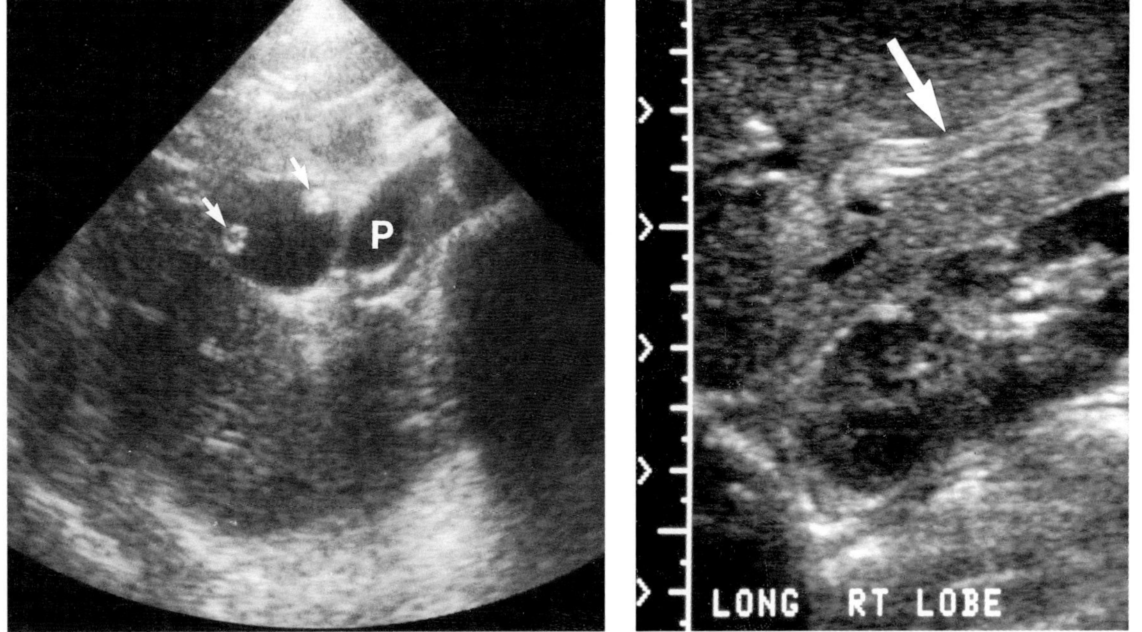

FIG. 3.60. Biliary ascariasis in two patients. **A:** Transverse scan of common duct demonstrates *Ascaris* coiled in dilated common bile duct (*arrows*). P, portal vein. **B:** In another patient, *Ascaris* in right intrahepatic ducts (*arrows*) is noted as tubular echogenic structure.

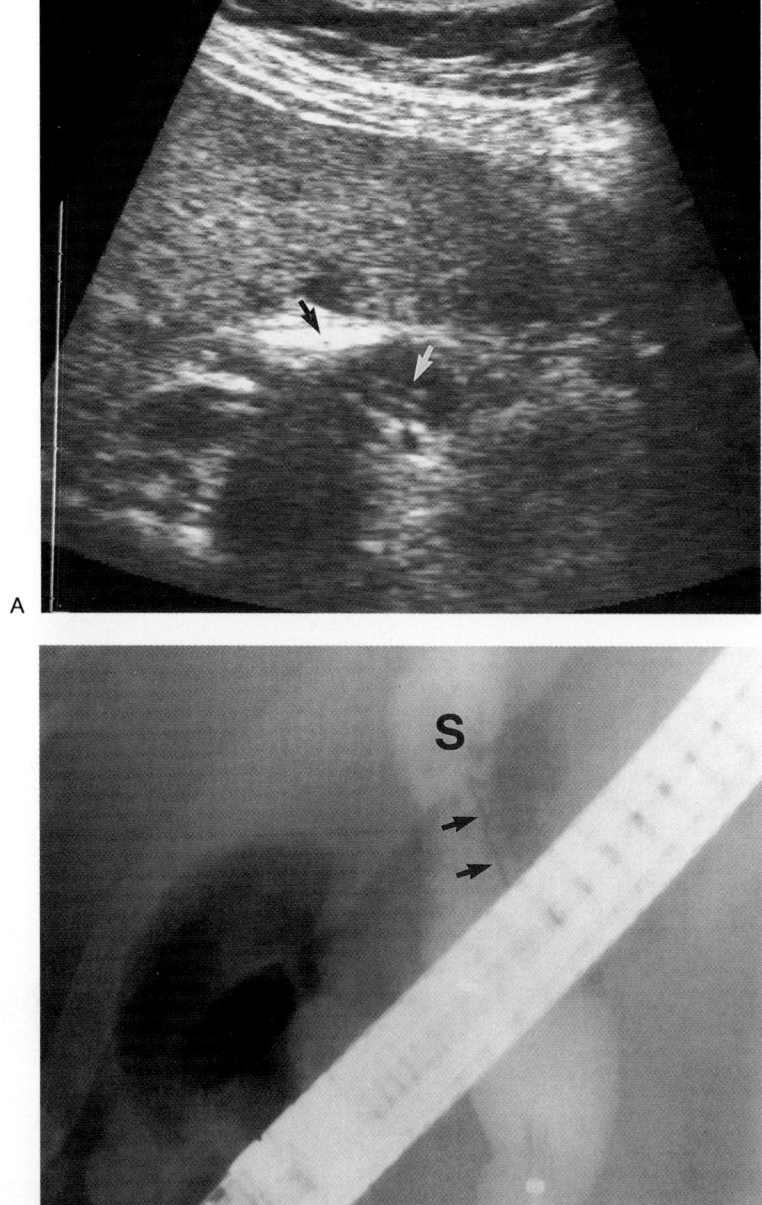

FIG. 3.61. Linear filling defects in bile duct due to mucus strands. **A:** Sagittal scan of bile duct on same patient as in Fig. 3.59. Note linear strands of mucus (*white arrow*) mimicking *Ascaris* and large amount of gas (*black arrow*). **B:** Retrograde cholangiogram demonstrates mucus strands (*arrows*) and common duct stone (S).

ever, guided needle aspiration biopsy is often required for definitive diagnosis.

Cholangiocarcinomas have distinctive clinical and imaging features. They are generally slow-growing adenocarcinomas. There are several different pathologic subtypes of cholangiocarcinoma, including papillary, nodular, sclerosing, and diffuse forms (61). Cholangiocarcinoma has a strong association with primary sclerosing cholangitis secondary to inflammatory bowel disease. There is also an increased incidence of cholangiocarcinoma in patients with *Clonorchis sinensis,* choledochal cysts, and Caroli's disease (63). Unless an obstructing mass is clearly identified, it may be exceedingly difficult to distinguish early cholangiocarcinoma from sclerosing cholangitis.

Approximately 20 percent of cholangiocarcinomas are of the hilar type often known as Klatskin tumors (Fig. 3.62) (63). Klatskin tumors often cause subtle infiltration of the wall of the bile duct. Not infrequently, both sonography and CT fail to demonstrate a mass associated with hilar obstruction. There may be discontinuity or "nonunion" of the dilated right and left biliary ducts. Hilar obstruction not associated with an obvious mass in patients with a normal extrahepatic biliary tree is highly suggestive of a Klatskin tumor. In a review of 51 Klatskin tumors with sonography and CT, Choi et al. (63) were able to detect a mass at the level of biliary obstruction in only 21 percent with sonography but 40 percent with CT. Often on contrast CT there may be intense enhancement of the fibrous tissues surrounding the tumor.

Sonography alone is inadequate for complete staging of Klatskin tumors. Color Doppler sonography may aid in appreciating a small extrahepatic mass (Fig. 3.63). Often the tumors appear sonographically as subtle focal thickening of the bile ducts and without a definable mass. Rarely, a polypoid or nodular intraluminal echogenic mass is noted sonographically. Because of the higher incidence of cholangiocarcinoma in patients with choledochal cysts, any polypoid mass identified within the bile duct requires biopsy (Fig. 3.64).

Miscellaneous Biliary Tract Abnormalities

Biliary Parasites

Biliary parasites such as *Ascaris* or *Clonorchis sinensis* may infest the biliary tree and cause secondary biliary tract obstruction (64). Ascariasis is typically found in Latin America, Asia, and Africa. The adult worm may be visualized as a tubular structure with echogenic outer margins (Fig. 3.60). *Clonorchis sinensis* parasites are significantly smaller in size than the adult *Ascaris* and may not be directly visible with sonography. However, aggregates or clumps of parasites may be identified within the extrahepatic bile duct or within the gallbladder. *Clonorchis* is endemic in Asia and may be associated with the development of recurrent pyogenic cholangitis and cholangiocarcinoma (65).

Mirizzi Syndrome

Mirizzi syndrome is caused by a gallstone impacted in the neck of the gallbladder, which secondarily obstructs the common hepatic duct. It is important to identify this entity preoperatively due to the potential for surgical injury to the common hepatic duct (66,67). In many instances, the cystic duct has an abnormally low-lying insertion into the common hepatic duct. Sonography may suggest the diagnosis of Mirizzi syndrome by demonstrating a large stone impacted in the neck of the gallbladder with secondary intrahepatic ductal dilatation (Figs. 3.65 to 3.67). An important clue to the diagnosis is that the distal common bile duct is normal in size.

Choledochal Cysts

One observation explaining the development of choledochal cysts is the high percentage of patients with an anomalous insertion of the distal common bile duct into the pancreatic duct. This common channel may predispose to chronic reflux of activated pancreatic enzymes into the bile and cause stricture formation (68). A choledochal cyst then develops proximal to the stricture. Choledochal cysts may involve only the extrahepatic duct or cause intra- or extrahepatic biliary obstruction.

There are four main types of choledochal cysts (68). Approximately 90 percent of cases involve dilatation of the extrahepatic bile duct and are classified as Type I. There are three distinct subcategories of Type I: Type IA is a cystic dilatation of the common bile duct; Type IB is a segmental or focal dilatation of the common bile duct; Type IC refers to fusiform dilatation of the bile duct. A Type II choledochal cyst is quite rare and represents a true choledochal diverticula. Type III (representing only 1 to 5 percent of cases) is a choledochocele involving only the intraduodenal portion of the duct. Type IV choledochal cysts have multiple intra- or extrahepatic cysts (68). Although sonography can suggest the diagnosis of choledochal cysts, often cholangiography is required to subtype the exact form of cyst to aid in treatment planning. Patients with choledochal cysts have a higher incidence of cholangiocarcinoma (Fig. 3.64). In general, choledochal cysts are more common in Asian women. Choledochal cysts may develop stones or sludge if there is associated biliary stasis from distal strictures (Figs. 3.68 and 3.69).

Caroli's Disease

Caroli's disease is a congenital anomaly resulting in cystic dilatation of intrahepatic bile ducts (69). The bile

(text continues on page 230)

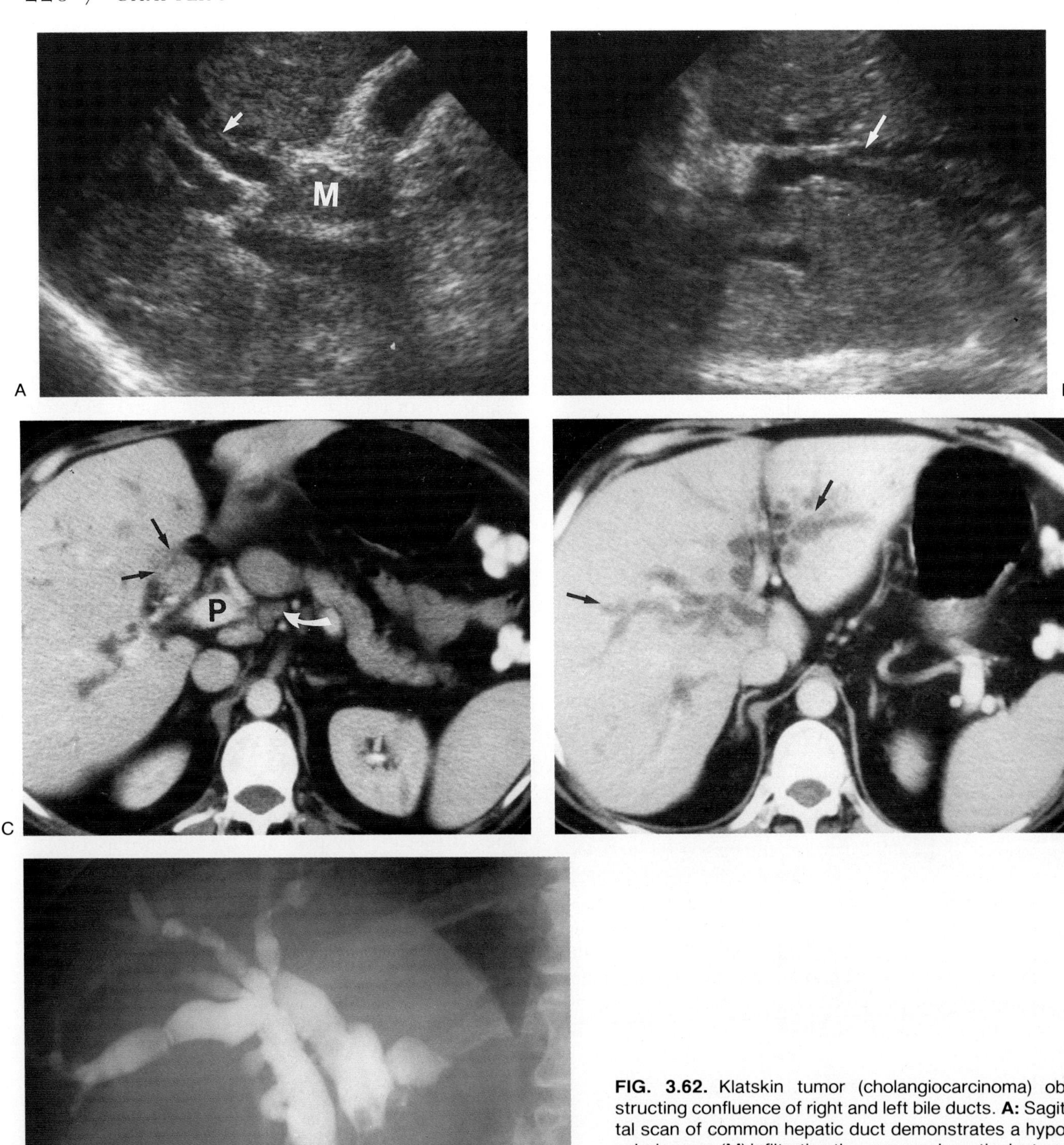

FIG. 3.62. Klatskin tumor (cholangiocarcinoma) obstructing confluence of right and left bile ducts. **A:** Sagittal scan of common hepatic duct demonstrates a hypoechoic mass (M) infiltrating the common hepatic duct and obstructing more proximal bile ducts (*arrow*). **B:** Dilated left intrahepatic ducts are demonstrated (*arrow*). **C:** Contrast CT scan demonstrates small mass (*arrow*) infiltrating extrahepatic duct. P, portal vein. Note celiac adenopathy (*curved white arrow*). **D:** Intrahepatic ductal dilatation is noted (*arrows*). **E:** ERCP demonstrates intraluminal filling defects from cholangiocarcinoma infiltrating the hilar confluence (*arrow*).

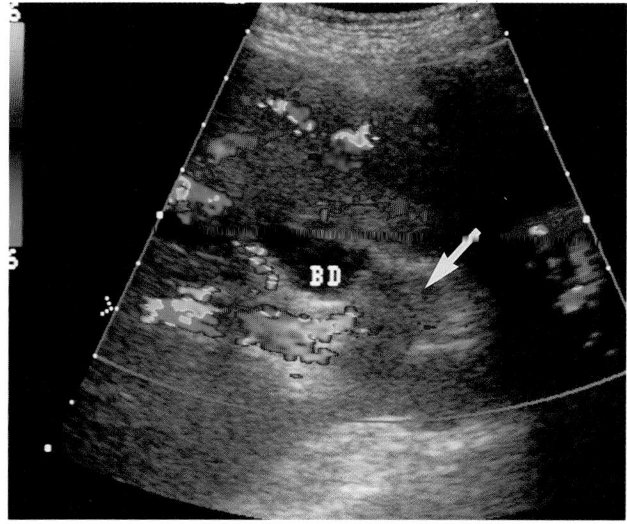

FIG. 3.63. Color Doppler sonogram demonstrating obstructing cholangiocarcinoma. Note hypoechoic mass (*arrow*) obstructing common hepatic duct (B). Cholangiocarcinoma was found at surgery.

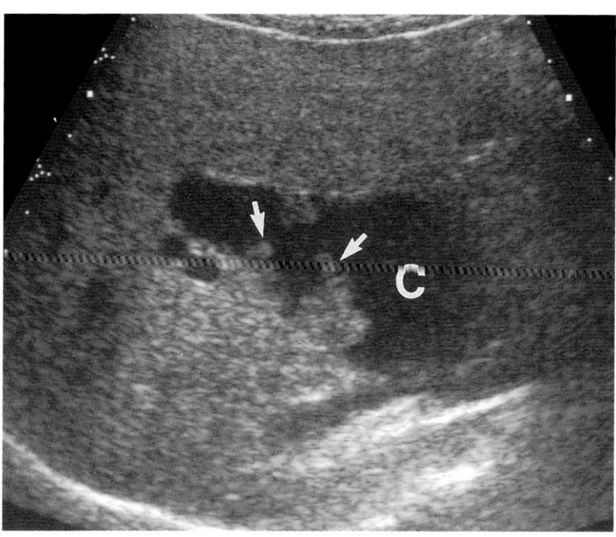

FIG. 3.64. Choledochal cyst with associated cholangiocarcinoma. Sagittal scan of choledochal cyst (C) demonstrates polypoid echogenic masses (*arrows*) representing cholangiocarcinoma.

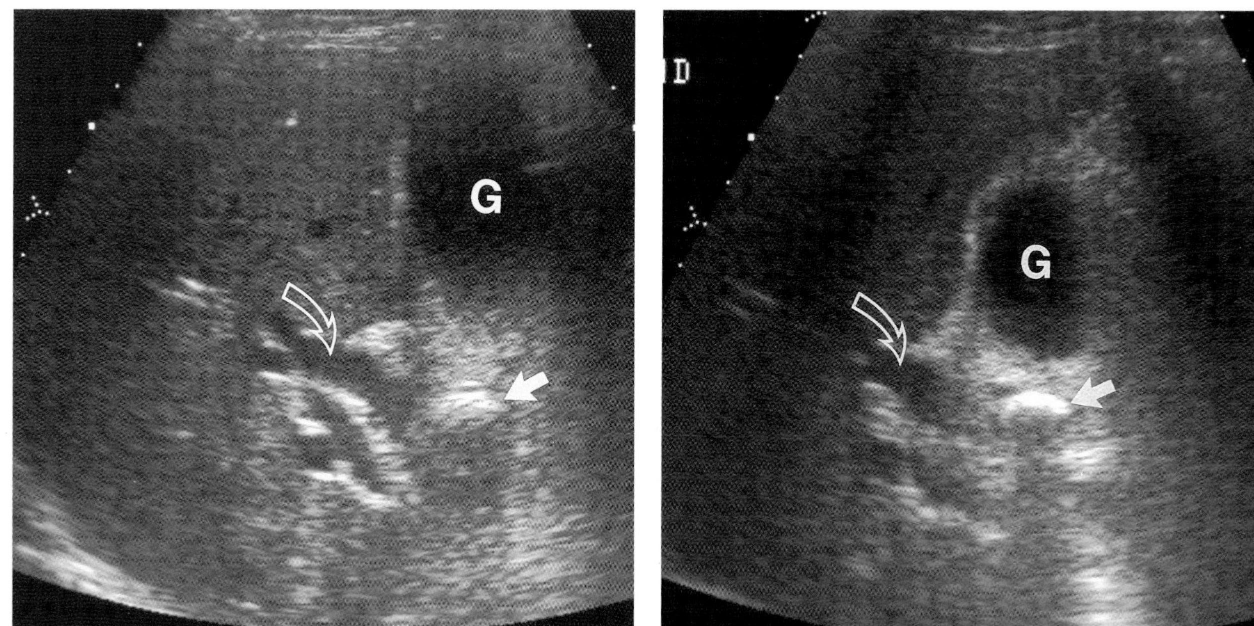

FIG. 3.65. Mirizzi syndrome. Oblique scans (**A, B**) of porta hepatis demonstrate impacted stone (*arrow*) in neck of gallbladder (G). Note secondary dilatation of common hepatic ducts (*curved arrows* in **B**).

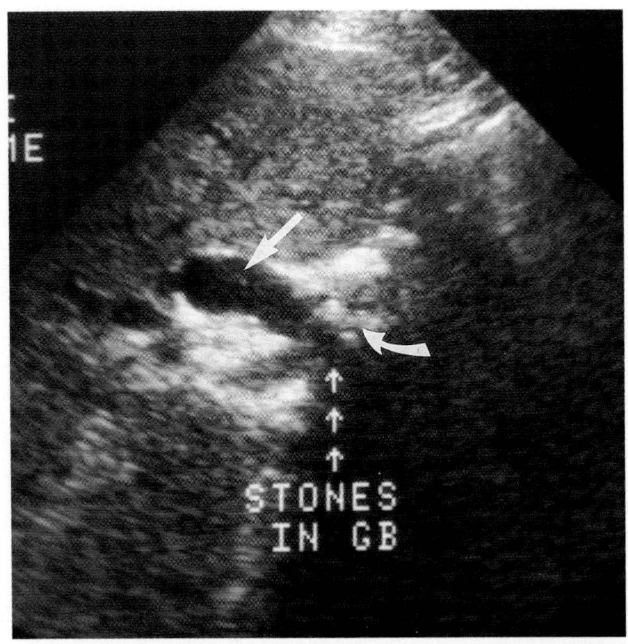

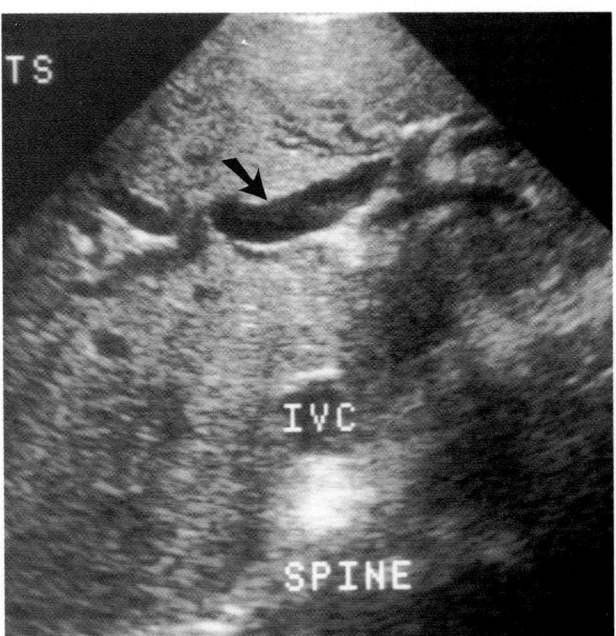

FIG. 3.66. Mirizzi syndrome with proximally dilated intrahepatic ducts. **A:** Oblique scan of common hepatic duct (*arrow*) demonstrates obstructing stones in gallbladder neck (*curved arrow*). **B:** Note prominent dilated intrahepatic ducts (*arrow*). IVC, inferior vena cava.

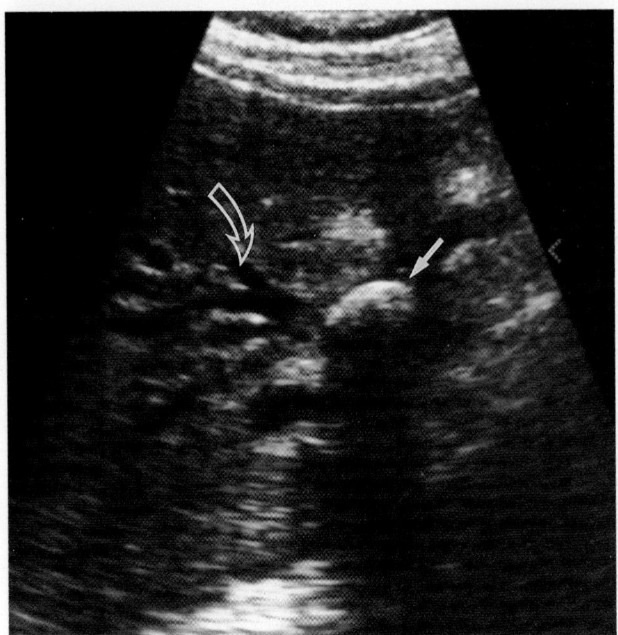

FIG. 3.67. Mirizzi syndrome. Transverse sonogram demonstrates stone in gallbladder neck (*arrow*). Note intrahepatic ductal obstruction (*curved arrow*). (Case courtesy of Peter Cooperburg, MD, Vancouver, BC, Canada.)

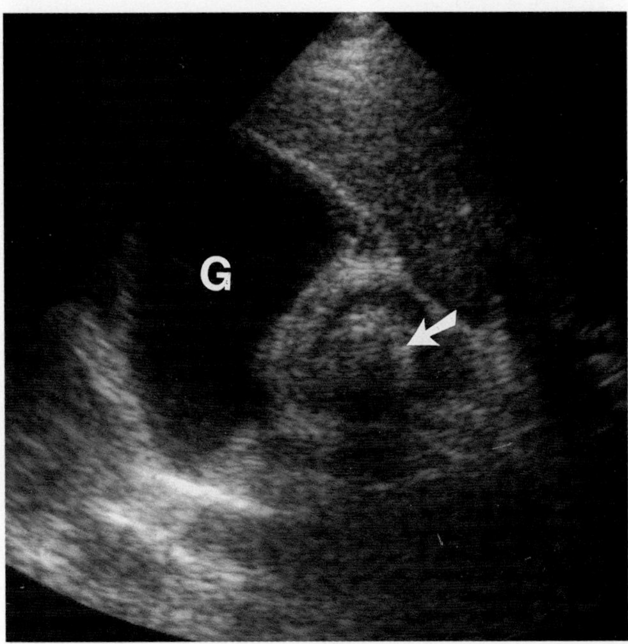

FIG. 3.68. Choledochal cyst filled with sludge. Transverse scan demonstrates sludge-filled choledochal cyst (*arrow*). G, gallbladder.

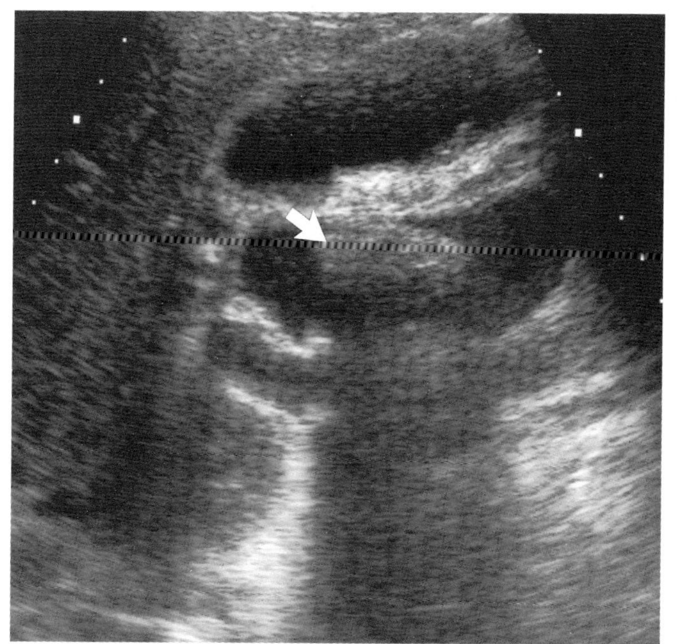

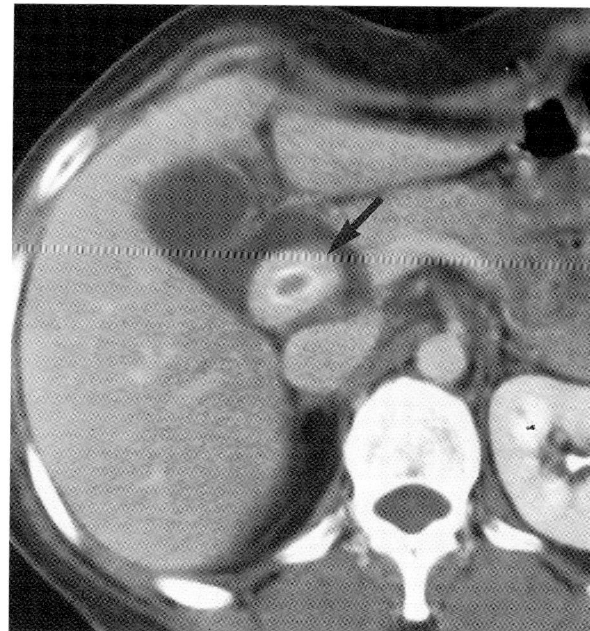

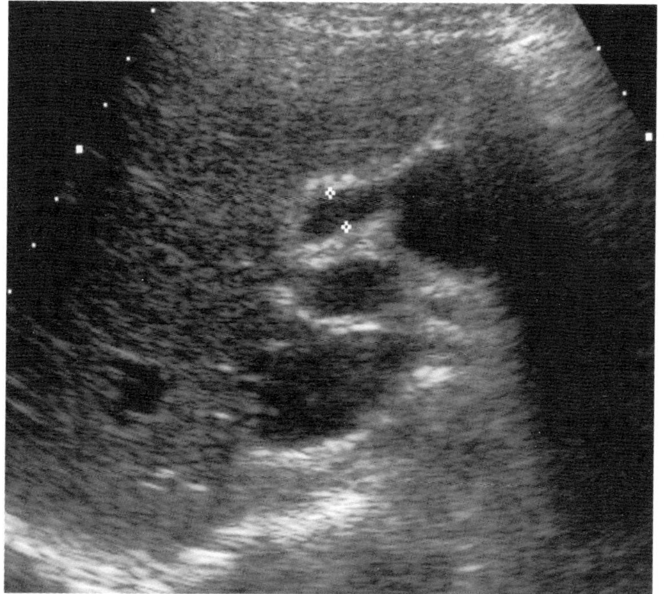

FIG. 3.69. Stone within choledochal cyst. **A:** Large stone within choledochal cyst (*arrow*) is evident. **B:** Stone is calcified on CT scan (*arrow*). **C:** Note normal caliber common hepatic duct (*cursors*).

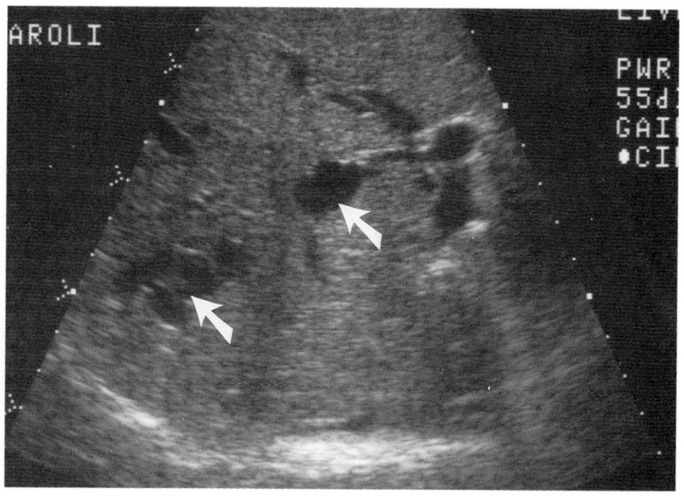

FIG. 3.70. Caroli's disease. Transverse sonogram of right hepatic lobe demonstrates multiple areas of cystic dilatation of bile ducts (*arrows*).

ducts do not communicate. It may be seen diffusely throughout the liver or isolated to one lobe. Bile stasis may lead to stone formation and subsequent biliary sepsis (Fig. 3.70). Caroli's disease may be associated with infantile polycystic liver disease and congenital perihepatic fibrosis (69).

REFERENCES

1. Way LW. Pathogenesis of gallstones. In: Way LW, ed. *Current surgical diagnosis & treatment,* 9th ed. Norwalk, CT: Appleton & Lange; 1991:535–537.
2. Nahrwold DL. Acute cholecystitis. In: Sabiston DC, ed. *Textbook of surgery: the biological basis of modern surgical practice,* 13th ed. Philadelphia: Saunders; 1986:1137–1146.
3. Laing FC, Federle MP, Jeffrey RB, Brown TW. Ultrasonic evaluation of patients with acute right upper quadrant pain. *Radiology* 1981;140:449–455.
4. Ralls PW, Colletti PM, Halls JM, Siemsen JK. Prospective evaluation of ^{99m}Tc-IDA cholescintigraphy and gray-scale ultrasound in the diagnosis of acute cholecystitis. *Radiology* 1982;144:369–371.
5. Shuman WP, Mack LA, Rudd TG, Rogers JV, Gibbs P. Evaluation of acute right upper quadrant pain: sonography and ^{99m}Tc-PIPIDA cholescintigraphy. *AJR* 1982;139:61–64.
6. Mauro MA, McCartney WH, Melmed JR. Hepatobiliary scanning with ^{99m}Tc-PIPIDA in acute cholecystitis. *Radiology* 1982;142:193–197.
7. Freeman LM, Sugarman LA, Weissmann HS. Role of cholecystokinetic agents in ^{99m}Tc-IDA cholescintigraphy. *Semin Nucl Med* 1981;11:186–193.
8. Weissmann HS, Badia J, Sugarman LA, Kluger L, Rosenblatt R, Freeman LM. Spectrum of 99m-Tc-IDA cholescintigraphic patterns in acute cholecystitis. *Radiology* 1981;138:167–175.
9. Ralls PW, Colletti PM, Lapin SA, et al. Real-time sonography in suspected acute cholecystitis: prospective evaluation of primary and secondary signs. *Radiology* 1985;155:767–771.
10. Laing FC, Jeffrey RB. Choledocholithiasis and cystic duct obstruction: difficult ultrasonographic diagnosis. *Radiology* 1983;146:475–479.
11. Simeone JF, Brink JA, Mueller, et al. The sonographic diagnosis of acute gangrenous cholecystitis: importance of the Murphy sign. *AJR* 1989;152:289–290.
12. Ralls PW, Quinn MF, Juttner HU, Halls JM, Boswell WD. Gallbladder wall thickening: patients without intrinsic gallbladder disease. *AJR* 1981;137:65–68.
13. Raghavendra BN, Feiner HD, Subramanyam BR, et al. Acute cholecystitis: sonographic–pathologic analysis. *AJR* 1981;137:327–332.
14. Herlin P, Ericsson M, Holmin T, Jönsson PE. Acute acalculous cholecystitis following surgical trauma. *Br J Surg* 1982;69:475–476.
15. Shlaer WJ, Leopold GR, Scheible FW. Sonography of the thickened gallbladder wall: a nonspecific finding. *AJR* 1981;136:337–339.
16. Teefey SA, Baron RL, Radke HM, Bigler SA. Gangrenous cholecystitis: new observations on sonography. *J Ultrasound Med* 1991;10:603–606.
17. Teefey SA, Baron RL, Bigler SA. Sonography of the gallbladder: significance of striated (layered) thickening of the gallbladder wall. *AJR* 1991;156:945–947.
18. Shuman WP, Gibbs P, Rudd TG, Mack LA. PIPIDA scintigraphy for cholecystitis: false positives in alcoholism and total parenteral nutrition. *AJR* 1982;138:1–5.
19. Johnson LB. The importance of early diagnosis of acute acalculous cholecystitis. *Surg Gynecol Obstet* 1987;164:197–203.
20. Savoca PE, Longo WE, Zucker KA, et al. The increasing prevalence of acalculous cholecystitis in outpatients: results of a 7-year study. *Ann Surg* 1990;211:433–437.
21. Becker CG, Dubin T, Glenn F. Induction of acute cholecystitis by activation of factor XII. *J Exp Med* 1980;151:81–90.
22. Shuman WP, Rogers JV, Rudd TG, Mack LA, Plumley T, Larson EB. Low sensitivity of sonography and cholescintigraphy in acalculous cholecystitis. *AJR* 1984;142:531–534.
23. Howard RJ. Acute acalculous cholecystitis. *Am J Surg* 1981;141:194–198.
24. Blankenberg F, Wirth R, Jeffrey RB, Mindelzun R, Francis I. Computed tomography as an adjunct to ultrasound in the diagnosis of acute acalculous cholecystitis. *Gastrointest Radiol* 1991;16:149–153.
25. Mirvis SE, Vainright JR, Nelson AW, et al. The diagnosis of acute acalculous cholecystitis: a comparison of sonography, scintigraphy, and CT. *AJR* 1986;147:1171–1175.
26. McGahan JP, Lindfors KK. Acute cholecystitis: diagnostic accuracy of percutaneous aspiration of the gallbladder. *Radiology* 1988;167:669–671.
27. Teplick SK, Harshfield DL, Brandon JC, Broadwater JR, Cone JB. Percutaneous cholecystostomy in critically ill patients. *Gastrointest Radiol* 1991;16:154–156.
28. Lee MJ, Saini S, Brink JA, et al. Treatment of critically ill patients with sepsis of unknown cause: value of percutaneous cholecystostomy. *AJR* 1991;156:1163–1166.
29. Morfin E, Ponka JL, Brush BE. Gangrenous cholecystitis. *Arch Surg* 1968;96:567–572.
30. Wall CA, Weiss RM. Early operation for acute cholecystitis. *Arch Surg* 1958;77:433–438.
31. Strohl EL, Diffenbaugh WG, Baker JH, et al. Gangrene and perforation of the gallbladder. *Int Abstracts Surg* 1962;114:1–7.
32. Jeffrey RB, Laing FC, Wong W, Callen PW. Gangrenous cholecystitis: diagnosis by ultrasound. *Radiology* 1983;148:219–221.
33. Miyazaki K, Uchiyama A, Nakayama F. Use of ultrasonographic risk score in the timing of operative intervention for acute cholecystitis. *Arch Surg* 1988;123:487–489.
34. Chinn DH, Miller EI, Piper N. Hemorrhagic cholecystitis: sonographic appearance and clinical presentation. *J Ultrasound Med* 1987;6:313–317.
35. Madrazo BL, Francis I, Hricak H, Sandler MA, Hudak S, Gitschlag K. Sonographic findings in perforation of the gallbladder. *AJR* 1982;139:491–496.
36. Brunetti JC, Van Heertum RL. Preoperative detection of gallbladder perforation. *Clin Nucl Med* 1980;5:347–348.
37. Takada T, Yasuda H, Uchiyama K, Hasegawa H, Asagoe T, Shikata J. Pericholecystic abscess: classification of US findings to determine the proper therapy. *Radiology* 1989;172:693–697.
38. Teefey SA, Wechter DG. Sonographic evaluation of pericholecystic abscess with intrahepatic extension. *J Ultrasound Med* 1987;6:659–662.
39. Andreu J, Pérez C, Cáceres J, Llauger J, Palmer J. Computed tomography as the method of choice in the diagnosis of emphysematous cholecystitis. *Gastrointest Radiol* 1987;12:315–318.
40. Nemcek AA, Gore RM, Vogelzang RL, Grant M. The effervescent gallbladder: a sonographic sign of emphysematous cholecystitis. *AJR* 1988;150:575–577.
41. Quinn SF, Fazzio F, Jones E. Torsion of the gallbladder: findings on CT and sonography and role of percutaneous cholecystostomy. *AJR* 1987;148:881–882.
42. Hanada K, Nakata H, Nakayama T, et al. Radiologic findings in xanthogranulomatous cholecystitis. *AJR* 1987;148:727–730.
43. Raghavendra BN, Subramanyam BR, Balthazar EJ, Horii SC, Megibow AJ, Hilton S. Sonography of adenomyomatosis of the gallbladder: radiologic–pathologic correlation. *Radiology* 1983;146:747–752.
44. Fowler RC, Reid WA. Ultrasound diagnosis of adenomyomatosis of the gallbladder: ultrasonic and pathological correlation. *Clin Radiol* 1988;39:402–406.
45. Price RJ, Stewart ET, Foley WD, Dodds WJ. Sonography of polypoid cholesterolosis. *AJR* 1982;139:1197–1198.
46. Lane J, Buck JL, Zeman RK. Primary carcinoma of the gallbladder: a pictorial essay. *Radiographics* 1989;9:209–228.
47. Franquet T, Montes M, Ruiz de Azua Y, Jimenez FJ, Cozcolluela R. Primary gallbladder carcinoma: imaging findings in 50 patients with pathologic correlation. *Gastrointest Radiol* 1991;16:143–148.
48. Bret PM, de Stempel JV, Atri M, Lough JO, Illescas FF. Intrahepatic bile duct and portal vein anatomy revisited. *Radiology* 1988;169:405–407.

49. Davies RP, Downey PR, Moore WR, Jeans PL, Toouli J. Contrast cholangiography versus ultrasonographic measurement of the "extrahepatic" bile duct: a two-fold discrepancy revisited. *J Ultrasound Med* 1991; 10:653–657.
50. Wu CC, Ho YH, Chen CT. Effect of aging on common bile duct diameter: a real-time ultrasonographic study. *J Clin Ultrasound* 1985; 12:473–478.
51. Laing FC. The gallbladder and bile ducts. In: Rumack CM, Wilson SR, Charboneau JW, eds. *Diagnostic ultrasound*. St Louis: Mosby–Year Book; 1991:131.
52. Laing FC, Jeffrey RB Jr, Wing VW, Nyberg DA. Biliary dilatation: defining the level and cause by real-time US. *Radiology* 1986; 160: 39–42.
53. Muhletaler CA, Gerlock AJ, Fleischer AC, James AE. Diagnosis of obstructive jaundice with nondilated bile ducts. *AJR* 1980; 134: 1149–1152.
54. Simeone JF, Butch RJ, Mueller PR, et al. The bile ducts after a fatty meal: further sonographic observations. *Radiology* 1985; 154: 763–768.
55. Willson SA, Gosink BB, vanSonnenberg E. Unchanged size of a dilated common bile duct after a fatty meal: results and significance. *Radiology* 1986; 160:29–31.
56. Darweesh RMA, Dodds WJ, Hogan WJ, et al. Fatty-meal sonography for evaluating patients with suspected partial common duct obstruction. *AJR* 1988; 151:63–68.
57. Dolmatch BL, Laing FC, Federle MP, Jeffrey RB. AIDS-related cholangitis: radiographic findings in nine patients. *Radiology* 1987; 163:313–316.
58. Schulman A. Non-western patterns of biliary stones and the role of ascariasis. *Radiology* 1987; 162:425–430.
59. Chen HH, Zhang WH, Wang SS, Caruana JA. Twenty-two year experience with the diagnosis and treatment of intrahepatic calculi. *Surg Gynecol Obstet* 1984; 159:519–524.
60. Lim JH, Ko YT, Lee DH, Hong KS. Oriental cholangiohepatitis: sonographic findings in 48 cases. *AJR* 1990; 155:511–514.
61. Teixidor HS, Godwin TA, Ramirez EA. Cryptosporidiosis of the biliary tract in AIDS. *Radiology* 1991; 180:51–56.
62. Laing FC, Jeffrey RB, Wing VW. Improved visualization of choledocholithiasis by sonography. *AJR* 1984; 143:949–952.
63. Choi BI, Lee JH, Han MC, Kim SH, Yi JG, Kim CW. Hilar cholangiocarcinoma: comparative study with sonography and CT. *Radiology* 1989; 172:689–692.
64. Schulman A, Loxton AJ, Heydenrych JJ, Abdurahman KE. Sonographic diagnosis of biliary ascariasis. *AJR* 1982; 139:485–489.
65. Lim JH, Ko YT, Lee DH, Kim SY. Clonorchiasis: sonographic findings in 59 proved cases. *AJR* 1989; 152:761–764.
66. Jackson VP, Lappas JC. Sonography of the Mirizzi syndrome. *J Ultrasound Med* 1984; 3:281–283.
67. Becker CD, Hassler H, Terrier F. Preoperative diagnosis of the Mirizzi syndrome: limitations of sonography and computed tomography. *AJR* 1984; 143:591–596.
68. Savader SJ, Benenati JF, Venbrux AC, et al. Choledochal cysts: classification and cholangiographic appearance. *AJR* 1991; 156: 327–331.
69. Sherlock S. Cysts and congenital biliary abnormalities. In: *Diseases of the liver and biliary system*. Oxford: Blackwell Scientific Publications; 1981:406–412.

CHAPTER 4

The Pancreas

TECHNIQUE

Optimal pancreatic visualization requires that intervening gastrointestinal tract gas be displaced by filling the gut with water or by compressing gas out of the intervening loop. Large footprint 3- to 5-MHz curved array transducers with favorable near-field imaging characteristics are suitable for this. After water administration, upright scanning is often best, as gas rises to the gastric fundus. Alternatively, a left anterior oblique position may be useful, since water will frequently fill the duodenum in this position. It may be difficult to obtain adequate pancreatic images when the left hepatic lobe is small or when gas distends the transverse colon.

Useful scan planes include transverse, sagittal, and medially angled right anterior oblique (RAO) scans (similar to the scan plane used in imaging the common bile duct). The pancreatic head is often best seen in transverse scans performed by placing the transducer to the left of the midline and angling back toward the right, thus avoiding gas within the duodenal sweep. The tail of the pancreas near the splenic hilus and left kidney is frequently the most difficult region of the pancreas to image. Coronal and axial images using the spleen and left kidney as an acoustic window should be routine. The normal pancreatic tail is usually not seen on this view, but lesions in the tail, invisible on other views, are occasionally delineated.

Attention to technical detail and persistence will usually yield adequate images of the pancreas. In many patients, however, computed tomography (CT) yields additional information.

PANCREATITIS

Pancreatitis is a common, but still poorly understood, illness. Its pathogenesis is undetermined. Its clinical course is varied and unpredictable. Its natural history has not been adequately studied. There are no controlled trials comparing radically different approaches to therapy of acute necrotizing pancreatitis, pancreatic abscess, and pseudocyst.

In this setting, the "correct" use of imaging is difficult to assess. The precise role of imaging and image-guided intervention varies considerably at different institutions.

Acute Pancreatitis

According to the 1984 Marseilles classification (1), acute pancreatitis causes acute abdominal pain and elevated levels of pancreatic enzymes in the blood or urine. Edematous pancreatitis, with minor areas of fat necrosis, is most frequent, but hemorrhage and extensive intra- and extrapancreatic necrosis may occur. The clinical course of acute pancreatitis is extremely variable. It is usually a mild, self-limited disease. Most patients recover fully and uneventfully. Less commonly, major complications occur. Pancreatic necrosis may result in extensive abdominal, pelvic, and retroperitoneal pathology, including hemorrhage, fluid collections, and inflammation (phlegmonous change). Other local complications include venous thrombosis, arterial pseudoaneurysms, and gastrointestinal fistulas. Systemic complications include hypovolemia, acute compromise of pulmonary, cardiac, and renal functions, hyperglycemia, and, occasionally, disseminated intravascular coagulation.

Gallstones and alcoholism cause about 75 percent of pancreatitis; the relative frequency varies in different patient populations. Trauma and miscellaneous causes (hereditary, lipid abnormalities, drugs, etc.) account for about 15 percent (2,3). No cause is known for the remaining 10 percent, although biliary sludge, sometimes undetectable by sonography, may account for most of these previously unclassified cases (4).

There is no definitive therapy for acute pancreatitis; management is supportive. All patients must be followed closely, as clinical outcome is best when potential complications, especially abscess, are detected and treated early. Various clinical (Ranson criteria, etc.) and imaging criteria have been used to attempt to identify patients at higher risk for complications of pancreatitis. CT classification of pancreatitis based on pancreatic or peripancreatic fluid collections (5) has little useful predictive value (6). Dynamic contrast-enhanced CT (CECT) has been proposed as a method to diagnose pancreatic necrosis (7–10). Indeed, prognosis appears to parallel the extent of nonenhancing, presumably necrotic, pancreatic parenchyma. Nonenhancing areas are targeted for aspiration or used as an indication for early (after 3 days of intensive care unit therapy) surgical debridement of necrotic retroperitoneal tissue (11).

No prospective clinical trial has shown whether early surgical debridement (necrosectomy) or treatment of complications as they arise is superior. Early necrosectomy results in a laparotomy rate of nearly 30 percent (11); only about 5 percent of patients are operated on otherwise (3). In institutions where early surgical debridement is considered appropriate, early dynamic contrast-enhanced CT is useful. In our practice, CT is used only when complications are suspected.

Both CT and sonography are useful in patients with acute pancreatitis. Imaging goals include determining the cause of pancreatitis and detecting (as well as treating) complications. All patients with acute pancreatitis, even alcoholics, should have sonography to detect gallstones and evaluate bile duct obstruction (usually from a distal stone). If duct obstruction is present, urgent surgical or endoscopic decompression may be needed to forestall severe complications (Fig. 4.1). Color flow sonography and mechanically injected bolus contrast-enhanced CT are useful in detecting vascular complications such as pseudoaneurysms or venous thrombosis.

Although sonography may reveal local complications (12), contrast-enhanced CT is the most effective technique to detect complications or guide appropriate percutaneous intervention. Because of its superiority as a survey tool, CT is best to evaluate the entire abdomen and pelvis, or when the diagnosis is uncertain. CT, with aggressive diagnostic needle aspiration, is required if infected pancreatic fluid collections are to be detected early. Early detection is the only way to minimize mortality from pancreatic abscess. Sonography can be used to follow selected fluid collections cost effectively, even those detected with CT (13). When access is straightforward, sonography can guide aspiration or catheter drainage of pseudocysts and abscesses.

Sonographic Findings in Acute Pancreatitis

The pancreas may be obscured in patients with acute pancreatitis by gas within the distended gastrointestinal tract. Pain may make compression difficult. While the pancreas may be imaged in as many as 90 percent of patients with acute pancreatitis (14), the frequency of successful visualization depends on the examiner's experience and the persistence with which the exam is pursued. In our practice, sonography in the acute clinical phase is performed to detect gallstones or biliary obstruction, not to evaluate the pancreas itself. We depend on contrast-enhanced CT for that purpose. While intrinsic and nonpancreatic abnormalities can be identified sonographically, CT should be performed, when indicated, to more completely delineate the extent of disease.

The pancreas often appears normal in acute pancreatitis, although there is wide variance in the reported frequency of sonographic abnormalities, ranging from 33 (15) to 90 percent (14). The most frequent sonographic abnormalities in acute pancreatitis are enlargement and diffusely decreased glandular echogenicity (Figs. 4.1 and 4.2). Both may be difficult to assess confidently. Pancreatic size varies markedly with age and other parameters. Echogenicity is usually determined by comparison to the liver (Figs. 4.1 and 4.2). This is unreliable when liver echogenicity is increased by fatty infiltration or fibrosis/cirrhosis (Fig. 4.3). Acute intrapancreatic masses may be caused by focal edema (Fig. 4.4), acute fluid collections (Fig. 4.5), hemorrhage, or necrosis. Echogenic masses should suggest the possibility of hemorrhage.

Vascular complications of pancreatitis are not unusual. Inflammation around portal veins ("vascular cloaking") can be identified with grayscale sonography (Fig. 4.6) (12). When the vessels themselves are affected, hemorrhage, usually into the gastrointestinal tract or peripancreatic soft tissues, may occur. Thrombosis may occur in any splanchnic vein (Fig. 4.7) but is most common in the splenic vein. On occasion, the entire portal venous system may be clotted (Fig. 4.8). Splenic vein clot may lead to bleeding from isolated gastric varices. This type of bleeding (left-sided or "sinestral" portal hypertension) is cured by splenectomy. Bleeding from esophageal varices may occur when other portal veins are thrombosed. Portal vein thrombosis may be diagnosed effectively with color flow sonography (16). Arterial pseudoaneurysms, which should be sought when hemorrhagic pancreatitis is diagnosed or suspected, may be identified with color flow sonography (Fig. 4.9) or dynamic contrast-enhanced CT. Arteries most frequently affected are (in order) splenic, gastroduodenal, pancreaticoduodenal, gastric, and hepatic (17). Arteriography should be considered in these patients, both to confirm the diagnosis and treat the pseudoaneurysm by embolization.

Extrapancreatic abnormalities may be identified sonographically, usually as hypoechoic enlargement of the tissue planes about the pancreas (Figs. 4.10 to 4.12). The lateral anterior pararenal spaces are usually easiest to visualize by using a lateral flank acoustic window (Fig. 4.13). The more central areas are often obscured by gas. If increased echogenicity is present in the extrapancreatic

(*text continues on page 242*)

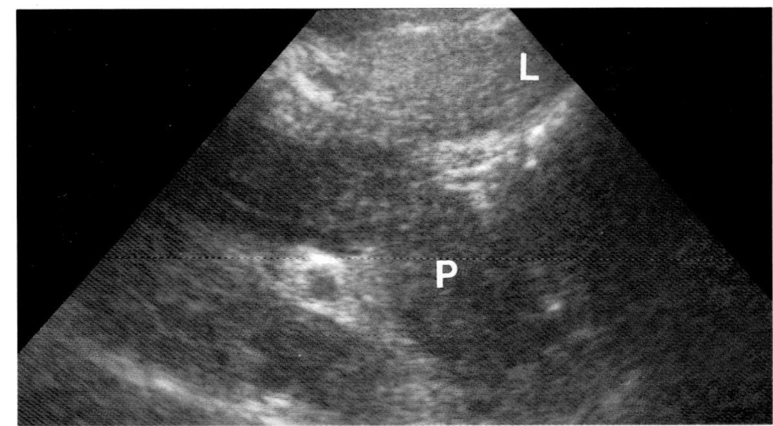

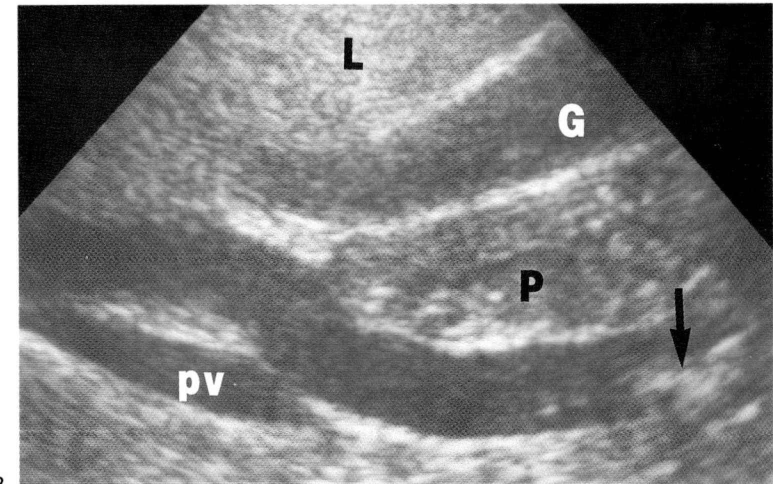

FIG. 4.1. Acute pancreatitis, stone obstructing common bile duct. **A:** Transverse sonogram of the region of the body and tail of the pancreas reveals decreased echogenicity of the pancreas (P) compared to the liver (L). Most often, mild pancreatitis results in no alteration of the pancreatic echogenicity. A relatively hypoechoic pancreas, as noted in this case, is somewhat unusual. This patient's pancreatitis was caused by calculous obstruction of the common bile duct. **B:** The longitudinal image of the bile duct reveals extrahepatic bile duct dilatation and a distal stone (*arrow*). L, liver; G, gallbladder; PV, portal vein.

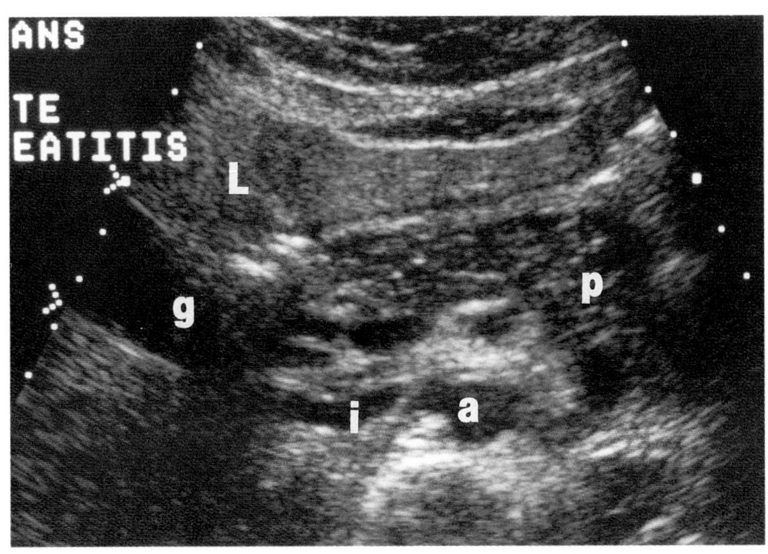

FIG. 4.2. Acute pancreatitis with decreased pancreatic echogenicity. Transverse sonogram at the level of the upper head and body of the pancreas. Although the pancreas is often normal in acute pancreatitis, glandular echogenicity may be diffusely decreased. Echogenicity is usually judged by comparing the echogenicity of the liver (L) to that of the pancreas (p). a, aorta; i, IVC; g, gallbladder.

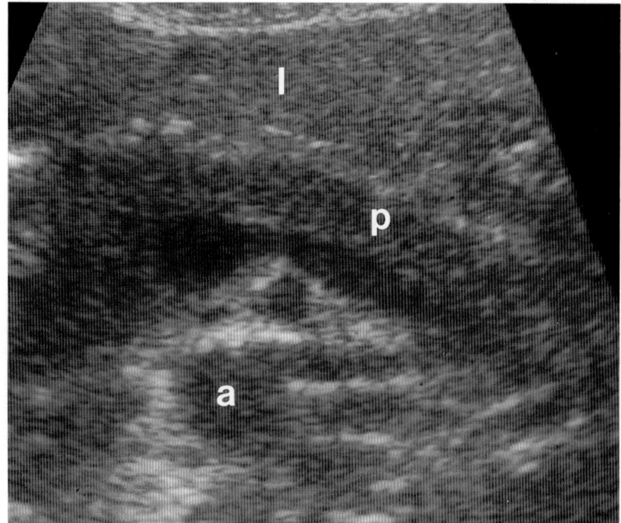

FIG. 4.3. Pseudopancreatitis. Transverse sonogram at the level of the body and tail of the pancreas. When there is increased liver echogenicity, the normal pancreas may be relatively hypoechoic, simulating the findings sometimes associated with edematous acute pancreatitis. l, liver; p, pancreas; a, aorta.

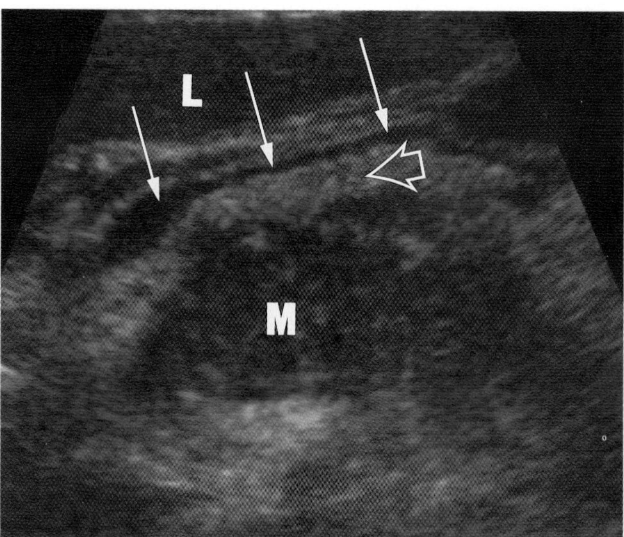

FIG. 4.4. Hypoechoic mass, acute pancreatitis. Transverse sonogram in the region of the body of the pancreas. Acute pancreatitis may occasionally result in focal hypoechoic masses, such as this (M). Note the higher echogenicity of the normal pancreas (*open arrow*). On occasion, masses like this may simulate neoplasm. L, liver; *small arrows,* fluid in stomach.

A

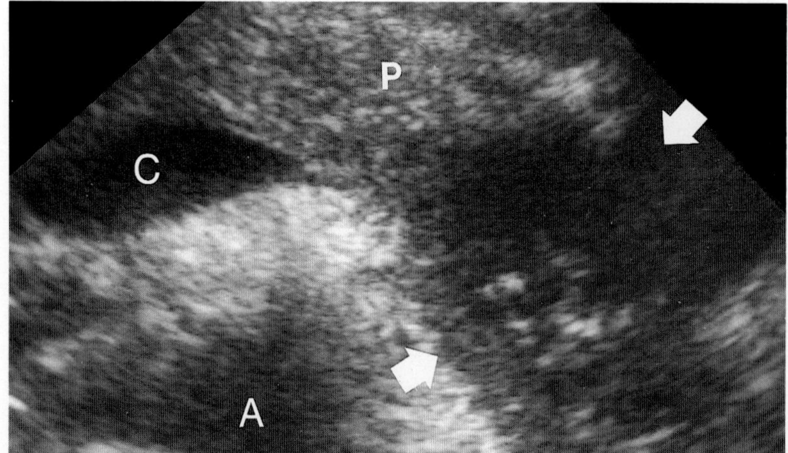

B

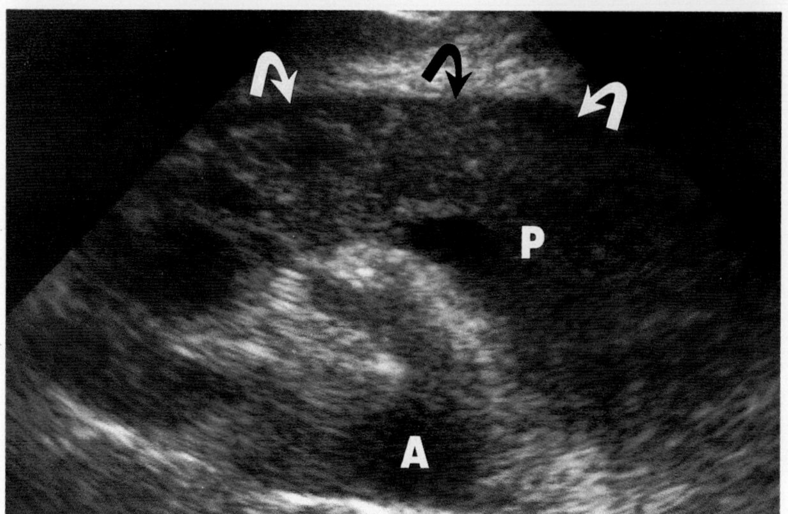

FIG. 4.5. Acute pancreatitis, focal fluid collection. **A:** Transverse sonogram reveals a fluid collection in the tail of the pancreas (*arrows*). Fluid collections such as this often occur in patients with moderate to severe pancreatitis. These collections are often transient. **B:** Transverse sonogram of the body and tail of the pancreas reveals a thin pancreatitis-associated fluid collection (*curved arrows*). In this patient, both the peripancreatic and intrapancreatic fluid collections resolved on conservative management. A, aorta; C, splenic vein/superior mesenteric vein (SMV) confluence; P, pancreas.

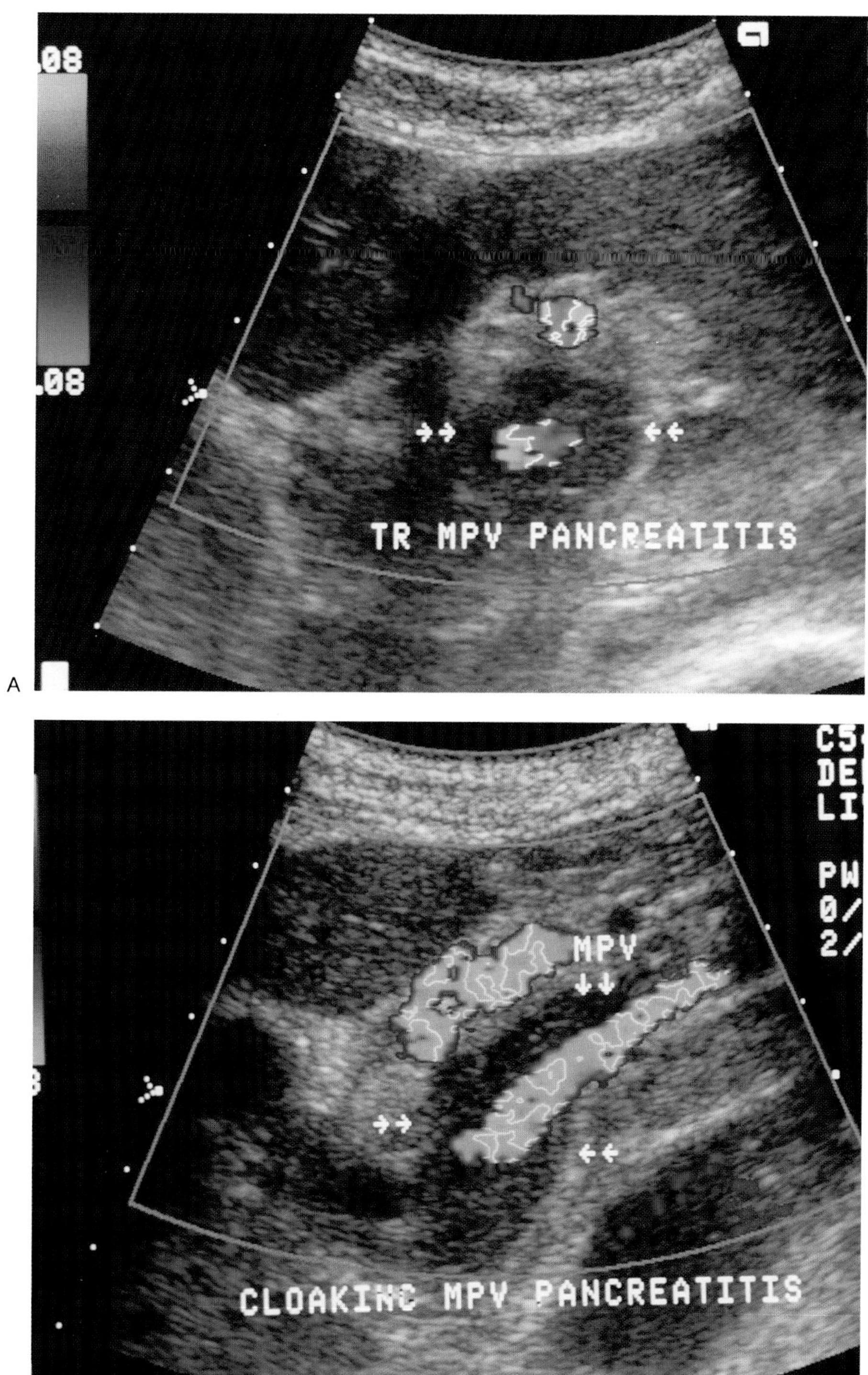

FIG. 4.6. Pancreatitis, perivascular cloaking. Transverse (**A**) and longitudinal (**B**) color Doppler sonograms of the main portal vein (MPV). Pancreatic inflammation may surround blood vessels, resulting in hypoechoic area that tracks along the vessels (*arrows*) near and around the pancreas. This is called perivascular cloaking.

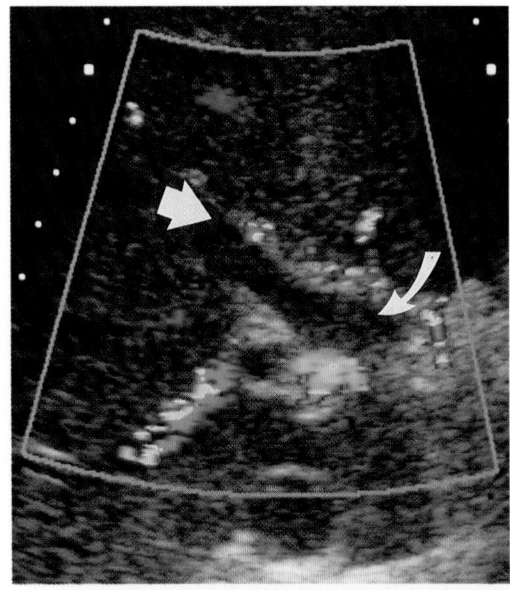

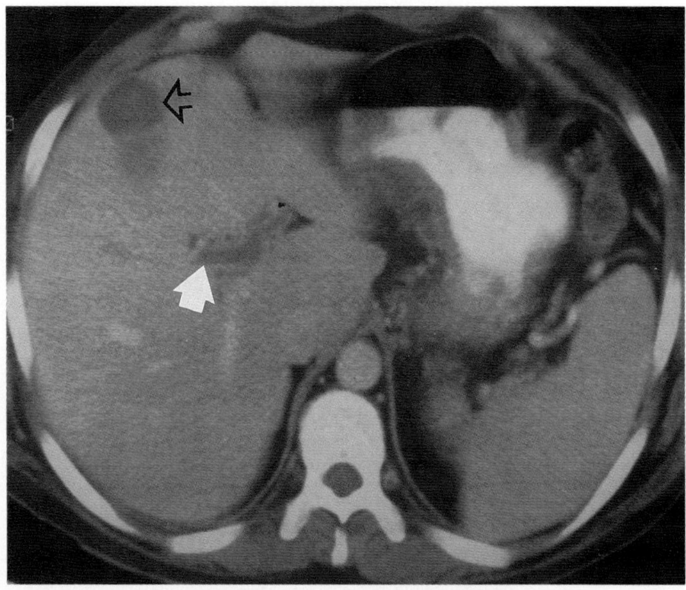

A B

FIG. 4.7. Thrombosis, right portal vein. **A:** Transverse color Doppler sonogram of the right portal vein. **B:** CT scan, level of right portal vein. Pancreatitis may lead to partial or complete thrombosis of the portal venous system. This patient developed complete venous thrombosis of the anterior segmental branch of the right portal vein (*arrow*), with partial clot of the main right portal vein (*curved arrow*). This is demonstrated on both color Doppler sonography and contrast-enhanced CT. This patient developed septic portal venous thrombosis (pylephlebitis) that led to a hepatic abscess (*open arrow*), visible on the CT scan.

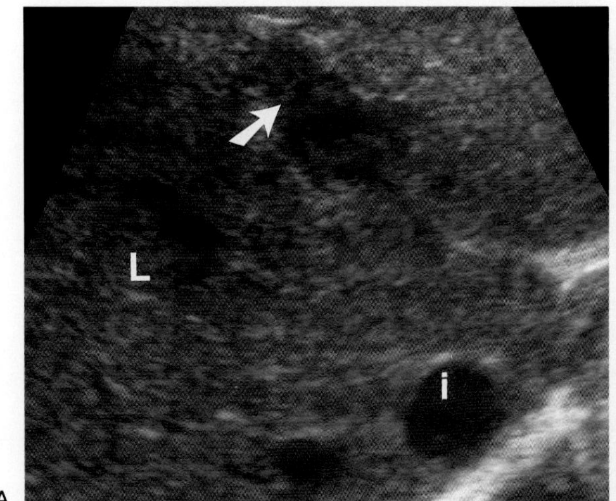

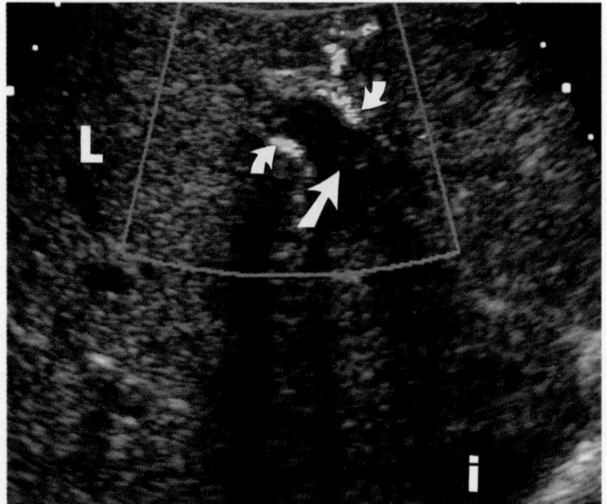

A B

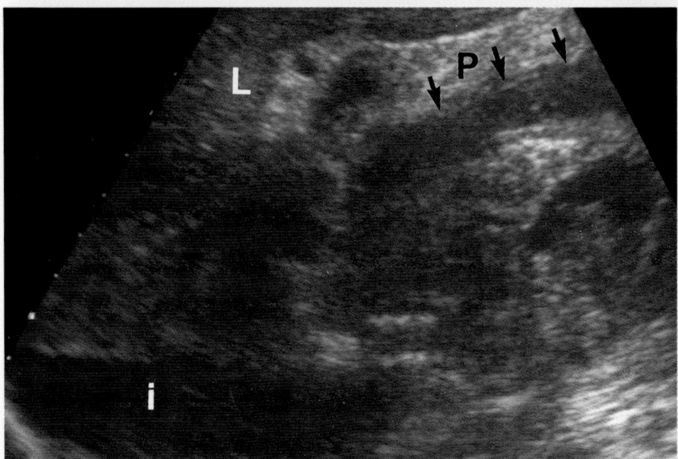

C

FIG. 4.8. Complete portal venous thrombosis. Complete thrombosis of all the major splanchnic veins may occur in some patients with pancreatitis. Left portal venous thrombosis (*arrow*) is demonstrated on both the transverse grayscale (**A**) and color Doppler (**B**) images. The longitudinal grayscale image (**C**) reveals complete superior mesenteric vein thrombosis (*black arrows*). Note the increased arterial flow (*curved arrows*) demonstrated on the color Doppler sonogram (**B**). Increased arterial flow often results when portal venous thrombosis is present. i, inferior vena cava; L, liver; P, pancreas.

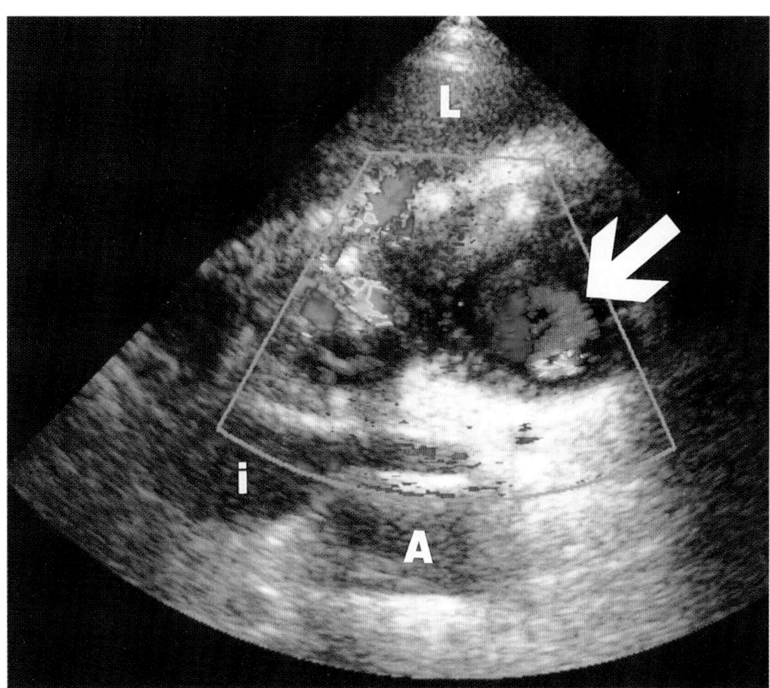

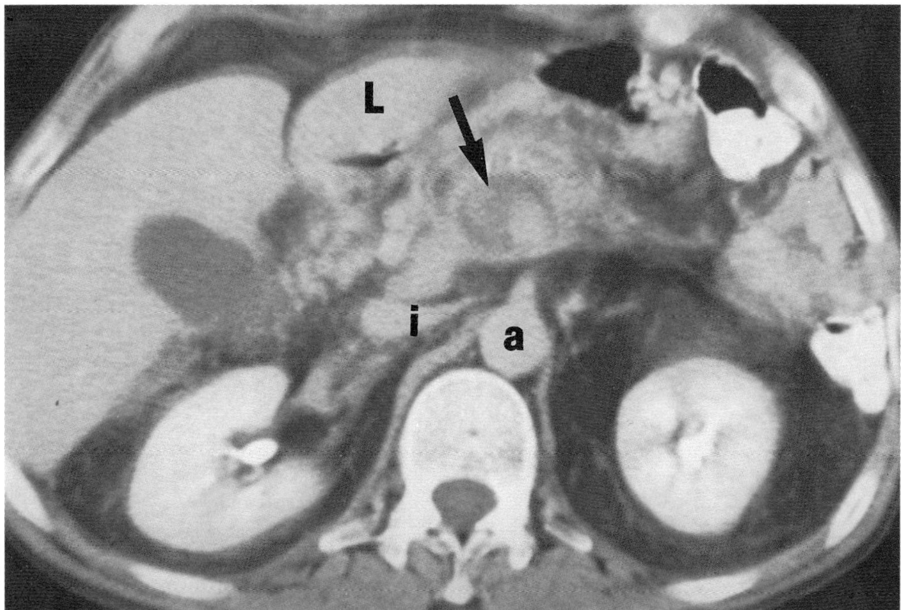

FIG. 4.9. Splenic artery pseudoaneurysm. **A:** Transverse color Doppler sonogram revealed a splenic artery pseudoaneurysm (*arrow*) in this patient with hemorrhagic pancreatitis. Note the swirling red/blue color within the pseudoaneurysm. Subsequent to therapeutic embolization, a small persistent pseudoaneurysm was detected by color Doppler sonography. **B:** A CT scan performed at this time also demonstrated the persistent pseudoaneurysm (*arrow*). Repeat embolization was successful. The pseudoaneurysm was obliterated on follow-up color Doppler sonography. a, aorta; L, liver; i, inferior vena cava.

A

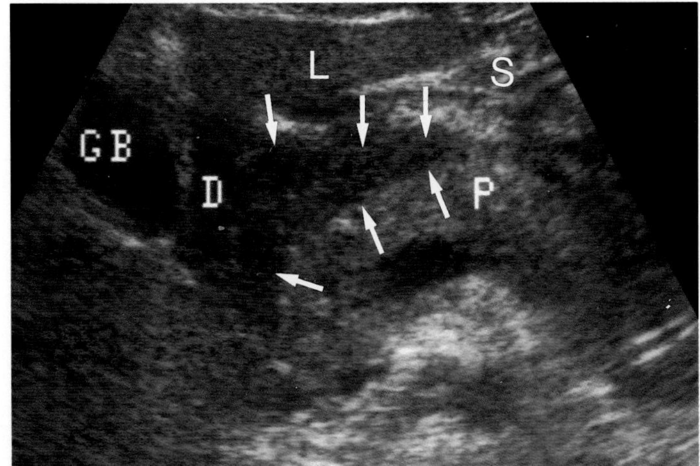

B

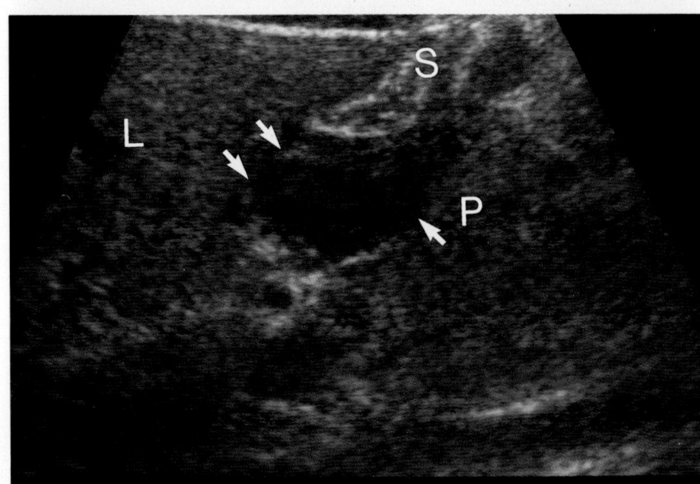

FIG. 4.10. Peripancreatic phlegmonous change. Peripancreatic abnormality is noted on both the transverse (**A**) and the longitudinal (**B**) sonograms. Hypoechoic enlargement of the peripancreatic tissue planes is a sign of phlegmon (*arrows*). Abnormalities such as this may resolve spontaneously with conservative management or progress to fluid collections or abscess. P, pancreas; D, duodenum; G, gallbladder; L, liver; S, stomach.

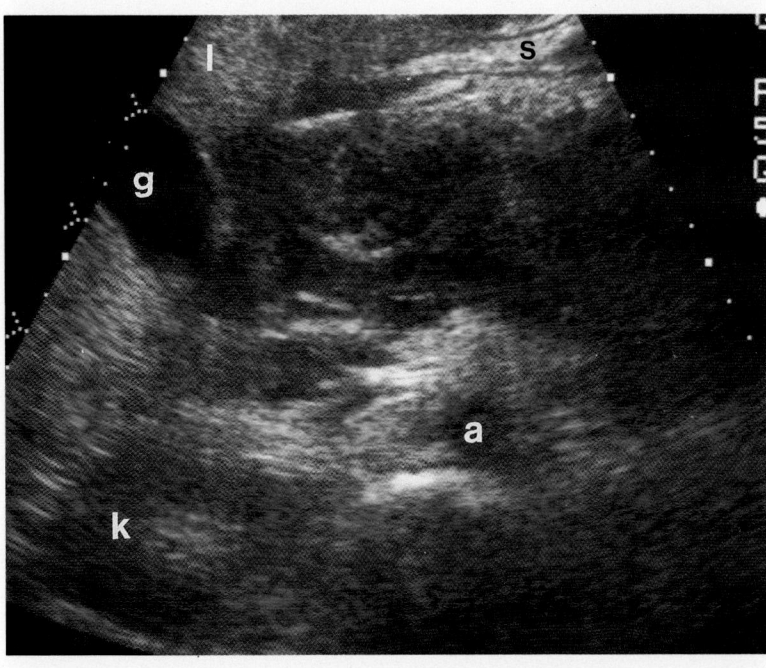

FIG. 4.11. Intra- and peripancreatic inflammatory changes, acute pancreatitis. A transverse sonogram (**A**) reveals both intrapancreatic (*open arrows*) and peripancreatic (*arrows*) abnormalities. In severe cases, definition of the pancreas itself may be lost. s, stomach; g, gallbladder; k, right kidney; a, aorta; l, liver.

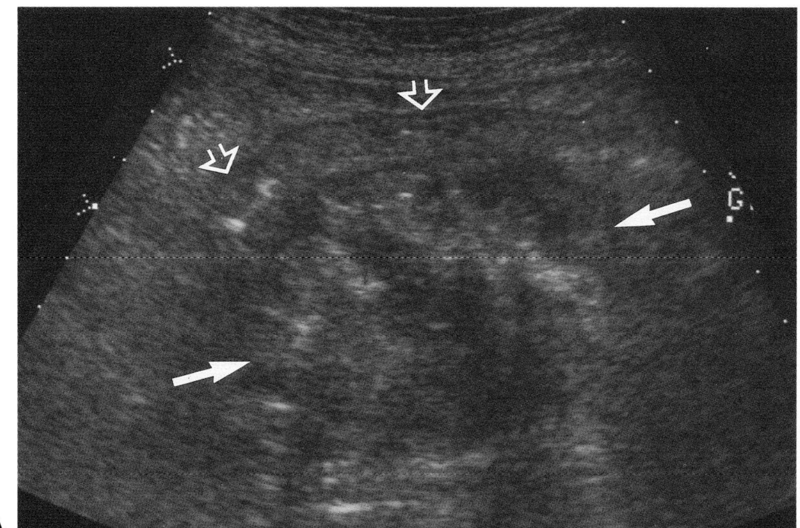

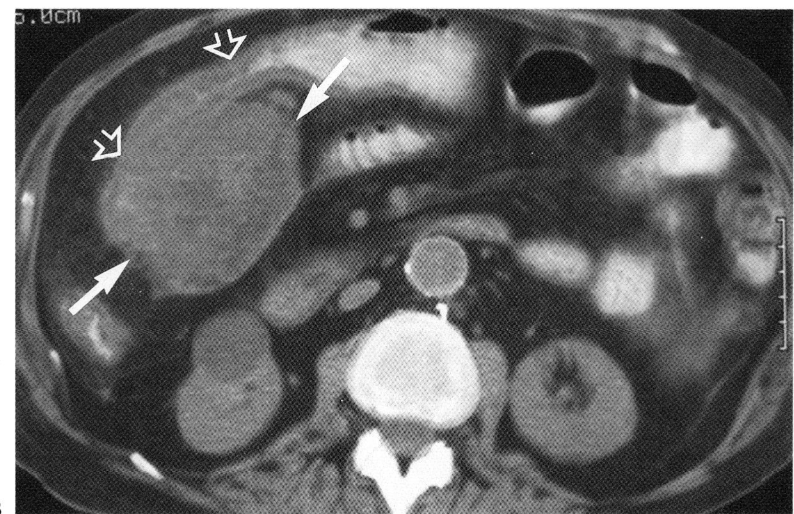

FIG. 4.12. Phlegmonous pancreatitis adjacent to stomach and duodenum. **A:** Transverse sonogram in the region of the pancreatic head. **B:** CT scan in same location. Phlegmonous change related to acute pancreatitis may have a mixed echogenicity pattern, as noted in this case (*arrows*). The phlegmonous mass displaces the stomach and duodenum (*open arrows*).

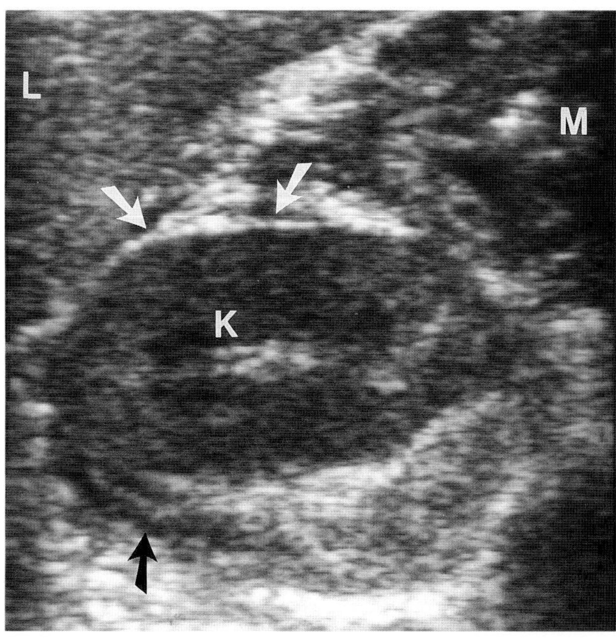

FIG. 4.13. Perirenal phlegmonous change, acute pancreatitis. Transverse sonogram through the region of the right kidney (K). Pancreatic inflammation often crosses multiple tissue planes. Note the decreased perirenal echogenicity caused by perirenal phlegmon (*arrows*). A large predominantly hypoechoic mixed echogenicity phlegmonous mass (M) is seen ventromedial to the right kidney. L, liver.

abnormality, hemorrhagic pancreatitis should be suspected and confirmed with a noncontrast CT scan. Ascitic fluid should be aspirated to distinguish bland ascites from infected ascites, pancreatic ascites, or hemorrhagic fluid (15).

Chronic Pancreatitis

By the 1984 Marseilles classification, chronic pancreatitis is usually characterized by recurrent or persistent abdominal pain. Pancreatic insufficiency is often present. Exocrine insufficiency is more common than endocrine insufficiency (1). Image findings are poor predictors of the clinical severity of chronic pancreatitis (18), although patients with severe exocrine insufficiency are more likely to have abnormal pancreatic size and contour irregularities (19). It is important to understand the diverse findings that occur in chronic pancreatitis, largely to avoid confusion with other conditions. Detecting multiple pancreatic calcifications (Figs. 4.14 and 4.15) allows a confident diagnosis of chronic pancreatitis, usually alcohol related. These calcifications are caused by stones within the main or branch pancreatic ducts (Figs. 4.16 and 4.17). Sonography is less sensitive than CT in detecting pancreatic calcifications (20). On occasion, a diffusely hyperechoic pancreas may be an indicator of chronic pancreatitis. Abnormally increased echogenicity may be difficult to judge sonographically, as the normal pancreas is already more echogenic than adjacent parenchymal organs like the liver. Chronic pancreatitis may cause dilatation of the pancreatic (Figs. 4.14 and 4.16) or common bile duct. Bolondi et al. (20) feel that dilatation of the main pancreatic duct is the most reliable sign of chronic pancreatitis. The "double duct sign" (dilatation of both ducts) is nonspecific, occurring in both chronic pancreatitis and pancreatic carcinoma (21). Duct dilatation within a mass generally means that the mass is caused by chronic pancreatitis (Fig. 4.14), although carcinoma may occasionally have internal hypoechoic regions as well. Glandular atrophy or fatty infiltration may occur, making evaluation of the pancreas difficult sonographically. Chronic asymptomatic pseudocysts may be found in patients with chronic pancreatitis. Pseudocysts also occur in association with pancreatic carcinoma.

Acute pancreatitis may occur in patients with known chronic pancreatitis. On occasion, findings of chronic pancreatitis are discovered in a first-time acute pancreatitis patient. Clinical information, coupled with the image findings, should allow correct diagnosis.

Approximately one-third of patients with chronic pancreatitis have focal masses that must be differentiated from neoplasm. Calcification within the mass makes the diagnosis of chronic pancreatitis almost certain (Figs. 4.14, 4.15, and 4.18). Hyperechoic masses, even those without discrete calcifications, are usually caused by chronic pancreatitis, even though hyperechoic carcinoma is not rare. Uncalcified isoechoic or hypoechoic masses may be difficult to differentiate from pancreatic carcinoma (Fig. 4.19). About one-third of chronic pancreatitis-associated masses have this appearance (18); retrograde pancreatography or biopsy may be required to exclude malignancy.

Pancreatic Pseudocysts

Surprisingly, the distinction between pancreatitis-associated fluid collections and pseudocysts is arbitrary and based on conventional surgical treatment considerations. Pseudocysts are differentiated from other fluid collections largely on the basis of chronicity and the presence of mass effect. After 6 weeks, pseudocysts generally have a well-formed fibrous pseudocapsule necessary for surgical drainage. At times, this pseudocapsule may be imaged. Acute pancreatic and peripancreatic fluid collections occur in more than half of patients with significant acute pancreatitis (22). They are nonencapsulated and usually lack significant mass effect, generally conforming to retroperitoneal and other fascial compartments (Fig. 4.20). Acute fluid collections are evanescent; only a minority ultimately persist as well-defined pseudocysts after 6 weeks (23). It is surprising that the true prevalence and natural history of pseudocysts are unknown, especially in chronic pancreatitis. Prevalence is variously reported to range from 2 to 40 percent (20,24,25). Well-formed pseudocysts 5 cm or larger are said to have a high prevalence of complications (26). This conclusion is questionable, as pseudocyst complications have never been evaluated in a controlled longitudinal study using modern imaging techniques.

Sonographically, pseudocysts are well defined and have variable internal echogenicity (Fig. 4.21). Internal hyperechogenicity suggests hemorrhage (Figs. 4.22 and 4.23). Pseudocysts may be septated or contain debris (Fig. 4.23). A pseudocyst may be confidently diagnosed when a persistent fluid collection is detected in the clinical setting of pancreatitis (Fig. 4.24). There is often mass effect on adjacent bowel loops and solid viscera, and occasionally a definable fibrous pseudocapsule. Biliary obstruction may be caused by a pseudocyst (Fig. 4.25). Percutaneous pseudocyst drainage may be successful; cure rates ranging from 60 to 90 percent are reported (24,27–29) approaching the level of success with surgical drainage.

Several pitfalls related to neoplasm should be kept in mind. Occasionally, a cystic pancreatic neoplasm may be mistaken for a pancreatic pseudocyst. The absence of clinical and laboratory findings of pancreatitis should prevent misdiagnosis. Conversely, a complex pseudocyst may simulate a cystic neoplasm (Fig. 4.26). Pancreatic

(*text continues on page 249*)

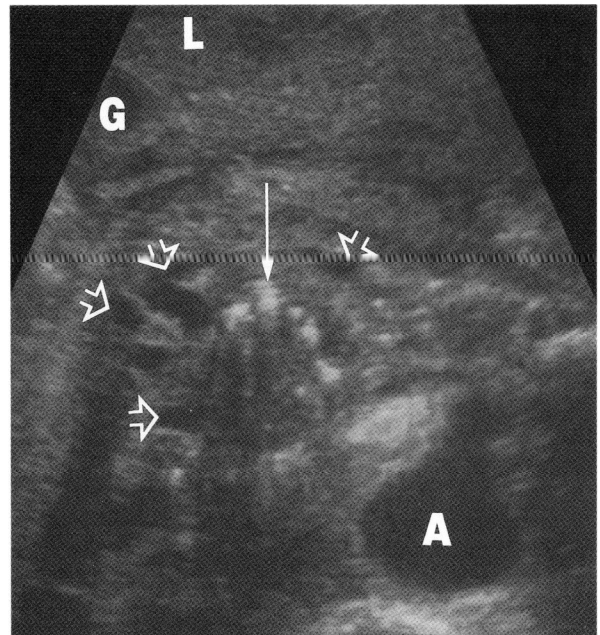

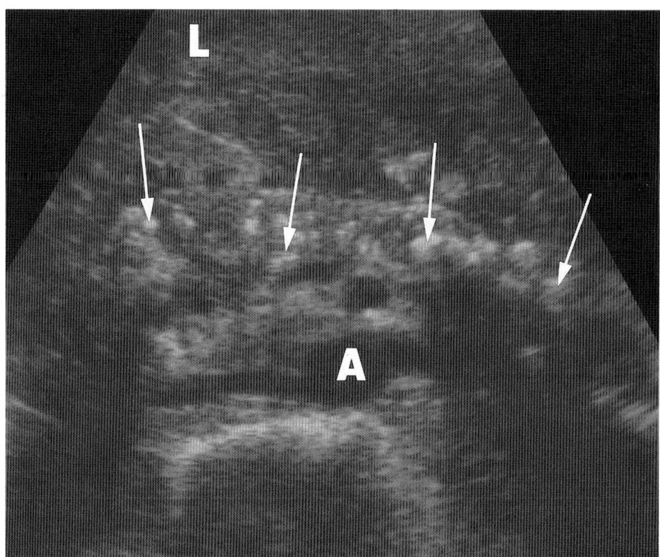

FIG. 4.14. Chronic calcific pancreatitis. Transverse sonograms of the pancreatic head (**A**) and pancreatic body and tail (**B**). Multiple large, echogenic shadowing pancreatic calculi like these are virtually diagnostic of chronic calcific pancreatitis. Calcifications such as this are typically located in the major pancreatic ducts. A few of the many calcifications are indicated by *thin arrows*. The ducts themselves may not be identifiable when they are filled with stones. Stones fill the main pancreatic duct in the body of the pancreas. Small dilated pancreatic ducts (*open arrows*) are another feature that suggests the diagnosis of chronic pancreatitis. Note the enlargement of the pancreatic head (**A**). Masses related to chronic pancreatitis are frequent, occurring in as many as one-third of patients. A, aorta; G, gallbladder; L, liver.

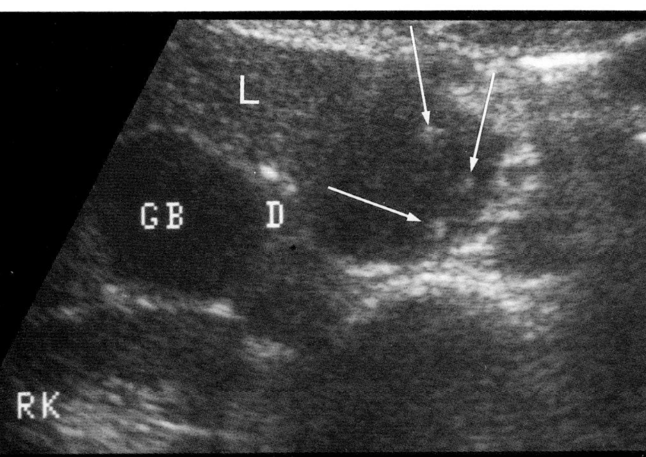

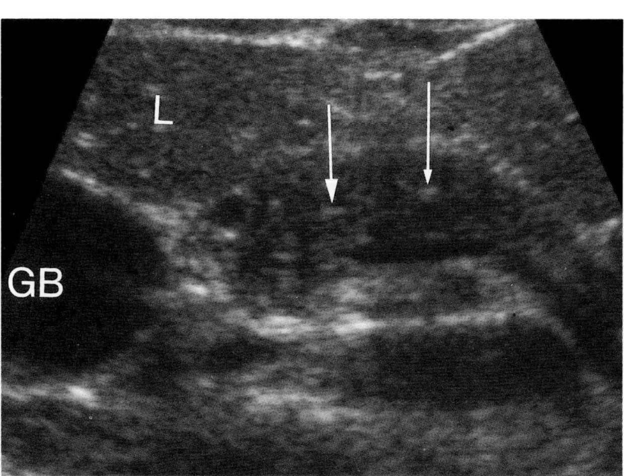

FIG. 4.15. Chronic calcific pancreatitis with faint calcifications. Transverse sonograms of the head (**A**) and body/tail (**B**) region of the pancreas. The presence of multiple echogenic foci (*arrows*) is strong evidence for chronic pancreatitis even though shadowing is not present. Often, chronic pancreatitis-related calculi do not shadow. GB, gallbladder; RK, right kidney; A, aorta; L, liver; D, duodenum.

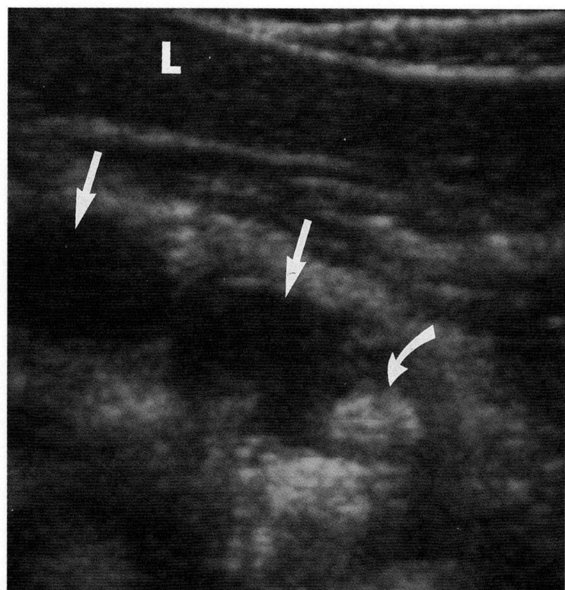

FIG. 4.16. Chronic pancreatitis, markedly dilated ducts. Transverse sonogram of body of pancreas. This markedly dilated pancreatic duct (*arrows*) is noted in a patient with severe chronic pancreatitis. A large intraductal calculus (*curved arrow*) is present. L, liver.

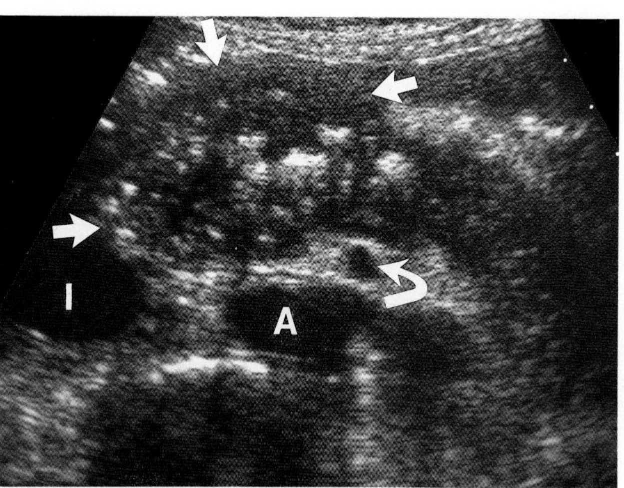

FIG. 4.18. Pancreatic head mass, chronic pancreatitis. Transverse sonogram in the region of the upper head and body of the pancreas. Chronic calcific pancreatitis often results in focal enlargement of the pancreas (about one-third of patients). This mass (*arrows*) is easily differentiable from pancreatic carcinoma as it contains multiple echogenic calcifications, some of which shadow. A, aorta; *curved arrow,* superior mesenteric artery; I, inferior vena cava.

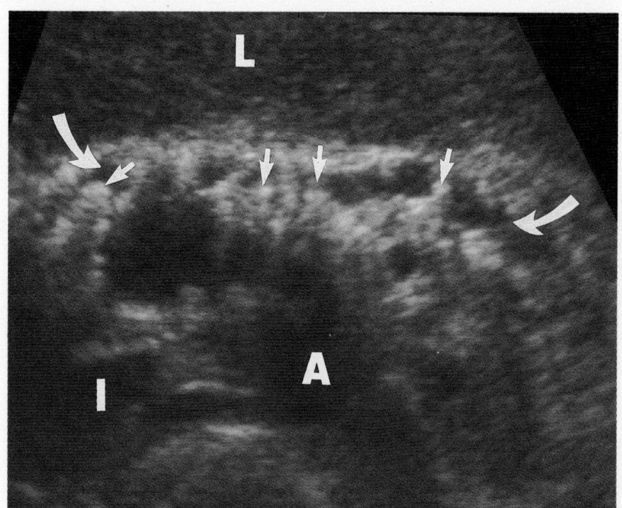

FIG. 4.17. Chronic pancreatitis. This pancreas is increased in echogenicity relative to the liver (L). Multiple small calculi (some indicated by *small arrows*) are present in a dilated pancreatic duct (*curved arrows*). Some of these stones exhibit echogenic comet tail artifact deep to the stone. On occasion, diffuse increased pancreatic echogenicity is the only sonographic sign that indicates chronic pancreatitis. A, aorta; I, inferior vena cava.

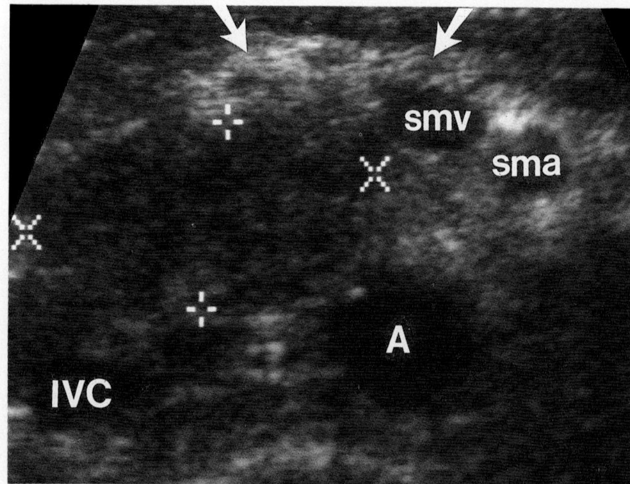

FIG. 4.19. Chronic head mass, chronic pancreatitis. A hypoechoic pancreatic head mass (*cursors*) may be difficult or impossible to differentiate from pancreatic carcinoma. Note the normal, more echogenic pancreas (*arrows*). About one-third of chronic pancreatitis-associated masses are hypoechoic. Biopsy or ERCP may be needed in patients like this. Most resolve spontaneously. Fluid collections that persist 6 weeks are generally called pseudocysts. This is a somewhat arbitrary definition, based on traditional surgical practice. It takes 6 weeks for a pseudocyst to develop a fibrous capsule to which a cyst enterostomy for surgical drainage can be attached. A, aorta; IVC, inferior vena cava; sma, superior mesenteric artery; smv, superior mesenteric vein.

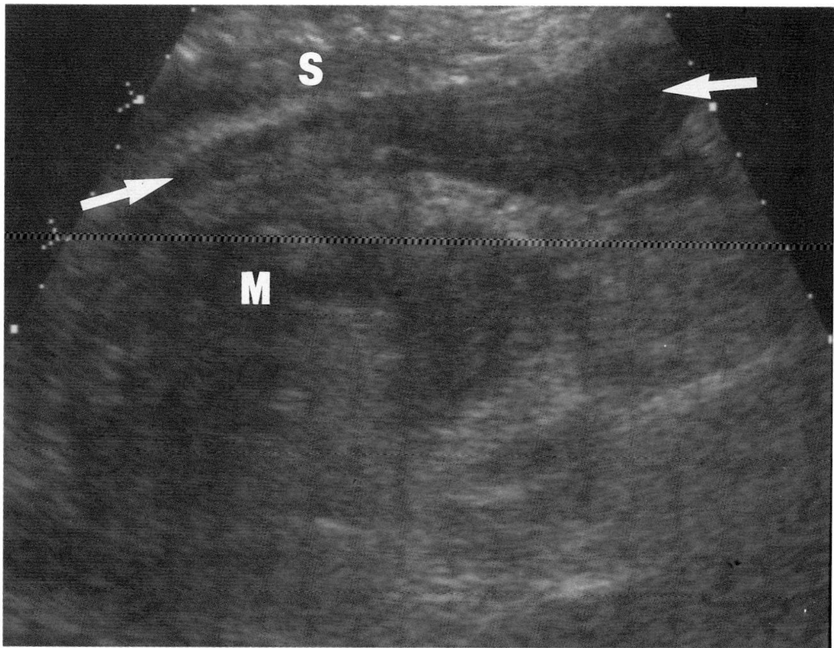

FIG. 4.20. Acute pancreatitis-related fluid collection. Transverse sonogram of region of the pancreatic body. Acute pancreatitis-associated fluid collections (*arrows*) generally conform to the tissue planes. Only a minority of these acute fluid collections persist to become well-defined pseudocysts. Most resolve spontaneously. An inhomogeneous phlegmonous mass (M) is seen dorsal to the fluid collection. S, stomach.

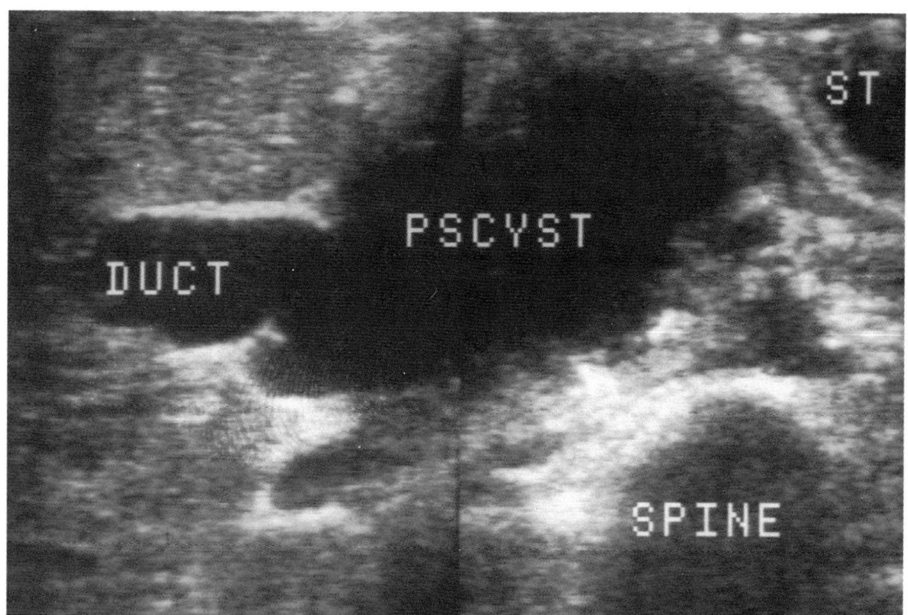

FIG. 4.21. Pseudocyst causing biliary obstruction. Oblique transverse compound sonogram, region of pancreatic head. A large, predominantly anechoic pseudocyst (PsCyst) is obstructing the common bile duct. Internal echogenicity of pseudocysts varies considerably from virtually anechoic, as seen here, to moderate internal echogenicity, especially when hemorrhage is present (see Figs. 4.22 and 4.23). Biliary obstruction, present here, is an infrequent complication.

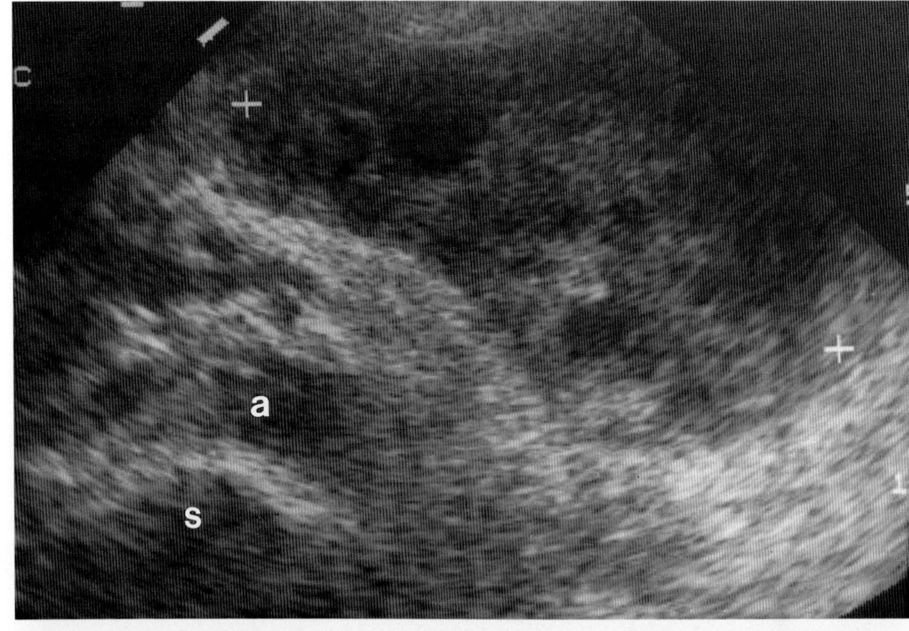

A

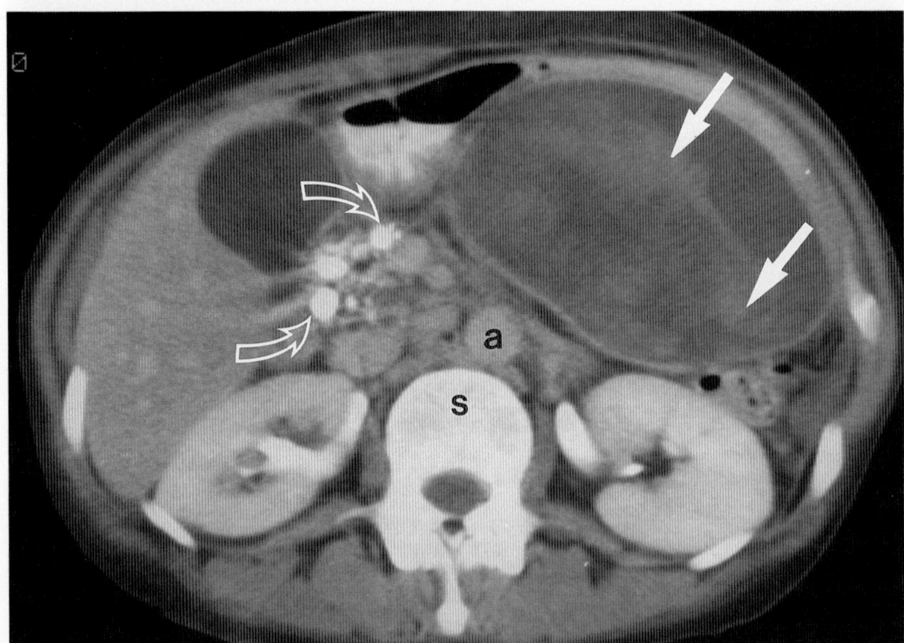

B

FIG. 4.22. Large hemorrhagic pseudocyst. **A:** Transverse sonogram of the region of the body of the pancreas. This large, mixed echogenicity mass (outlined by calipers) is heterogeneous and predominantly filled with medium level echoes. This is acute hemorrhage into the pseudocyst in a patient with chronic pancreatitis. **B:** The CT scan more clearly delineated the primarily cystic nature of the mass, although internal increased attenuation is present related to the hemorrhage (*arrows*). Note the calcifications in the head of the pancreas (*curved arrows*). Hemorrhage into pseudocysts may be life threatening. In unstable patients with hemorrhagic pancreatitis, angiography may be useful to seek a bleeding site. s, spine; a, aorta.

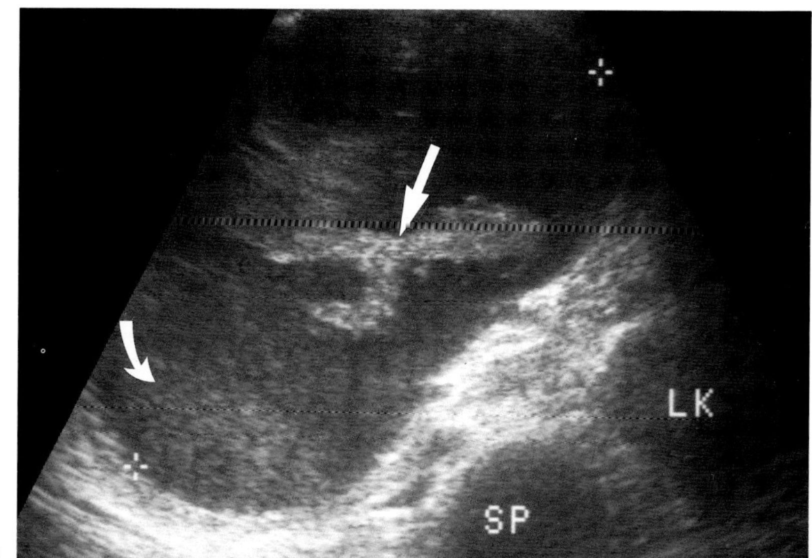

A

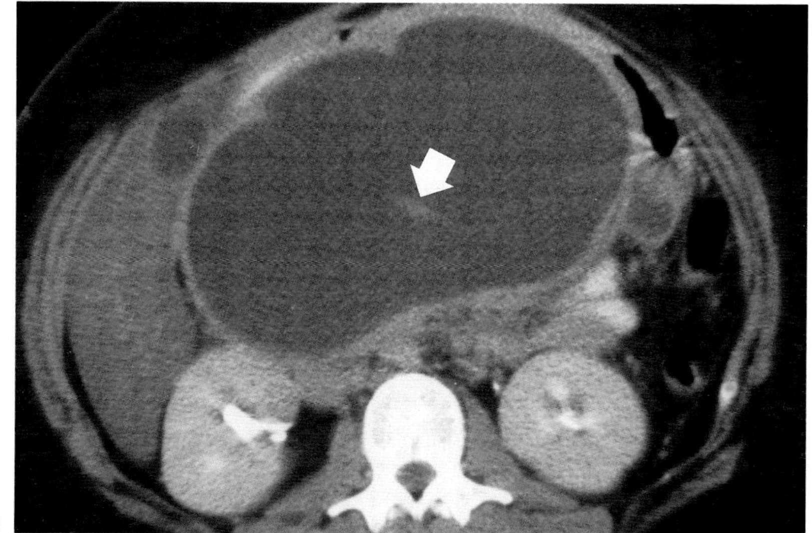

B

FIG. 4.23. Huge pseudocyst with internal clot. Transverse sonogram (**A**) in the region of the head of the pancreas. This large pseudocyst shows prominent irregular strand-like hyperechogenicity (*arrow*) representing fibrin from intracystic hemorrhage. Also noted is some dependent sludge-like debris (*curved arrow*). Sonography typically shows the internal architecture of cystic structures like this to better advantage than CT (**B**). The fibrin strands are barely demonstrated (*arrow*) on the CT scan. SP, spine; LK, left kidney.

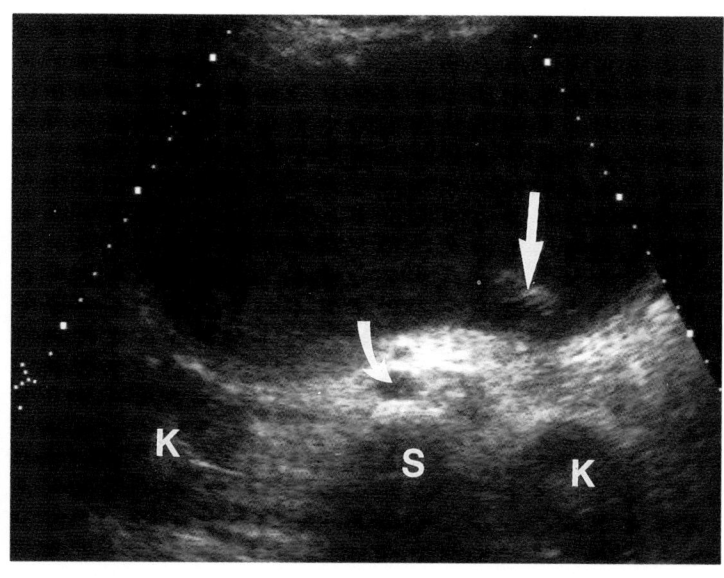

FIG. 4.24. Huge pancreatic pseudocyst. Transverse sonogram at the level of the pancreas. This 20-cm pseudocyst has some internal debris within it (*arrow*) possibly related to previous hemorrhage. This large pseudocyst was treated successfully with percutaneous drainage. K, kidneys; S, spine; curved arrow, aorta.

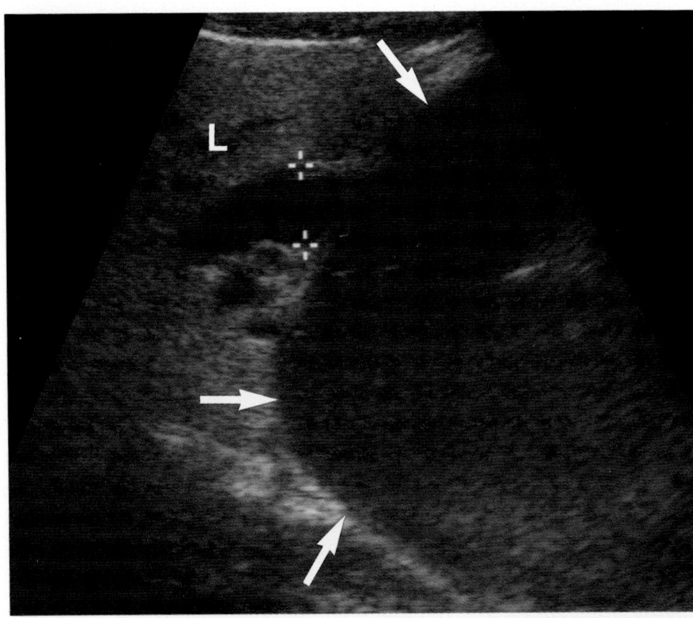

FIG. 4.25. Pseudocyst obstructing the common bile duct. Longitudinal oblique sonogram shows a dilated common bile duct (calipers) obstructed by a large sludge-containing pseudocyst. *Arrows* outline the pseudocyst. L, liver.

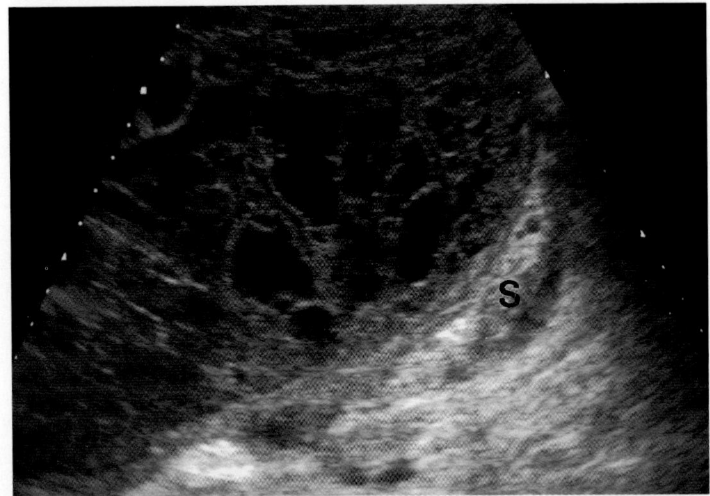

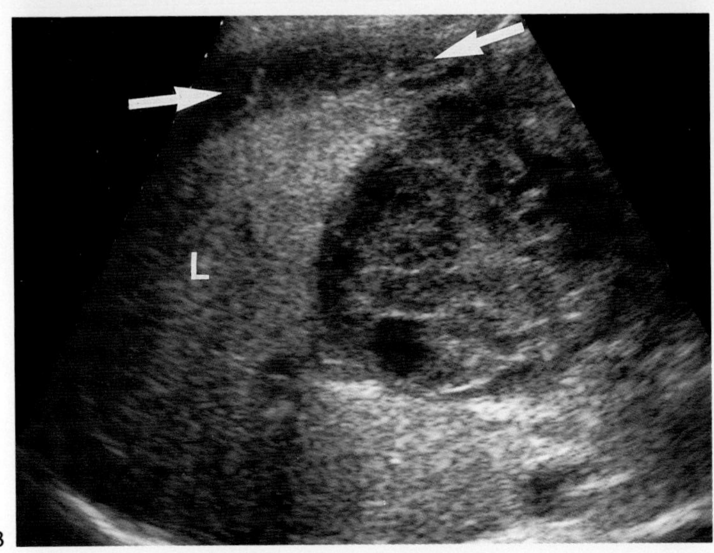

FIG. 4.26. Bizarre complex pseudocyst, simulating neoplasm. Transverse (**A**) and longitudinal (**B**) sonograms reveal a multicystic complex mass that is seen in the region of the pancreas. The preliminary image diagnosis in this case was mucinous pancreatic cystic neoplasm with probable carcinomatosis. Note the complex material (*arrows*) ventral to the liver (L) on the longitudinal sonogram. At surgery, all this material was easily resectable. Pathologically, the findings revealed a hemorrhagic fibrotic pseudocyst. S, stomach.

carcinoma may obstruct the pancreatic duct and thereby cause a pseudocyst.

Pancreatic Abscess

Pancreatic abscess is the most frequent life-threatening complication of pancreatitis. Abscess occurs in about 2.5 to 9 percent of patients with acute pancreatitis (3,30). Early diagnosis is essential for effective management. Of all abdominal and pelvic abscesses, pancreatic abscess is the most difficult to treat successfully, probably because pancreatic abscesses are often associated with extensive tissue necrosis in the retroperitoneum and elsewhere.

There are two distinct pathophysiologic types of pancreatitis-associated abscesses. The first results when a preexisting uninfected fluid collection becomes infected. This type of abscess is generally successfully treated by percutaneous catheter drainage. Recovery is usually relatively quick when the abscess does not communicate with the pancreatic duct and no gastrointestinal fistula is present. The second type of abscess, that arising *de novo* from necrotic pancreatic and peripancreatic tissue, is much more difficult to diagnose and treat. Infected necrosis tends to be more poorly defined on CT and much less well vascularized. Our experience suggests that percutaneous drainage is often ineffective in treating infected necrosis (31), although cure rates approaching 90 percent (32) have been reported. Some feel drainage may be used as a temporizing measure prior to surgery (33). Surgical treatment, even early extensive surgical debridement (necrosectomy), is also imperfect (3). Necrosectomy is advocated by some pancreatic surgeons as a means of preventing infected necrosis. It is not yet clear whether this aggressive approach, which may lead to significant surgical mortality (3), is superior to supportive management, with treatment of abscesses as they arise.

FOCAL PANCREATIC DISEASE

In the past two decades, innovations in pancreatic imaging have led to remarkable advances in the detection and characterization of focal pancreatic masses. Early hopes that imaging might detect small curable pancreatic carcinomas have not been fulfilled; survival of these patients has not improved. Despite this, imaging, especially CT, has become an integral tool in the diagnosis and management of patients with pancreatic masses. Initial lesion detection, diagnosis by guided percutaneous biopsy, assessment of resectability, and evaluation of response to therapy are all facilitated by imaging.

Sonography in Focal Lesion Detection

Sonography and CT are the primary modalities used to detect focal pancreatic disease, especially pancreatic carcinoma. CT is generally superior because it routinely images the entire pancreas. Sonography is superb when the entire pancreas can be imaged. At times, sonography may delineate pancreatic masses better than contrast-enhanced CT (Fig. 4.27). Unfortunately, even with optimal equipment and scanning technique (upright, water-filled stomach and duodenum), the entire pancreas can be visualized in only about 25 percent of patients (34–36). Sonography is sometimes superior to CT in distinguishing nodes adjacent to the pancreas from masses arising within the parenchyma (Figs. 4.28 and 4.29). The collapsed duodenum may simulate peripancreatic adenopathy or cause a pancreatic pseudomass dorsal to the pancreatic head (Fig. 4.30). On occasion, enlarged intrapancreatic lymph nodes may simulate a neoplasm (Fig. 4.31).

We use sonography to guide biopsy of easily imaged pancreatic masses. CT guidance is preferred when sonography fails to image the mass or when the mass is visualized only with difficulty, that is, seen only with the use of upright water technique or significant compression. As there is some risk of spreading tumor with biopsy, we do not biopsy lesions that are potentially resectable for cure. Sometimes biopsy of associated lesions, such as liver metastases, rather than the presumed pancreatic primary tumor, is preferable.

Sonography is the primary imaging method to screen patients with jaundice. Sonography usually detects pancreatic carcinoma that obstructs the bile duct (Fig. 4.32). Sonography may also reveal a pancreatic mass in a patient scanned for abdominal pain. Sonography is occasionally useful to characterize abnormalities noted with CT, determining, for example, whether a lesion is cystic or solid. Sonography may prove useful when CT is negative or equivocal for pancreatic mass, since a carcinoma may be detected as an area of altered, usually decreased, echogenicity within the gland when no morphologic or attenuation abnormality is noted with CT (34) (Fig. 4.27).

Pancreatic Ductal Adenocarcinoma

Pancreatic ductal adenocarcinoma is by far the most common primary pancreatic neoplasm, comprising approximately 80 percent of all pancreatic neoplasms and about 90 percent of malignant epithelial tumors. All other pancreatic tumors are relatively rare (37). Pancreatic carcinoma, whose prevalence has tripled during the last 40 years, is one of the commonest causes of cancer death in the United States. Fortunately, its incidence seems to have leveled off recently (38). Pancreatic ductal adenocarcinoma is one of the most lethal of all malignancies. Overall 5-year survival is poor—2 percent or less (39). Most (60 percent) pancreatic carcinomas arise in the pancreatic head, 35 percent arise in the body and tail, and about 5 percent are diffuse (Fig. 4.33).

(*text continues on page 255*)

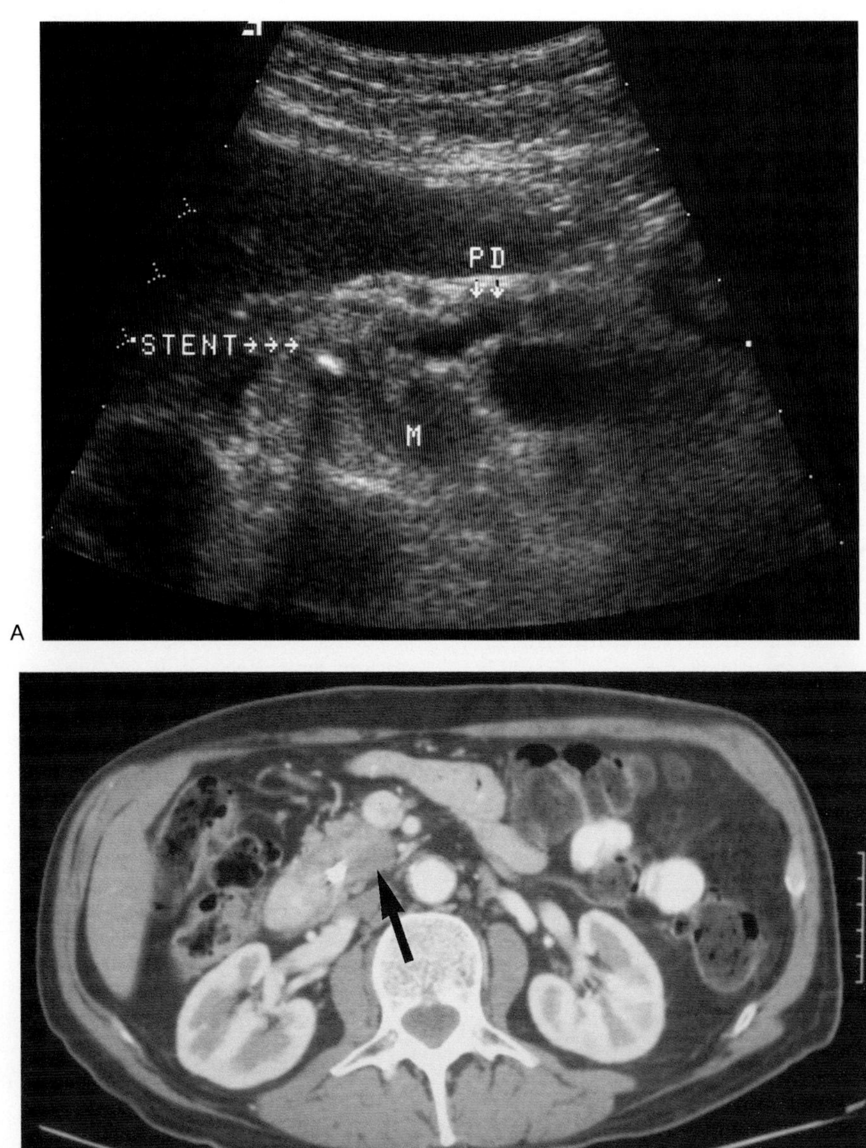

FIG. 4.27. Pancreatic carcinoma seen better with ultrasound than CT. **A:** Transverse sonogram in the region of the head of the pancreas. **B:** CT scan at the same level. Sonography occasionally delineates pancreatic masses better than contrast-enhanced CT. The transverse sonogram delineates the pancreatic mass (M) in this patient much better than the CT scan. The CT scan reveals only a subtle area of decreased attenuation, partially obscured by artifact and biliary stent (*arrow*). Although sonography often delineates pancreatic carcinoma well, the extent of disease is generally better assessed using CT. PD, pancreatic duct.

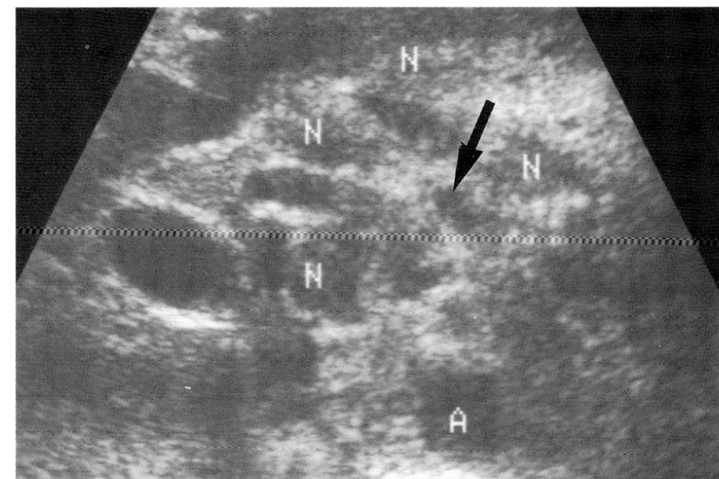

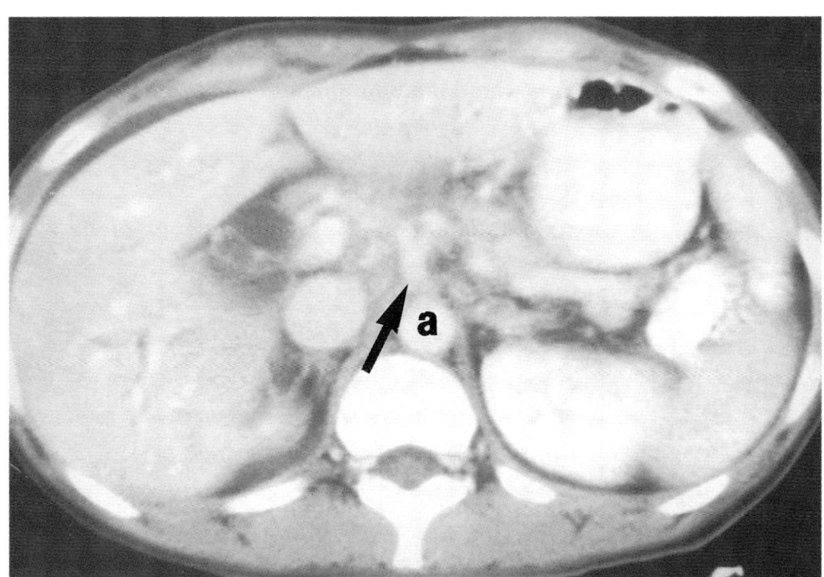

FIG. 4.28. Pancreatic carcinoma, peripancreatic nodes. **A:** Transverse sonogram at the level of the celiac axis. **B:** CT scan at the same level. It is not unusual for sonography to display peripancreatic lymph nodes more clearly than CT. In this patient, the sonogram reveals discrete lymphadenopathy (N) about the celiac axis (*arrow*). The CT scan reveals a similar abnormality but does not demonstrate the nodes as distinct from the primary mass. Although sonography may sometimes detect or display peripancreatic lymph nodes more clearly than CT, CT usually provides a better overall picture of the stage of pancreatic carcinoma. A, aorta.

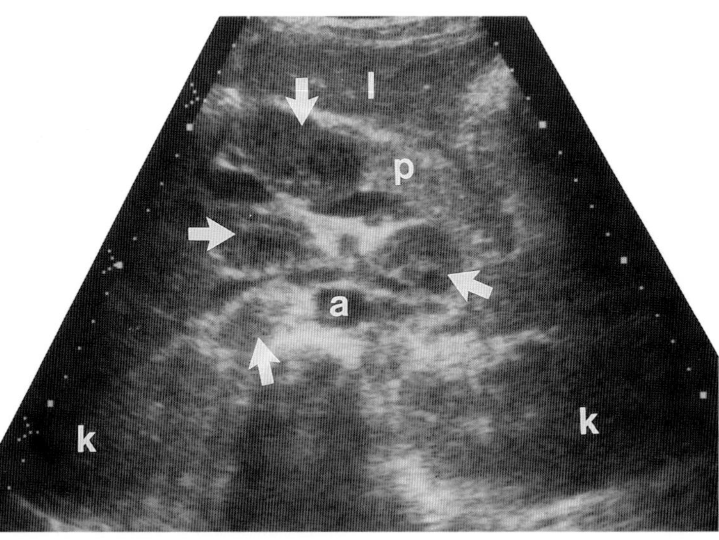

FIG. 4.29. Peripancreatic nodes, tuberculous adenopathy. Transverse sonogram at the level of the body of the pancreas. Multiple peripancreatic lymph nodes (*arrows*) are shown as distinct from the pancreas (p). Sonography is often useful in distinguishing peripancreatic adenopathy from masses arising within the pancreas. l, liver; a, aorta; k, kidneys.

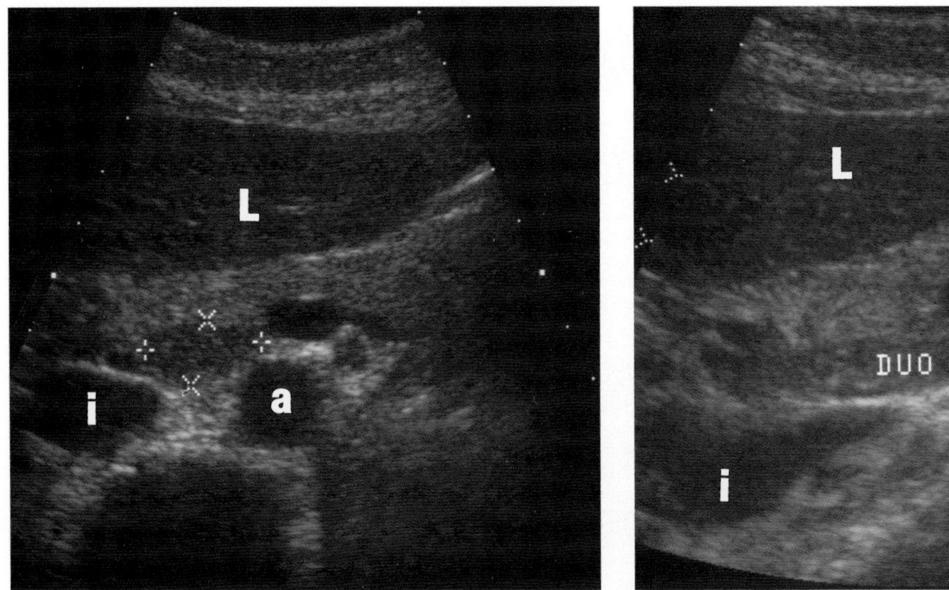

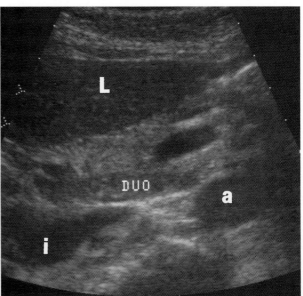

FIG. 4.30. Pancreatic pseudomass, caused by adjacent duodenum. Transverse sonograms in the region of the head of the pancreas (**A**), slightly cephalad to (**B**). On occasion, the duodenum may simulate an intrapancreatic mass or peripancreatic lymphadenopathy. These transverse sonograms show a hypoechoic area (calipers, DUO) that is difficult to distinguish from the pancreatic head. Cognizance of this pitfall can allow differentiation by careful scanning or by administering water to confirm the duodenal nature of the pseudomass. L, liver; a, aorta; i, inferior vena cava.

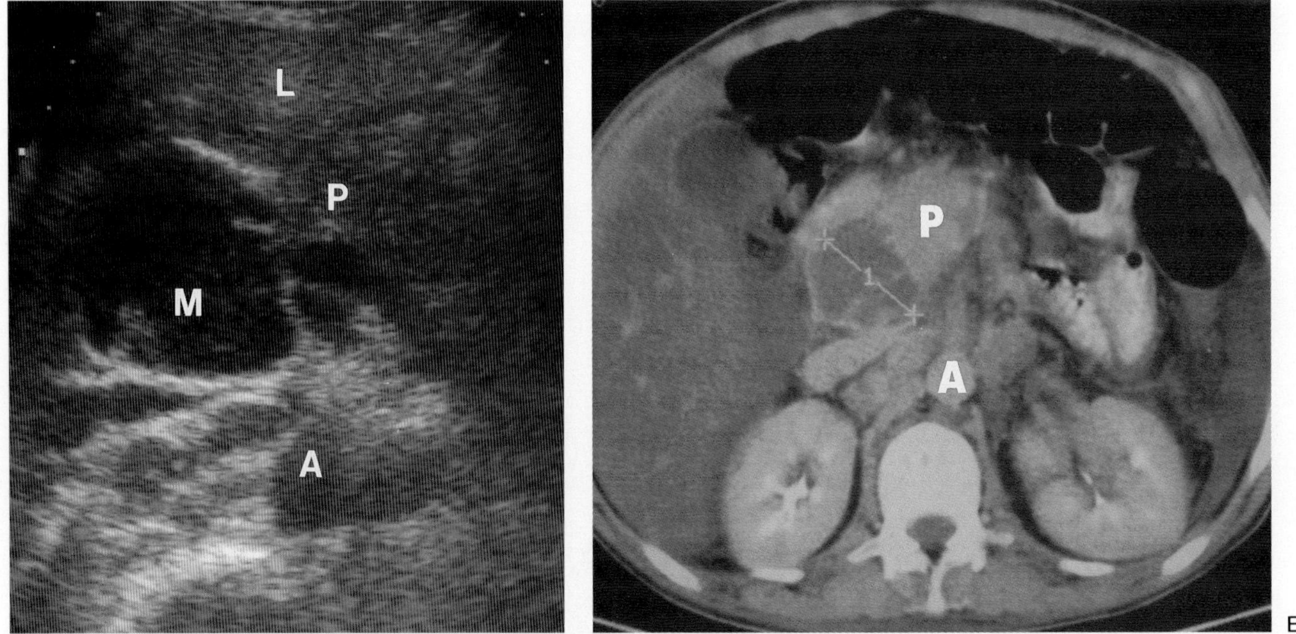

FIG. 4.31. Intrapancreatic lymph node, tuberculosis. Transverse sonogram (**A**) and CT scan (**B**) both reveal an intrapancreatic mass (M) that, respectively, is hypoechoic and shows decreased attenuation. Pancreatic carcinoma was suspected clinically. Laparotomy revealed an intrahepatic tuberculous node in this HIV-positive patient. A, aorta; P, pancreas; I, inferior vena cava; L, liver.

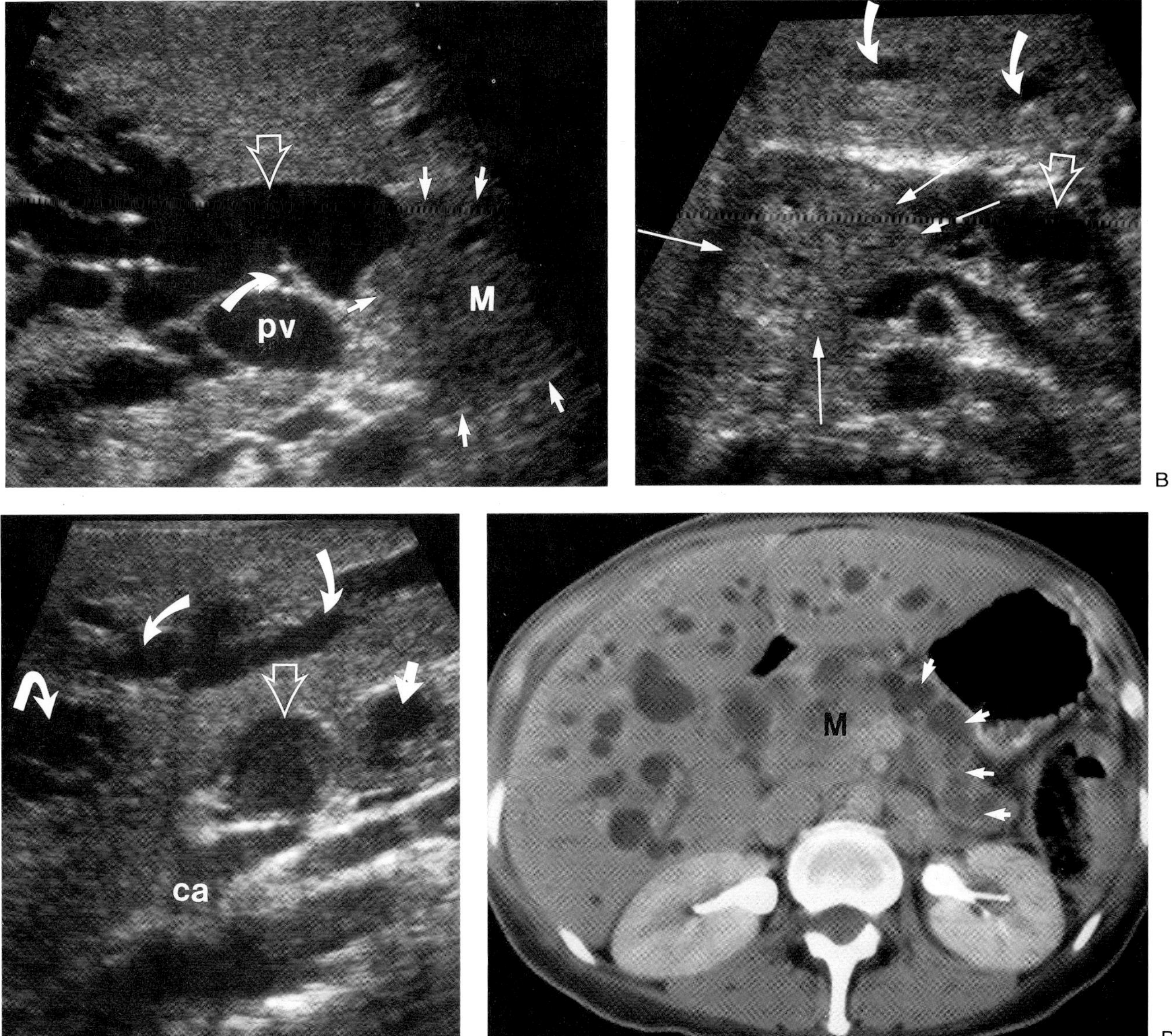

FIG. 4.32. Pancreatic carcinoma, double duct sign. Sonography is often the first modality to detect a pancreatic carcinoma that obstructs the common bile duct. **A:** A longitudinal oblique sonogram reveals a markedly dilated common bile duct (*large arrow*) that is obstructed by a large mass (M) representing a pancreatic carcinoma (*small arrows*). A *curved arrow* depicts the proper hepatic artery, which is just ventral to the main portal vein (PV). **B:** The transverse sonogram shows a dilated pancreatic duct (*arrow*), obstructed by the large pancreatic head mass (*thin arrows*). Dilated intrahepatic ducts (*curved arrows*) are shown in the left lobe of the liver. **C:** A longitudinal sagittal sonogram reveals a juxtapancreatic node (*open arrow*) just ventral to the celiac axis (CA) and just cephalad to the pancreas. Note the dilated pancreatic duct within the pancreas (*arrow*). Dilated intrahepatic bile ducts (*curved arrows*) are seen within the liver. Sonography is often effective in detecting peripancreatic lymph nodes. **D:** The CT scan reveals dilated intrahepatic ducts and the dilated pancreatic duct (*thin arrows*), confirming the presence of a "double duct" sign. M, mass.

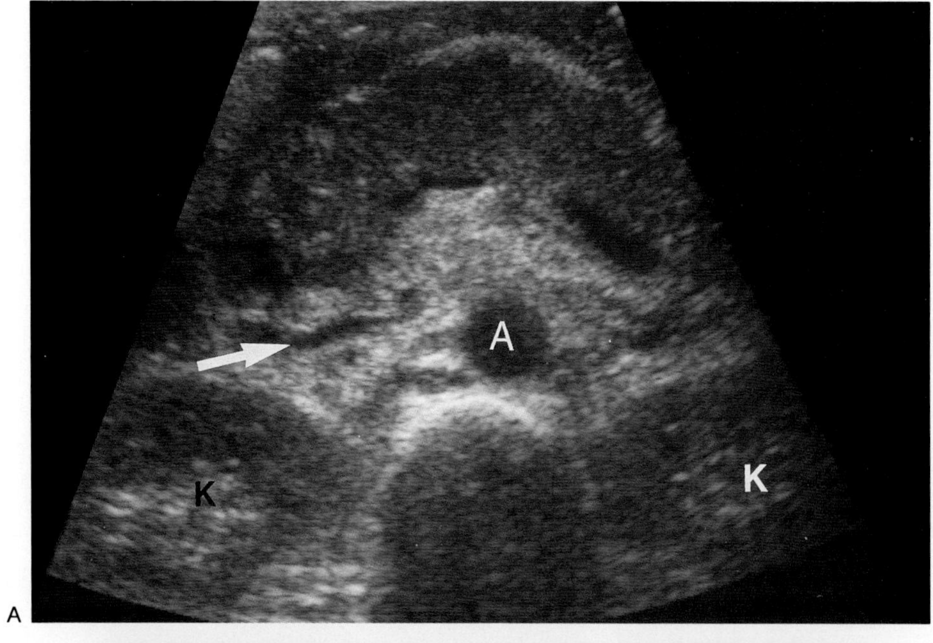

A

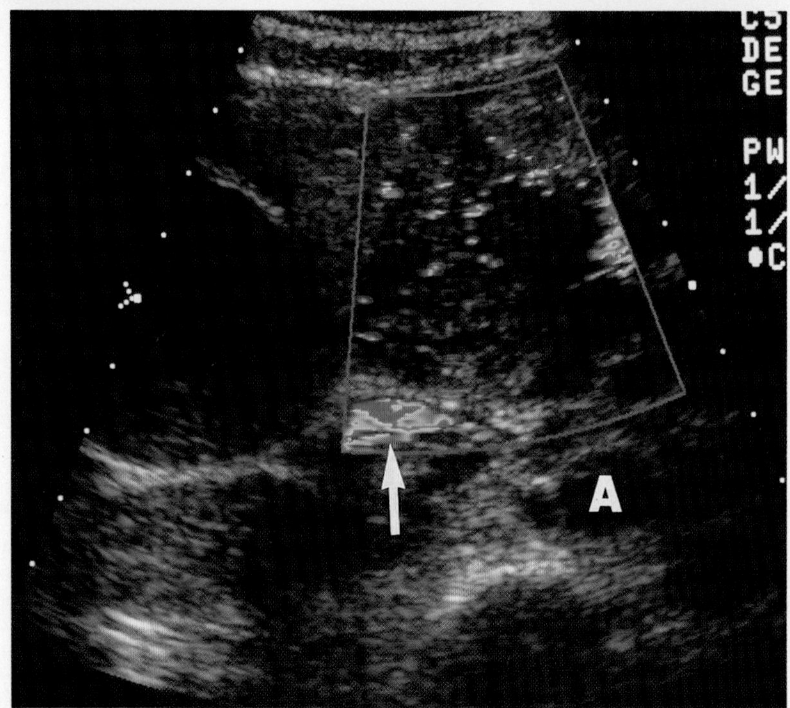

B

FIG. 4.33. Diffuse pancreatic carcinoma. **A:** Transverse sonogram reveals diffuse enlargement and hypoechoic abnormality of the body and tail of the pancreas. Diffuse carcinoma of the pancreas is unusual, comprising only 5 percent of all ductal adenocarcinomas. Ductal adenocarcinoma arises in the pancreatic head in 60 percent of cases. **B:** A color Doppler sonogram of the hypoechoic pancreatic head reveals another unusual feature of this particular tumor, where increased internal color flow is demonstrated. Most pancreatic ductal adenocarcinomas exhibit no internal flow on color Doppler imaging. A, aorta; *arrow,* inferior vena cava; K, kidneys.

Sonographically, pancreatic carcinoma is typically a hypoechoic mass that deforms the gland's morphology (Figs. 4.34 and 4.35). Occasionally, pancreatic carcinoma is echogenic (40,41) (Figs. 4.32 and 4.36). Masses with increased echogenicity are common in chronic pancreatitis (more than 50 percent) and unusual in carcinoma. Calcification, though unusual in typical histology ductal adenocarcinoma, occurs in a few percent of tumors, usually as a few scattered calcifications (Fig. 4.37). Cystic areas occasionally occur in typical histology carcinomas (Fig. 4.38). Cystic areas also occur in masses caused by variants of ductal adenocarcinoma, cystic pancreatic neoplasms, and chronic pancreatitis. Secondary findings of carcinoma include ductal dilatation (biliary and pancreatic) (Fig. 4.39), vascular and extraglandular invasion, and metastatic disease. Pseudocysts, related to obstruction of a pancreatic duct, have been reported in as many as 11 percent of patients (Figs. 4.35 and 4.40) (42), although in our experience carcinoma-related pseudocysts are less frequent.

Some investigators have reported that sonography is sufficiently sensitive and efficacious in staging pancreatic carcinoma that other tests are rarely needed (35). Our experience favors the use of CT to determine resectability. The following findings suggest unresectability: tumor larger than 2 cm, extracapsular extension, vascular invasion (venous or arterial), lymphadenopathy, or metastatic disease. Color flow sonography can be useful in identifying vascular invasion, encasement, or contiguity (Figs. 4.41 to 4.43). It has largely replaced angiography for that purpose in our practice. Image findings of unresectability are reliable; only rarely can such a tumor be resected at the time of surgery. Conversely, many tumors believed resectable because of their image appearance on CT scans or sonograms cannot be resected for cure at surgery. Furthermore, the 5-year survival of patients undergoing attempted curative resection is only 5 to 8 percent. Despite these discouraging facts, surgery represents the only real, albeit small, hope for cure (43).

Masses Associated with Chronic Pancreatitis

Focal pancreatic enlargement occurs in approximately 30 percent of patients with chronic pancreatitis (18). Carcinoma and masses secondary to pancreatitis can usually be differentiated clinically. In addition, the presence of calcification within a mass makes the diagnosis of pancreatitis much more likely (18,35) (Figs. 4.14, 4.15, and 4.18). Although calcification may also be noted in some carcinomas (Fig. 4.37), hyperechoic masses, even without discrete calcifications, are usually related to chronic pancreatitis (Fig. 4.19). An uncalcified iso- or hypoechoic mass is nonspecific. In this instance, biopsy or endoscopic retrograde cholangiopancreatography (ERCP) is indicated to differentiate carcinoma from chronic pancreatitis. Carcinoma and pancreatitis may both cause obstruction of the pancreatic duct or extrahepatic bile duct. Obstruction of both ducts, the "double duct sign," is nonspecific, occurring in both pancreatitis and pancreatic carcinoma (21). On occasion, adenopathy may also cause the double duct sign. Pseudocysts, while more frequent in pancreatitis, occur in both conditions.

Cystic Pancreatic Lesions

Cystic pancreatic tumors are relatively uncommon, comprising fewer than 15 percent of pancreatic cystic lesions and only a few percent of pancreatic tumors (44). Cystic pancreatic neoplasms include serous (microcystic) cystic neoplasms (Figs. 4.44 and 4.45) and mucinous (macrocystic) cystic neoplasms (Figs. 4.46 to 4.49). Serous cystic neoplasms are almost universally benign, although a malignant variant has been reported (45). This may be important; when typical image findings are present, asymptomatic or poor risk patients need not undergo surgery. Serous cystic neoplasm (microcystic adenoma) is slightly more common in females and tends to occur in older individuals.

Morphologically, serous microcystic neoplasms comprise many tiny cysts, most smaller than 2 cm. Occasionally, a few larger cysts are present. The most distinctive, although one not always present, is a central stellate fibrotic scar that frequently calcifies (about one-half of tumors) (Fig. 4.44). Sonographically, microcystic adenomas have a somewhat variable appearance. In regions where there are many tiny cysts, increased echogenicity from the myriad cyst walls is noted (Figs. 4.44 and 4.45). Through transmission is frequent. When larger cysts predominate, hypoechoic regions are often imaged (Fig. 4.45). The central stellate scar and calcification may be identified, suggesting the diagnosis. Calcifications are imaged more often with CT than sonography (Fig. 4.45). The lesion's suggestive morphology is also demonstrated by CT. The tiny cysts are imaged less well with CT than sonography, although CT is often better in showing the central scar and calcification.

Mucinous cystic neoplasms consist of large cysts that are usually easily imaged with CT or sonography (Figs. 4.46 and 4.49). Most tumors are located in the tail or body of the pancreas and are much more common in females, approaching 10:1 predominance. Because differentiation between benign and malignant mucinous cystic neoplasms is often impossible even pathologically, all tumors are considered malignant and surgical removal is indicated. Calcifications occur in approximately 20 percent of these neoplasms (compared to about one-half of serous/microcystic neoplasms).

Sonography usually reveals a mass with internal cysts of variable size (Fig. 4.47). Unilocular lesions may occur (Fig. 4.49). The septations may be few or many, quite thin or thick, and polypoid. The internal architecture is

(text continues on page 267)

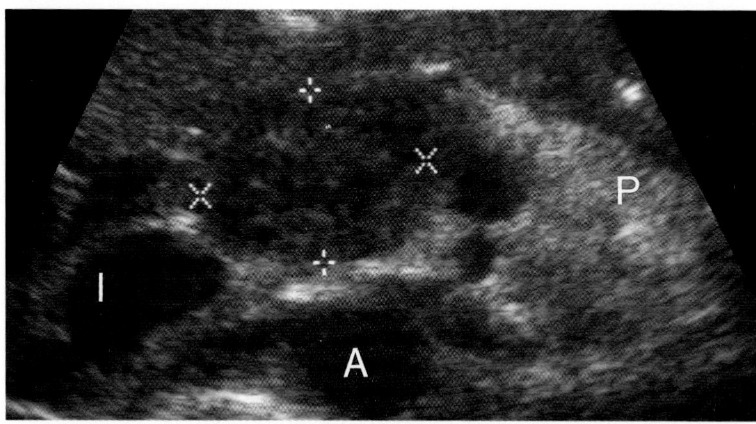

FIG. 4.34. Ductal adenocarcinoma of the pancreatic head. This transverse sonogram shows a typical predominantly hypoechoic, slightly heterogeneous pancreatic head carcinoma. Note that the echogenicity is significantly less than that of the normal distal pancreas (P). A, aorta; I, inferior vena cava.

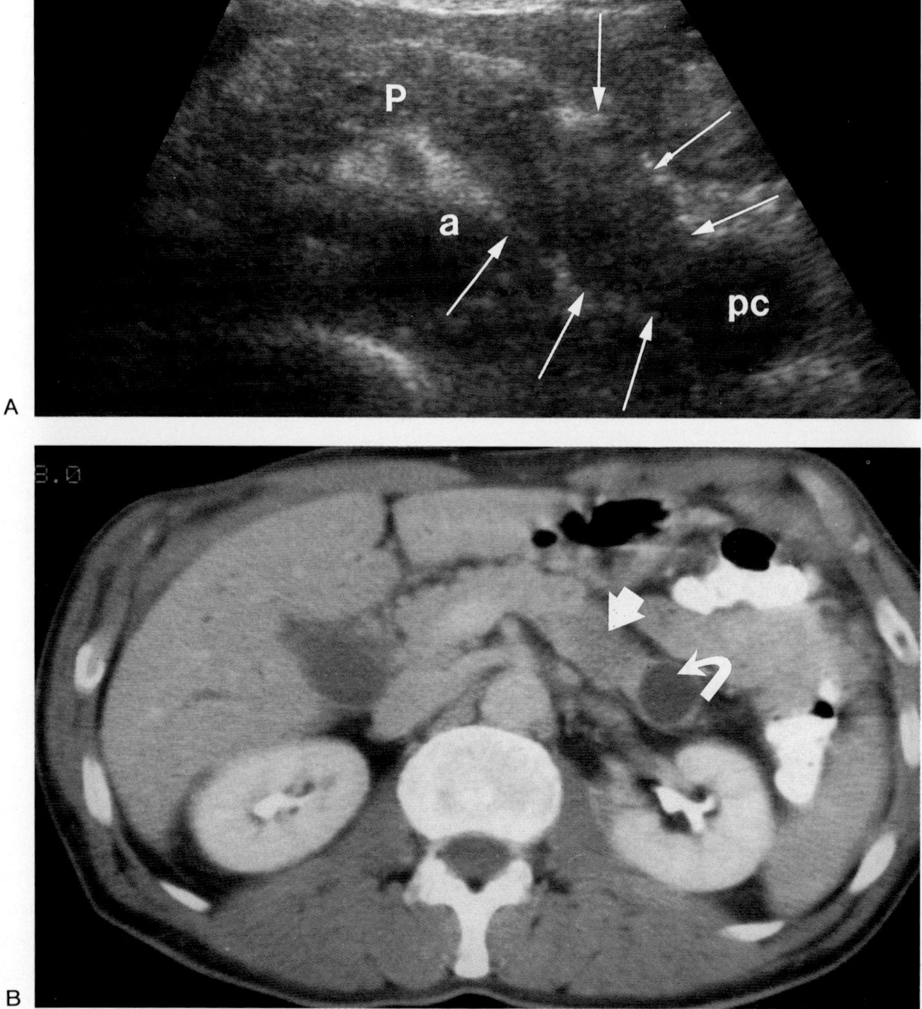

FIG. 4.35. Subtle pancreatic carcinoma causing pseudocyst. **A:** The transverse sonogram reveals subtle enlargement of the tail of the pancreas (*thin arrows*). Note that the pancreatic mass is mildly hypoechoic compared to the more normal pancreas (P). A distal obstructive pseudocyst (pc) is present. a, aorta. **B:** The CT scan reveals similar subtle findings with mild decreased attenuation (*arrow*), representing the pancreatic carcinoma. No morphologic enlargement of the pancreas is noted on the CT scan. A pseudocyst (*curved arrow*), presumably related to duct obstruction, is noted. Although pancreatic carcinoma-related obstructive pseudocysts are reported in as many as 11 percent of cases, our experience suggests a lower prevalence.

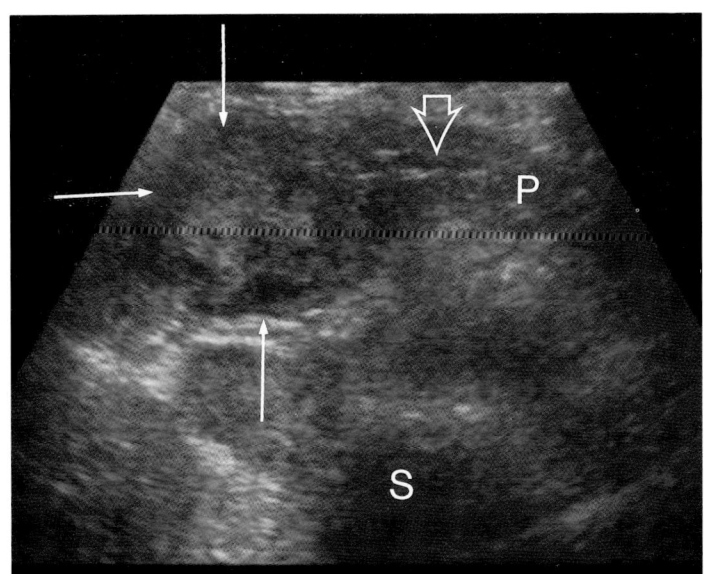

FIG. 4.36. Echogenic pancreatic ductal adenocarcinoma. This transverse sonogram reveals pancreatic carcinoma (*thin arrows*) that is predominantly of higher echogenicity than the normal pancreas (P). Note the dilated pancreatic duct in this patient (*open arrow*). S, spine.

A

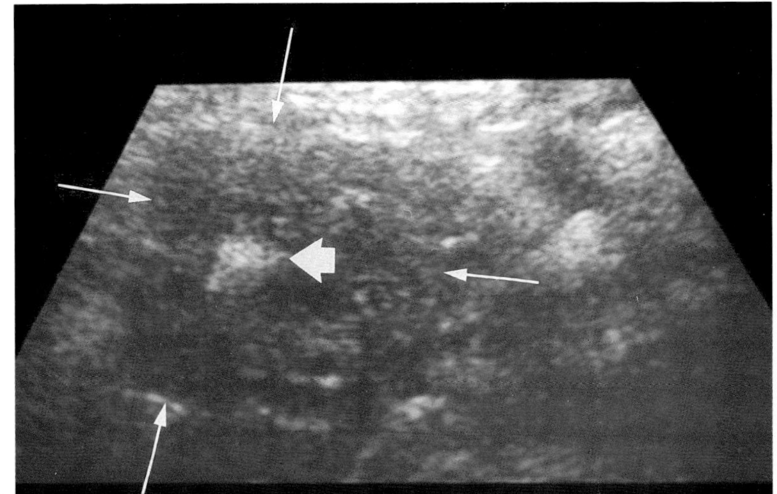

B

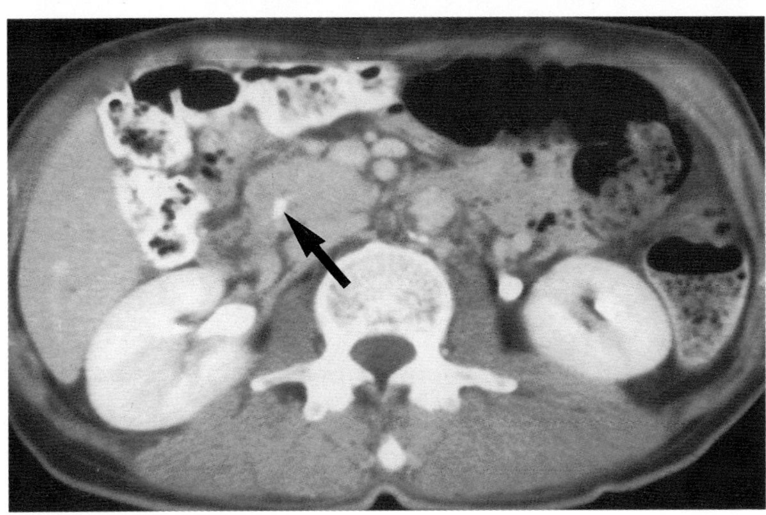

FIG. 4.37. Pancreatic ductal adenocarcinoma, focal calcification. The transverse sonogram (**A**) and CT scan (**B**) reveal a discrete calcification (*arrow*) within this pancreatic ductal adenocarcinoma (*thin arrows*). Previously considered a virtually definitive sign of chronic pancreatitis, calcifications within a pancreatic ductal adenocarcinoma are actually not unusual. Compare this with Fig. 4.15.

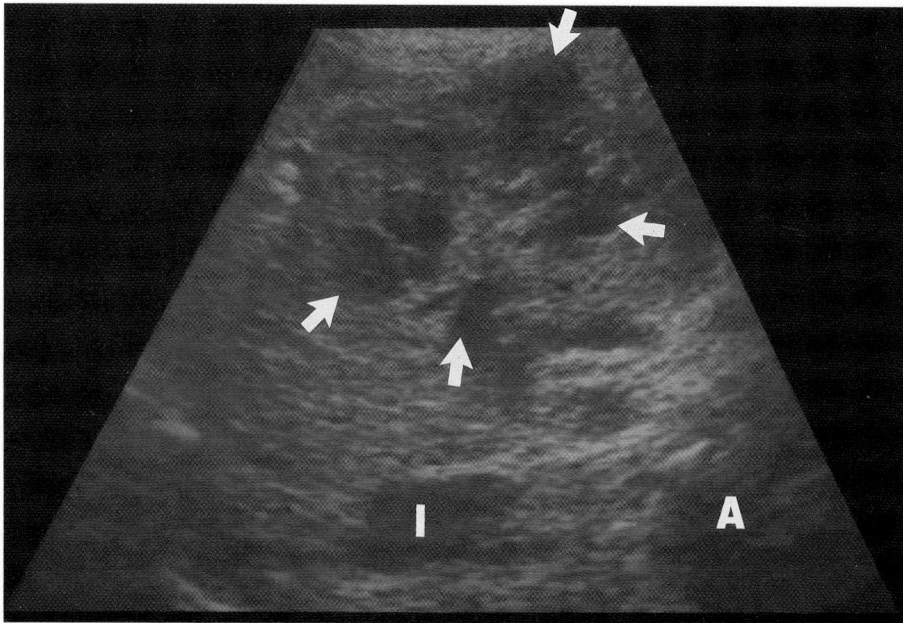

FIG. 4.38. Pancreatic ductal adenocarcinoma with internal cystic areas. Small cystic structures (presumed to represent ducts) within a pancreatic mass have been proposed as a sign of chronic pancreatitis, rather than pancreatic carcinoma. Unfortunately, cystic change, as demonstrated in this case (*arrows*), is not rare in typical histology ductal adenocarcinoma, or in variants of carcinoma. Compare with Figs. 4.14 and 4.59. A, aorta; I, inferior vena cava.

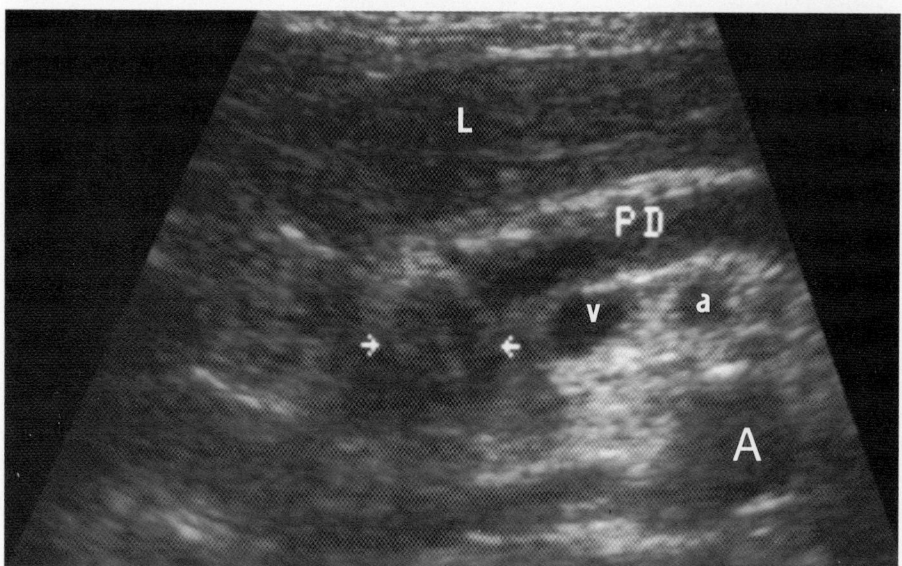

FIG. 4.39. Small pancreatic ductal adenocarcinoma, dilated pancreatic duct. This transverse sonogram reveals a small 1.5-cm hypoechoic pancreatic carcinoma (*arrows*) that obstructs the pancreatic duct (PD). Pancreatic ductal adenocarcinoma may obstruct both the pancreatic and common bile ducts (double duct sign), or either the pancreatic or common bile duct in isolation. A, aorta; v, superior mesenteric vein; a, superior mesenteric artery; L, liver.

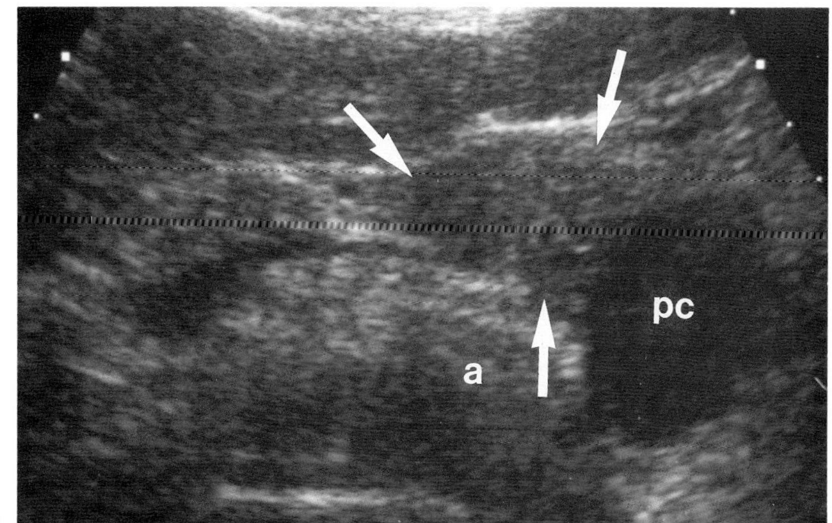

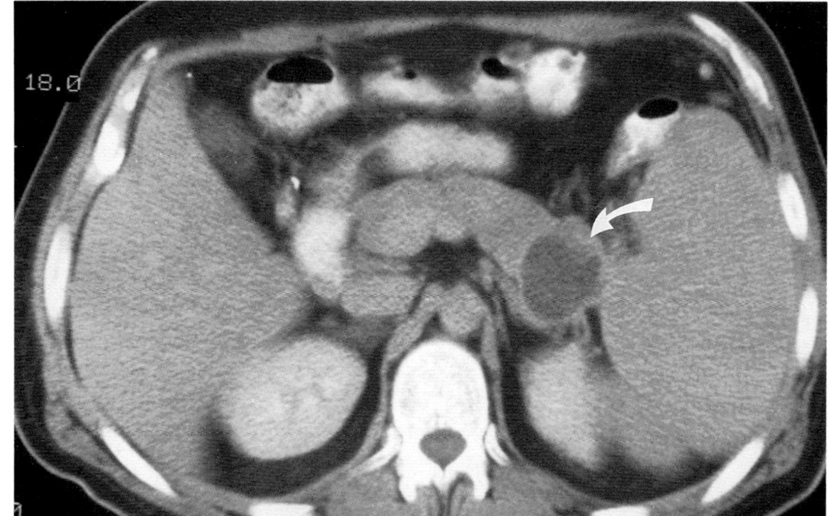

FIG. 4.40. Postobstructive pseudocyst from ductal adenocarcinoma. The transverse sonogram (**A**) and CT scan (**B**) reveal a pseudocyst in the tail of the pancreas (PC). The hypoechoic mass that represents the pancreatic carcinoma (*arrows*) is much less well seen on the CT scan than on the sonogram in this instance. A small mass in the wall of the pseudocyst is shown on the CT scan (*curved arrow*) but not on the sonogram. Peripheral splenic vein thrombosis and isolated gastric varices were present in this individual, but not demonstrated by either color Doppler sonography or CT. a, aorta.

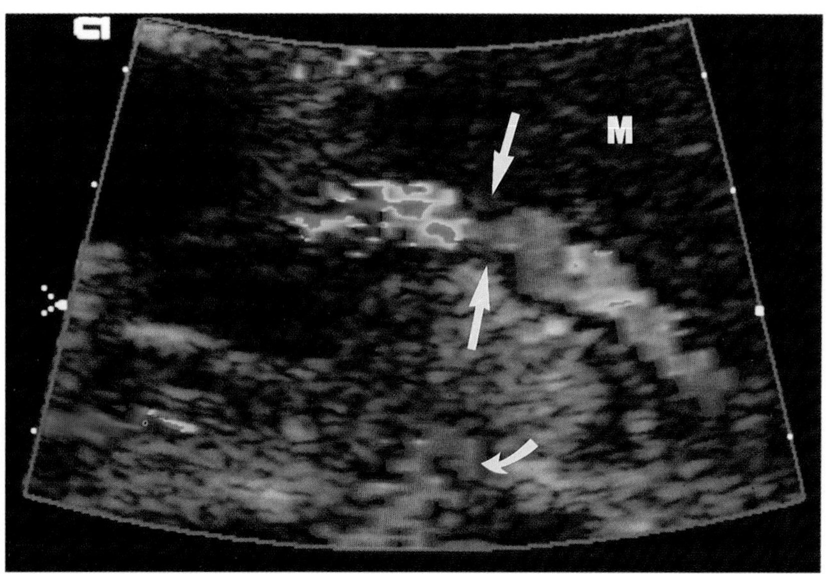

FIG. 4.41. Unresectable carcinoma, encasement of splenic vein. Transverse color Doppler sonogram of the splenic vein reveals encasement (*arrows*) by the hypoechoic tumor mass (M), a sign of unresectability. Venous encasement and invasion are more frequent causes of unresectability than arterial encasement. *Curved arrow*, superior mesenteric artery.

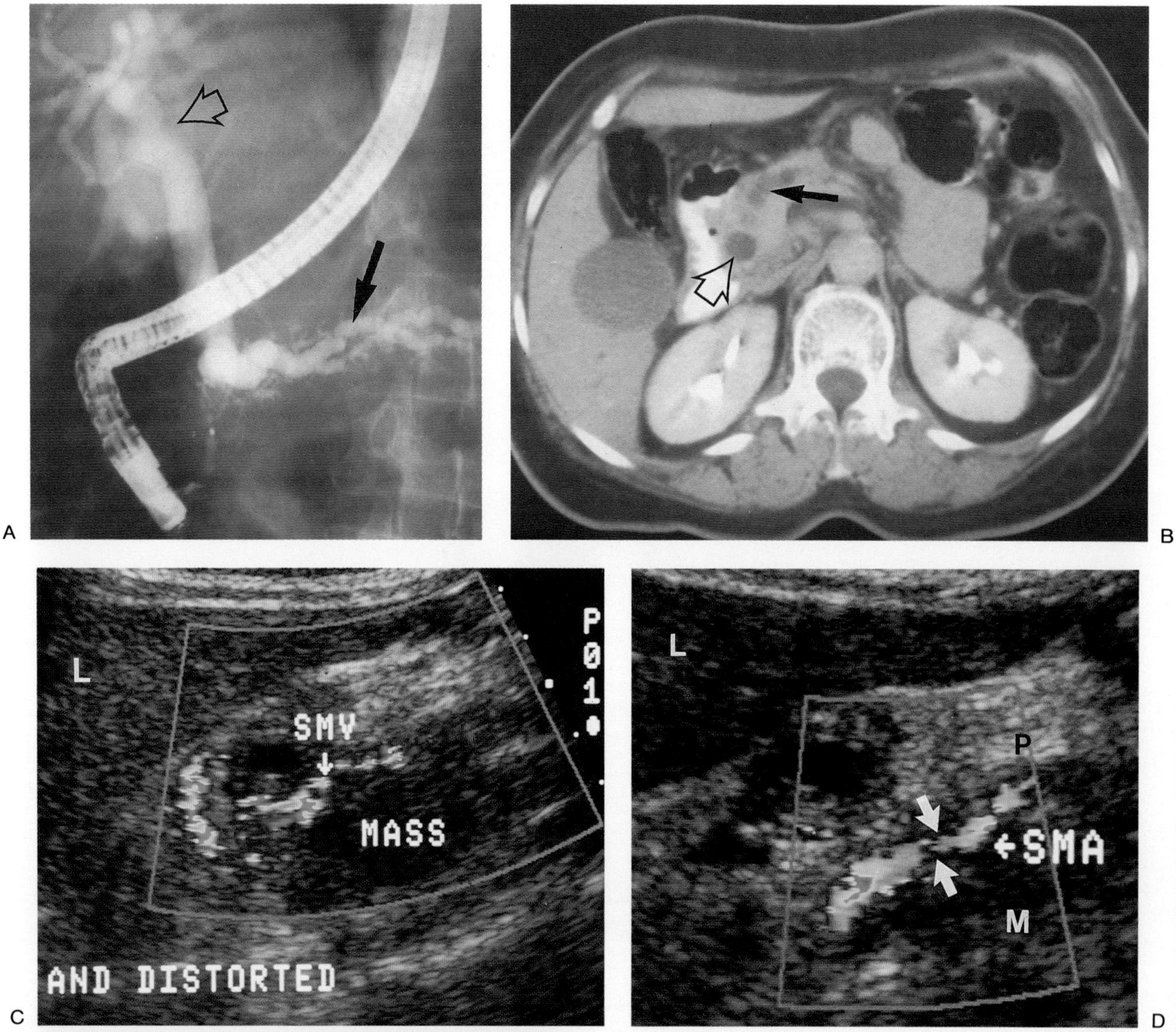

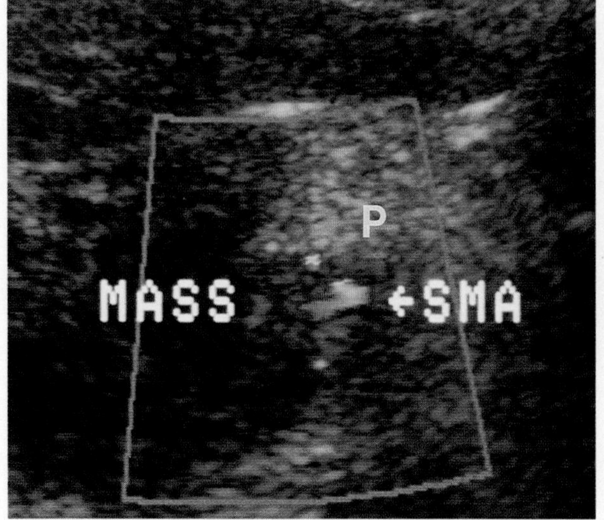

FIG. 4.42. Unresectable pancreatic carcinoma. An ERCP (**A**) and CT scan (**B**) reveal a double duct sign, dilatation of both the pancreatic duct (*arrow*) and common bile duct (*open arrow*). The results of color Doppler sonography suggested that this tumor was not resectable. A longitudinal color Doppler sonogram (**C**) reveals encasement of the superior mesenteric vein (SMV) by the mass. The superior mesenteric artery, as shown on longitudinal (**D**) and transverse (**E**) sonograms, is displaced and encased by tumor (*arrows*). Color Doppler sonography has largely replaced angiographic techniques as a means of detecting vascular abnormality and assessing resectability in our lab. L, liver; P, pancreas; M, mass.

A

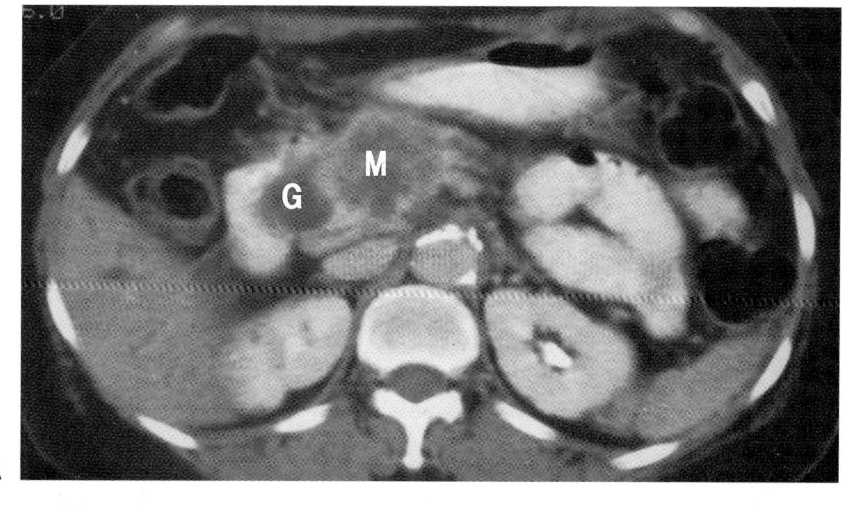

B

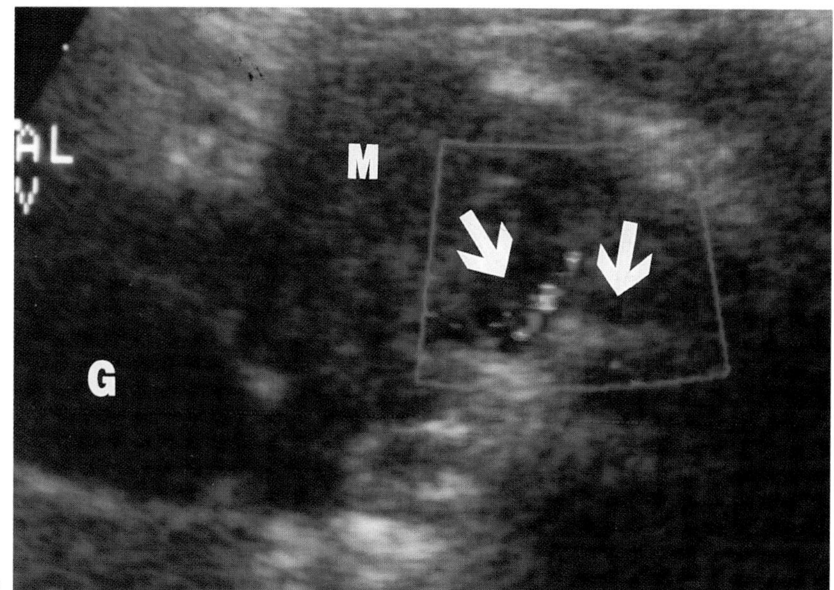

C

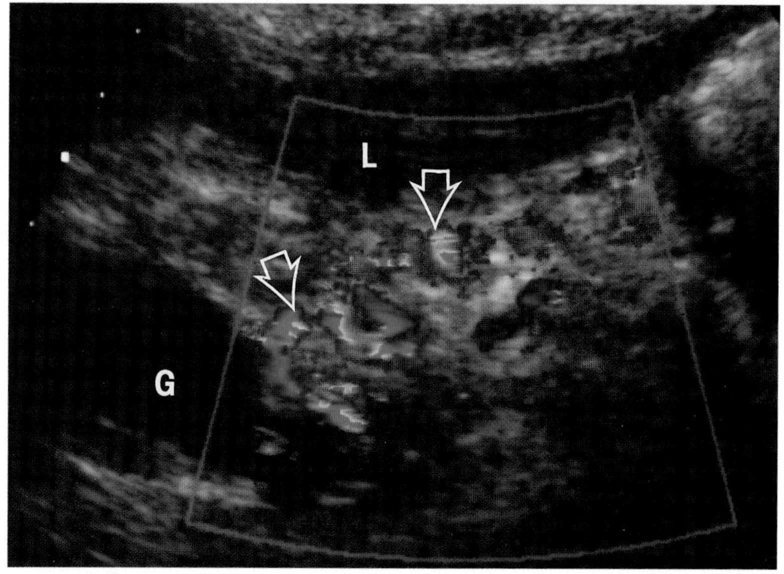

FIG. 4.43. Portal collaterals, splenic vein occlusion by pancreatic carcinoma. **A:** CT scan reveals a moderate sized pancreatic mass (M) related to pancreatic carcinoma. **B:** A transverse color Doppler sonogram reveals that the mass invades and occludes the splenic vein (*arrows*). This led to gastric varices and suprapancreatic coronary vein collaterals that convey portal flow to the liver (hepatopetal flow). **C:** A transverse color Doppler sonogram just above the level of the pancreas reveals these hepatopetal coronary vein collaterals (*open arrows*). Splenic vein thrombosis almost always causes gastric varices and hepatopetal coronary vein collaterals. In this patient, color flow sonography confirms splenic vein involvement, a sign of unresectability. Also noted are collaterals (C) associated with the splenic vein occlusion. L, liver; G, gallbladder.

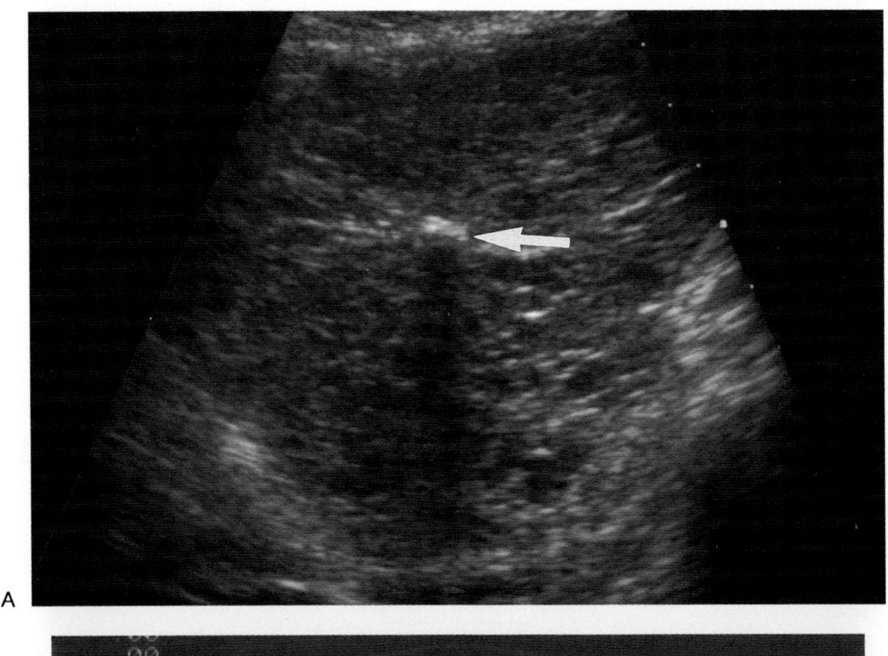

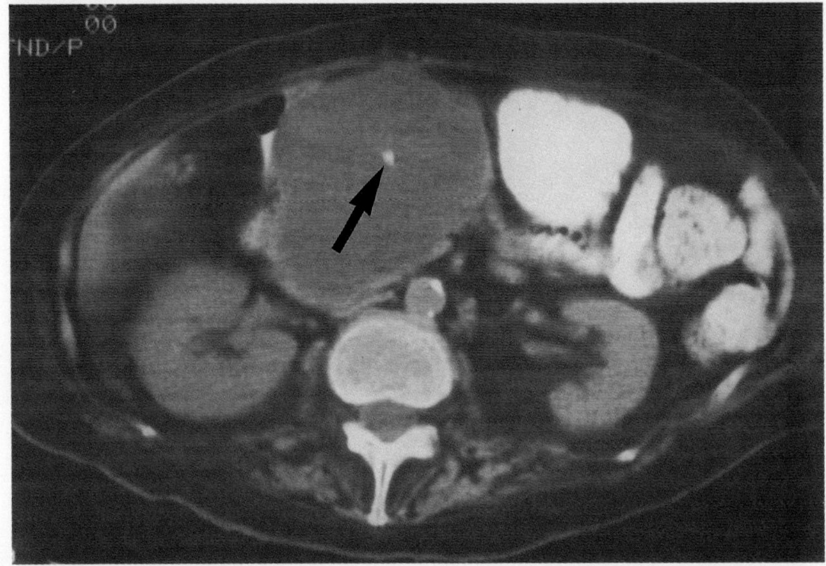

FIG. 4.44. Serous cystic neoplasm (microcystic adenoma). **A:** Transverse sonogram of the pancreatic head reveals multiple small cysts and echogenic areas. These echogenic areas are microcysts too small to be resolved individually. A central shadowing calcification (*arrow*) is noted in the central stellate scar that often characterizes these masses. **B:** The CT scan reveals the central calcification (*arrow*), but the internal architecture is less well delineated. Sonography shows the internal architecture of predominantly cystic masses to better advantage than does CT.

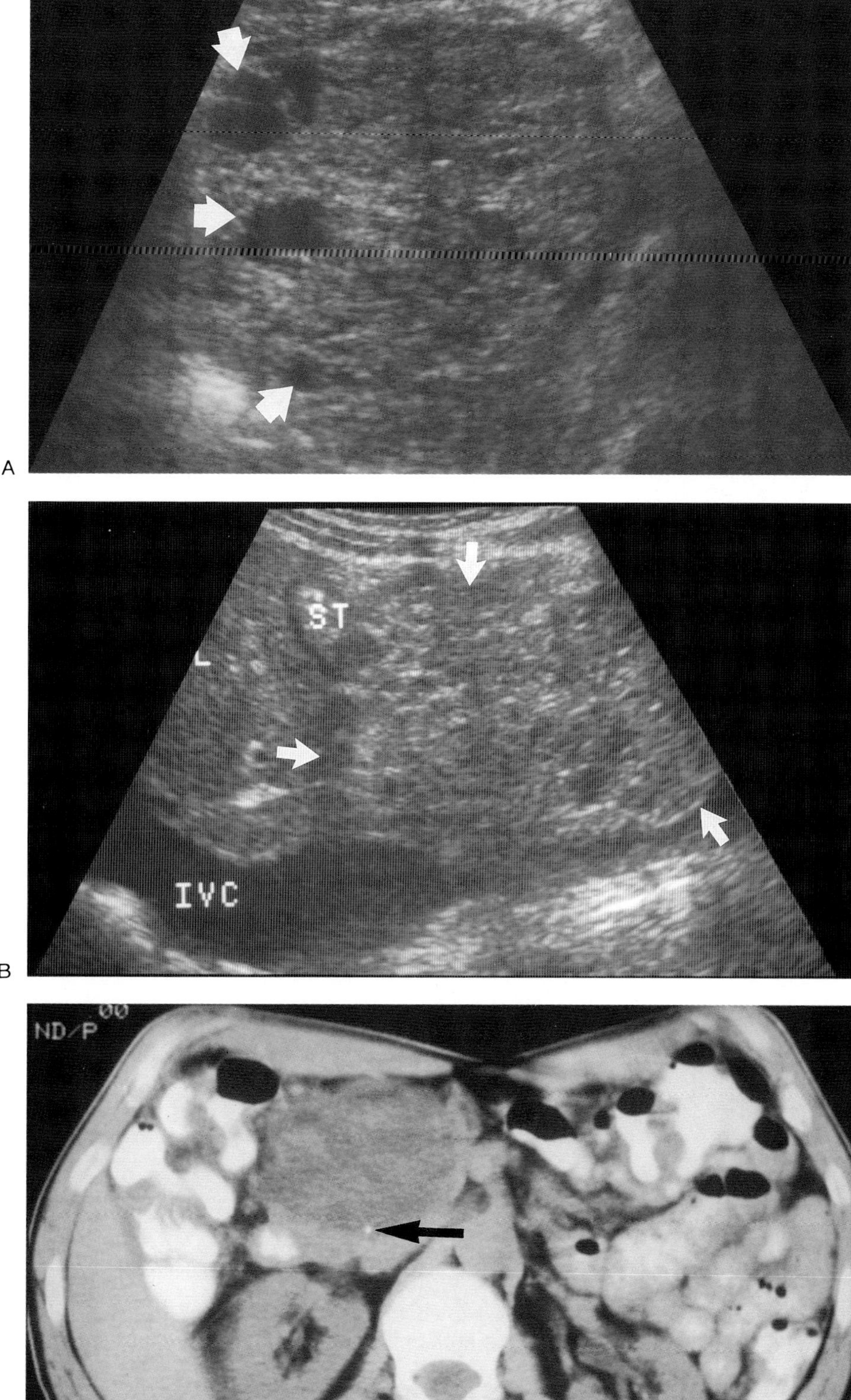

FIG. 4.45. Serous cystic neoplasm (microcystic adenoma). **A:** The transverse sonogram of the pancreatic head reveals a larger cystic area (*arrows*) and echogenic areas that represent microcysts too small to be resolved sonographically. **B:** The longitudinal sonogram reveals the relationship of this pancreatic head neoplasm (*arrows*) to the inferior vena cava (IVC), the liver (L), and the stomach (ST). **C:** The CT scan reveals a small calcification in the dorsal aspect of the neoplasm (*arrow*) but does not show the internal architecture as well as the sonographic images. No stellate scar is identified in this lesion. Serous cystic neoplasm is an almost universally benign tumor.

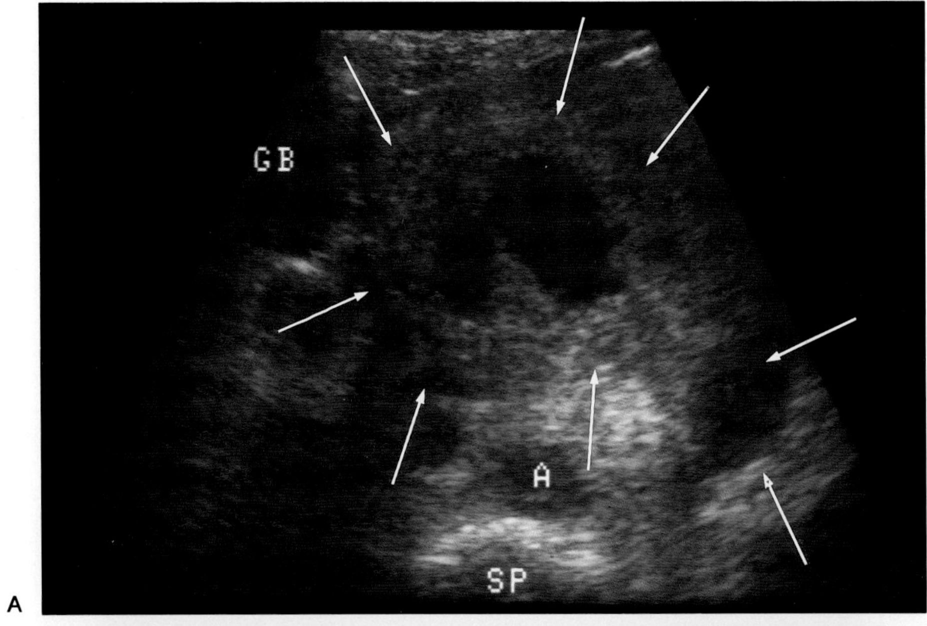

A

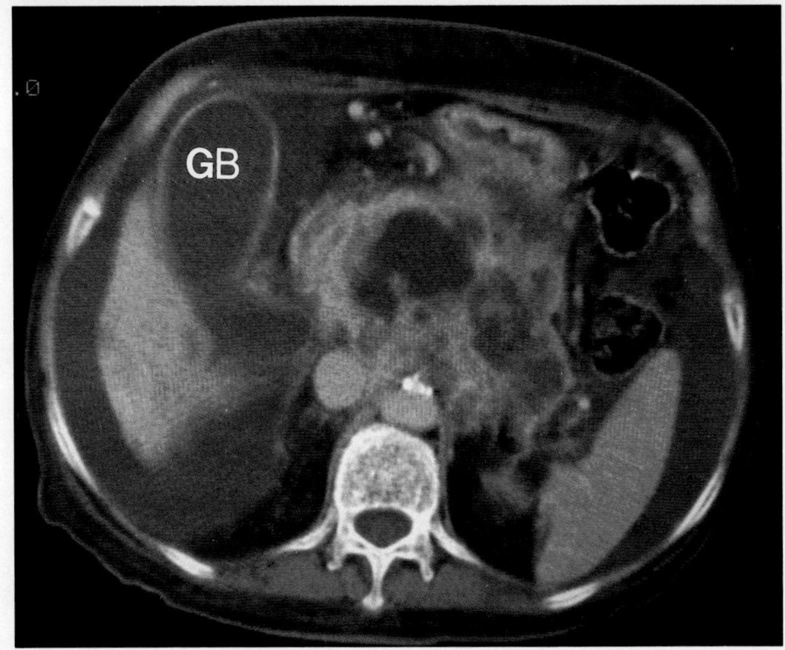

B

FIG. 4.46. Malignant mucinous cystic neoplasm. **A:** The transverse sonogram shows the multiloculated predominantly cystic neoplasm (*arrows*) within the pancreas. **B:** The CT scan reveals the extrapancreatic involvement more clearly than the sonogram. Ascites, caused by carcinomatosis, was present at the time of clinical presentation. Unless secondary signs of advanced malignancy are present, as in this patient, it may be impossible to differentiate benign from malignant mucinous cystic neoplasms. The image appearance of the primary lesion alone is nonspecific. GB, gallbladder; A, aorta; SP, spine.

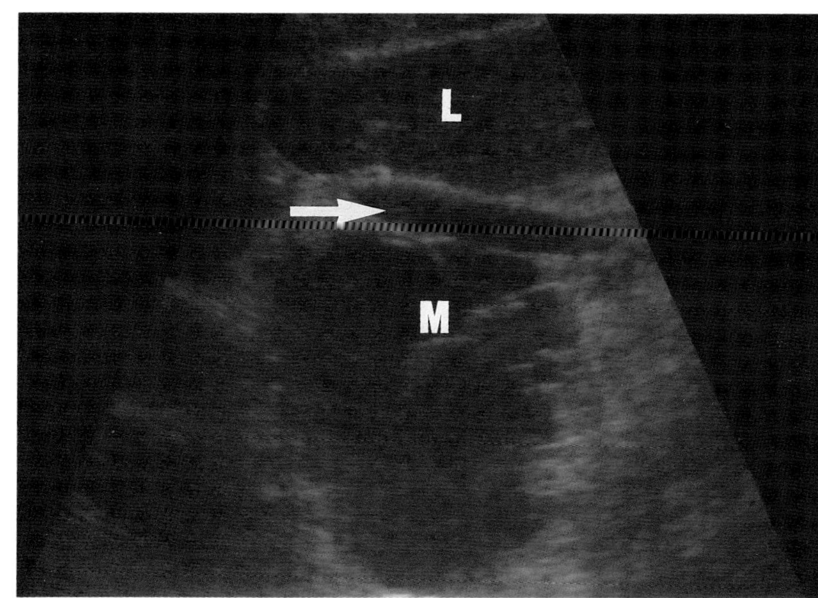

FIG. 4.47. Mucinous cystic neoplasm, benign. The transverse sonogram reveals a multiseptate predominantly cystic neoplasm (M, mass) involving the head of the pancreas. L, liver; *arrow,* common hepatic artery.

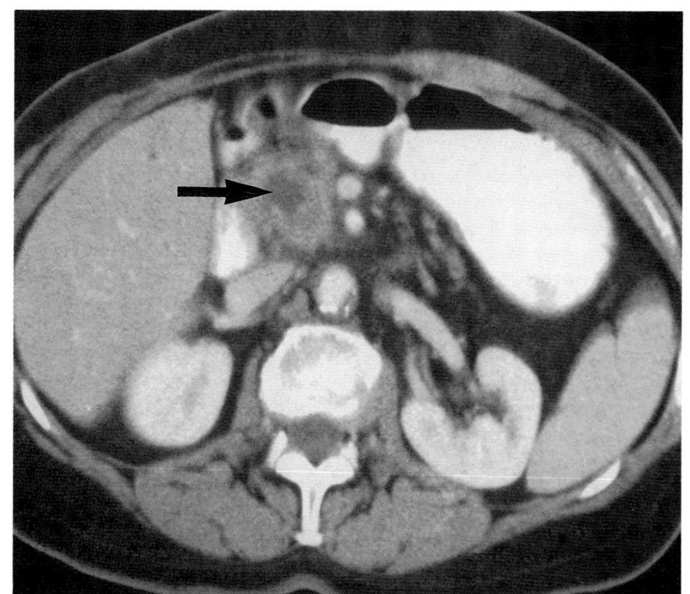

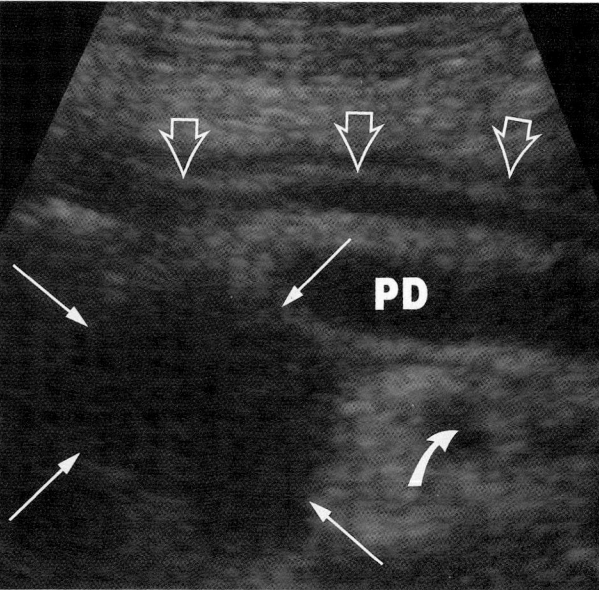

FIG. 4.48. Mucinous cystic adenocarcinoma. It is difficult to distinguish this mucinous cystic neoplasm from a necrotic pancreatic ductal adenocarcinoma. The low-attenuation area (*arrow*) seen on the CT scan (**A**) in this mucinous cystic tumor can also be present in ductal adenocarcinoma. The transverse sonogram (**B**) reveals pancreatic ductal (PD) dilatation. The mass itself is featureless and hypoechoic (*thin arrows*), making the correct diagnosis problematic. *Open arrows,* stomach; *curved arrow,* superior mesenteric artery.

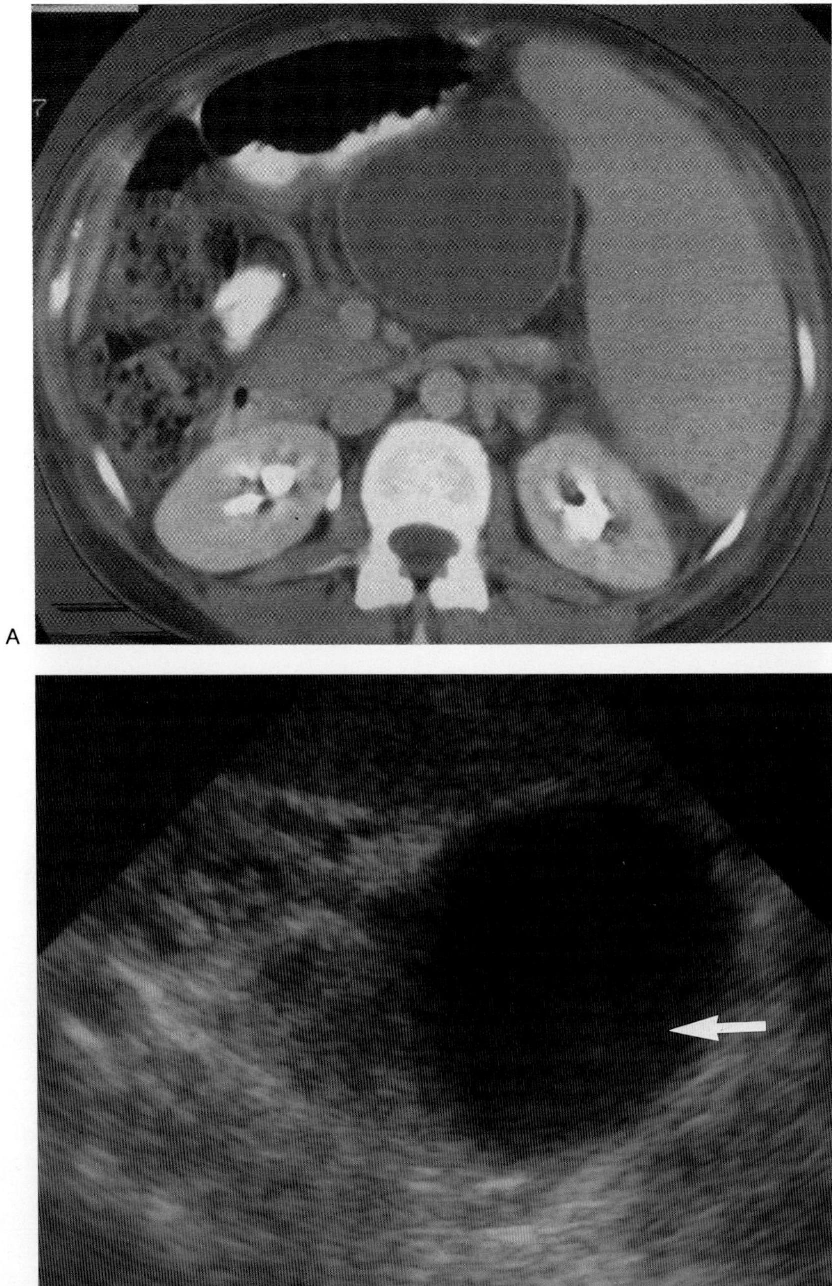

FIG. 4.49. Mucinous cystic adenocarcinoma. CT scan (**A**) and transverse sonogram (**B**) in the region of the body and tail of the pancreas. It may be impossible to distinguish a pseudocyst from a unilocular mucinous cystic neoplasm. This patient had a questionable history of pancreatitis. The large cystic mass was featureless on the CT scan and contained only some debris (*arrow*) on the sonogram. Splenic vein occlusion was present and isolated gastric varices were noted on endoscopy. It is treacherous to diagnose a cystic pancreatic mass as a pseudocyst in the absence of a firm history of pancreatitis. In such instances, mucinous cystic neoplasm should be considered a possibility.

often shown to better advantage by sonography than CT. CT findings are similar, except that the low attenuation masses are more internally featureless and calcification is more frequently identified (46–48). These lesions may be confused with rarer cystic neoplasms such as papillary cystic tumor, cystic islet cell tumor, lymphangioma (Fig. 4.50) and cystic metastases, or non-neoplastic lesions such as pseudocyst, abscess, and echinococcal disease (48). Simple cysts of the pancreas are rare. They may occur in association with von Hippel–Lindau disease (Figs. 4.51 and 4.52) and, rarely, in renal polycystic disease (Fig. 4.53).

Endocrine Tumors

Endocrine tumors are a small but important group of pancreatic neoplasms that generally originate in pancreatic islet cells. Insulinomas and gastrinomas are the commonest endocrine tumors. Other tumors are glucagonoma, somatostatinoma, VIPoma, carcinoid tumors, pheochromocytoma, and combined histology tumors. These tumors tend to be small and, with the exception of insulinoma, malignant. It is difficult to image islet cell tumors; they are usually small when the patient presents with hormonal abnormalities. Insulinomas and gastrinomas are frequently less than 2 cm in diameter. Thin section dynamic incremental CECT or angiography sometimes reveals these lesions. Intraoperative sonography is useful in localizing occult neoplasms (49–52) (Figs. 4.54 and 4.55).

Sonographic detection rates for insulinomas ranging from 25 to 60 percent have been reported (50,53). The results for gastrinomas are worse; approximately 20 percent are detected (52). Sonographically, islet cell tumors are usually well defined and round or oval in shape. They generally appear hypoechoic compared to the normal parenchyma (Fig. 4.56). On occasion, the only detectable abnormality may be an alteration of the pancreatic contour. Increased echogenicity from calcification has been reported (49).

Metastasis to the Pancreas

In autopsy series, metastasis to the pancreas is the commonest pancreatic neoplasm (37,39) (Figs. 4.57 and 4.58). Primary tumors that commonly metastasize to the pancreas include breast, lung, melanoma, colon, and stomach. Pancreatic metastases are rarely detected clinically as they generally occur late, in patients with widespread metastasic disease.

Unusual and Rare Pancreatic Neoplasms

Many histologic variants of pancreatic ductal adenocarcinoma are indistinguishable on images from tumors with the usual histologic features. These include adenosquamous cell carcinoma, anaplastic carcinoma, and pleomorphic giant cell carcinoma. Acinar center cell carcinoma and pleomorphic giant cell carcinoma, although often indistinguishable from ductal adenocarcinoma, can be larger and exhibit central necrosis (54).

Lesions with more distinctive ultrasound patterns include mucinous ductectatic/mucin hypersecreting neoplasm (54–56) and solid and papillary epithelial neoplasm (54,57).

Ductectatic carcinoma and mucin hypersecreting carcinoma are variants of ductal adenocarcinoma. A premalignant form may exist (45). These lesions are characterized by cystically dilated mucin-filled pancreatic branch ducts, usually in the uncinate process and pancreatic head (Fig. 4.59). These dilated ducts are lined with abnormal mucin hypersecreting epithelium. Some feel that the benign and malignant lesions in this group represent the spectrum of a single process. Others feel that mucin hypersecreting and ductectatic carcinoma are distinct entities. Sonographically, ductectatic carcinomas show multiple sonolucent dilated ducts within the uncinate process. A discrete mass may not be evident. Mucin hypersecreting carcinoma usually has more extensive ductal dilatation.

Solid and papillary epithelial neoplasm is found most frequently in young females. It is a low-grade malignancy, often curable by resection. The tumor tends to be large and well encapsulated. Tumors can be mostly solid, mixed cystic and solid, or almost entirely cystic. Images reveal a well-defined, round or oval mass with thick irregular walls. Varying areas of echogenic mass and cystic areas are seen depending on the morphology of the individual tumor (Fig. 4.60). Hemorrhage and necrosis may be present.

Less common cystic neoplastic tumors include papillary cystic tumor, cystic islet cell tumors, and acinar cell cystadenocarcinoma. Sarcomas of the pancreas are prohibitively rare, accounting for less than 1 percent of all pancreatic neoplasms. No specific radiologic findings have been reported.

Pancreatic Infarction

Pancreatic infarction is rare and generally caused by iatrogenic vascular insult (Fig. 4.61).

REFERENCES

1. Singer MV, Gyr K, Sarles H. Revised classification of pancreatitis. *Gastroenterology* 1985;89:683–690.
2. Steer ML. Classification and pathogenesis of pancreatitis. *Surg Clin North Am* 1989;69(3):467–480.
3. Potts JR III. Acute pancreatitis. *Surg Clin North Am* 1988;68(2): 281–299.
4. Lee SP, Nicholls JF, Park HZ. Biliary sludge as a cause of acute pancreatitis. *N Engl J Med* 1992;326:589–593.
5. Balthazar EJ, Ranson JHC, Naidich DP, Caccavale R, Cooper

(*text continues on page 276*)

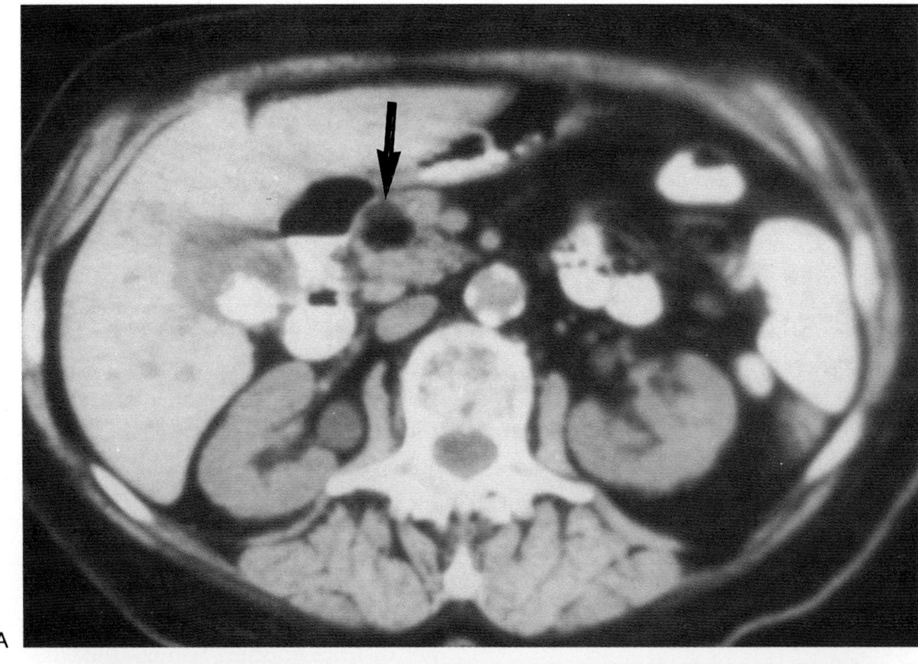

A

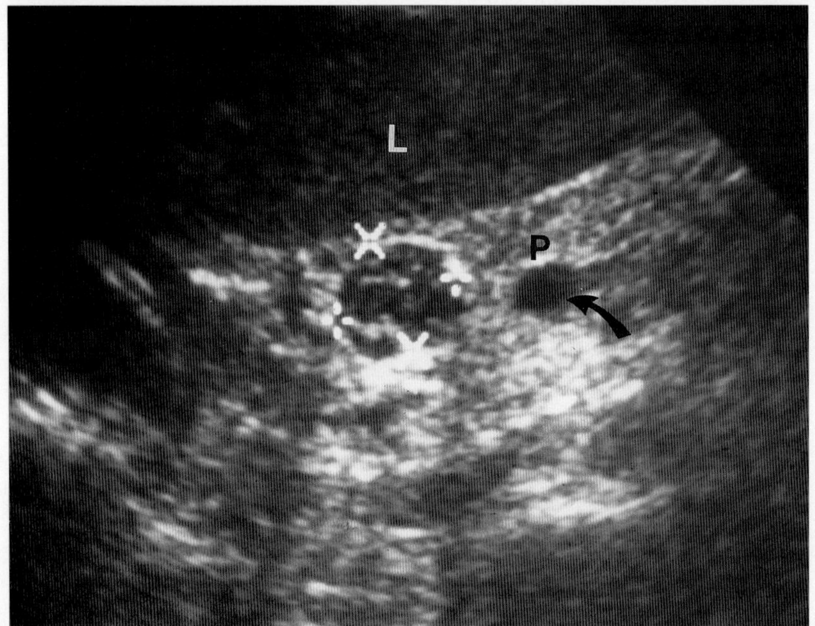

B

FIG. 4.50. Presumed cystic lymphangioma of the pancreas. This small mass (*arrow*) had Hounsfield numbers that were negative on the CT scan (**A**). The transverse pancreatic sonogram (**B**) revealed a predominantly cystic mass (calipers) with through transmission and few internal septations. The septations were poorly appreciated on the CT scan. Because of the negative CT numbers, this lesion was presumed to be a cystic lymphangioma, a rare benign pancreatic neoplasm. L, liver; P, pancreas; *curved arrow,* superior mesenteric vein. (Case courtesy of Dr. Edward Behnke.)

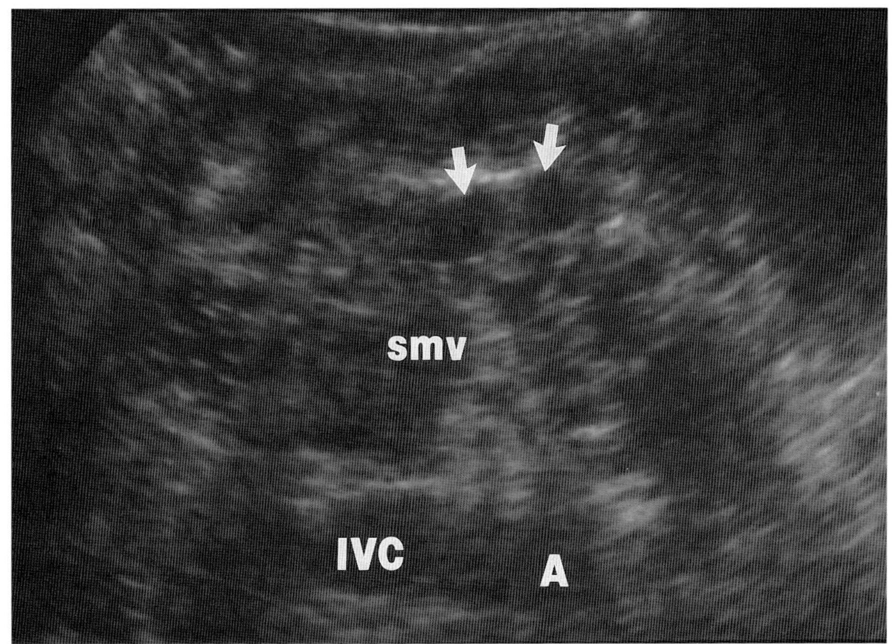

A

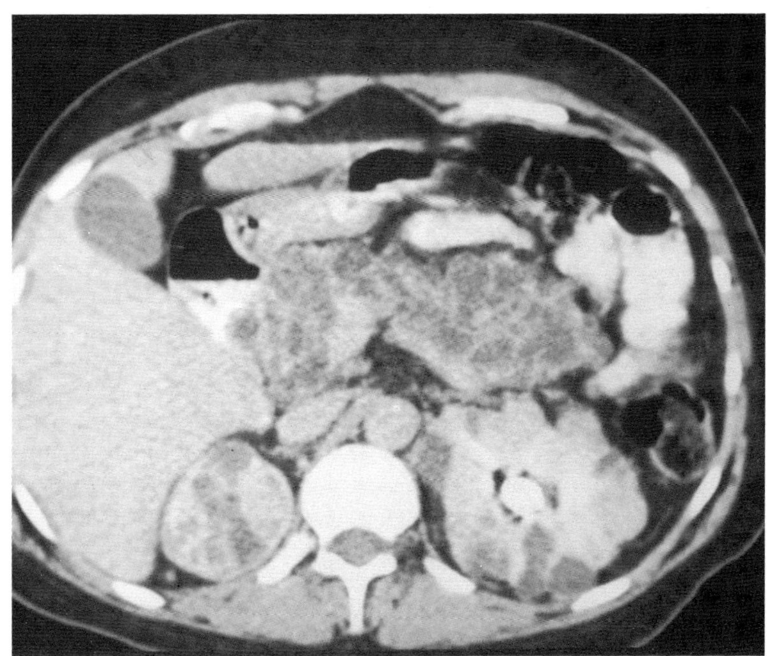

B

FIG. 4.51. Multiple pancreatic cysts, von Hippel–Lindau disease. The pancreas is virtually replaced by multiple pancreatic cysts in this patient with von Hippel–Lindau disease. **A:** The ultrasound reveals several larger cysts (*arrows*) and increased pancreatic echogenicity representing smaller cysts. **B:** The CT scan reveals lower attenuation throughout the gland, indicating cystic replacement of the pancreas. Multiple renal cysts are present as well. A, aorta; IVC, inferior vena cava; smv, superior mesenteric vein.

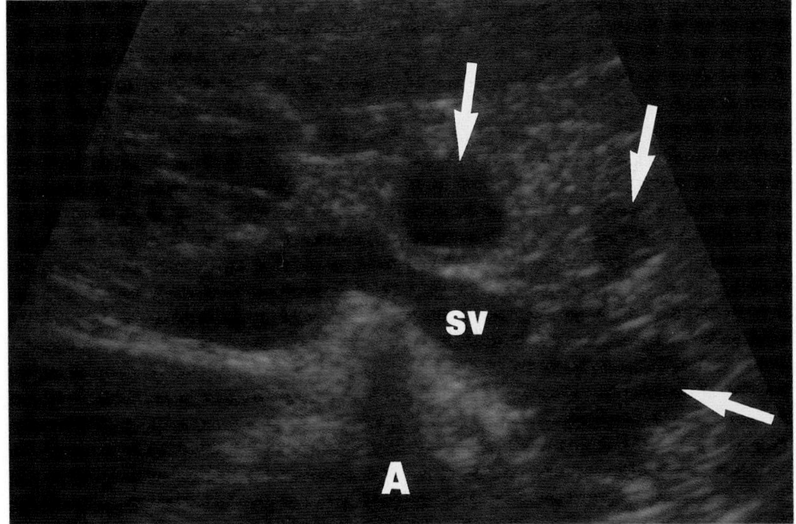

FIG. 4.52. Von Hippel–Lindau disease, pancreatic cysts. This transverse sonogram reveals several pancreatic cysts (*arrows*). Pancreatic cysts related to renal polycystic disease, supposedly common, are rare in our experience. Pancreatic cysts should suggest the diagnosis of von Hippel–Lindau disease, rather than polycystic disease. A, aorta; L, liver; SV, splenic vein.

A

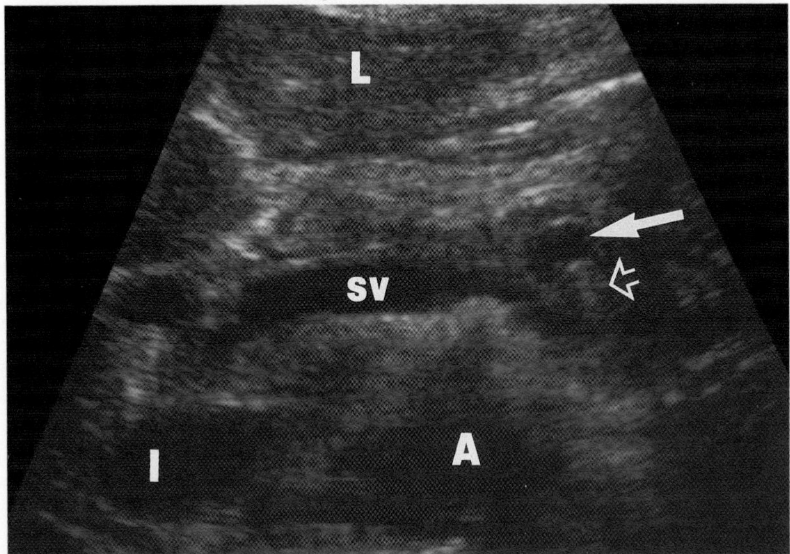

B

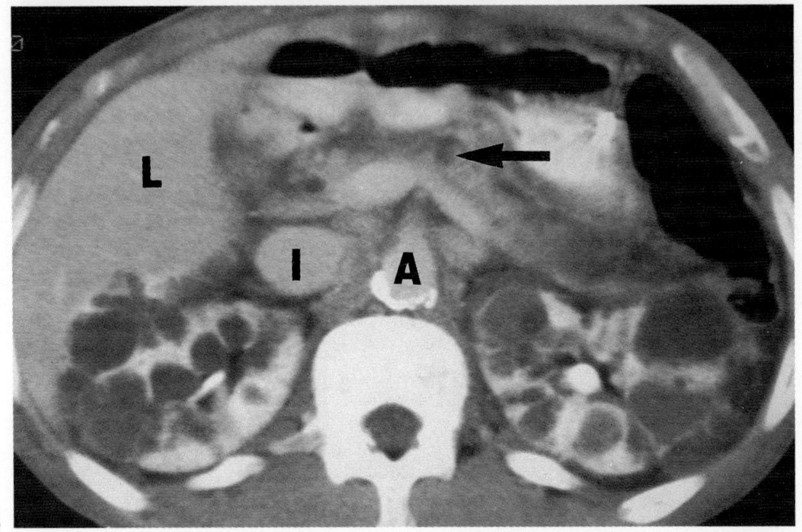

FIG. 4.53. Small pancreatic cyst, renal polycystic disease. **A:** Transverse sonogram through the body of the pancreas. **B:** CT scan at the same level. Multiple renal cysts are noted in both kidneys on the CT scan in this patient with renal polycystic disease. A single, small pancreatic cyst (*arrow*) is noted. Note the through transmission deep to the cyst on sonography (*open arrow*). L, liver; SV, splenic vein; A, aorta; I, inferior vena cava. This is the only imageable pancreatic cyst we have ever detected in a patient with renal polycystic disease. Despite a reported prevalence of 5 to 10 percent, imageable pancreatic cysts are, in fact, very rare in polycystic disease.

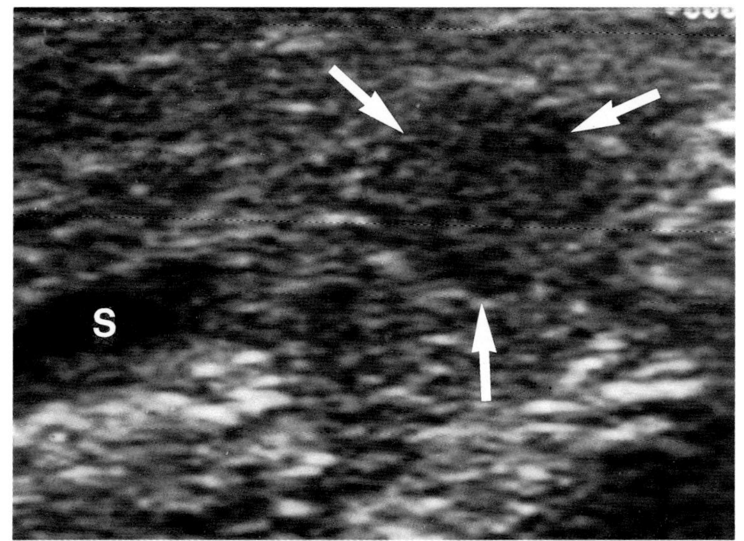

FIG. 4.54. Insulinoma, intraoperative sonogram. This high-resolution transverse intraoperative sonogram reveals a subtle small hypoechoic insulinoma (*arrows*) in the pancreatic tail. This mass was not detected on other imaging modalities. Intraoperative sonography is the most sensitive means to detect pancreatic islet cell neoplasms. It is even more sensitive than palpation at surgery. S, splenic vein.

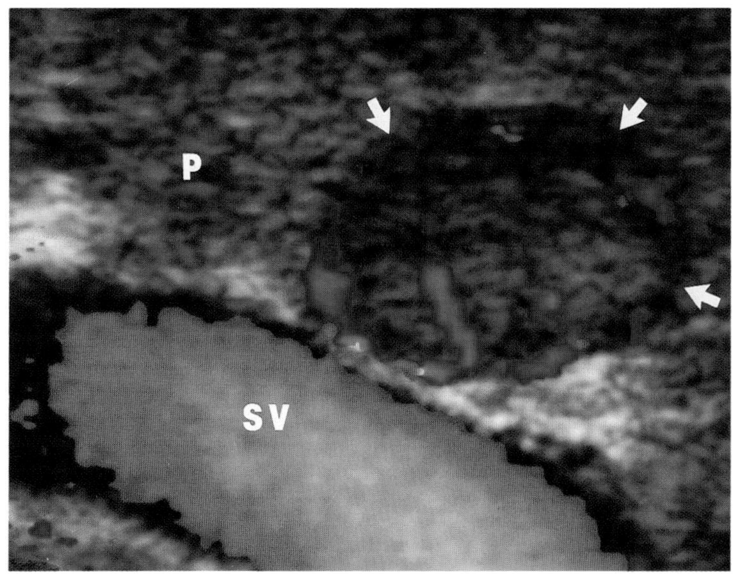

FIG. 4.55. Insulinoma, intraoperative sonogram. This insulinoma (*arrows*), which was suspected because of laboratory abnormalities, was not identified on preoperative high-resolution CT or ultrasound. Intraoperative sonography readily reveals the mass, which has increased color flow compared to the remainder of the pancreas. SV, splenic vein; P, pancreas.

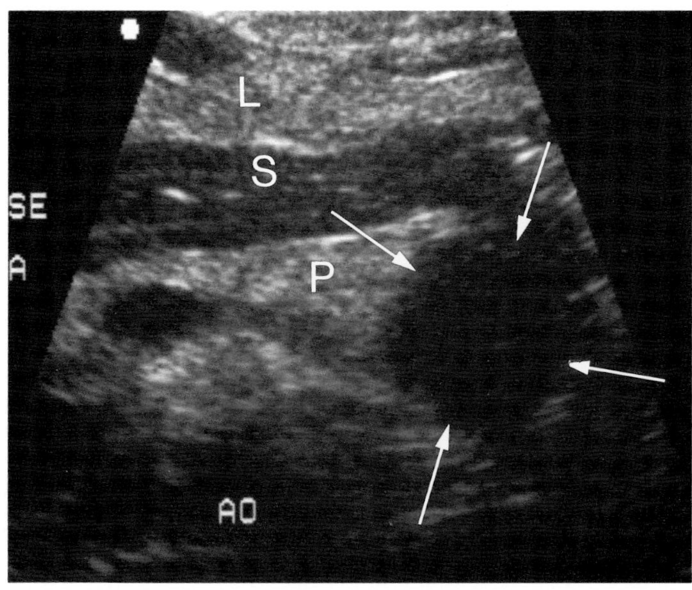

FIG. 4.56. Insulinoma. Transverse transabdominal sonogram reveals this relatively large, 2-cm insulinoma (*thin arrows*). Insulinomas are typically the largest of pancreatic islet cell tumors. Of islet cell tumors, insulinomas are the type most often detected with transabdominal ultrasound. AO, aorta; S, stomach; L, liver; P, pancreas.

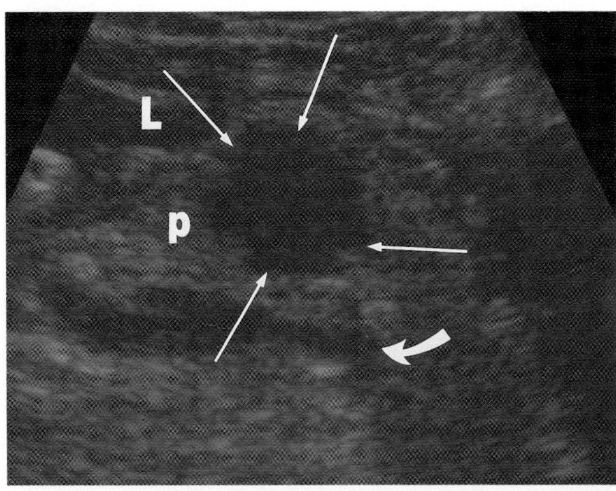

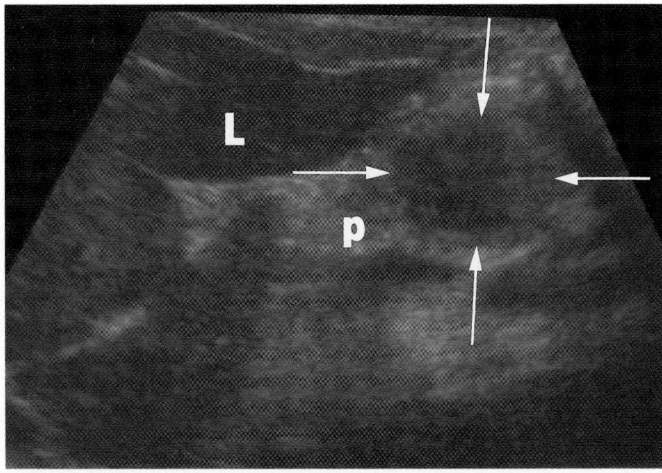

FIG. 4.57. Pancreatic metastasis from lung carcinoma. **A:** Transverse sonogram reveals a round hypoechoic mass (*small arrows*) within the pancreas. **B:** The longitudinal sonogram shows the same findings. Although common in autopsy series, pancreatic metastases are rarely detected clinically. L, liver; p, pancreas; *arrow,* superior mesenteric artery; *curved arrow,* splenic vein.

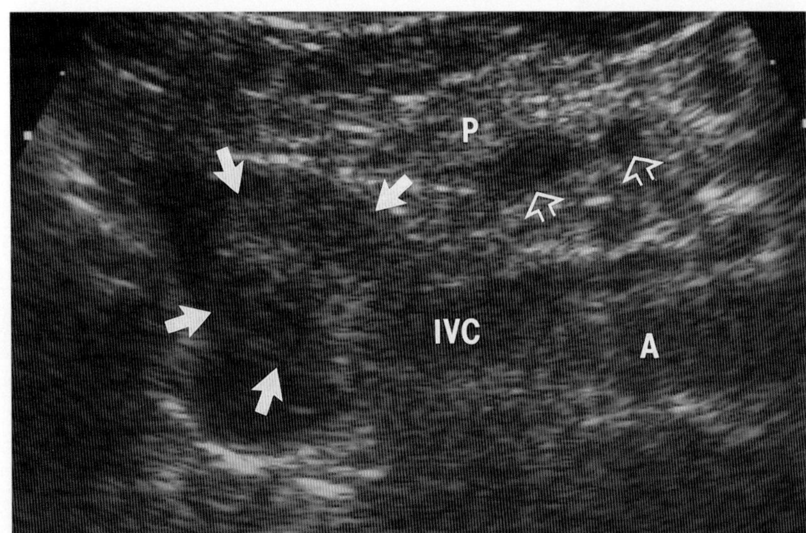

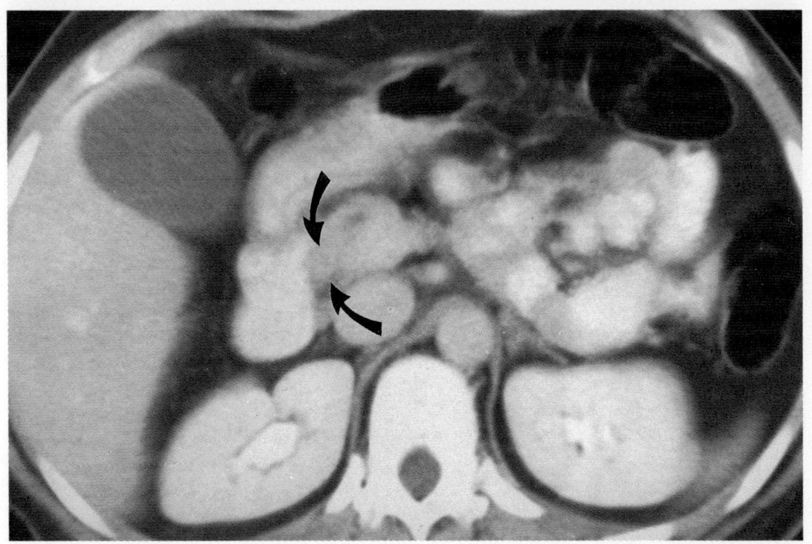

FIG. 4.58. Adenocarcinoma metastasis to the ampulla of Vater. This metastatic lesion from an adenocarcinoma of unknown primary caused findings indistinguishable from a periampullary neoplasm. **A:** The transverse sonogram of the region of the pancreatic head revealed a mass within the duodenum (*arrows*) immediately contiguous and perhaps involving the head of the pancreas (P). The superior mesenteric artery and vein (*open arrows*) are noted. **B:** A CT scan reveals similar findings, although the mass is more subtle (*curved arrow*). A, aorta; IVC, inferior vena cava.

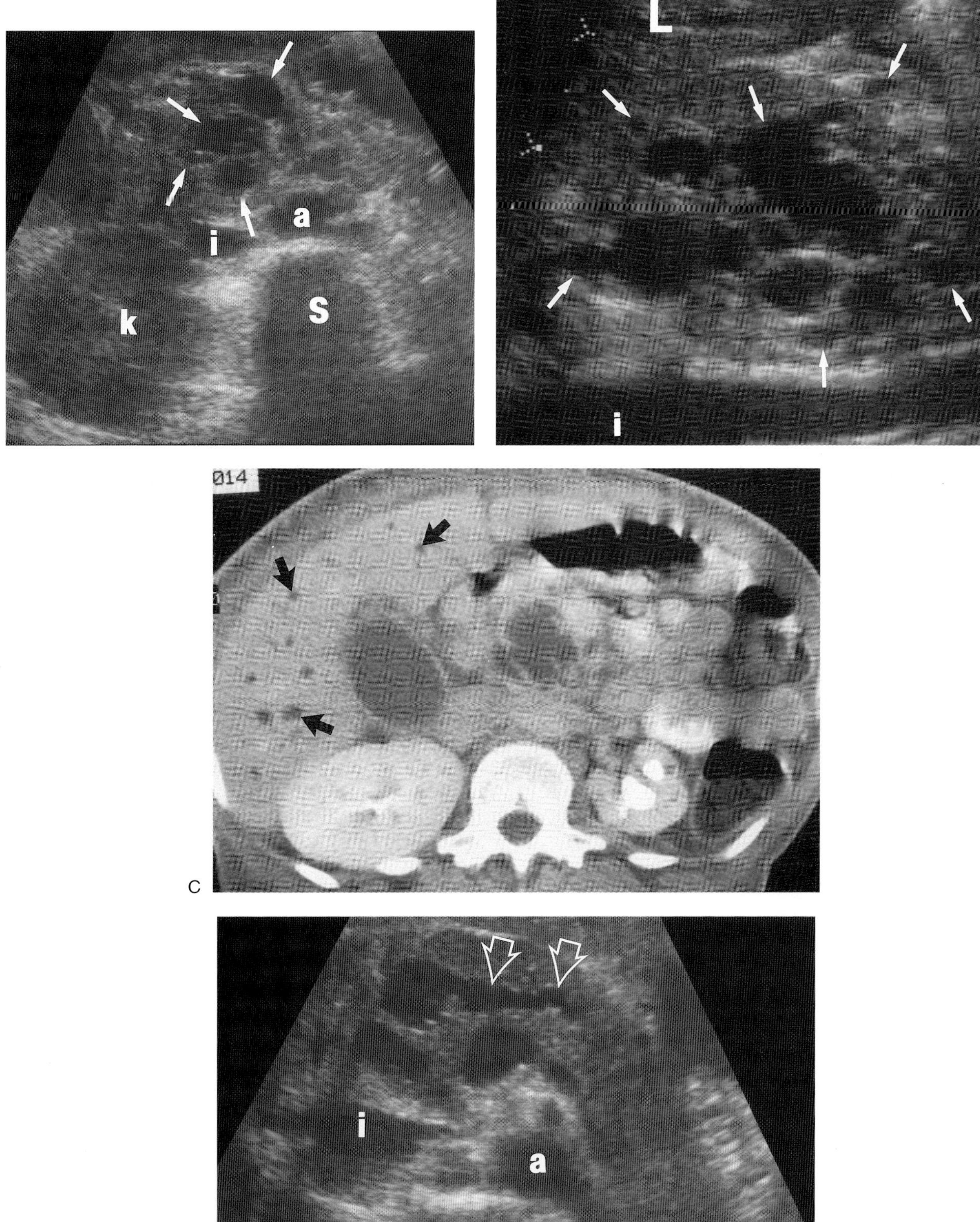

FIG. 4.59. Ductectatic/mucin hypersecreting carcinoma. **A:** Transverse sonogram through the head of the pancreas reveals enlargement of the pancreatic head with multiple internal ectatic ducts (*arrows*). **B:** A magnified longitudinal sonogram again reveals the internal cystic areas (*arrows*) representing dilated pancreatic ducts within this neoplasm. **C:** Similar findings are noted on the CT scan, which also demonstrates the dilated intrahepatic bile ducts (*black arrows*). **D:** A transverse sonogram of the body of the pancreas reveals the dilated main pancreatic duct (*open arrows*). This rare variant of ductal adenocarcinoma is characterized by dilated mucin-filled ducts. Potential confusion with regular histology adenocarcinoma (see Fig. 4.38) is possible. i, inferior vena cava; a, aorta; S, spine; K, right kidney; L, liver.

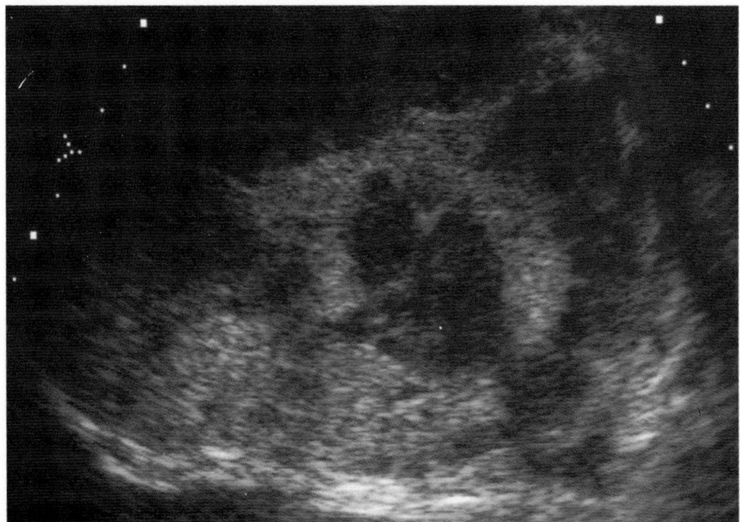

A

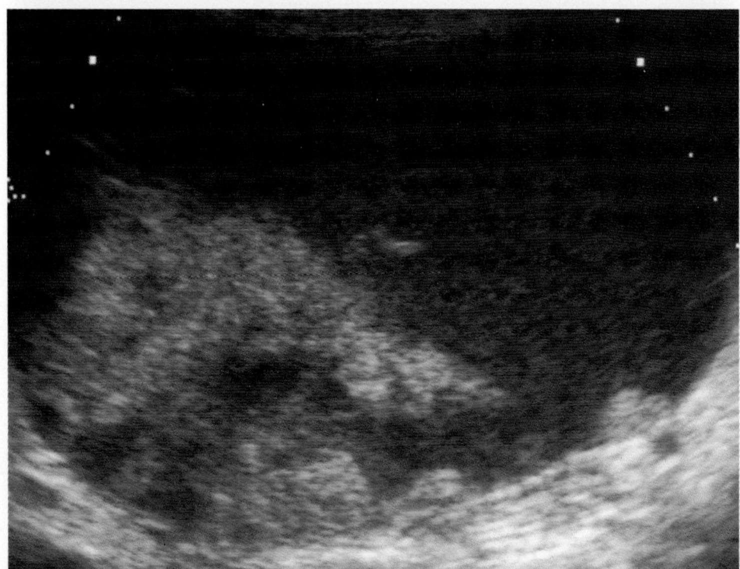

B

FIG. 4.60. Solid and papillary epithelial neoplasm of the pancreas. The transverse (**A**) and longitudinal (**B**) sonograms reveal a predominantly cystic mass with large internal papillary projections and solid material. The CT scan (**C**) displays similar internal structure, although less well than the sonograms. A T2-weighted MR scan (**D**) demonstrates the mural papillary excrescences (*arrows*) projecting into the high-signal, cystic interior of the tumor. This rare, spectacular neoplasm may be benign or malignant. Unlike most other pancreatic malignancies, resection is often curative. This tumor had malignant features pathologically.

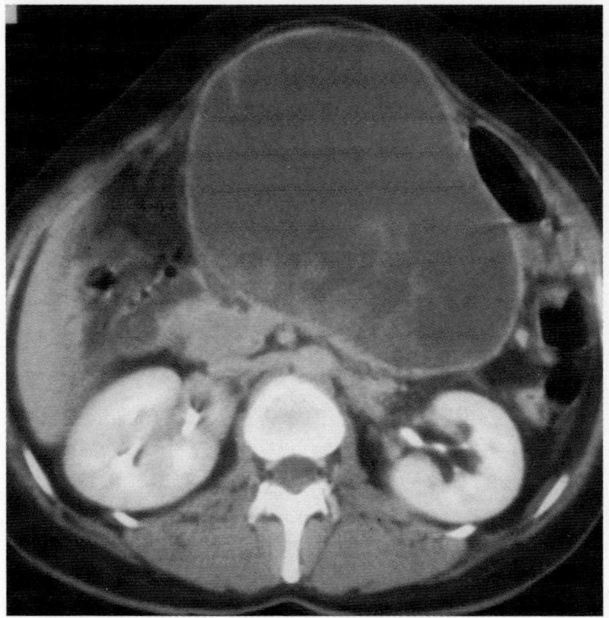

C

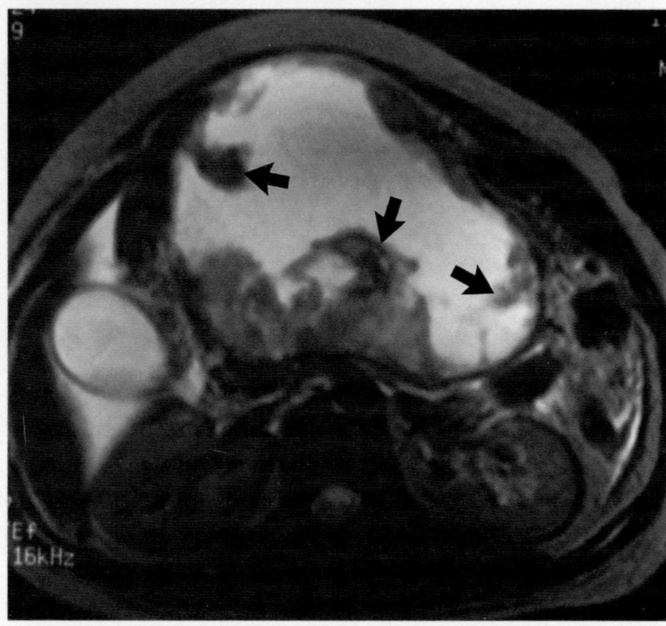

D

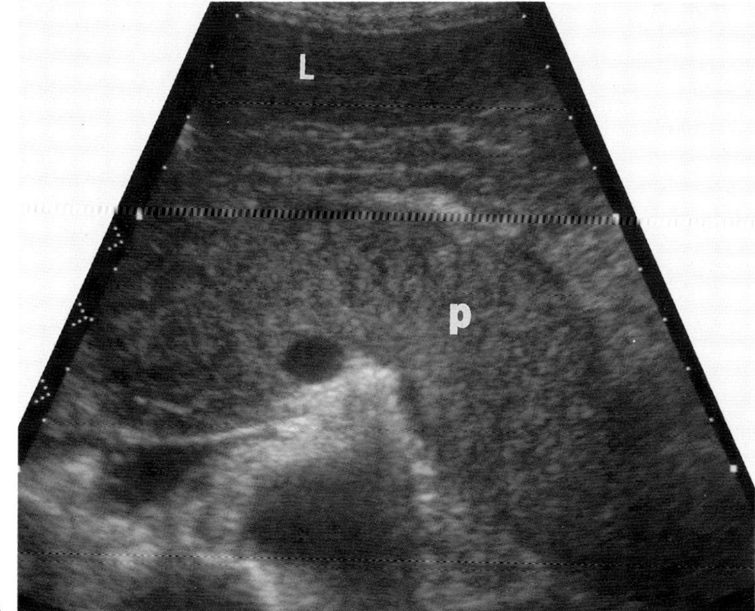

A

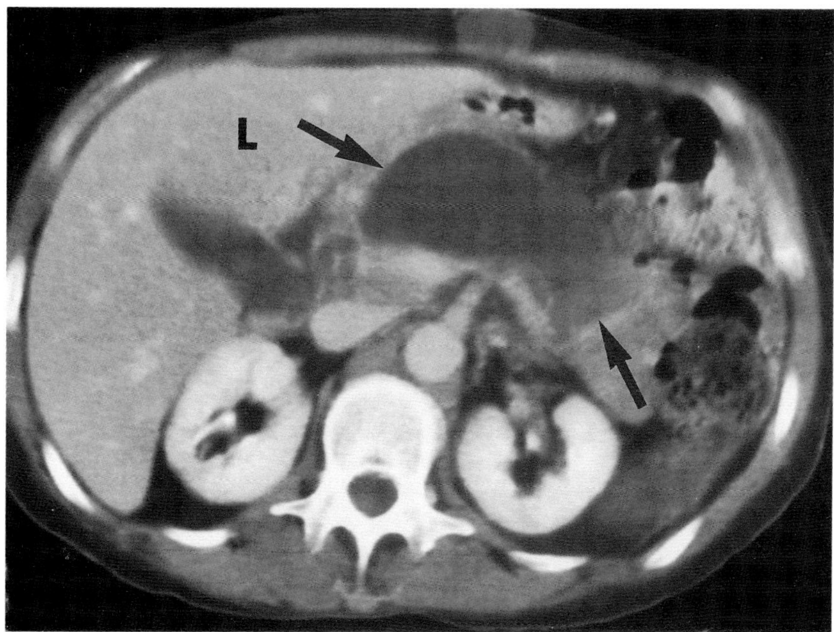

B

FIG. 4.61. Iatrogenic pancreatic infarct. After a therapeutic splenic artery embolization, this patient developed a pancreatic infarct. **A:** The transverse sonogram reveals an enlarged edematous pancreas (P) with accentuation of lobular architecture, caused by edema. **B:** A CT scan, performed a few days later, reveals liquefactive necrosis (*arrows*). This patient recovered on conservative management. L, liver.

MM. Acute pancreatitis: prognostic value of CT. *Radiology* 1985;156:767–772.
6. Vernacchia FS, Jeffrey RB Jr, Federle MP, et al. Pancreatic abscess: predictive value of early abdominal CT. *Radiology* 1987;162:435–438.
7. Kivisaari L, Somer K, Standertskjold-Nordenstam CG, Schroder T, Kivilaakso E, Lempinen M. A new method for the diagnosis of acute hemorrhagic-necrotizing pancreatitis using contrast-enhanced CT. *Gastrointest Radiol* 1984;9:27–30.
8. Block S, Maier W, Bittner R, Buchler M, Malfertheiner P, Beger HG. Identification of pancreas necrosis in severe acute pancreatitis: imaging procedures versus clinical staging. *Gut* 1986;27:1035–1042.
9. Nuutinen P, Kivisaari L, Schroder T. Contrast-enhanced computed tomography and microangiography of the pancreas in acute human hemorrhagic/necrotizing pancreatitis. *Pancreas* 1988;3(1):53–60.
10. Balthazar EJ, Robinson DL, Megibow AJ, Ranson JHC. Acute pancreatitis: value of CT in establishing prognosis. *Radiology* 1990;174:331–336.
11. Beger HG. Surgical management of necrotizing pancreatitis. *Surg Clin North Am* 1989;69(3):529–549.
12. Jeffrey RB Jr, Laing FC, Wing VW. Extrapancreatic spread of acute pancreatitis: new observations with real-time US. *Radiology* 1986;159:707–711.
13. Williford ME, Foster WL, Halvorsen RA, Thompson WM. Pancreatic pseudocyst: comparative evaluation by sonography and computed tomography. *AJR* 1983;140:53–57.
14. Freise J. Evaluation of sonography in the diagnosis of acute pancreatitis. In: Beger HG, Buchler M, eds. *Acute pancreatitis*. Berlin: Springer-Verlag; 1987:118–131.
15. Jeffrey RB Jr. Sonography in acute pancreatitis. *Radiol Clin North Am* 1989;27(1):5–17.
16. Ralls PW. Color Doppler sonography of the hepatic artery and portal venous system. *AJR* 1990;155:517–525.
17. Bradley EL III. Complications of chronic pancreatitis. *Surg Clin North Am* 1989;693:481–497.
18. Luetmer PH, Stephens DH, Ward EM. Chronic pancreatitis: reassessment with current CT. *Radiology* 1989;171:353–357.
19. Bolondi L, Priori P, Gullo L, et al. Relationship between morphological changes detected by ultrasonography and pancreatic exocrine function in chronic pancreatitis. *Pancreas* 1987;2:222–229.
20. Bolondi L, LiBassi S, Gaiani S, Barbara L. Sonography of chronic pancreatitis. *Radiol Clin North Am* 1989;27(4):815–833.
21. Ralls PW, Halls J, Renner I, Juttner H. Endoscopic retrograde cholangiopancreatography (ERCP) in pancreatic disease. *Radiology* 1980;134:347–352.
22. Siegelman SS, Copeland BE, Saba GP, Sanders RC, Zerhouni EA. CT of fluid collections associated with pancreatitis. *AJR* 1980;134:1121–1132.
23. Silverstein W, Isikoff MB, Hill MC, Barkin J. Diagnostic imaging of acute pancreatitis: prospective study using CT and sonography. *AJR* 1981;137:497–502.
24. Matzinger FRK, Ho CS, Yee AC, Gray RR. Pancreatic pseudocysts drained through a percutaneous transgastric approach: further experience. *Radiology* 1988;167:431–434.
25. Balthazar EJ. CT diagnosis and staging of acute pancreatitis. *Radiol Clin North Am* 1989;27(1):19–37.
26. Bradley EL, Clements JL, Gonzalez AC. The natural history of pancreatic pseudocysts: a unified concept of management. *Am J Surg* 1979;137:135–141.
27. vanSonnenberg E, Wittich GR, Casola G, et al. Complicated pancreatic inflammatory disease: diagnostic and therapeutic role of interventional radiology. *Radiology* 1985;155:335–340.
28. Grosso M, Gandini G, Cassinis MC, Regge D, Righi D, Rossi P. Percutaneous treatment (including pseudocystogastrostomy) of 74 pancreatic pseudocysts. *Radiology* 1989;173:493–497.
29. Steiner E, Mueller PR, Hahn PF, et al. Complicated pancreatic abscesses: problems in interventional management. *Radiology* 1988;167:443–446.
30. Warshaw AL. Management of pancreatic abscesses. In: Beger HG, Buchler M, eds. *Acute pancreatitis*. Berlin: Springer-Verlag; 1987:354–363.
31. Lee MJ, Rattner DW, Legemate DA, et al. Acute complicated pancreatitis: redefining the role of interventional radiology. *Radiology* 1992;183:171–174.
32. vanSonnenberg E, Casola G, Varney RR, Wittich GR. Imaging and interventional radiology for pancreatitis and its complications. *Radiol Clin North Am* 1989;27(1):65–72.
33. vanSonnenberg E, Wittich GR, Casola G, et al. Percutaneous drainage of infected and non-infected pancreatic pseudocysts: experience in 101 cases. *Radiology* 1989;170:757–761.
34. Ormson MJ, Charboneau JW, Stephens DH. Sonography in patients with a possible pancreatic mass shown on CT. *AJR* 1987;148:551–555.
35. Campbell JP, Wilson SR. Pancreatic neoplasms: how useful is evaluation with US? *Radiology* 1988;167:341–344.
36. DelMaschio A, Vanzulli A, Sironi S, et al. Pancreatic cancer versus chronic pancreatitis: diagnosis with CA 19-9 assessment, US, CT and CT-guided fine-needle biopsy. *Radiology* 1991;178:95–99.
37. Cubilla AL, Fitzgerald PJ. Tumors of the exocrine pancreas. In: *Atlas of tumor pathology*, 2nd series, Fascicle 19. Washington DC: Armed Forces Institute of Pathology; 1984:1.
38. Fontham ETH, Correa P. Epidemiology of pancreatic cancer. *Surg Clin North Am* 1989;69(3):551–567.
39. Friedman AC, Krudy AG Jr, Shawker TH, et al. Pancreatic neoplasms. In: *Radiology of the liver, biliary tract, pancreas and spleen*. Baltimore: Williams & Wilkins; 1987:735–837.
40. Carroll B, Sample WF. Pancreatic cystadenocarcinoma: CT body scan and gray scale ultrasound appearance. *AJR* 1978;131:339–341.
41. Kunzmann A, Bowie JD, Rochester D. Texture patterns in pancreatic sonograms. *Gastrointest Radiol* 1979;4:353–357.
42. Freeny PC. Radiologic diagnosis and staging of pancreatic ductal adenocarcinoma. *Radiol Clin North Am* 1989;27:121–128.
43. Jordan GL. Pancreatic resection for pancreatic cancer. *Surg Clin North Am* 1989;69(3):569–597.
44. Cubilla AL, Fitzgerald PJ. Classification of pancreatic cancer (nonendocrine). *Mayo Clin Proc* 1979;54:449–458.
45. George DH, Murphy F, Michalski R, Ulmer BG. Serous cystadenocarcinoma of the pancreas: a new entity? *Am J Surg Pathol* 1989;13(1):61–66.
46. Friedman AC, Lichtenstein JE, Dachman AH. Cystic neoplasms of the pancreas. *Radiology* 1983;149:45–50.
47. Johnson CD, Stephens DH, Carboneau JW, Carpenter HA, Welch TJ. Cystic pancreatic tumors: CT and sonographic assessment. *AJR* 1988;151:1133–1138.
48. Mathieu D, Guigui B, Valette PJ, et al. Pancreatic cystic neoplasms. *Radiol Clin North Am* 1989;27(1):163–176.
49. Gunther RW, Klose KJ, Ruckert K, Beyer J, Kuhn FP, Klotter JH. Localization of small islet-cell tumors. Preoperative and intraoperative ultrasound, computed tomography, arteriography, digital subtraction angiography, and pancreatic venous sampling. *Gastrointest Radiol* 1985;10:145–152.
50. Gorman B, Charboneau JW, James EM, et al. Benign pancreatic insulinoma: preoperative and intraoperative sonographic localization. *AJR* 1986;147:929–934.
51. Shawker TH, Doppman JL. Intraoperative US. *Radiology* 1988;166:568–569.
52. Rossi P, Allison DJ, Bezzi M, et al. Endocrine tumors of the pancreas. *Radiol Clin North Am* 1989;27(1):129–161.
53. Galiber AK, Reading CC, Charboneau JW, et al. Localization of pancreatic insulinoma: comparison of pre- and intraoperative US with CT and angiography. *Radiology* 1988;166:405–408.
54. Friedman AC, Edmonds PR. Rare pancreatic malignancies. *Radiol Clin North Am* 1989;27(1):177–190.
55. Bastid C, Bernard JP, Sarles H, Payan MJ, Sahel J. Mucinous ductal ectasia of the pancreas: a premalignant disease and a cause of obstructive pancreatitis. *Pancreas* 1991;6(1):15–22.
56. Agostini S, Choux R, Payan MJ, Sastre B, Sahel J, Clement JP. Mucinous pancreatic duct ectasia in the body of the pancreas. *Radiology* 1989;170:815–816.
57. Compagno J, Oertel JE, Krezmar M. Solid and papillary epithelial neoplasm of the pancreas, probably a small duct origin: a clinical pathologic study of 52 cases. *Lab Invest* 1979;40:248–249.

CHAPTER 5

Kidneys and Adrenal Gland

TECHNIQUE

Renal sonography should be initiated with curved linear 3- and 5-MHz transducers. The right kidney is often best imaged using the liver as an acoustic window. Images of the coronal axis of the kidney can be obtained in the decubitus position. When acoustic access is limited, a small footprint sector or annular array transducer may facilitate scans between ribs or around gas. Renal sonography is often more technically difficult than generally appreciated. A flexible, inventive approach provides best results.

Renal Doppler evaluation is often best performed with a lower insonant frequency, usually 2 or 3 MHz, than that used for grayscale imaging. Lower frequency ensures adequate tissue penetration needed to acquire the inherently fainter Doppler frequency shift signal. Proximal renal artery stenoses are best sought by evaluating the aorta while the patient is positioned in a decubitus or prone position. While curved linear transducers may be effective in some patients, small footprint sector transducers are often needed to obtain optimal Doppler information. A variety of patient positions and acoustic access windows are required to evaluate the renal veins, the more peripheral renal arteries, and the renal sinus vessels. Evaluation of the renal arteries is facilitated by color Doppler imaging and may be difficult or impossible without it (Fig. 5.1). When more detailed spectral Doppler analysis is required, color Doppler sonography is used to guide placement of the sample volume.

Color Doppler sonography is potentially useful in the evaluation of renal artery occlusion and stenosis, aneurysm, pseudoaneurysm, arteriovenous (AV) fistula, AV malformation, and venous thrombosis. Color flow sonography is also useful to differentiate normal anatomic variants from tumors and to evaluate ureteral jets in patients with suspected obstruction. Spectral analysis to assess peripheral arterial resistance is useful in renal parenchymal disease, hydronephrosis, and other diffuse renal diseases. Spectral analysis of neoplasms may be used to attempt to distinguish benign from malignant tumors.

RENAL VASCULAR DISEASE

Renal Artery Occlusion

Renal artery occlusion is generally caused by trauma, atherosclerosis, inadvertent ligation, or interventional embolization. Segmental occlusion may be related to atherosclerosis, embolism, or vasculitis (such as that occurring in renal transplant rejection). Color flow sonography can diagnose segmental or global renal artery occlusion, although it is infrequently requested clinically except to evaluate renal transplants. Computed tomography (CT) and arteriography are more frequently used. Of note is the fact that grayscale sonography may be normal in patients with segmental or global renal infarction.

Renal Artery Stenosis/Renal Vascular Hypertension

Focal or diffuse renal artery stenosis may result in renal vascular hypertension, a treatable cause of hypertension. Two-thirds of stenoses are caused by arteriosclerosis (Fig. 5.2) and the remainder are generally related to fibromuscular hyperplasia. Aneurysms (Fig. 5.3), pseudoaneurysms, vasculitis, Takayasu's arteritis (Fig. 5.4), neurofibromatosis, and Page kidney (renal compression related to subcapsular collections) are rare causes of hypertension.

Spectral Doppler analysis, often guided by color flow sonography, to directly detect renal artery stenosis has been reported as either efficacious (1–3) or difficult and of questionable usefulness (4). Renal artery stenosis may be diagnosed when renal artery velocities are greater than 1.5 to 1.9 m/sec, or a ratio of renal artery to aortic peak velocity of 3.5 to 1 or greater are documented (Figs. 5.2 and 5.4). Problems include technical difficulty, lengthy exam time, and the presence of multiple renal arteries (more than 20 percent of patients).

Another approach to detecting renal artery stenosis involves systolic waveform analysis in distal (downstream)

(text continues on page 280)

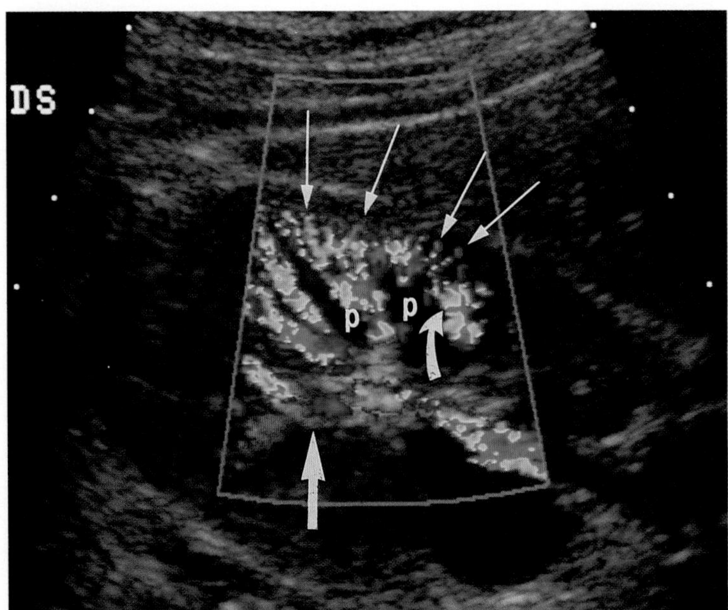

FIG. 5.1. Normal intrarenal flow. Transverse systolic color Doppler image of the kidney. Flow is noted around the medullary pyramids (p) and on into the periphery of the renal cortex—segmental artery (*large arrow*), arcuate artery (*curved arrow*), and intralobular artery (*thin arrows*). Color flow sonography delineates intrarenal vessels that are invisible on grayscale images and undetectable using other noninvasive vascular imaging techniques. Color Doppler sonography can be used to guide sample volume placement when spectral analysis is needed.

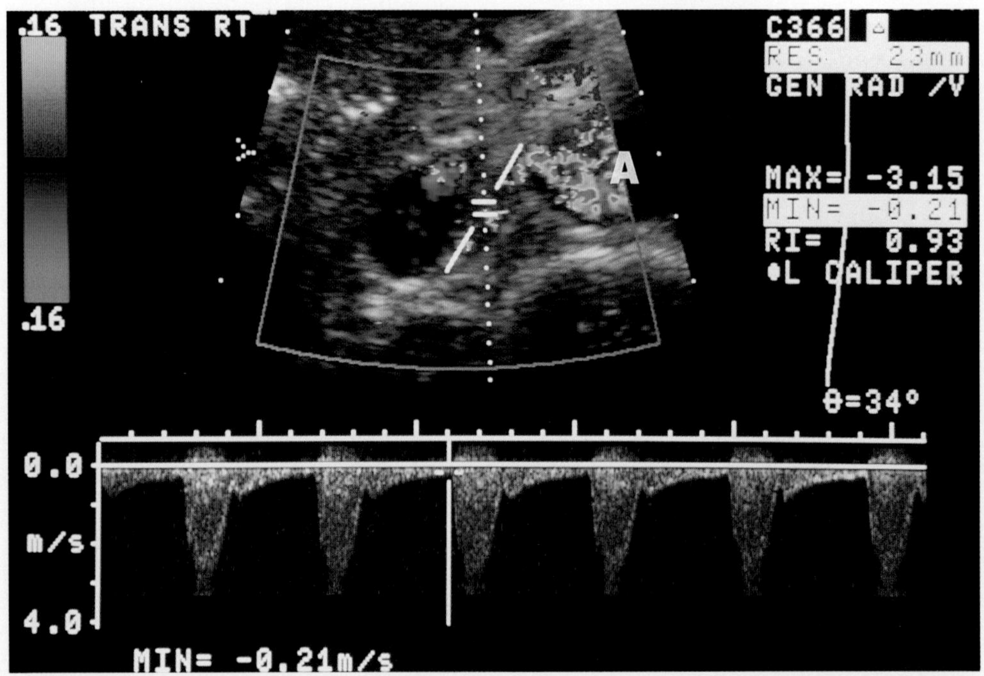

FIG. 5.2. Atherosclerotic renal artery stenosis. Transverse color and spectral Doppler sonogram. Flow velocity in this stenotic renal artery exceeded 3 m/sec, greater than the upper normal limit of 1.5 to 1.9 m/sec. The ratio of peak velocity in the renal artery compared to that in the aorta was greater than 5:1 (exceeding the 3.5:1 upper limit). Findings such as this have a very high predictive value for stenosis. Unfortunately, the sensitivity of detecting stenosis with this type of Doppler analysis is relatively low. A, aorta.

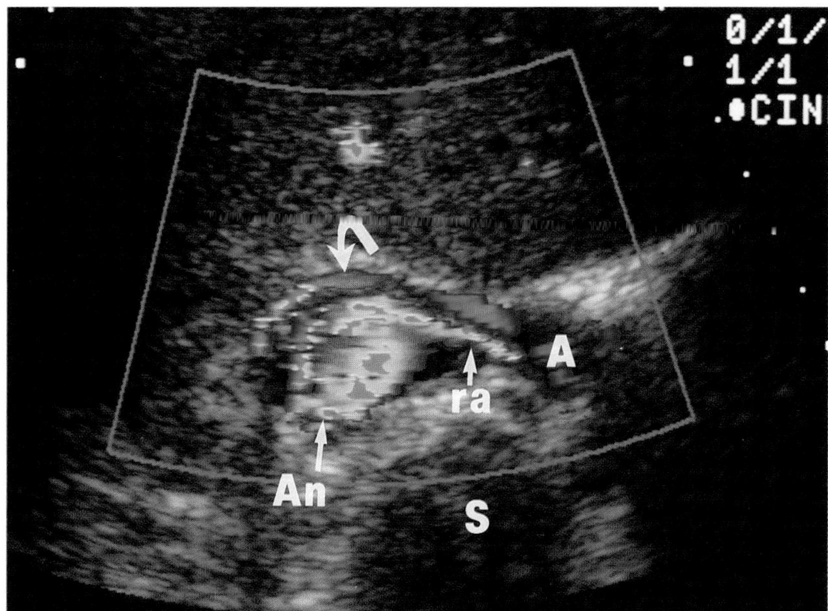

FIG. 5.3. Right renal artery aneurysm. Transverse color Doppler sonogram through the region of the right renal artery. Note the large right renal artery aneurysm (An) in this 20-year-old female who had a 4-year history of hypertension. The patient suffered from an unknown type of angiopathy that caused multiple aneurysms throughout her body. Aneurysmectomy and revascularization resulted in near normalization of her blood pressure. S, spine; A, aorta; *curved arrow,* inferior vena cava; ra, right renal artery.

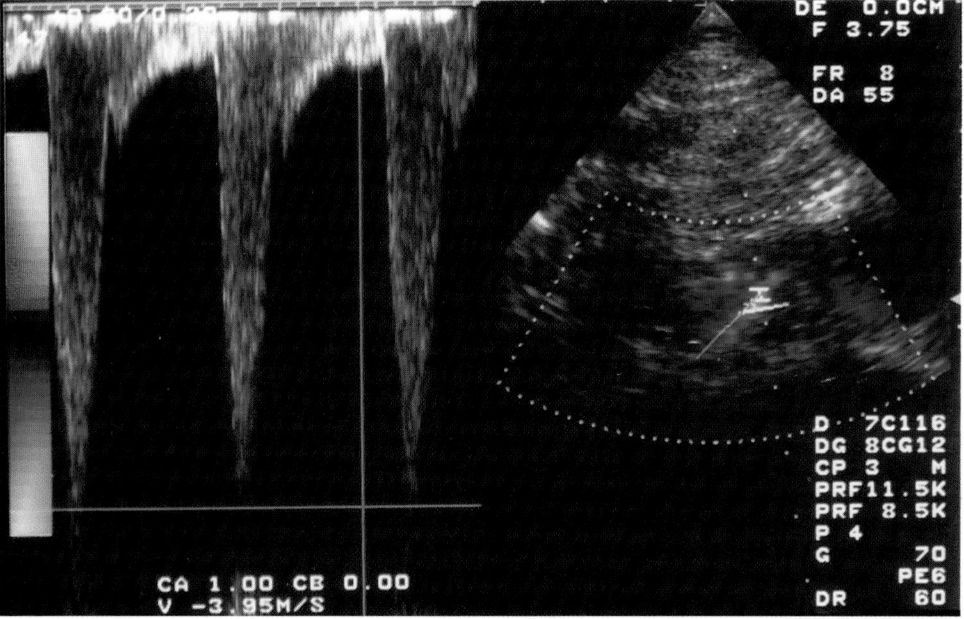

FIG. 5.4. Renal artery stenosis, Takayasu's arteritis. Transverse color and spectral Doppler sonogram reveals a peak renal artery velocity of nearly 4 m/sec, far exceeding the 1.5- to 1.9-m/sec normal limit. The color Doppler image (**right**) is used to facilitate placement of the sample volume.

renal arteries, peripheral to the stenosis. Several reports have indicated that decreased acceleration and height of the systolic upstroke (parvus/tardus waveform) are predictive of a 75 percent or greater renal artery stenosis in a proximal artery (5–7). In addition, Stavros et al. (6) have reported that loss of the early systolic peak/reflective waveform complex (ESP) (Fig. 5.5) may be the most sensitive indicator of a more proximal stenosis. The usefulness of all these techniques to detect renal artery stenosis depends heavily on the expertise of the operator. New advances, such as ultrasound vascular contrast agents, may make these techniques easier and more reliable.

Renal vascular disease accounts for less than 1 percent of all hypertension, although higher rates are often quoted. This low prevalence and the imperfections of diagnostic techniques suggest that evaluation for renal vascular hypertension should be restricted to patients with more severe hypertension, especially those unresponsive to pharmacologic control (8). Even detecting renal artery stenosis does not automatically mean that a patient's hypertension is stenosis related. Stenosis may be incidentally present without causing hypertension.

Nonsonographic techniques used to evaluate patients with suspected renal vascular hypertension include intra-arterial digital subtraction angiography, Captopril radionuclide renography, magnetic resonance (MR) angiography, and spiral CT angiography. The validity of Doppler techniques and the relative usefulness of Doppler sonography compared to other techniques are not yet established. Studies that correlate image/Doppler findings to clinical outcome are needed.

Other Arterial Lesions

Pseudoaneurysms, arteriovenous malformations (Fig. 5.6), and AV fistulas related to renal biopsy (Figs. 5.7 and 5.8), renal trauma, or neoplasm such as angiomyolipoma (see Fig. 5.76) may be diagnosed with color flow sonography. The sensitivity of color flow sonography in detecting these vascular abnormalities is not yet known.

Renal Vein Thrombosis

Renal vein thrombosis generally occurs as a complication of renal disease such as nephrotic syndrome (systemic lupus erythematosis [SLE], membranous glomerulonephritis) or neoplastic invasion. Primary renal vein thrombosis may be related to trauma, infection, or hypercoagulable states. While acute symptoms including flank pain hematuria, fever, and leukocytosis may occur, many patients are asymptomatic.

Sometimes, renal vein thrombus may be directly identified on grayscale images. Real-time color flow sonography is much more reliable, however; clot is highlighted in contrast to color-coded flow in uninvolved portions of the renal vein, the adjacent inferior vena cava, and in other nearby vessels (Figs. 5.9 and 5.10). Partial clot is easily diagnosed with color flow sonography (Fig. 5.11).

RENAL INFECTION

Renal infection is virtually always caused by bacterial reflux from the lower urinary tract, rather than hematogenous dissemination. Exceptions include staphylococcal infection, sepsis in intravenous drug abusers, and tuberculosis. Urinary tract obstruction or stasis, some anatomic variants and anomalies, vesicoureteral reflex, diabetes mellitus, and stones all predispose to pyelonephritis. In many patients, however, no predisposing condition is present.

Patients with pyelonephritis (renal parenchymal infection) usually do not require radiologic imaging. The diagnosis is easily established based on clinical symptoms of fever and flank pain, and laboratory findings of pyuria and bacteriuria. Radiologic imaging is reserved for those patients who have recurrent renal infection or renal infection unresponsive to antibiotic therapy. Imaging goals include detection of pathology or of physiologic conditions that predispose to infection (stones, reflux, anatomic anomalies) or identification of complications such as pyonephrosis, renal abscess, and perinephric abscess.

Intravenous urography, contrast-enhanced CT, and diagnostic sonography are useful, complementary techniques to evaluate patients with renal infection. The imaging modality chosen for diagnostic workup is largely based on institutional preference. Intravenous urography provides functional information and superior anatomic information about the ureters and bladder. Contrast-enhanced CT is far more sensitive than sonography or urography in detecting renal and perirenal abnormalities. Sonography's advantages include patient comfort, and that no intravenous contrast material or ionizing radiation are used.

Sonography has many limitations in the evaluation of patients with renal infection—poor contrast resolution, suboptimal detection of renal and perinephric infection, and suboptimal ability to detect renal calculi (9). Nevertheless, careful sonography generally detects clinically significant infections (10) that require surgery or percutaneous drainage (i.e., pyonephrosis or large abscess). It cannot be emphasized enough that meticulous sonographic technique is crucial to minimize the risk of missing significant infectious complications. When either intravenous urography or ultrasound reveal no significant abnormality in a patient who has persistent fever or other ominous symptoms, contrast-enhanced CT may be useful to rule out an undiagnosed complication (10,11).

(*text continues on page 285*)

A

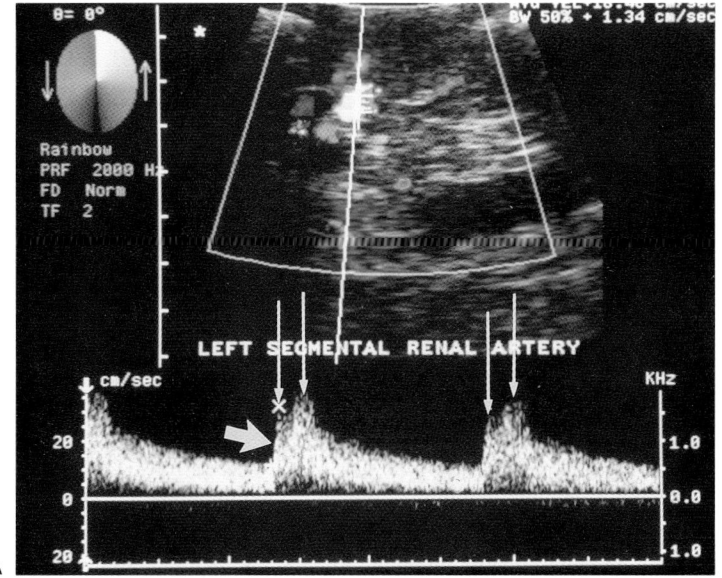

B

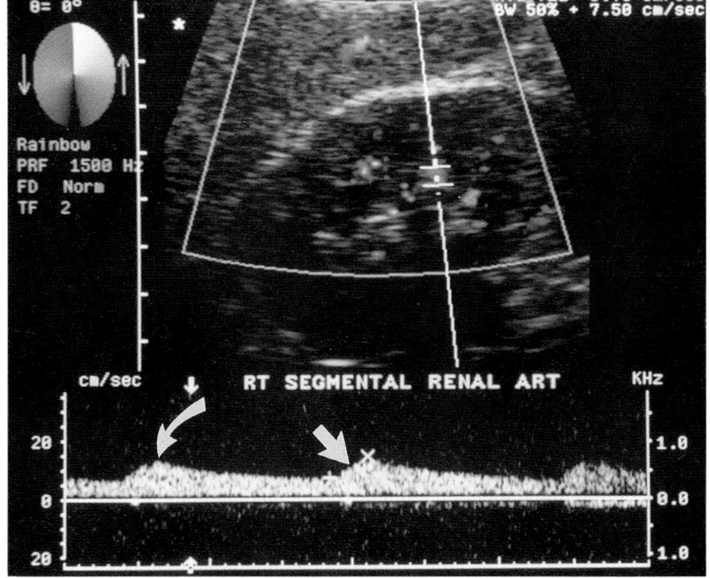

C

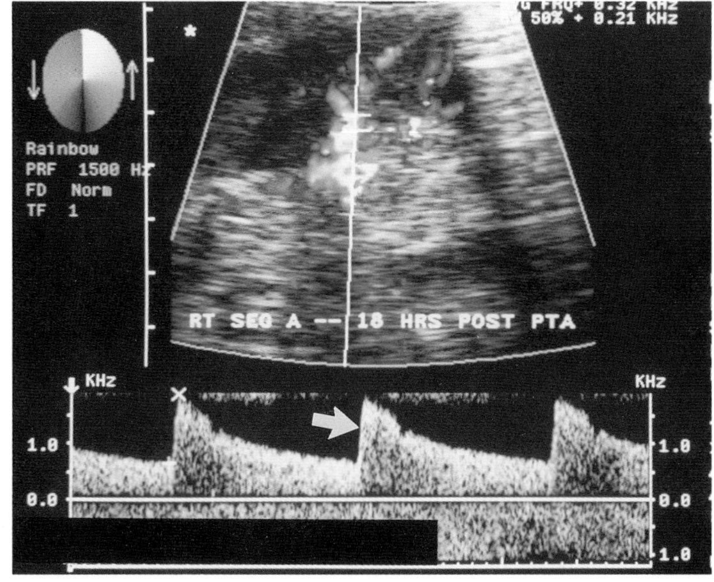

FIG. 5.5. Renal artery stenosis, downstream waveform analysis. **A:** Spectral Doppler sonogram of a left segmental renal artery reveals a normal waveform with a quick systolic upstroke (*arrow*) and a normal early systolic peak/reflective waveform complex (ESP, *thin arrows*). **B:** A right-sided segmental renal artery spectral Doppler image reveals a parvus/tardus waveform. In this abnormal waveform, the systolic upstroke is abnormally delayed (*arrow*). The notched ESP systolic waveform is lost (*curved arrow*). This pattern indicates proximal renal artery stenosis. **C:** Eighteen hours after right renal artery angioplasty, a spectral Doppler image of a right segmental artery reveals normalization of the fast systolic upstroke (*arrow*). This new technique in assessing renal artery stenosis may positively influence the ability to detect renal artery stenosis with sonography. Further clinical investigation is needed to assess the overall usefulness of this technique. (Case courtesy of Dr. A. Thomas Stavros.)

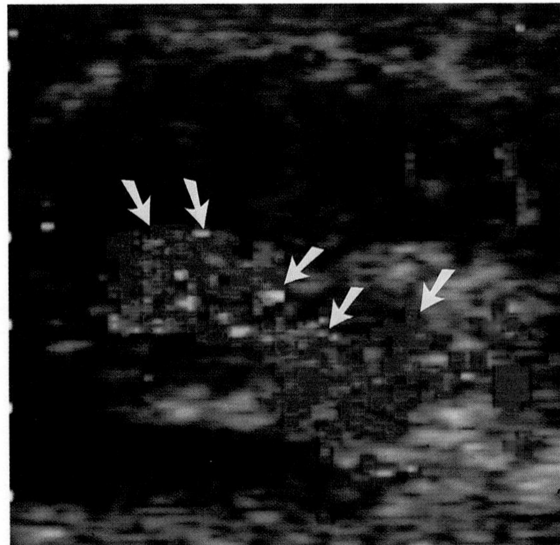

FIG. 5.6. Cirsoid arteriovenous malformation (AVM). Longitudinal color Doppler sonogram reveals a cirsoid AVM, involving the renal sinus and upper pole renal parenchyma (*angled arrows*). The mottled color pattern is partially related to "tissue hum." This patient, who had hematuria from the right kidney on ureteroscopy, had normal MRI, normal contrast-enhanced CT, and a normal conventional sonogram prior to discovery of the lesion with color Doppler sonography. (From ref. 7a, with permission.)

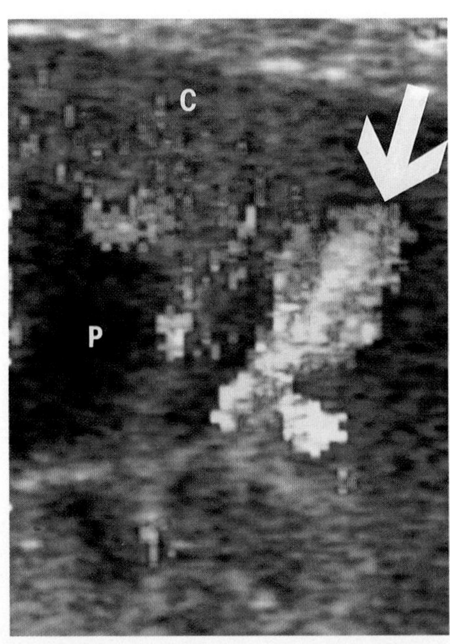

FIG. 5.7. AV fistula after renal biopsy. Magnified color Doppler sonogram of the lower pole of the kidney reveals enlarged arteries and veins indicative of an AV fistula (*arrow*) at the site of a renal biopsy. There is vascular enlargement owing to the increased flow caused by the fistula. Most biopsy-related AV fistulas resolve spontaneously. P, renal pyramid; C, renal cortex.

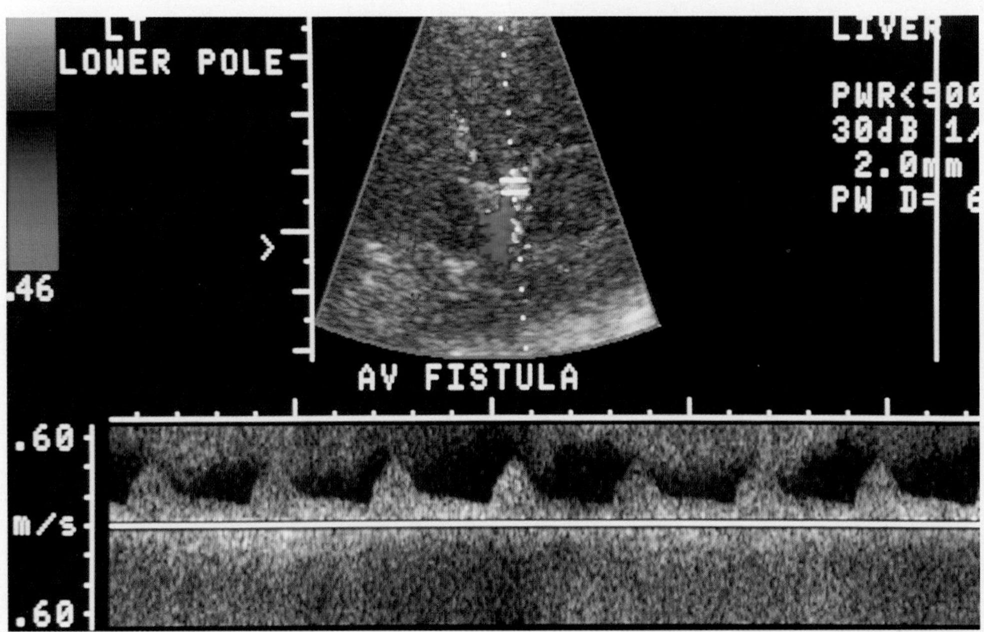

FIG. 5.8. AV fistula after renal biopsy. This color Doppler guided spectral Doppler image of a renal biopsy-related AV fistula reveals both arterial and venous components as well as high-velocity venous flow (aliased). Confirmation of AV fistulas with spectral Doppler sonography is useful when the diagnosis is unclear from the color Doppler image alone.

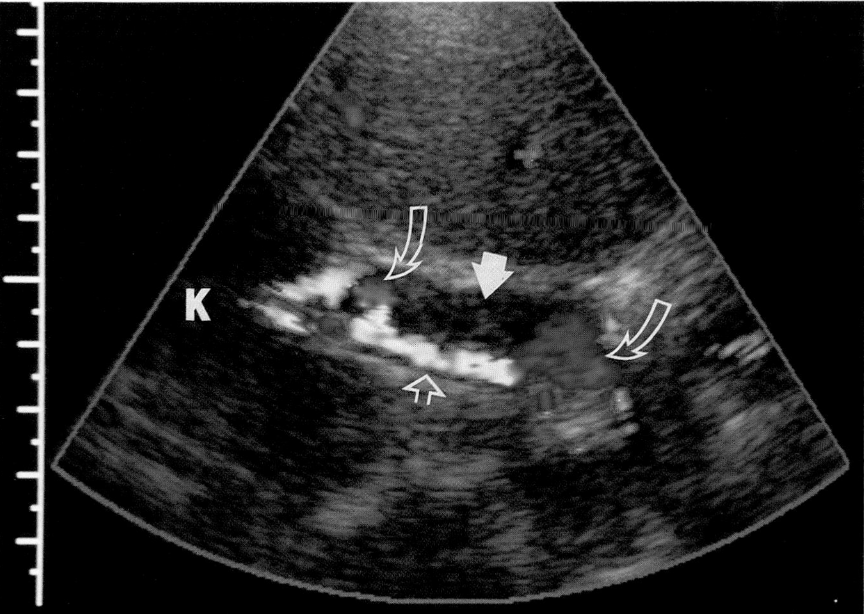

FIG. 5.9. Renal vein thrombosis, nephrotic syndrome. Transverse sonogram of the right renal artery and vein. The right renal vein clot (*arrow*) is echogenic but is highlighted by venous flow on either side of the clot (*curved open arrows*). The right renal artery (*open arrow*) is noted dorsal to the renal vein. Color facilitates detection of hypoechoic thrombus. When clot is anechoic, color Doppler may be the only means of detecting it successfully. K, right kidney.

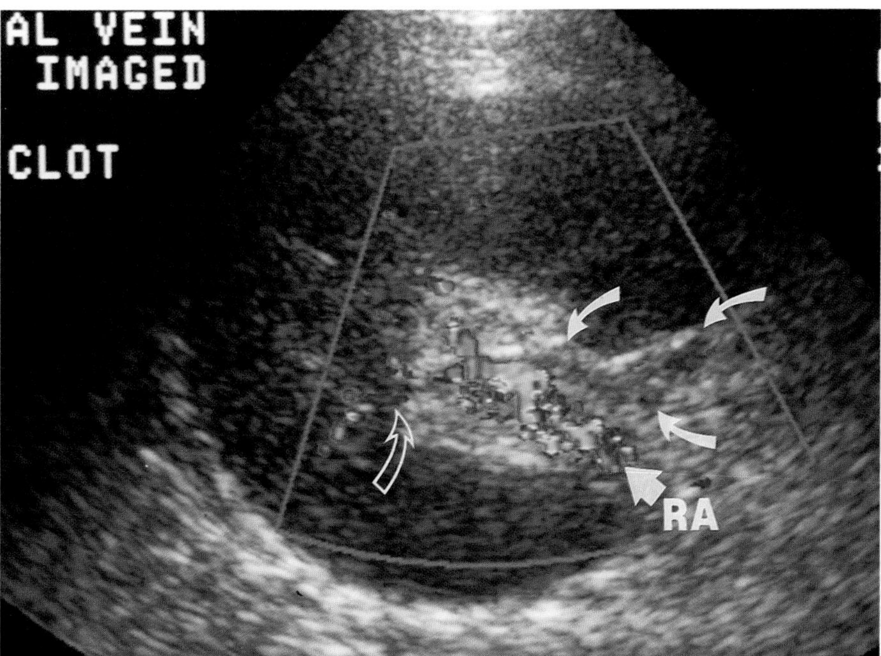

FIG. 5.10. Renal vein thrombus. A presumptive diagnosis of renal vein thrombus may be made if flow in the renal vein is not imaged when flow in other renal sinus vessels (renal artery—RA, *arrow*) and in more peripheral veins (*open curved arrow*) can be identified. In this setting, a presumptive diagnosis is possible, although identification of the vein itself with no flow within it is required for definitive diagnosis. Here, the vein (*curved arrows*) is only questionably identified.

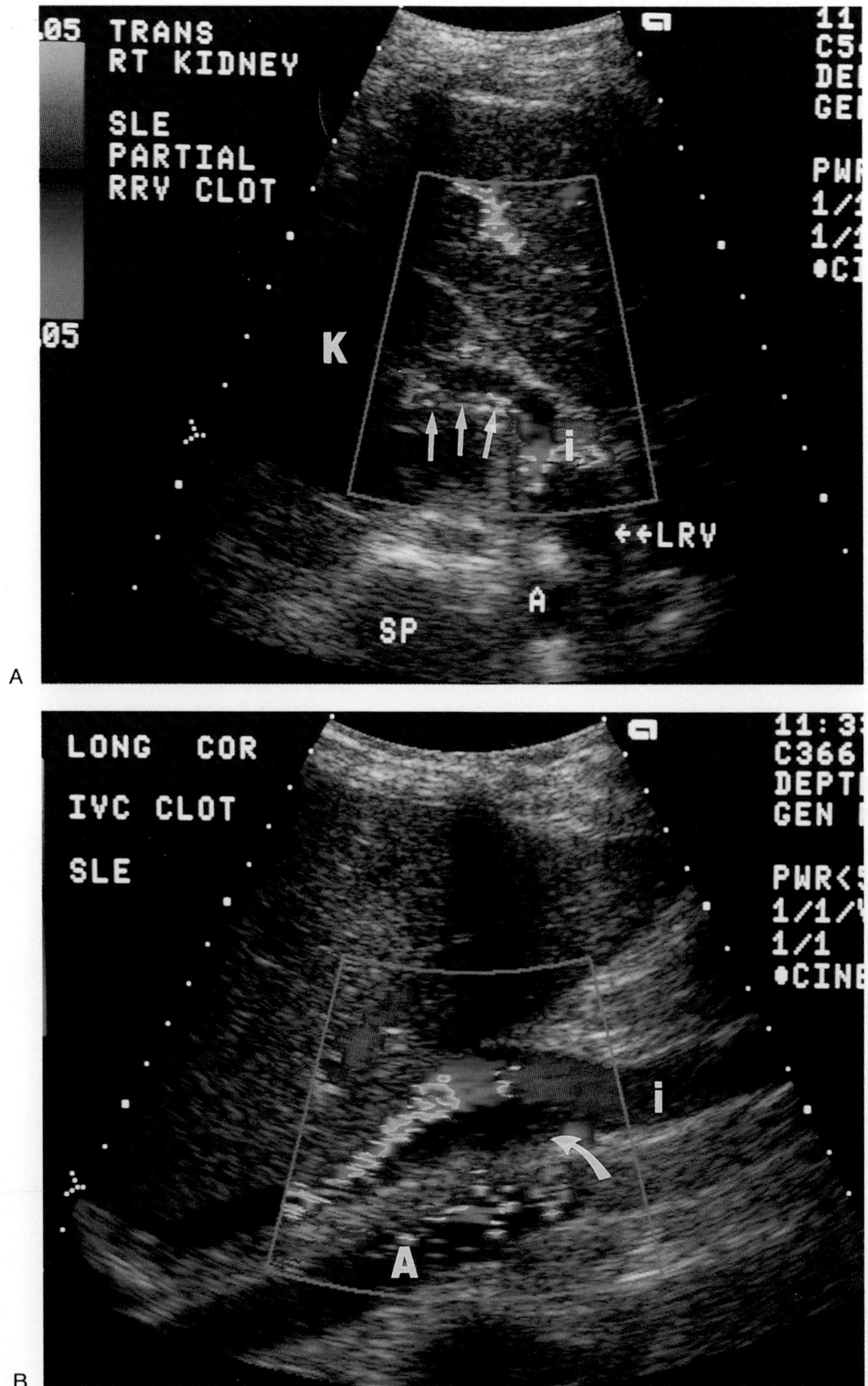

FIG. 5.11. Renal vein and IVC clot, systemic lupus erythematosus. **A:** This transverse color Doppler sonogram reveals partial thrombosis of the right renal vein. Note flow in the dorsal portion of the vein (*arrows*). The left renal vein (LRV) is completely thrombosed. **B:** The longitudinal coronal color Doppler sonogram reveals partial inferior vena caval clot (*curved arrow*). A, aorta; Sp, spine; K, right kidney; i, inferior vena cava.

Acute Pyelonephritis

Acute uncomplicated pyelonephritis usually causes no sonographic abnormalities. Findings, when present, include renal enlargement from edema, patchy (Fig. 5.12) or diffuse areas of increased or decreased echogenicity, and blurred corticomedullary junctions. CT is a more sensitive detector of parenchymal abnormalities (10). On occasion, acute pyelonephritis may cause thickening of the collecting system walls visible on sonographic images (Fig. 5.13).

Focal Pyelonephritis, Renal and Perirenal Abscess

Progression of acute pyelonephritis may lead to a series of complications that are stages of a continuum of disease leading to abscess. With progression of pyelonephritis, focally worse infection may occur, variously called focal pyelonephritis, acute bacterial nephritis, or focal lobar nephronia. Focal lesions may become necrotic and form renal abscesses.

Sonography in focal pyelonephritis often reveals localized hypoechoic regions (Fig. 5.14) that may exhibit increased color flow (Fig. 5.15). On occasion, focal pyelonephritis may be echogenic (Fig. 5.16) (12). With further progression, necrosis ensues and an abscess may form (Fig. 5.17). Color flow is absent or nearly absent in an abscess (Fig. 5.18). Sonographically, abscesses cause more mass effect than focal pyelonephritis and tend to deform the contour and normal anatomy of the kidney. Rarely, pyogenic renal abscess may involve adjacent organs or extend outside the perinephric space. This is more common with tuberculosis or xanthogranulomatous pyelonephritis. Abscesses are usually hypoechoic complex masses; anechoic liquefied areas may be identifiable. Occasionally, renal abscesses may be hyperechoic (Fig. 5.19). Focal pyelonephritis and renal abscess, both often hypoechoic with inhomogeneous internal echogenicity, may be difficult or impossible to distinguish. In fact, the distinction is somewhat artificial as both represent part of a continuum of disease. The only way to definitively differentiate abscess from focal pyelonephritis may be to aspirate pus from an abscess.

Subcapsular and perinephric abscesses may occur in conjunction with or independent of renal abscess. Sonographically, these collections are typically hypoechoic with variable internal echogenicity (Figs. 5.20 to 5.23). While CT is more sensitive in detecting these lesions (9,13), meticulous sonography generally detects those abscesses requiring drainage (Fig. 5.24). False positives for perinephric abscess may be caused by perirenal lymphoma (14,15), lymphangiectasia (16), or even hypoechoic perirenal fat (17). Again, CT should be employed in clinically problematic cases. Typically, subcapsular collections are focal and deform the adjacent parenchyma, while perinephric collections are more extensive and produce less mass effect on the kidney. As a practical matter, distinction may be more difficult. The differentiation of subcapsular from perinephric abscess is usually unimportant clinically.

In diabetic patients, renal infection is often more severe and rapidly progressive. Diabetics are more prone to develop more severe focal pyelonephritis, usually called acute bacterial nephritis. Emphysematous pyelonephritis, with gas in the renal parenchyma (Fig. 5.25), occasionally develops in diabetics. It is rare in other patients. Sonography can usually diagnose emphysematous pyelonephritis, but CT is more sensitive in detecting gas within the kidney (18) and in delineating the global extent of disease.

When required, percutaneous drainage is an effective means to treat renal and perirenal abscess (Fig. 5.24). Approximately two-thirds of renal and perirenal abscesses are cured with catheter drainage alone. Percutaneous abscess drainage generally results in clinical improvement even in patients who eventually require surgery (19,20). The subsequent surgical procedure is often simplified by preliminary percutaneous drainage.

Pyonephrosis

Pyonephrosis results from infection of an obstructed kidney, essentially creating an abscess within the renal pelvis and intrarenal collecting system. Sonography is useful both to screen patients with possible pyonephrosis and to guide emergency therapeutic percutaneous nephrostomy. Pyonephrosis may be difficult to diagnose. Some patients have a debris-filled dilated collecting system (Figs. 5.26 and 5.27). Unfortunately, pyonephrosis, particularly in patients with distal obstruction, may lack pelvicaliceal debris and be sonographically indistinguishable from bland hydronephrosis (Fig. 5.28) (21). In diabetics, emphysematous pyonephrosis (gas within the collecting system) occasionally occurs.

Chronic Pyelonephritis

Chronic pyelonephritis results from multiple acute infections. Although focal atrophic scarring is usual, cortical loss may be diffuse, resulting in a small echogenic kidney similar to kidneys found in end-stage renal parenchymal disease. Chronic atrophic pyelonephritis may also cause renal sinus lipomatosis. The sonographic diagnosis of chronic pyelonephritis usually depends on detecting cortical loss adjacent to renal pyramids (Figs. 5.29 and 5.30). Renal lobation (fetal lobulation) is associated with cortical indentation between medullary pyramids (Fig. 5.31). Pyelonephritis-related scar generally causes cortical loss that is adjacent to the pyramids. Cor-

(text continues on page 296)

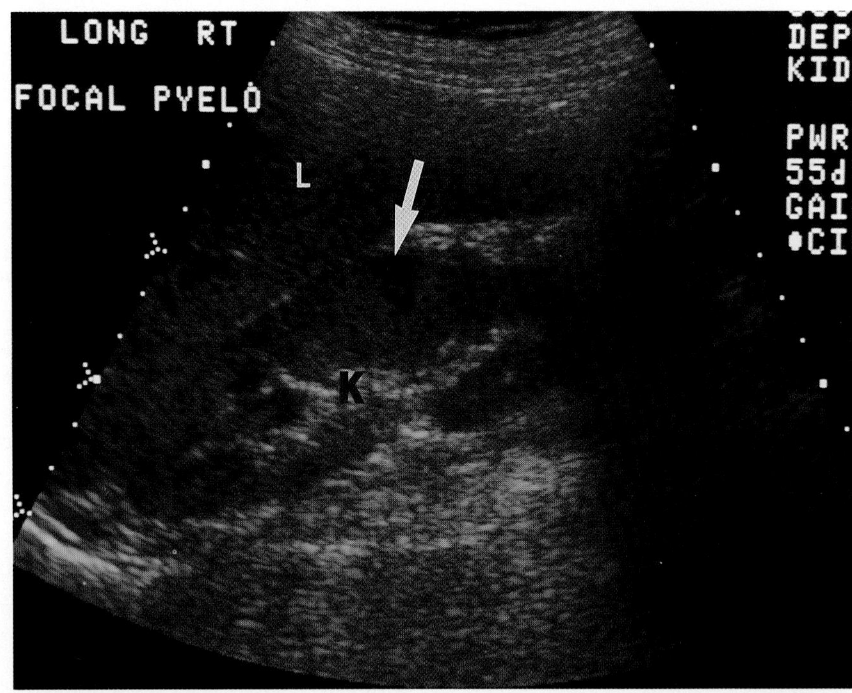

FIG. 5.12. Focal pyelonephritis. Longitudinal false color sonogram of the right kidney (K) reveals a small triangular shaped hypoechoic area (*arrow*) that represents an area of focal pyelonephritis. In most instances, uncomplicated acute pyelonephritis causes no sonographic abnormality. L, liver.

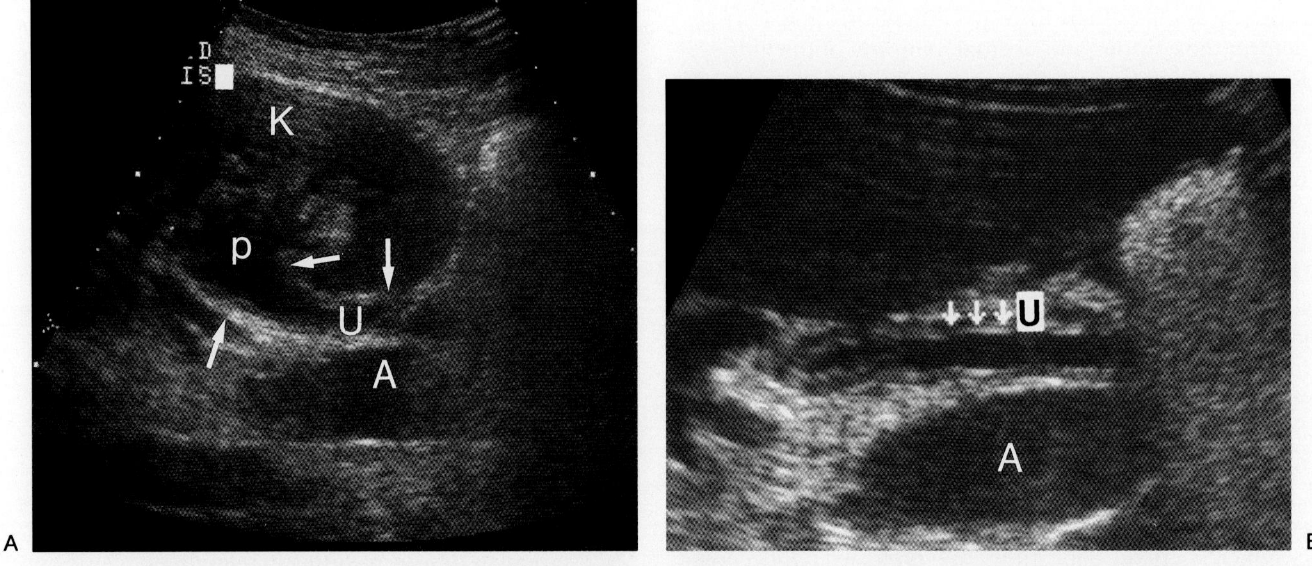

FIG. 5.13. Acute pyelonephritis, thickened collecting system walls. **A:** Longitudinal coronal sonogram of the left kidney reveals mucosal thickening (*arrows*) related to acute pyelonephritis. **B:** A magnified longitudinal coronal sonogram of the proximal left ureter reveals similar findings (*arrows,* U). Thickening of the mucosa in acute pyelonephritis is an uncommon finding. The diffuse nature of the thickening in an appropriate clinical setting should suggest the diagnosis. P, renal pelvis; K, left kidney; U, ureter; A, aorta.

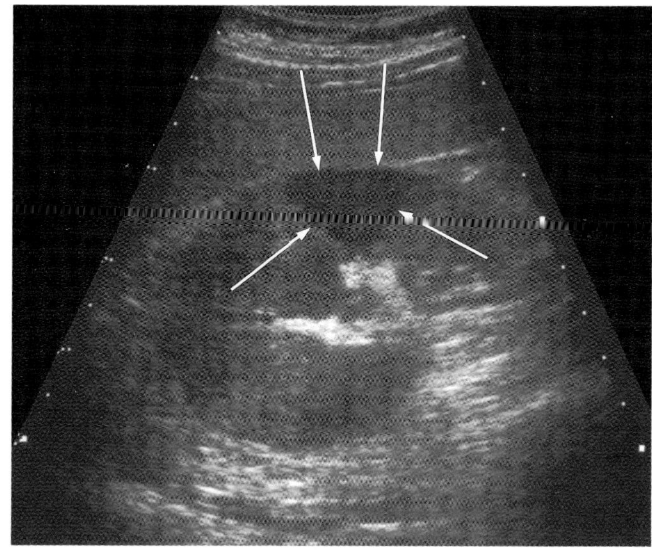

FIG. 5.14. Focal pyelonephritis. Transverse sonogram of the right kidney. A triangular shaped hypoechoic region (*thin arrows*) is noted in the ventral portion of the right kidney. This is a triangular area of focal pyelonephritis. Note that the morphology of the kidney is not altered, a finding that suggests focal pyelonephritis rather than abscess.

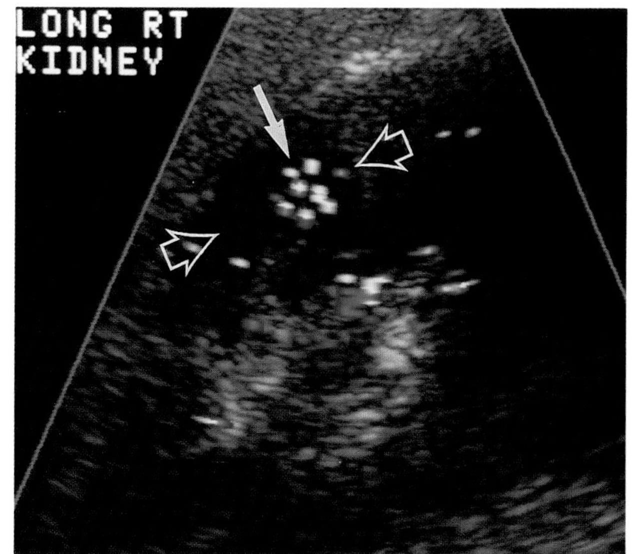

A

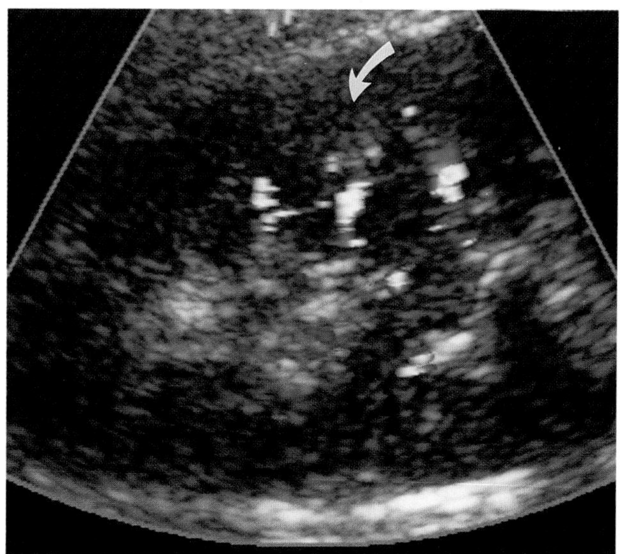

B

FIG. 5.15. Focal pyelonephritis, increased color flow. **A:** A longitudinal color Doppler sonogram of the right kidney reveals increased flow (*arrow*) within an area of decreased echogenicity (*open arrows*). This is an example of increased flow in an area of focal pyelonephritis (hypoechoic area). **B:** A repeat color Doppler sonogram after 3 days of antibiotic therapy reveals normal flow and normal renal parenchymal echo texture (*curved arrow*). Not all patients with focal pyelonephritis exhibit increased flow on color flow sonograms. Color Doppler findings depend on the stage of disease and individual host response. For example, renal abscesses typically have little or no internal flow.

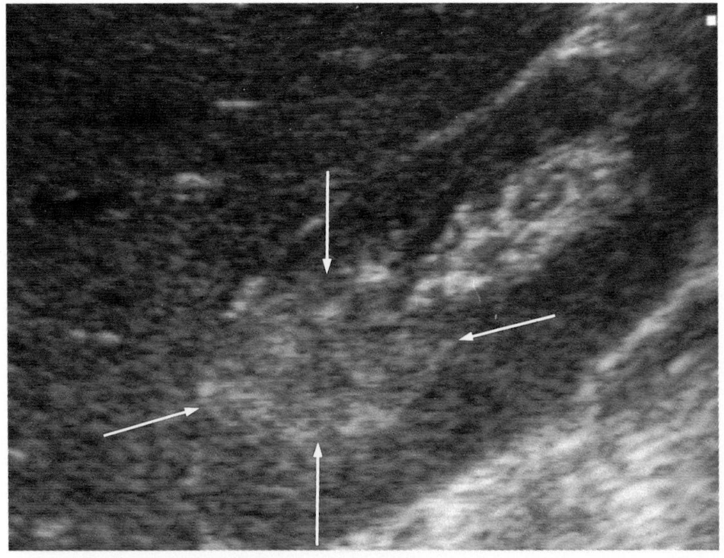

FIG. 5.16. Echogenic focal pyelonephritis. Longitudinal sonogram of the right kidney. An ill-defined area of increased echogenicity in the upper pole of the right kidney (*thin arrows*) is noted in this patient with acute focal pyelonephritis. After antibiotic therapy, this kidney returned to a normal appearance. Most patients with acute pyelonephritis have no sonographic abnormality. When focal abnormalities are present, they are generally hypoechoic. On occasion, hyperechoic abnormalities such as this may be encountered. Note that the contour of the kidney is unaltered. Abscesses generally produce a mass that distorts the kidney.

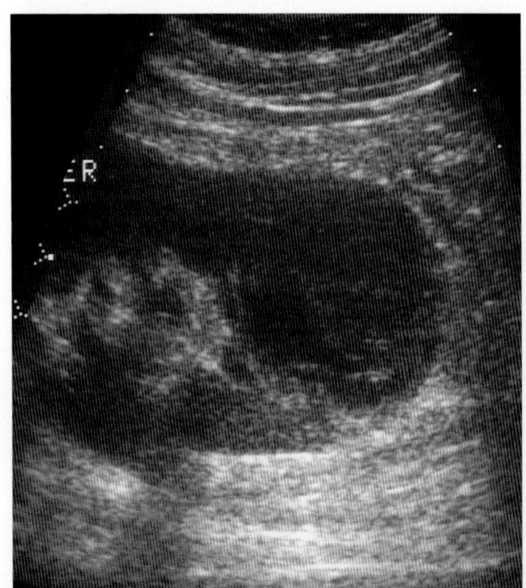

A

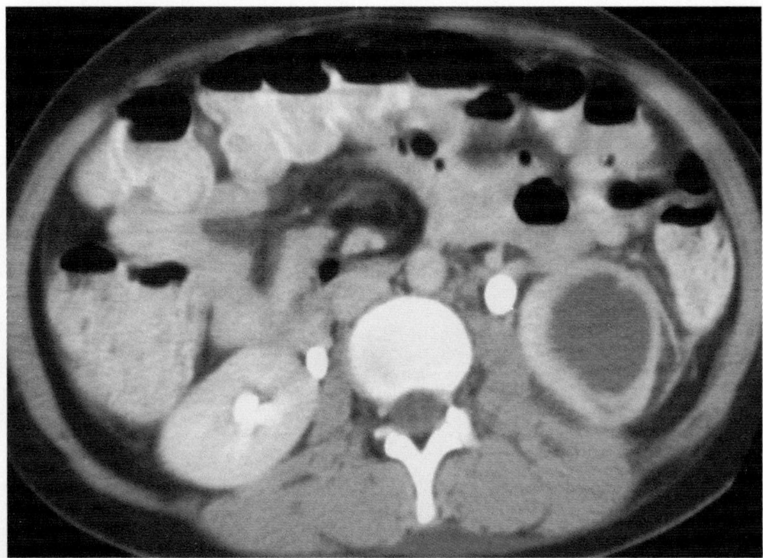

B

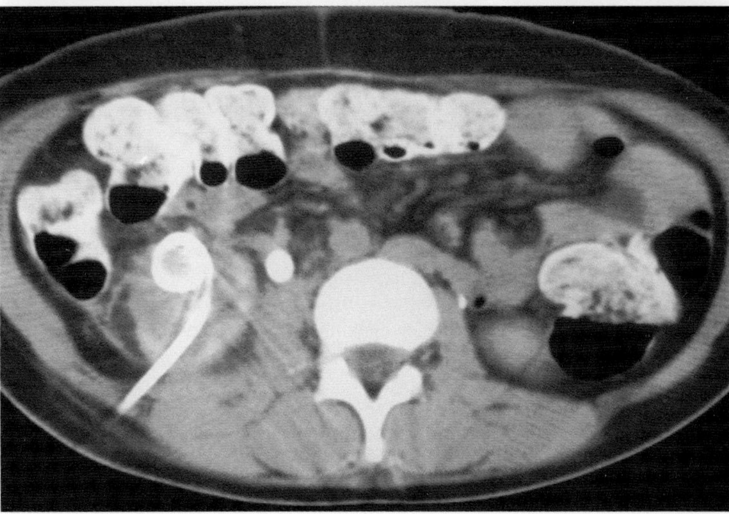

C

FIG. 5.17. Renal abscess, drained percutaneously. **A:** A longitudinal sonogram of the left kidney reveals a mixed echogenicity mass that deforms the shape of the kidney. In the appropriate clinical setting, these findings suggest renal abscess. Focal pyelonephritis or acute bacterial nephritis rarely cause significant anatomic distortion. Internally, the characteristics of abscesses and focal pyelonephritis may be indistinguishable. **B:** The presence of the abscess is confirmed on the CT scan. **C:** The abscess was subsequently drained percutaneously. Percutaneous drainage of renal and perirenal abscesses is an effective means of therapy.

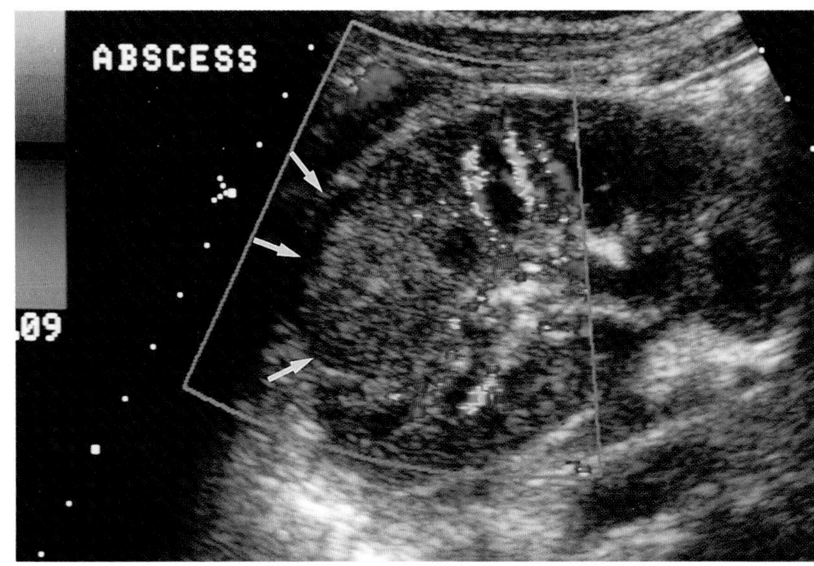

FIG. 5.18. Renal abscess. Longitudinal color Doppler sonogram reveals a slightly hyperechoic renal abscess that deforms the renal contour (*small arrows*). Very little flow is noted within this renal abscess. Absence of flow suggests renal abscess, rather than focal pyelonephritis. In instances where doubt persists, percutaneous aspiration may be required.

A
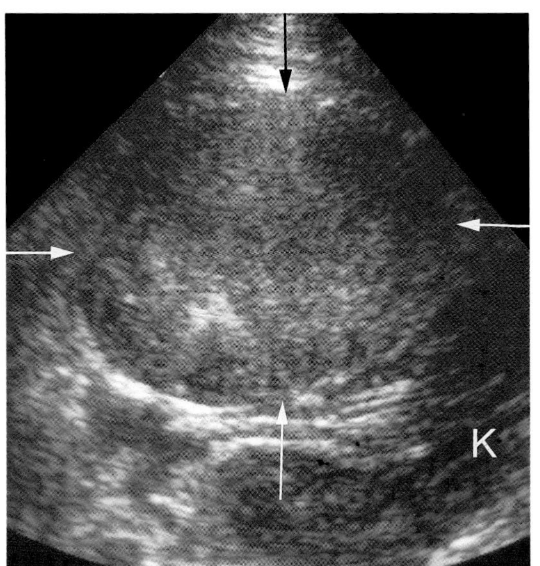

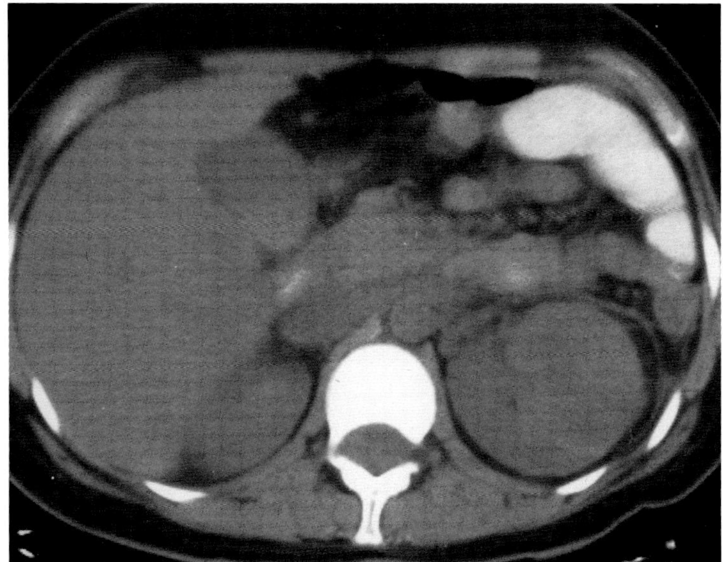
B

C
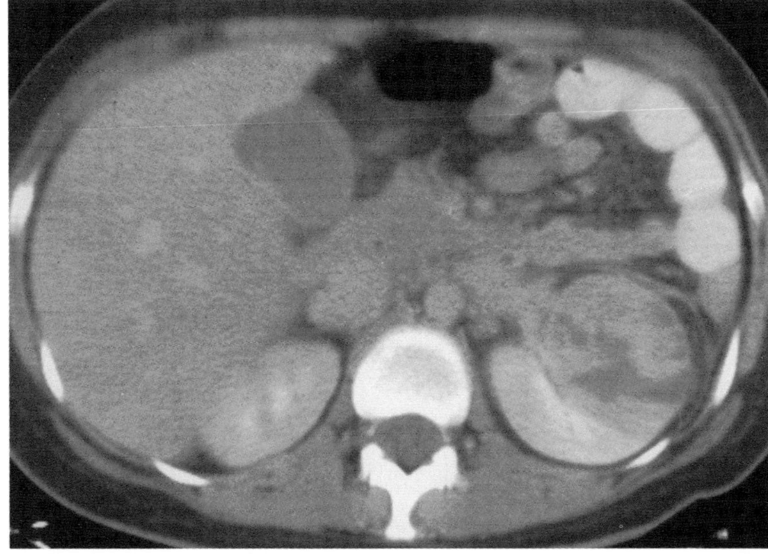

FIG. 5.19. Echogenic renal abscess. **A:** Transverse sonogram of the left kidney reveals a renal abscess (*arrows*) that is increased in echogenicity compared to the normal renal parenchyma (K). **B:** A transverse nonintravenous contrast-enhanced CT demonstrates higher attenuation within the mass, suggesting the possibility of intralesional hemorrhage. **C:** Contrast-enhanced CT shows a mixed attenuation mass that enhances more poorly than the normal parenchyma.

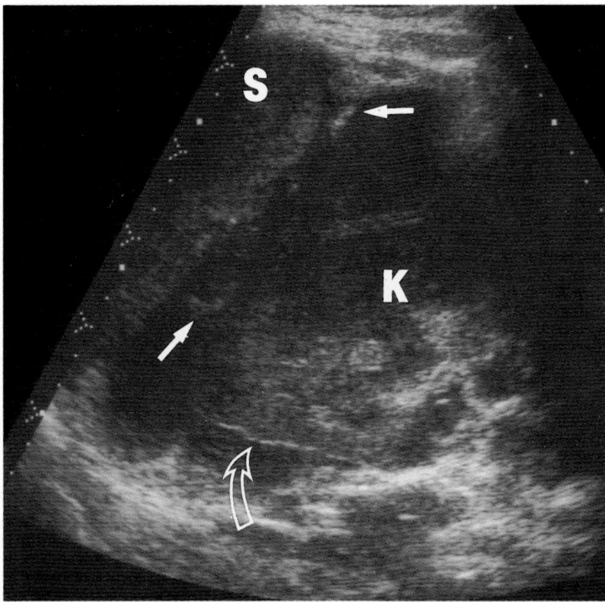

FIG. 5.20. Perinephric abscess. Longitudinal oblique sonogram of the left kidney and perirenal area. This large, ill-defined perinephric abscess slightly deforms the contour of the left kidney (K) (*open curved arrow*). Note the echogenic material within the abscess (*arrows*). S, spleen.

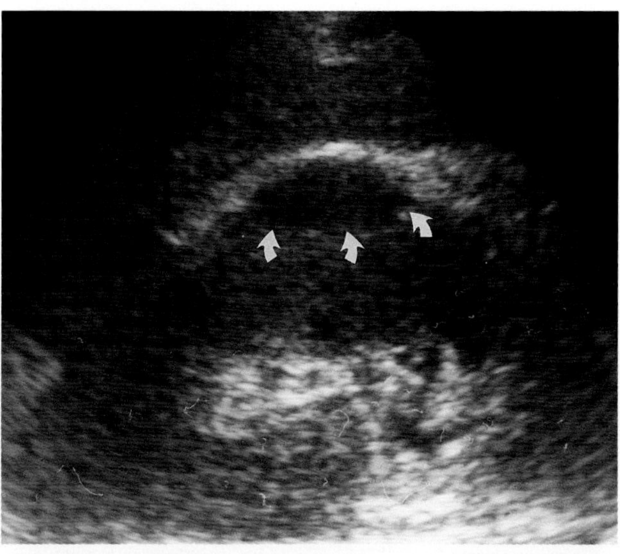

FIG. 5.21. Small perinephric abscess. Longitudinal coronal sonogram of the left kidney. This small abscess proved to be within the perinephric space at surgery. The relatively focal nature and significant displacement of the renal parenchyma (*small curved arrows*) suggested a subcapsular abscess. Differentiation of subcapsular and perinephric abscesses may be impossible based on image findings alone. Differentiation is usually clinically unimportant and rarely, if ever, affects management (surgery or percutaneous abscess drainage).

A

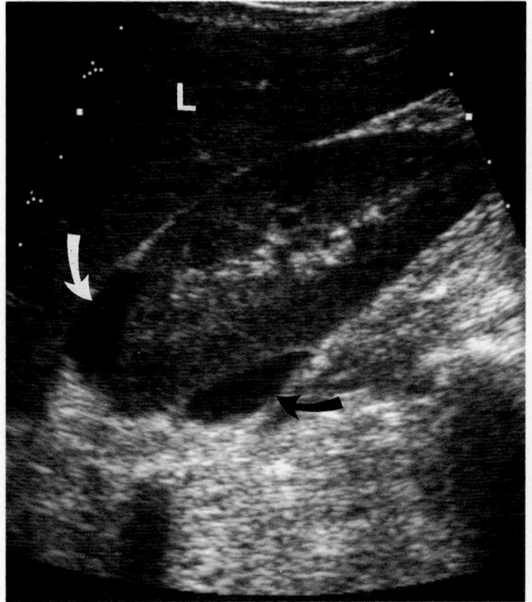

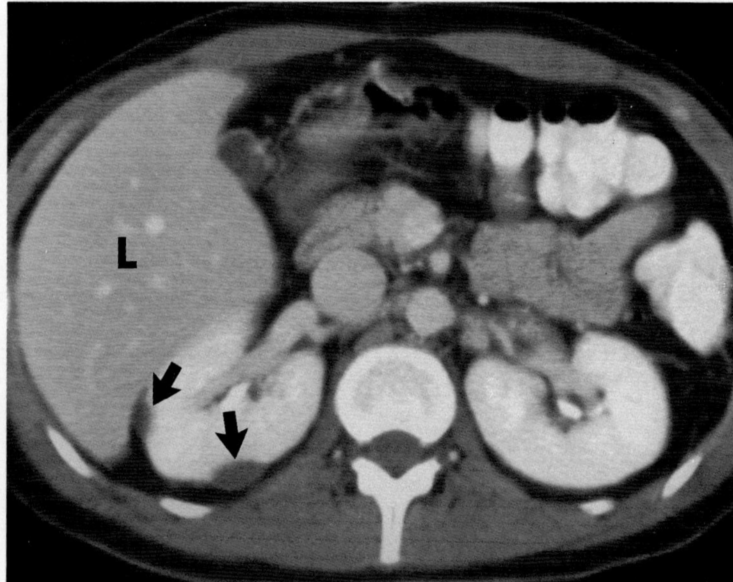

B

FIG. 5.22. Subcapsular abscess. **A:** Longitudinal sonogram reveals two small subcapsular abscesses (*curved arrows*). There is relatively little parenchymal deformity. Only a few internal echoes are present. **B:** The CT scan confirms the subcapsular location of the abscesses (*arrows*). L, liver.

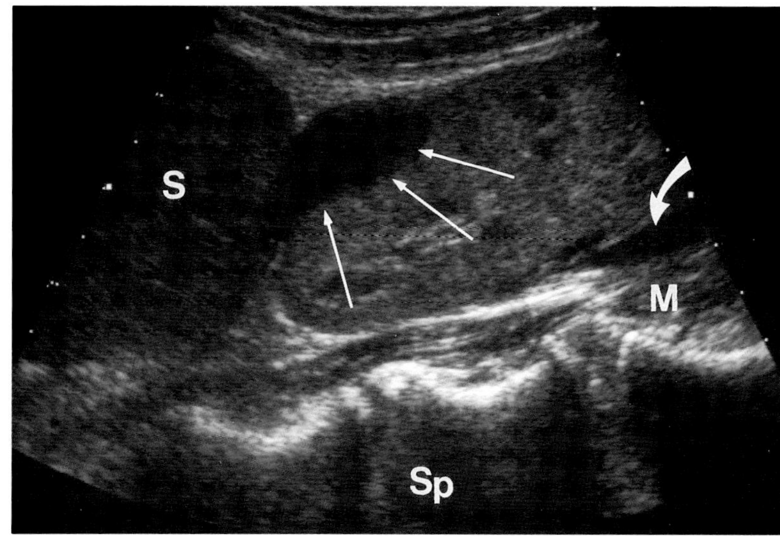

FIG. 5.23. Perinephric abscess. Longitudinal sonogram of the left kidney reveals an abscess in the perinephric space, even though there is significant deformity of the upper pole of the kidney (*small arrows*). The abscess was drained surgically. There are relatively few echoes inside the abscess. Note the abscess adjacent to the lower pole (*curved arrow*). Sp, spine; S, spleen; M, psoas muscle.

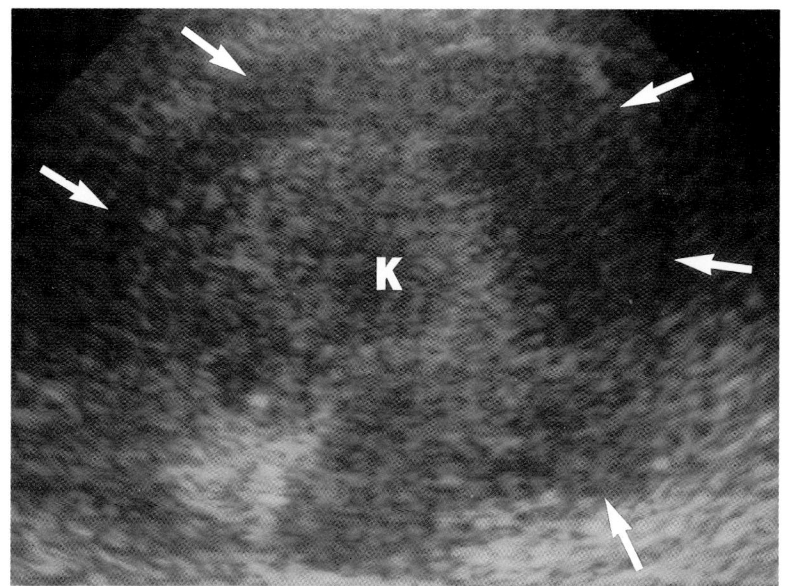

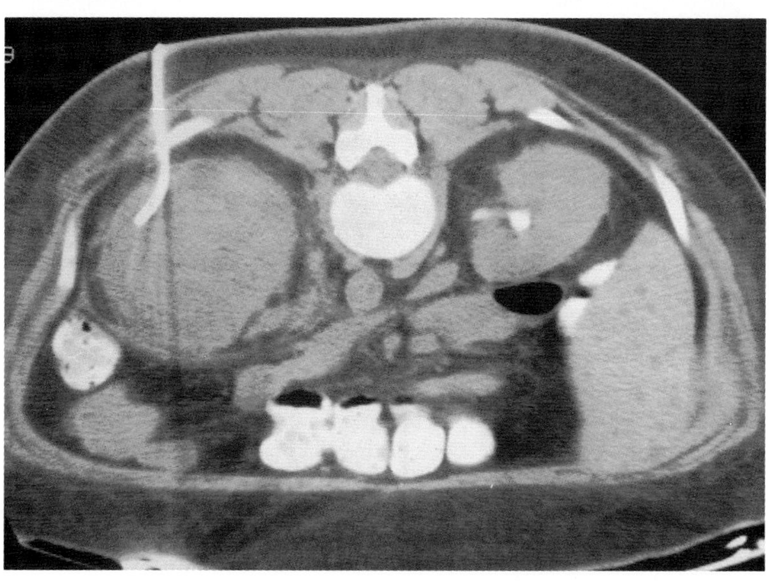

FIG. 5.24. Perinephric abscess, percutaneously drained. **A:** Transverse sonogram of the lower pole of the kidney reveals an ill-defined, echo-containing collection (*arrows*) around the lower pole of the left kidney (K). Even though this was a difficult sonogram in an obese diabetic patient, the perinephric abscess was detected. **B:** Under CT guidance, a percutaneous drain was placed. While CT is more sensitive in detecting renal and perirenal inflammatory abnormalities, careful sonography detects virtually all lesions, such as this perinephric abscess, that require intervention. For this reason, sonography can be used to screen patients for infectious complications of urinary tract disease.

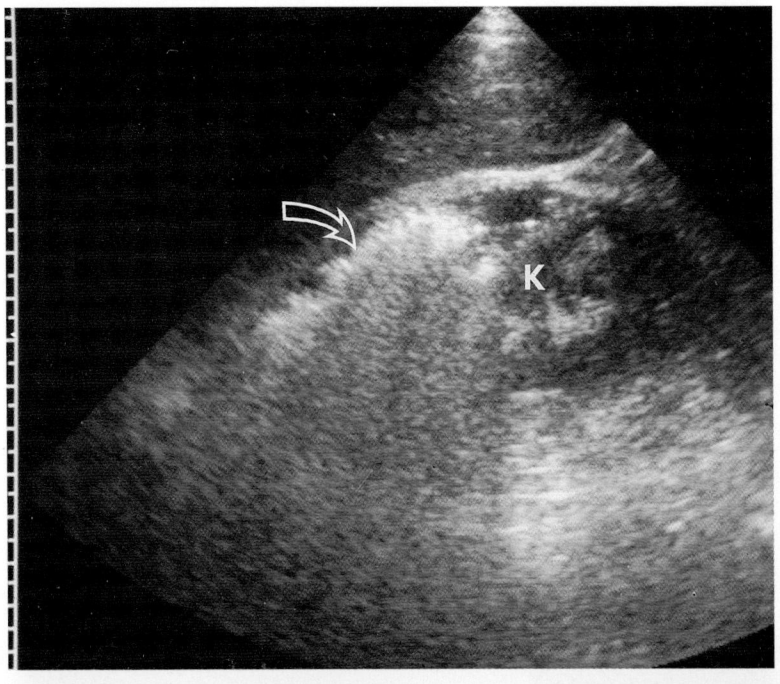

A

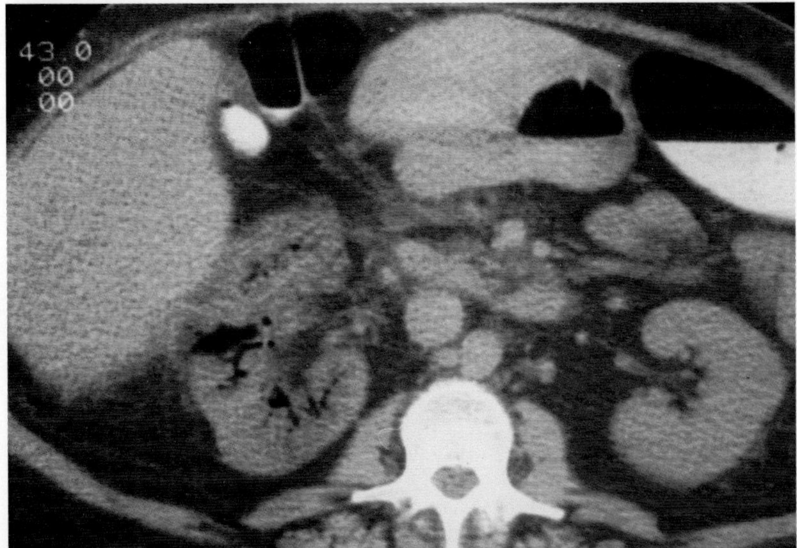

B

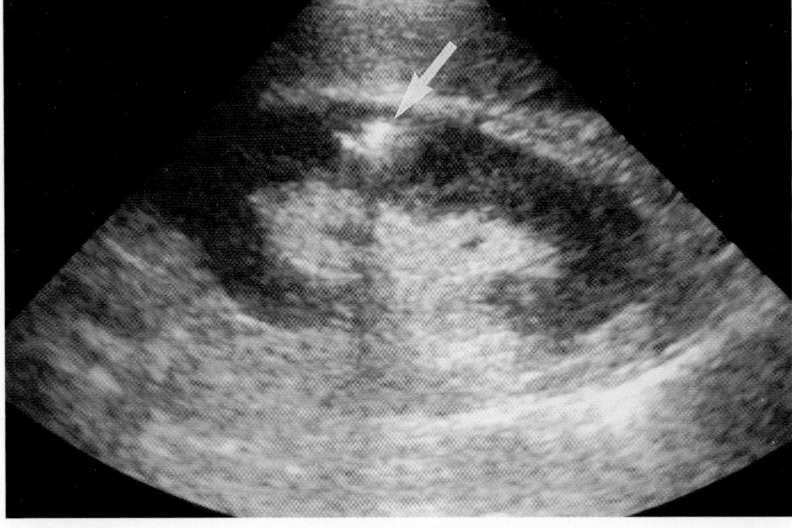

C

FIG. 5.25. Emphysematous pyelonephritis. **A:** Longitudinal sonogram reveals gas within the renal parenchyma (*open arrow*). **B:** The CT scan shows gas throughout much of the renal parenchyma. CT is generally a more sensitive means of detecting gas within the renal parenchyma, a prerequisite for the diagnosis of emphysematous pyelonephritis. K, right kidney. **C:** A follow-up longitudinal coronal sonogram performed 2 weeks later after therapy with intravenous antibiotics reveals improvement, although there is still some gas (*arrow*) within the renal cortex. (From ref. 17a, with permission.)

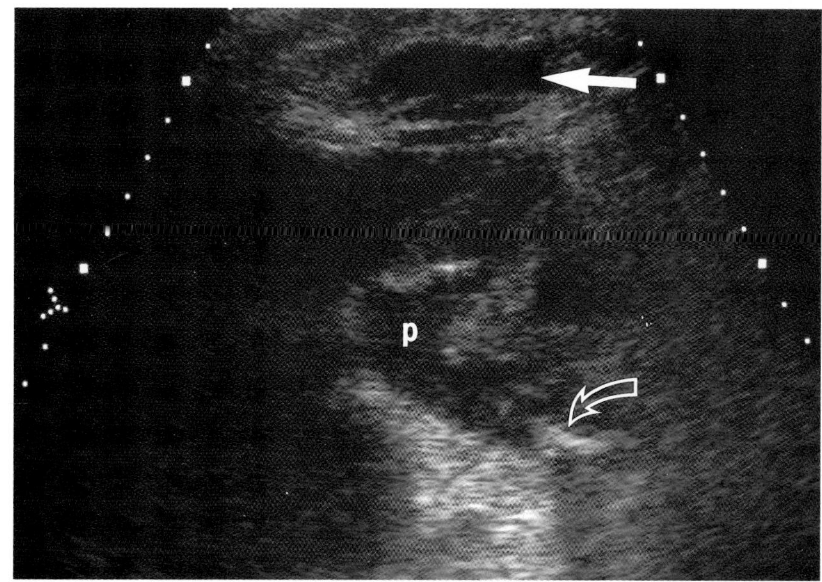

A

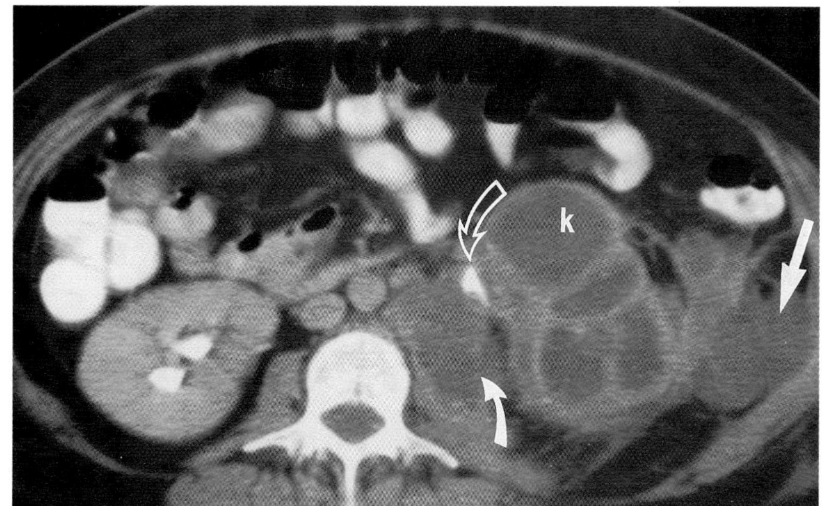

B

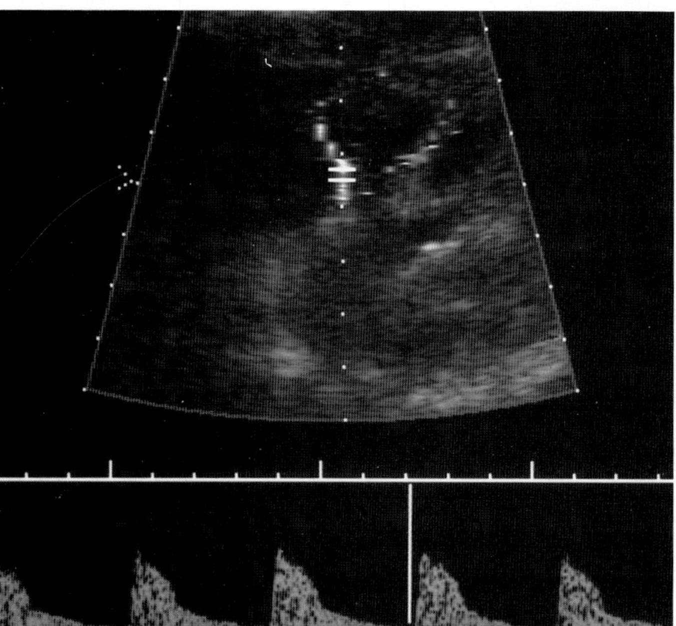

C

FIG. 5.26. Pyonephrosis, obstructing stone, flank and psoas abscess. **A:** Coronal longitudinal oblique sonogram of the left kidney reveals an obstructing calculus (*curved open arrow*) near the ureteropelvic junction (UPJ). Note the proximal dilatation of the pelvicaliceal system (p) and the internal echoes within it. These findings suggest pyonephrosis in this patient with symptoms of urosepsis. Note the more peripheral flank abscess (*arrow*). **B:** A CT scan shows the obstructing calculus (*open curved arrow*), the obstructed pyonephrotic kidney (k), as well as the flank (*arrow*) and psoas (*curved arrow*) abscesses. **C:** A color Doppler guided spectral Doppler sonogram reveals elevated peripheral resistance (RI = 0.96). The elevated peripheral resistance may have been related to the UPJ obstruction or,alternatively, related to the increased intracapsular renal pressure from the pyonephrosis. This patient required a nephrectomy.

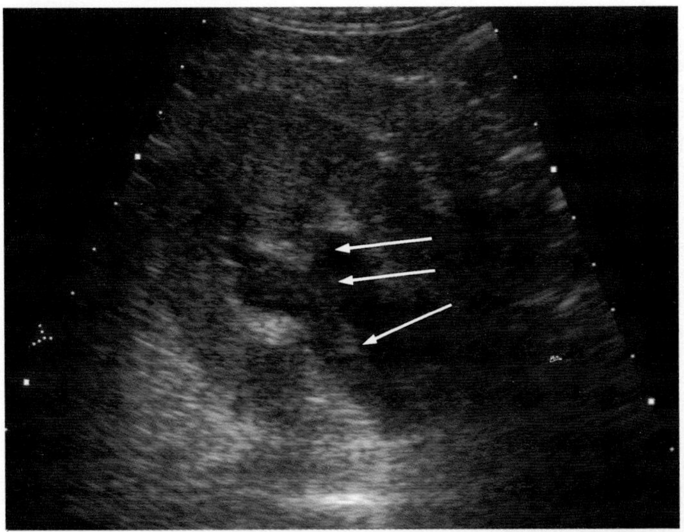

FIG. 5.27. Fungal pyonephrosis. Transverse coronal sonogram of the left kidney reveals debris within the dilated collecting system (*arrows*). This patient has fungal pyonephrosis. Not all patients with pyonephrosis have imageable echoes within the collecting system. If no echoes are present, it may be difficult to differentiate pyonephrosis from plain hydronephrosis.

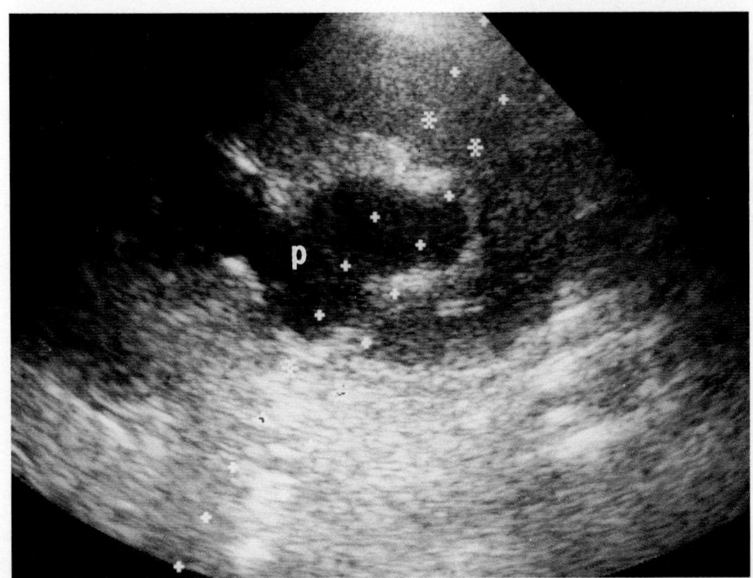

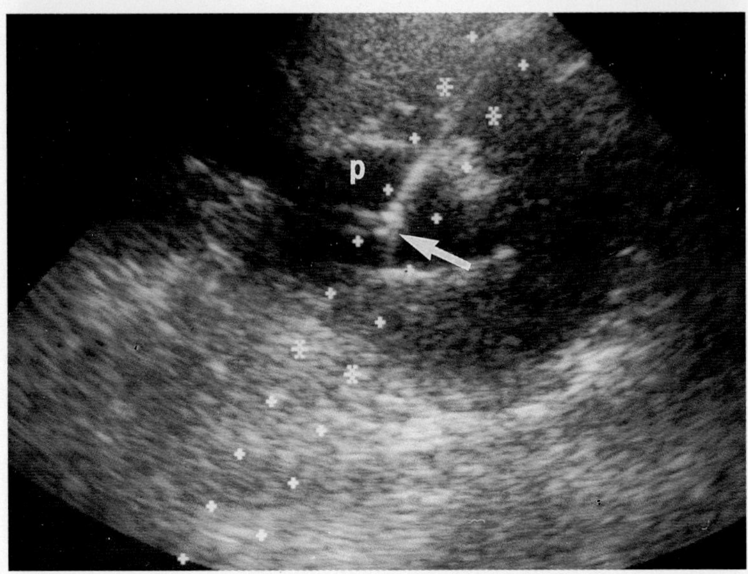

FIG. 5.28. Pyonephrosis, anechoic collecting system. **A:** Longitudinal sonogram in this patient with pyonephrosis reveals no obvious debris or internal echoes within the pelvicaliceal system (p). Note the cursors used to guide percutaneous aspiration. **B:** The presence of pyonephrosis was confirmed by aspiration. This patient had a distal obstructing ureteral stone. When patients with pyonephrosis have few or no echoes within the collecting system, as is noted here, it may difficult to diagnose pyonephrosis from the sonographic images alone. Note the needle tip (*arrow*). (From ref. 17a, with permission.)

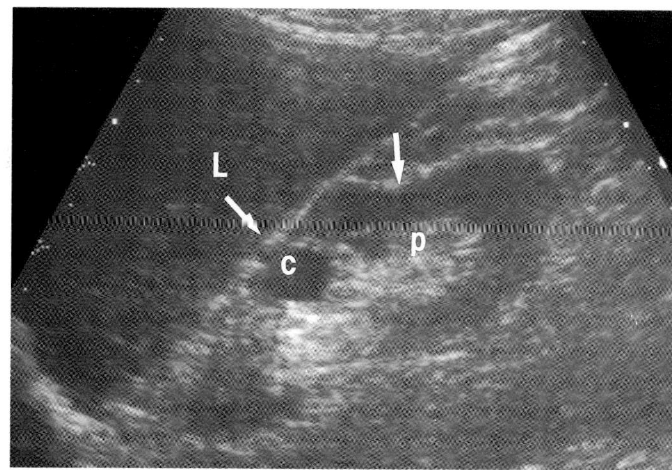

FIG. 5.29. Cortical scarring, chronic pyelonephritis. Longitudinal sonogram of the right kidney reveals several areas of cortical scarring (*arrows*) related to previous infection. Note how the scar is adjacent to the renal pyramid (p). A small cyst (c) is present. L, liver.

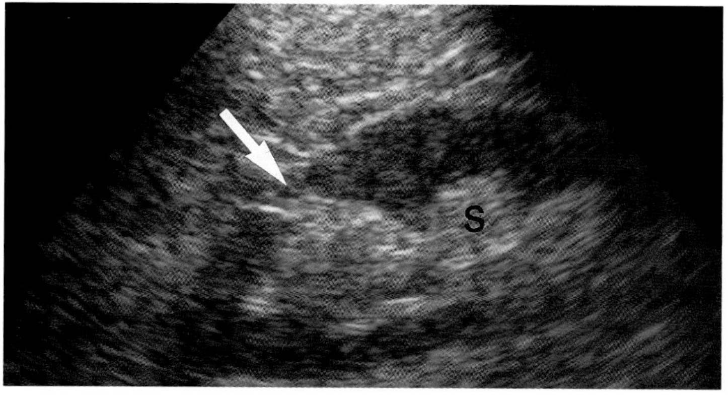

A

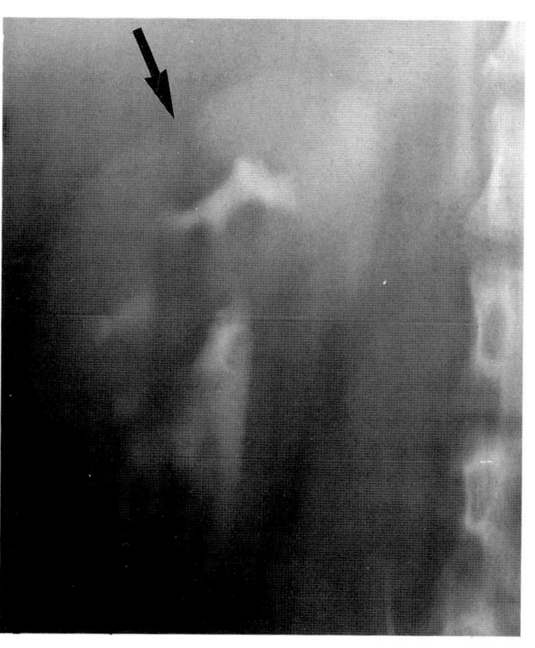

B

FIG. 5.30. Focal scar, previous pyelonephritis. **A:** A longitudinal sonogram of the right kidney reveals an area of focal scarring that is filled with echogenic fat (*arrow*) and continuous with the renal sinus (S). **B:** This same region is identified on the nephrotomogram. Fatty replacement of lost cortical tissue is unusual. Usually, atrophy, as noted in Fig. 5.29, results. This patient had a history of a single previous episode of right-sided pyelonephritis.

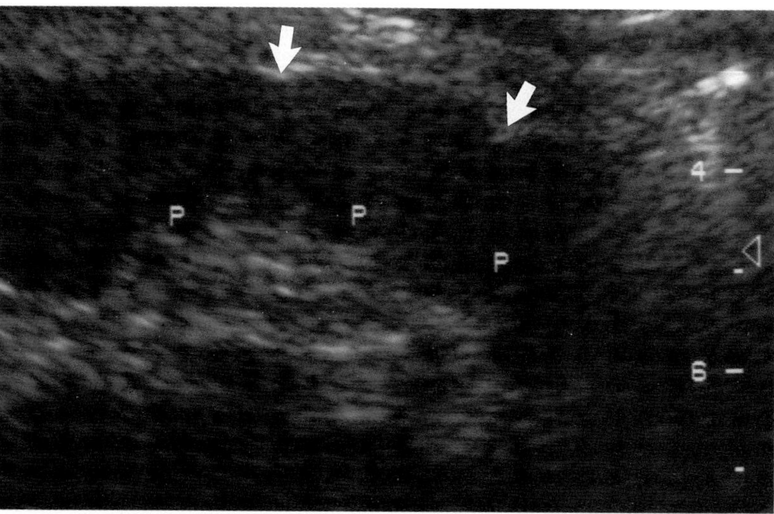

FIG. 5.31. Renal lobation (fetal lobulation). Longitudinal sonogram of the left kidney reveals prominent renal lobation (*arrows*). Note that the cortical indentation is between the medullary pyramids (P). This anatomic location allows distinction of fetal lobulation from infection-related scar. Pyelonephritis-associated scars cause indentation over or adjacent to the pyramids, not between them.

tical scarring is usually more easily detected and more readily distinguished from fetal lobation with urography (22) or CT than sonography.

Xanthogranulomatous Pyelonephritis

Xanthogranulomatous pyelonephritis (XGP) is a subtype of chronic renal infection associated with calculi and obstruction. Renal parenchyma is destroyed and replaced by lipid-filled macrophages. Sonographically, the kidney is usually enlarged and contains multiple hypoechoic and anechoic areas (Figs. 5.32 to 5.34). XGP may cause diffuse or focal enlargement of the kidney. Stones (including staghorn and other large calculi) and dilated collecting systems filled with echogenic debris are frequent (Fig. 5.35) (23). Extension of XGP outside the kidney is common. Retrofascial invasion into the psoas muscle, flank (Fig. 5.36), or even into the gastrointestinal tract may occur. Because of these unusual features, XGP can mimmic other diseases including tuberculosis or neoplasm.

While sonographic findings may suggest the diagnosis of XGP, CT often is more specific. Xanthogranulomatous pyelonephritis may be difficult to distinguish from pyonephrosis, although clinical differentiation is usually easy. Contrast CT reveals necrotic lower attenuation within the kidney, collecting system, and perirenal spaces. CT is also superior in delineating extrarenal involvement. Differentiation of XGP from tuberculosis, which is also characterized by calcifications, low attenuation areas, and dilated collecting systems, may prove difficult both clinically and radiographically (Figs. 5.35 and 5.37).

Renal Tuberculosis (TB)

Sonography is much less sensitive than urography or CT to the early changes caused by renal tuberculosis—subtle caliceal, infundibulopelvic, and ureteral abnormalities. Sonography is also less sensitive in detecting the calcifications often found in renal TB. In addition, it is difficult or impossible for sonography to demonstrate the relationship of caliceal inflammatory masses proximal to an obstructed infundibulum and the more distal collecting system (24).

Sonographically, focal tuberculous lesions may be hypoechoic or echogenic. Sonography in patients with early tuberculosis is normal in about 80 percent of patients (25). Tuberculous lesions may be indistinguishable from XGP (Fig. 5.37), acute focal pyelonephritis, pyogenic abscess, and other conditions. Sonographically guided needle aspiration cytology can facilitate early diagnosis, without having to wait weeks for culture (26).

RENAL CYSTIC DISEASE

Simple renal cysts are benign lesions that occur more frequently with increasing age. Approximately half of individuals older than 50 years have renal cysts. Simple renal cysts are found only in a small percentage of children (27,28). Sonographic criteria for simple renal cysts include a clearly defined thin or imperceptible cyst wall, no internal echos, and increased through transmission of sound (Figs. 5.38 and 5.39). Simple cysts may have thin septations or a lobulated shape (Fig. 5.40). If criteria for a simple cyst are met, no further evaluation is required.

Cysts that are atypical on either sonography or CT should generally be evaluated with the other modality. Cysts that do not fulfill classic criteria are more frequent on sonographic examination than on CT scans. Simple cysts that appear atypical on sonograms may have internal echogenicity caused by debris or artifact (Fig. 5.41); they may lack through transmission of sound. Cyst wall calcifications are not rare. About 20 percent of cysts with calcification harbor malignancy, usually renal cell carcinoma. While fine wall calcification is almost always benign (Fig. 5.42), all calcified cysts should be evaluated with CT to exclude malignancy. Thin septations are frequent in simple cysts. Thick or irregular/nodular septations should suggest neoplasm; such a lesion should be removed. High attenuation within cysts on CT is usually caused by intracystic hemorrhage. These hemorrhagic cysts may fulfill sonographic criteria for simple cyst (Fig. 5.43). Rarely, simple renal cysts become infected (Fig. 5.44) or cause obstruction. When definitive diagnostic criteria for simple cyst cannot be demonstrated on either CT or sonography, cyst aspiration or resection may be required.

Most simple renal cysts are cortical and do not communicate with the collecting system. Parapelvic cysts may be single or multiple and are sometimes confused on sonograms for hydronephrosis (Fig. 5.45) (29–32). Care must be taken to identify the renal pelvis if parapelvic cysts are to be distinguished from hydronephrosis sonographically. Either contrast-enhanced CT or intravenous urography can clearly delineate the pelvicaliceal structures and facilitate differentation of hydronephrosis from parapelvic cysts.

Cystic structures that arise from the renal collecting system (most frequently a caliceal diverticulum) may have an ultrasound appearance identical to that of simple cysts (Fig. 5.46) (33). Again, excretory urography or CT can facilitate this distinction when required clinically.

Discovery of several simple cysts in a child or young adult should suggest the possibility of a syndrome such as renal polycystic kidney disease, von Hippel–Lindau disease, or Turner's syndrome. Von Hippel–Lindau disease is associated with a higher risk for renal cell carci-

(*text continues on page 306*)

A 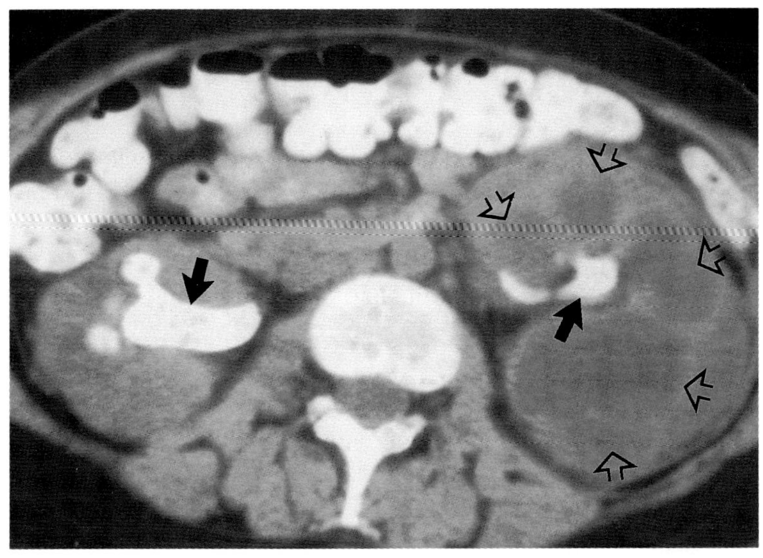

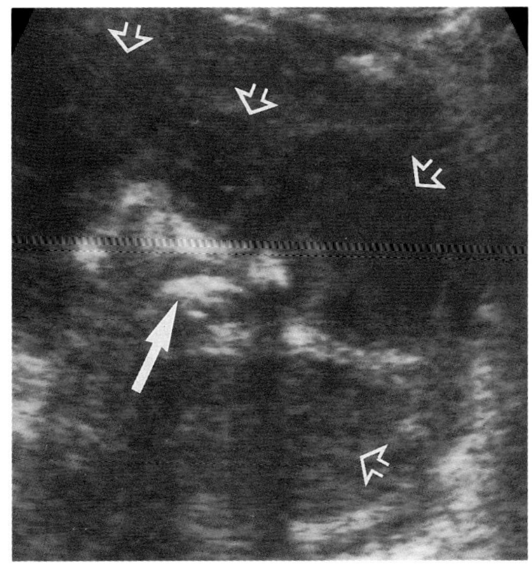 B

C 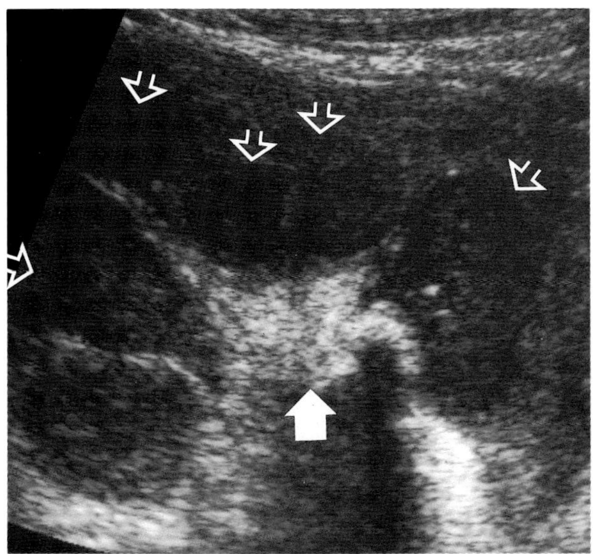

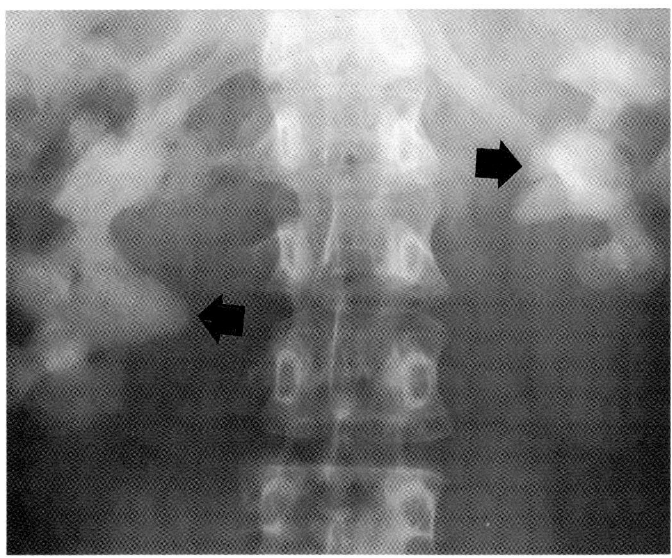 D

E 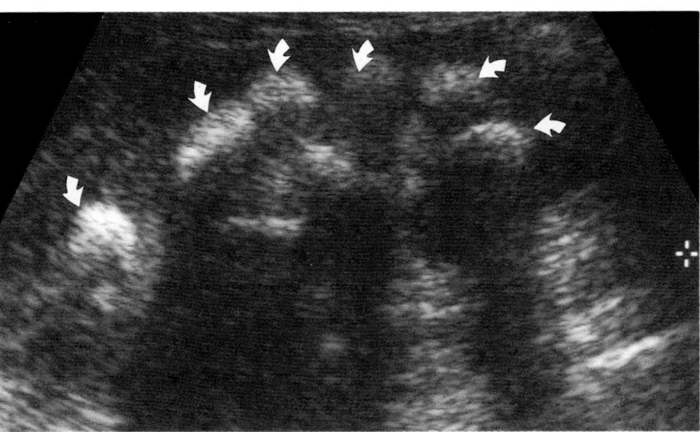

FIG. 5.32. Xanthogranulomatous pyelonephritis, staghorn calculus. The CT scan (**A**) reveals bilateral staghorn calculi (*arrows*). Left-sided xanthogranulomatous pyelonephritis is present. Note the dilated medium attenuation collecting system elements (*open arrows*). Coronal transverse (**B**) and coronal longitudinal (**C**) sonograms reveal similar findings. Note the obstructing calculus in the renal pelvis (*arrow*). The debris-filled dilated caliceal elements (*open arrows*) are clearly delineated. A plain radiograph (**D**) of the upper abdomen clearly depicts the staghorn calculi bilaterally (*arrows*). A longitudinal coronal sonogram (**E**) through the left kidney also reveals the caliceal components of the staghorn calculi (*arrows*). Note that sonography often tends to underestimate stone burden compared to plain radiographs. Staghorn calculi such as this are commonly found in patients with xanthogranulomatous pyelonephritis.

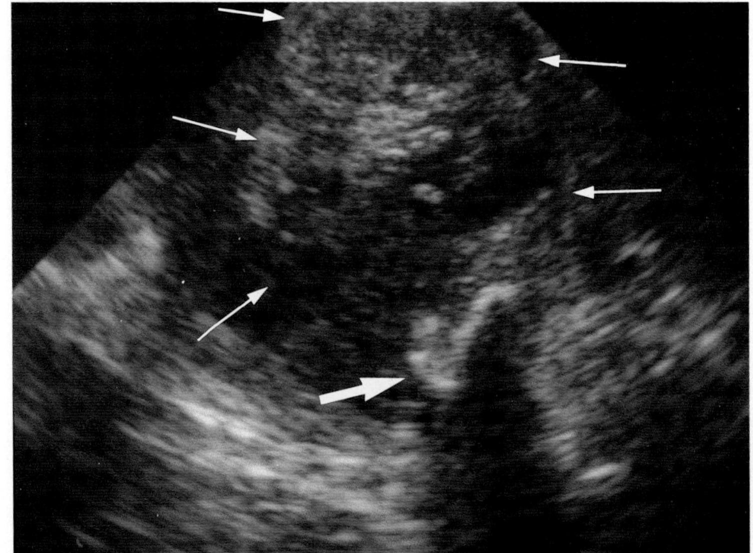

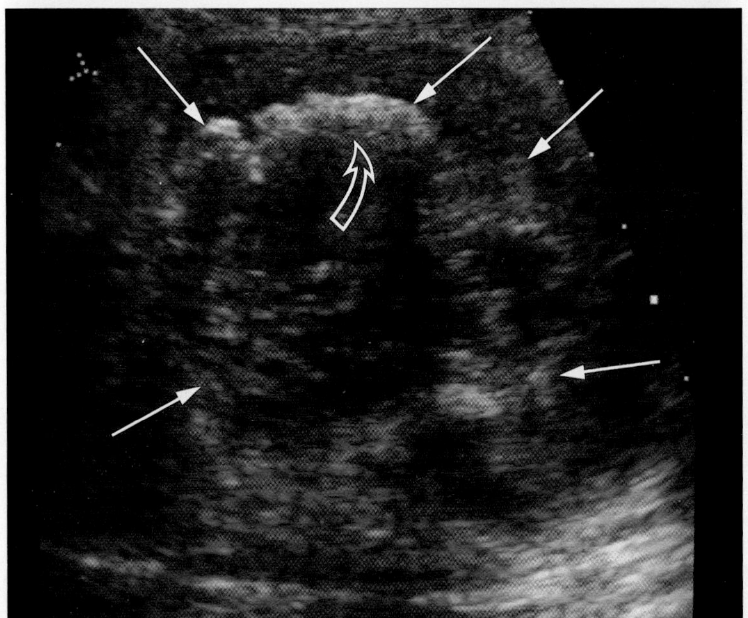

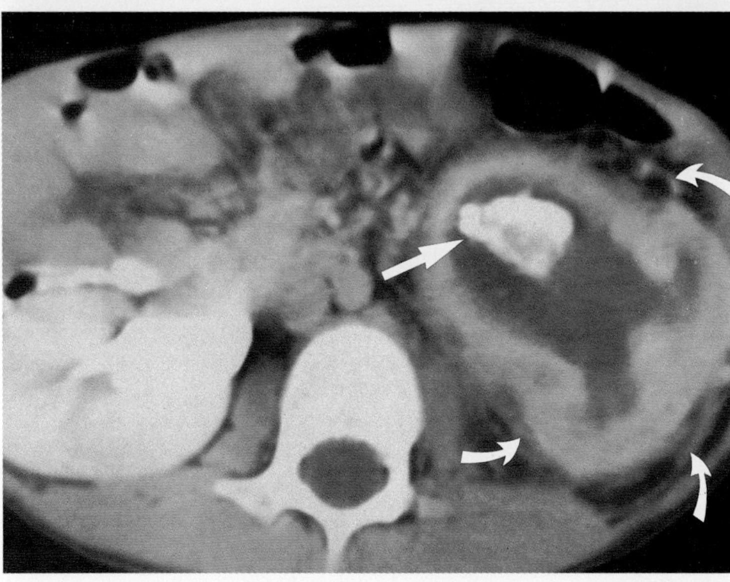

FIG. 5.33. Xanthogranulomatous pyelonephritis. **A:** Longitudinal coronal sonogram of the left kidney reveals a renal pelvic calculus (*arrow*) that causes obstruction and hydronephrosis. Note the dilated collecting system (*thin arrows*) that is filled with heterogeneous echogenicity debris. **B:** A transverse sonogram also reveals a dilated debris-filled collecting system. A large amount of echogenic debris (*open curved arrow*) is present. **C:** A CT scan also shows the large ureteropelvic junction calculus (*arrow*) and the dilated debris-filled collecting system. Note that there is some perinephric abnormality (*curved arrows*), shown to better advantage by CT than sonography. All the features of xanthogranulomatous pyelonephritis are shown in this patient—large calculi, a dilated debris-filled collecting system, abnormal renal parenchyma, and perinephric abnormality.

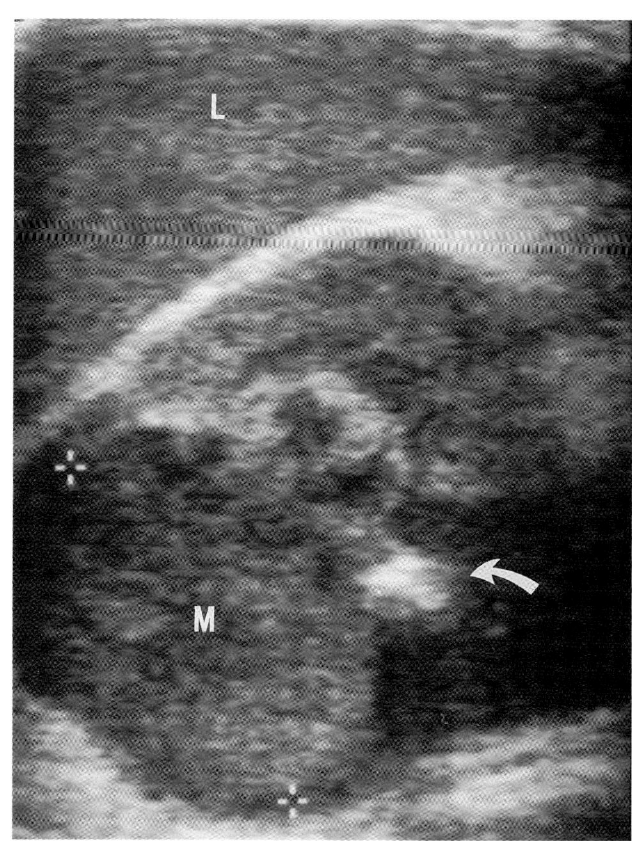

FIG. 5.34. Xanthogranulomatous pyelonephritis. Transverse sonogram of the right kidney reveals a central renal calculus (*curved arrow*). Lateral to the stone is a medium echogenicity mass (mass—m, calipers) that replaces much of the kidney. Some mixed echogenicity debris is seen in the renal sinus, ventral to the stone and the mass. L, liver. Xanthogranulomatous pyelonephritis can cause masses, such as the one seen here, that may simulate neoplasm.

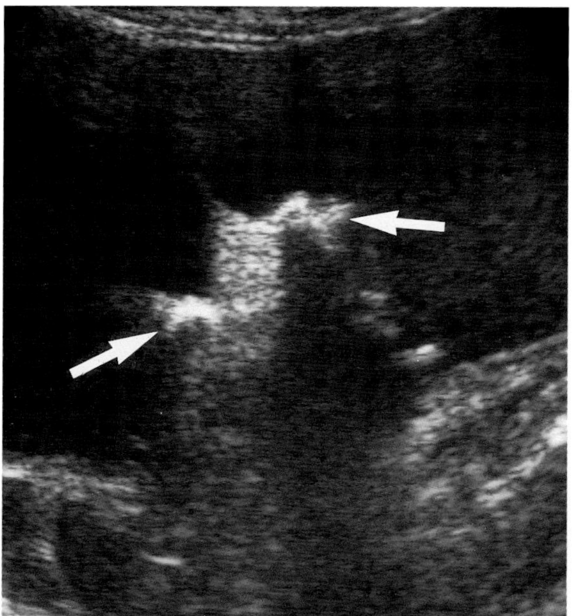

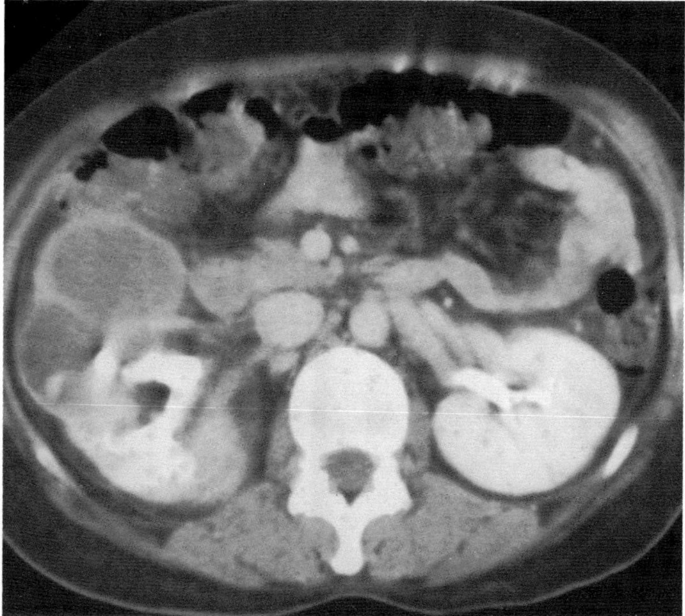

FIG. 5.35. Xanthogranulomatous pyelonephritis. **A:** Longitudinal sonogram reveals markedly dilated, debris-filled collecting system elements. Several central calcifications (*arrows*) indicative of a large renal calculus are noted. **B:** The CT scan reveals similar findings, though it is difficult to differentiate contrast within the collecting system from the renal calculi. The diagnosis from the clinical and image findings was indeterminate between xanthogranulomatous pyelonephritis and tuberculosis. Pathologically, this proved to be xanthogranulomatous pyelonephritis.

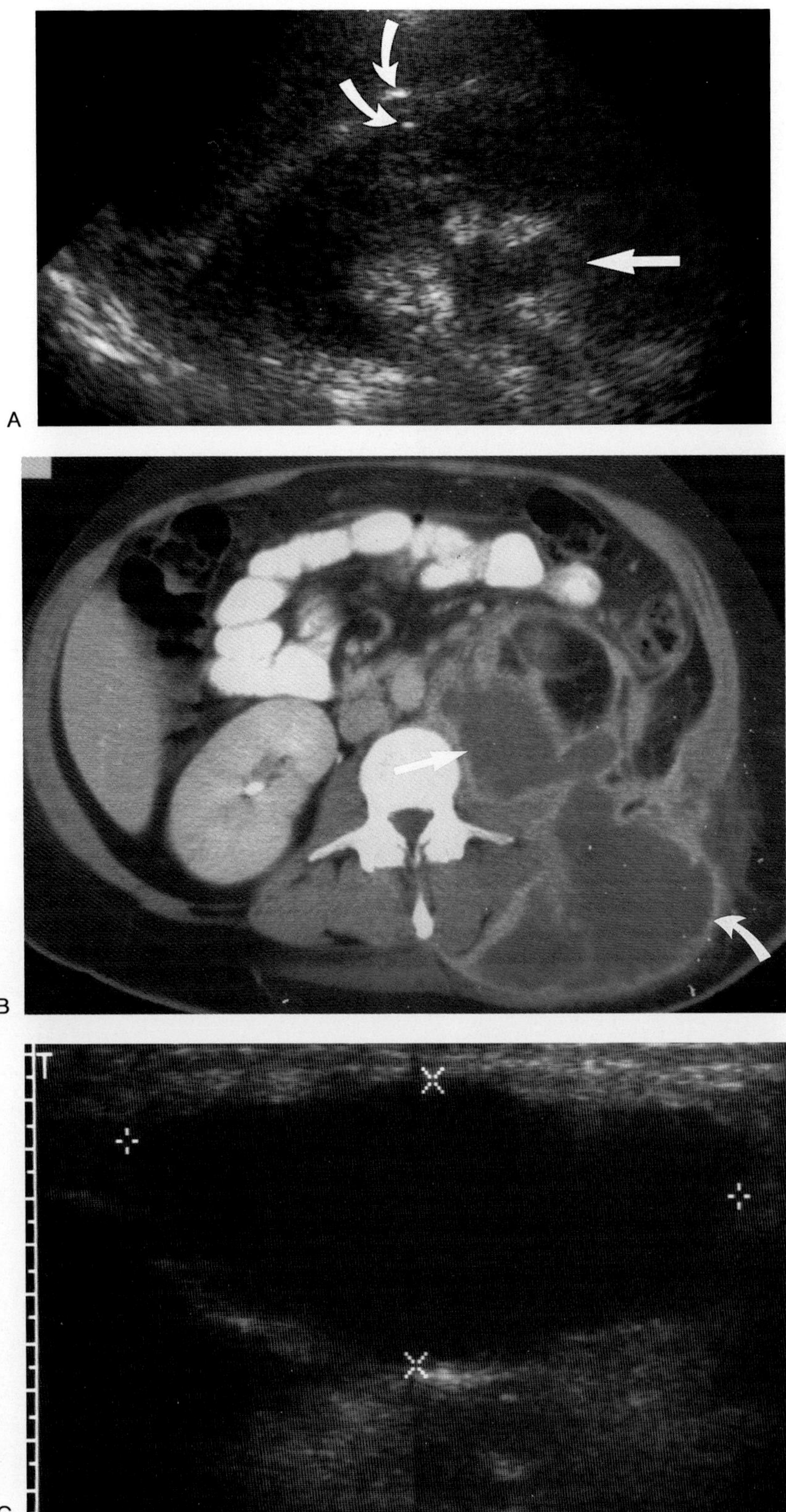

FIG. 5.36. Xanthogranulomatous pyelonephritis with retrofascial and flank involvement. **A:** Longitudinal coronal sonogram of the left kidney reveals a somewhat enlarged kidney with a dilated renal pelvis that is filled with debris (*arrow*). A small amount of gas is noted at the periphery of the kidney (*curved arrows*). The presence of gas was confirmed on a CT scan (not shown). **B:** The CT scan reveals retrofascial (*arrow*) and flank (*curved arrow*) extension of the inflammation related to the xanthogranulomatous pyelonephritis. **C:** A longitudinal compound sonogram illustrates the flank mass. While this mass is low attenuation on CT and low echogenicity on ultrasound, masses related to XGP can occasionally simulate malignancy.

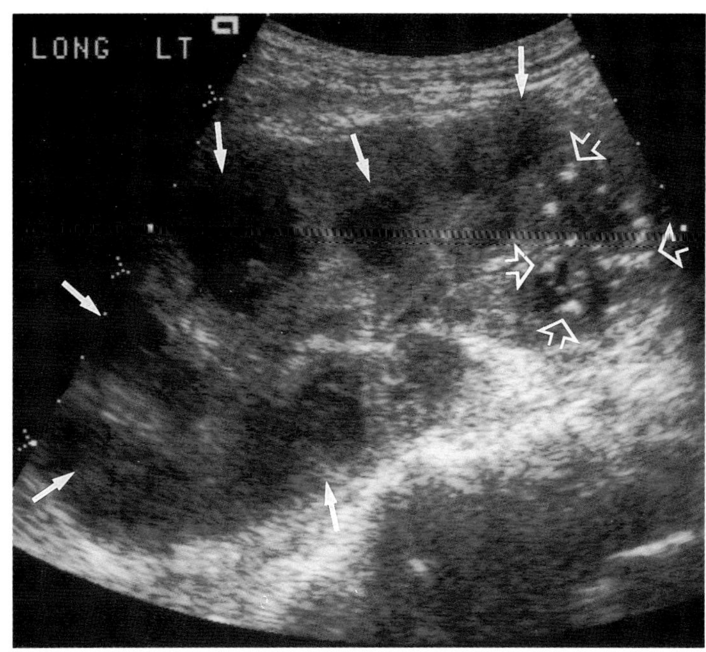

FIG. 5.37. Renal tuberculosis. Longitudinal coronal sonogram of the left kidney. There are multiple dilated debris-filled caliceal elements (*arrows*). Multiple small calcifications (*open arrows*) are noted in the lower pole. Tuberculosis and xanthogranulomatous pyelonephritis can be difficult or impossible to differentiate from one another, both clinically and on images.

A

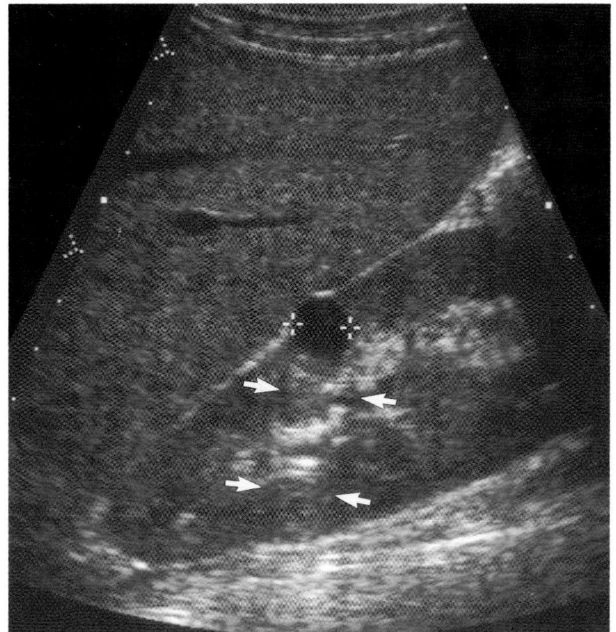

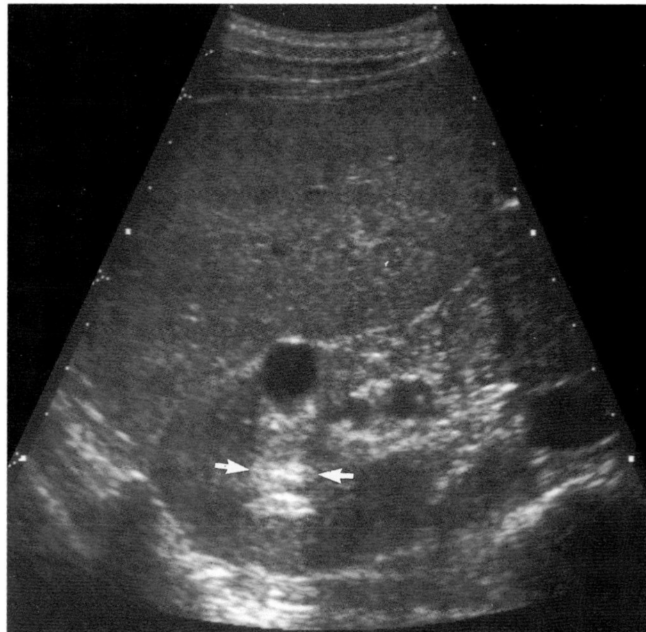

B

FIG. 5.38. Simple cyst. Longitudinal (**A**) and transverse (**B**) sonograms of the right kidney reveal a small, approximately 1-cm simple renal cyst. This lesion fulfills classic criteria for simple cyst as it has no perceptible walls, no internal echoes, and has through transmission (*arrows*). Note that the through transmission is more pronounced on the transverse image. It is not unusual for different scan orientation and even different acoustic access windows to demonstrate different degrees of enhanced through transmission.

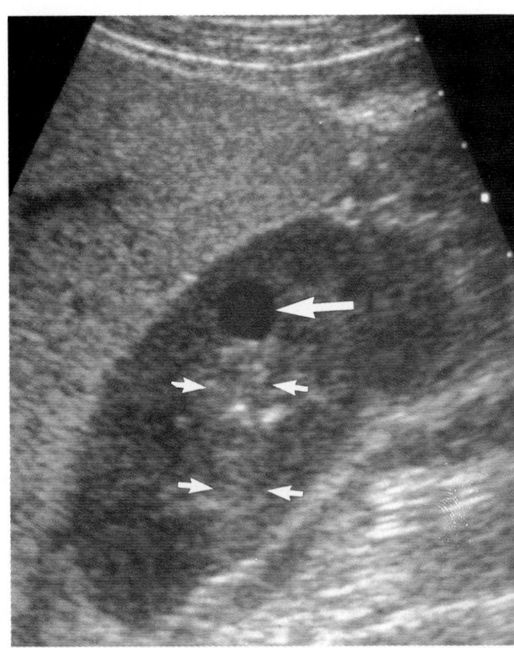

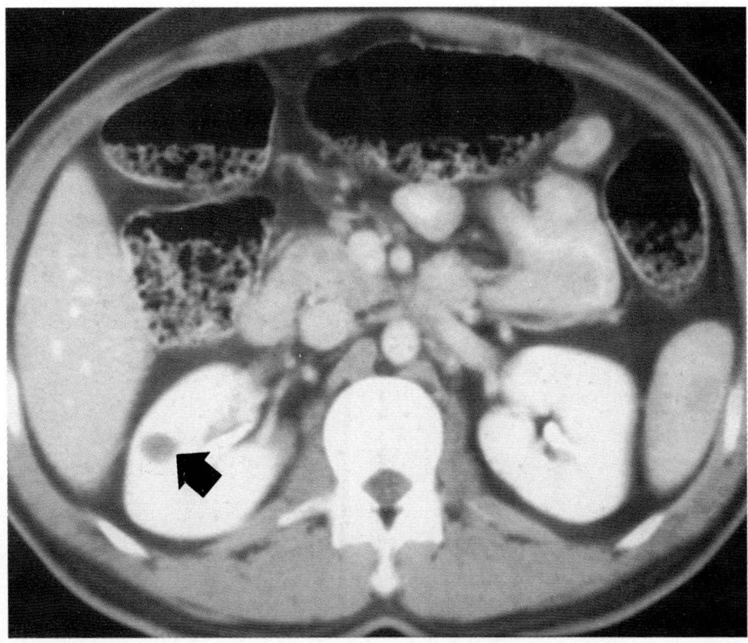

FIG. 5.39. Simple renal cyst. **A:** Longitudinal sonogram reveals a 1-cm simple cyst (*arrow*) in the right kidney. This cyst has fairly subtle through transmission (*small arrows*). It fulfills the other classic criteria as it has no internal echoes and imperceptible walls. **B:** The CT scan reveals a small, low-attenuation lesion (*arrow*). On CT, this lesion does not fulfill classic simple cyst criteria as the Hounsfield numbers are greater than 15. It is not unusual for small renal cysts to have attenuation values higher than this on CT performed with 10-mm thick slices. Sonography is useful to evaluate probable cysts that fail to meet classic criteria on CT. Conversely, CT can be used to confirm the diagnosis of simple cyst when sonography is not diagnostic. Failure to meet classic criteria is more frequent with sonography than with CT.

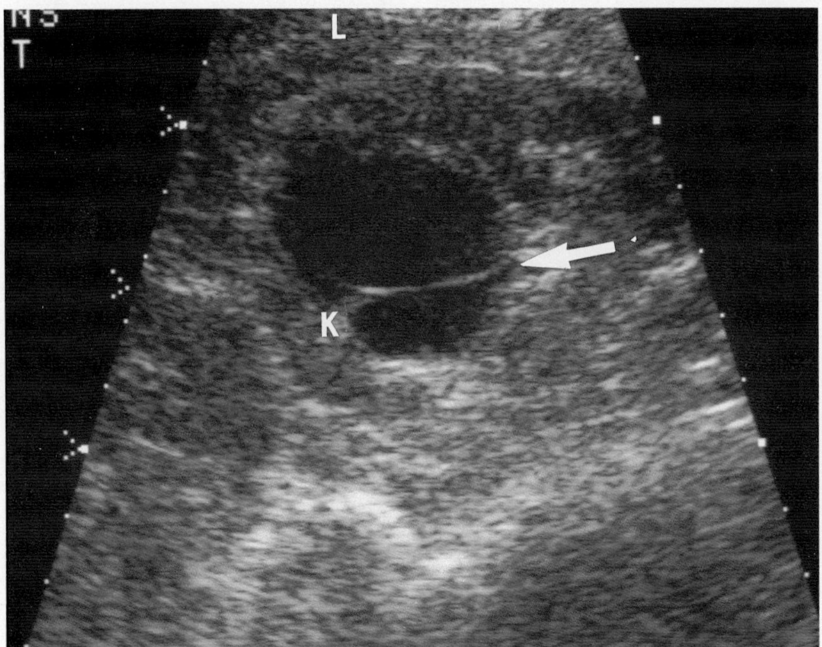

FIG. 5.40. Simple cyst with septation. Transverse oblique sonogram of the right kidney reveals a 3-cm cyst that contains a thin septation (*arrow*). Simple cysts may have thin septations. Enhanced through transmission of sound was shown to better advantage on another image (not illustrated). L, liver; K, kidney.

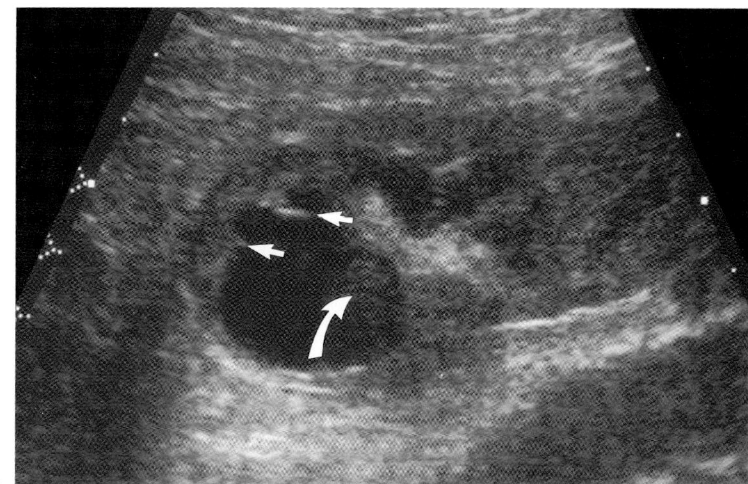

A

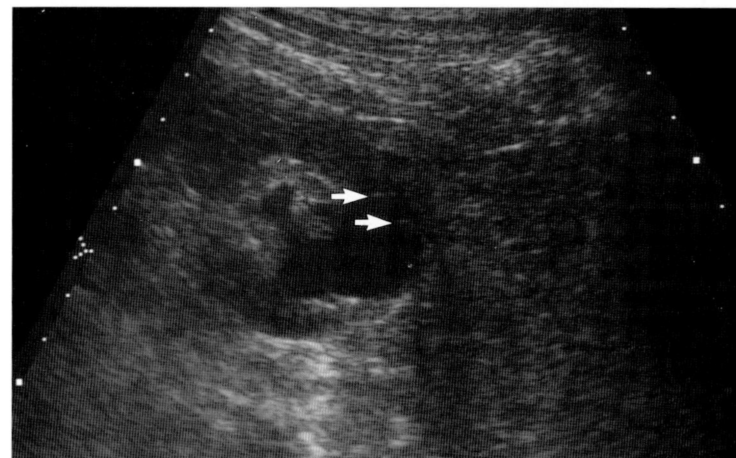

B

FIG. 5.41. Lobulated simple cyst, septations and artifact. Longitudinal (**A**) and transverse (**B**) sonograms of the left kidney. A lobulated simple cyst that has a few thin septations (*arrows*) is present in the upper pole of this kidney. On the longitudinal image, some internal echoes (*curved arrow*) are noted. With careful scanning, it was possible to determine that these echoes were related to artifact. This lesion met all criteria for simple cyst. Lobulation and thin septations are acceptable in a lesion diagnosed as simple cyst. Internal echogenicity, even though often caused by artifact, precludes the diagnosis of simple cyst. In such instances, further evaluation, most often with CT, is required to ensure that such a lesion is a simple cyst.

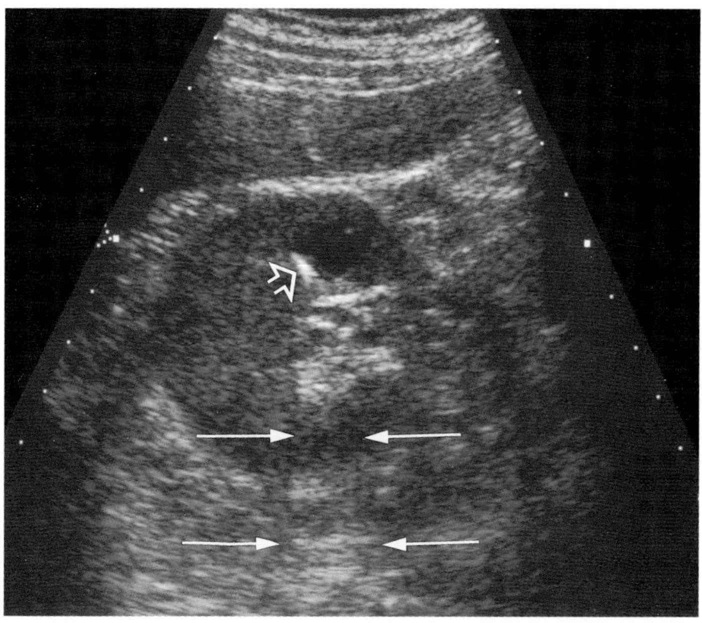

FIG. 5.42. Benign renal cyst with thin mural calcification. Transverse sonogram of the right kidney. This small, 13-mm renal cyst has a thin mural calcification (*open arrow*). While thin mural calcification almost always signifies a benign lesion, all calcified cysts should undergo CT scanning to ensure that no malignancy is present. This lesion has all the other features of a simple cyst including subtle through transmission (*small arrows*).

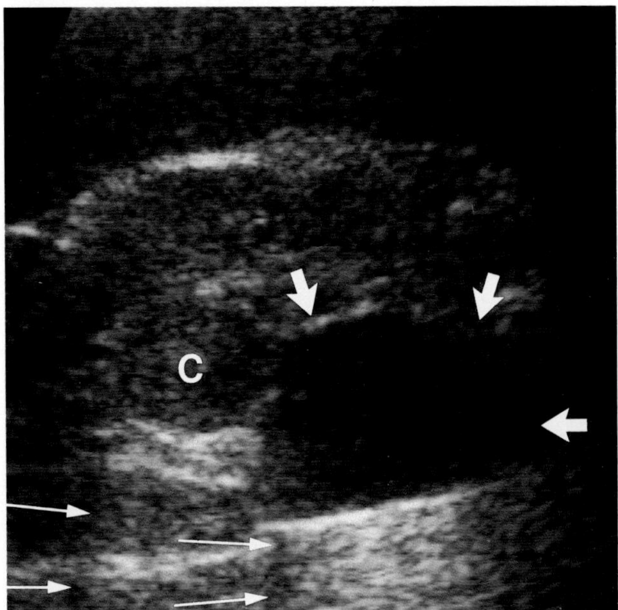

FIG. 5.43. Hemorrhagic renal cysts. Longitudinal sonogram of the right kidney. CT scan revealed high attenuation in the two cysts demonstrated here. The smaller cyst (C) is filled with debris that is essentially equivalent in echogenicity to the remainder of the kidney. The larger cyst (*arrows*) has fewer internal echoes. On aspiration, both of these proved to be benign hemorrhagic cysts. Note the prominent through transmission deep to both hemorrhagic cysts (*small arrows*).

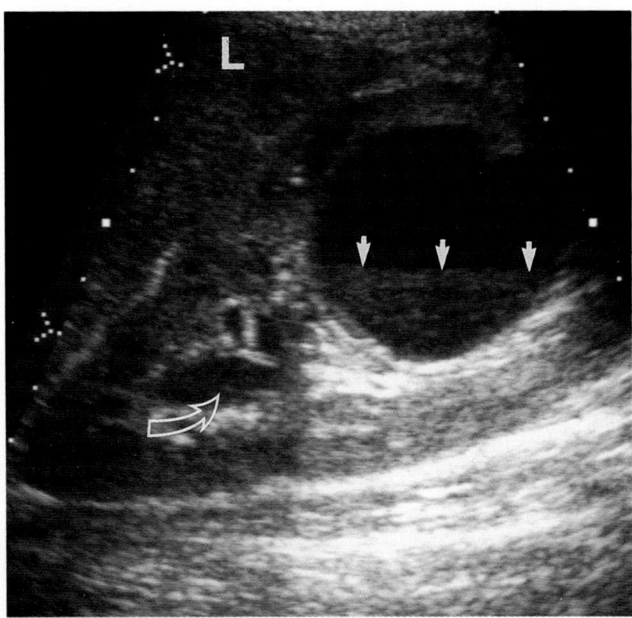

FIG. 5.44. Infected renal cyst. Longitudinal sonogram of the right kidney. This 4-cm renal cyst is infected, resulting in a debris/fluid level (*small arrows*). Prominent through transmission is noted deep to the cyst. Note the mild to moderate dilatation of the upper pole collecting system (*open curved arrow*). L, liver.

A

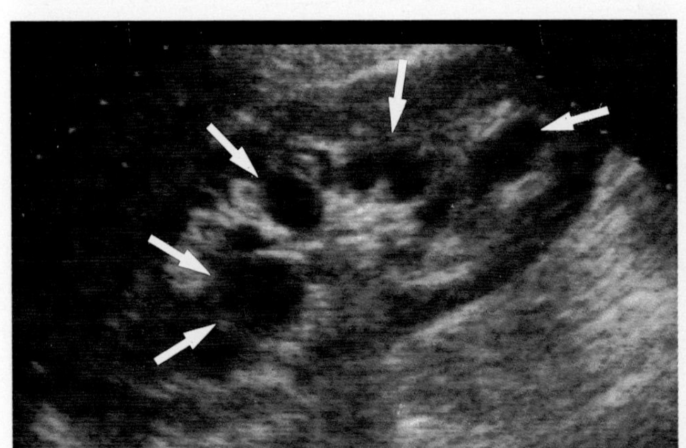

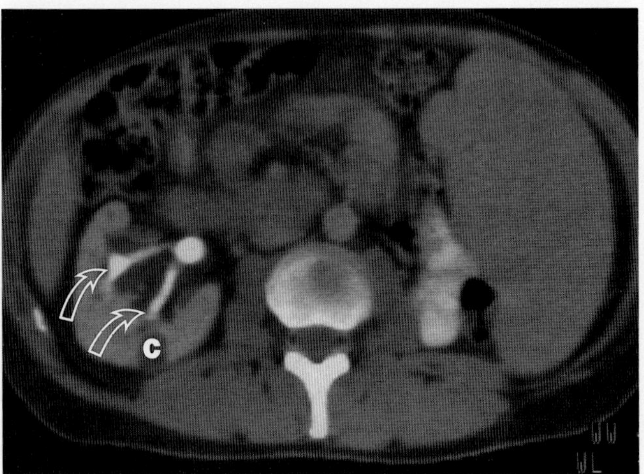

B

FIG. 5.45. Parapelvic cysts. **A:** Longitudinal sonogram of the right kidney reveals multiple hypoechoic areas within the renal sinus (*arrows*). The key to ensuring that multiple parapelvic cysts are not confused with hydronephrosis is identification of the renal pelvis. In this instance, the renal pelvis is not dilated, and thus the diagnosis of multiple parapelvic cysts is secure. **B:** Diagnosis of parapelvic cysts is simpler on a CT scan as the collecting system elements are opacified with high attenuation urine (*curved open arrows*) highlighting the water attenuation cysts as distinct from the collecting system elements. Note the cortical cyst (C) that is also present.

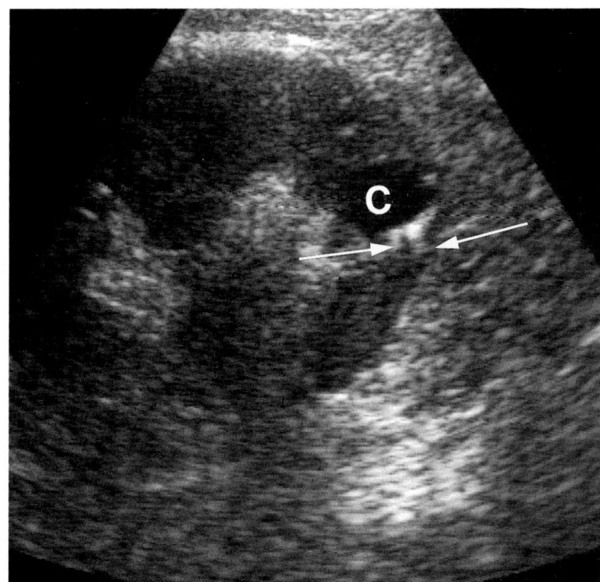

FIG. 5.46. Caliceal diverticulum with small stones. Transverse oblique sonogram of the left kidney reveals a small cyst-like structure (C) with several echogenic dependent foci that exhibit a small comet-tail artifact (*thin arrows*). On this image alone, it would be difficult to differentiate a cyst with mural calcification from a caliceal diverticulum that contains several small stones. With change in position of the patient, the stones moved to a dependent location. This made caliceal diverticulum the most likely diagnosis. Communication with the collecting system could not be shown sonographically. Communication can usually be reliably demonstrated only by contrast-enhanced CT or, as in this patient, by intravenous urography.

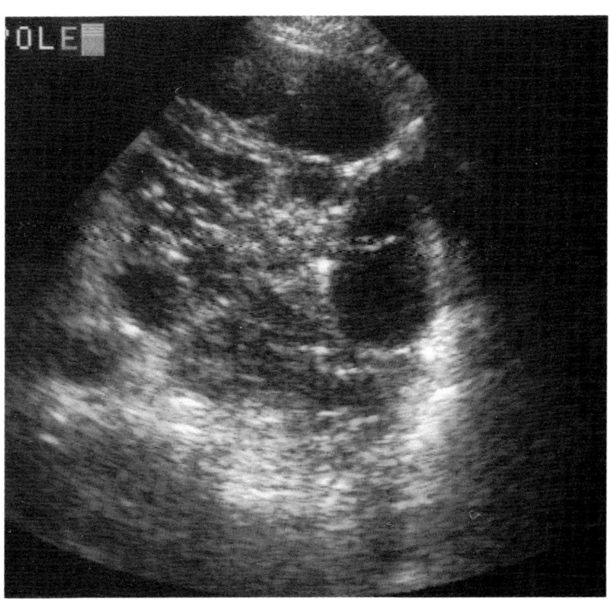

FIG. 5.47. Renal polycystic disease. Transverse sonogram of the lower pole of the right kidney reveals virtual total replacement of the normal renal parenchyma by multiple cysts of varying sizes. Note that, in contrast to simple cysts, the margins of cysts in polycystic disease are often irregular. Formerly called autosomal dominant polycystic kidney disease, it is not known that this entity and polycystic liver disease are merely different phenotypes of the same genetic defect.

A

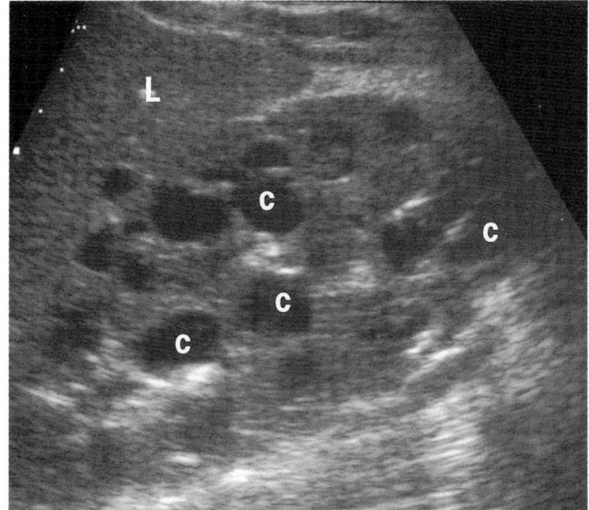

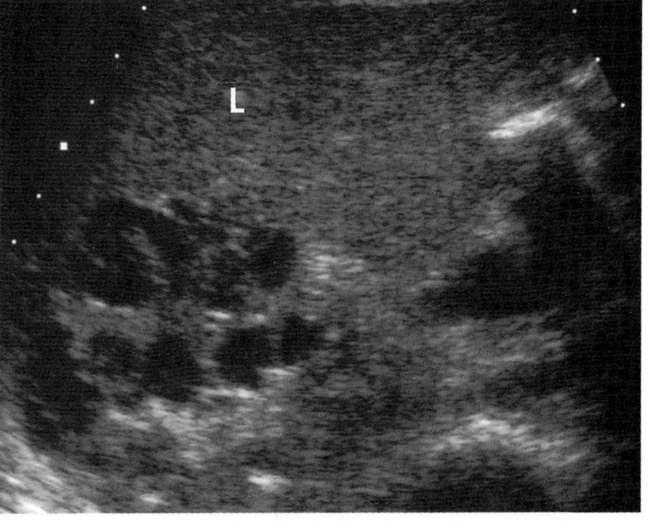

B

FIG. 5.48. Renal polycystic disease. **A:** Longitudinal sonogram of the right kidney reveals multiple, relatively small, renal cysts, some of which are indicated by (c). **B:** A transverse sonogram through the right kidney reveals similar findings. Note that only moderate irregularity of the cyst walls is present. In this patient, no hepatic cysts were identified. L, liver.

noma (34). Some feel that renal (autosomal dominant) polycystic disease (35) may also be associated with increased risk for renal cell carcinoma.

Renal (Autosomal Dominant) Polycystic Disease

Recent research has shown that renal (autosomal dominant) polycystic disease, which often has both hepatic and renal cysts, results from the same genetic abnormality as hepatic polycystic disease (36). Sonography easily diagnoses renal polycystic disease by revealing numerous cortical cysts of varying sizes, often with irregular margins (Figs. 5.47 and 5.48). This last feature is distinct from multiple simple cysts, where smooth margins are usual. Incomplete phenotypic penetrance or renal polycystic disease in a child may result in a sonographic pattern indistinguishable from multiple simple cysts. Liver cysts (Fig. 5.49) are found in as many as 50 percent of patients with renal polycystic disease (37). Hepatic and renal enlargement from cysts may progress to uncomfortably distend the entire abdominal/pelvic cavity. Intracystic infection or hemorrhage may cause symptoms. It also may cause echogenic debris on sonograms (Fig. 5.50) and increased attenuation on CT scans. Often, several different cysts in asymptomatic individuals are abnormal, probably caused by previous episodes of intracystic hemorrhage. In patients with symptoms, it may be difficult to identify which of several abnormal cysts is causing the acute symptoms. The symptomatic cyst can often be identified with real-time sonography by linking focal tenderness to a specific abnormal cyst. Percutaneous aspiration or drainage may prove useful to relieve symptoms and treat infected cysts.

Renal polycystic disease may be associated with slowly progressive renal failure, hypertension, and intracranial berry aneurysms (present in about 15 percent of patients) (33). Despite these potential complications, many patients with renal cystic disease live normal life spans, although average life expectancy is diminished compared to the general population. Some have suggested that renal polycystic disease is associated with a higher prevalence of renal cell carcinoma (35).

Although pancreatic cysts are said to be common in renal polycystic disease, we have encountered only one patient with an imageable pancreatic cyst (Fig. 5.51). Thus finding renal and pancreatic cysts should suggest von Hippel–Lindau disease rather than renal polycystic disease. When renal polycystic disease is detected, immediate family members who are at risk should be screened with sonography. Affected children may be detected early in this way.

Other Renal Cystic Diseases

Medullary sponge kidney is a fairly common, usually insignificant disease. Dilated ectatic collecting tubules are easily imaged on intravenous urography. Sonography is almost totally insensitive to this finding. The medullary calcifications and stones often present in medullary sponge kidney may be detected sonographically (Figs. 5.52 and 5.53) but are more sensitively detected by CT and intravenous urography (28,33).

Medullary cystic disease (nephronophthisis) is a very rare disease that occurs in young adults and children (38,39). These patients often have profound renal failure, salt wasting, and anemia. While small, sonographically invisible cysts are the rule, discrete cysts up to 2 cm in size in the medullary pyramids or at the corticomedullary junction may be identified. Increased echogenicity indistinguishable from other diffuse renal parenchymal diseases may be present (30).

Multicystic dysplastic kidney is often discovered in infants as a palpable mass. On occasion, a multicystic dysplasic kidney is discovered, often incidentally, in an adult. Cystic and disorganized solid elements are found sonographically.

Multilocular cystic nephroma is a very rare cystic neoplasm generally imaged as a well-circumscribed multicystic, septated mass. Cystic renal cell carcinoma, cystic Wilms' tumor, and renal lymphangioma may be indistinguishable from multilocular cystic nephroma (40,41).

Dialysis-Related Acquired Cystic Disease of the Kidney (ACDK)

Patients on long-term hemodialysis or peritoneal dialysis develop cysts in their native kidneys. Although present sooner pathologically, cysts are not commonly imageable by CT or sonography prior to 3 years of dialysis (42–46). Sonographically, the kidneys in ACDK are often small and have multiple cysts. Progression often occurs with continued dialysis, resulting in renal enlargement and findings indistinguishable from renal polycystic disease (Figs. 5.54 and 5.55). Intracystic hemorrhage is common. It appears as high attenuation on CT scan and increased echogenicity sonographically. ACDK patients are at increased risk for renal cell carcinoma. Because it is uncertain if these neoplasms adversely affect the patient's longevity, it is not clear that patients with ACDK should be followed for the development of renal cell carcinoma.

RENAL NEOPLASIA

Renal Cell Carcinoma

In adults, renal cell carcinoma (RCC) is by far the commonest solid renal neoplasm. Although generally a disease of middle aged and older individuals, RCC oc-

(*text continues on page 311*)

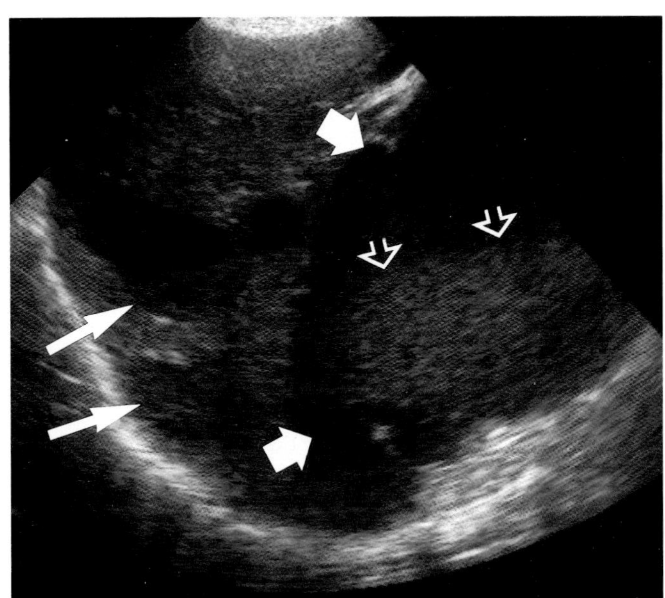

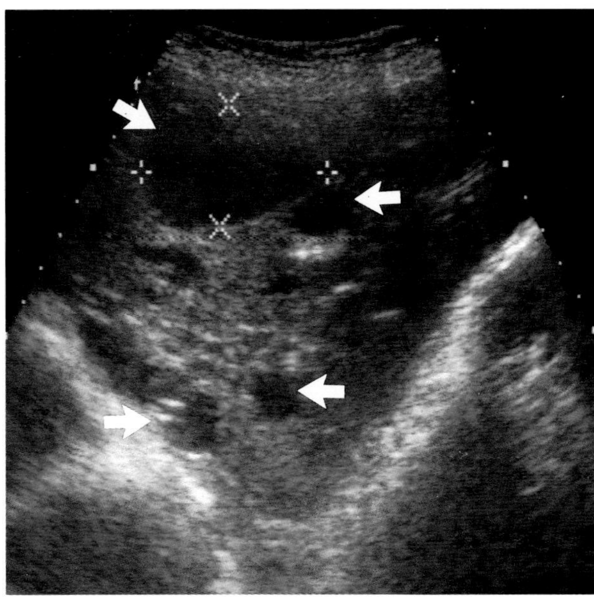

FIG. 5.49. Renal polycystic disease with hepatic cysts. **A:** Longitudinal sonogram on the right reveals a hemorrhagic renal cyst (*large arrows*) with a debris–fluid level within it (*open arrows*). Several hepatic cysts are also noted, two of which also have internal debris (*arrows*), presumably related to previous hemorrhage or infection. **B:** A transverse sonogram through the left lobe of the liver shows multiple hepatic cysts of varying size (*arrows*). Note that these cysts are more irregular than typical simple liver cysts. About 50 percent of patients with renal polycystic disease also have hepatic cysts. This patient was asymptomatic at the time of the study. The debris within the large renal cyst was probably related to previous hemorrhage.

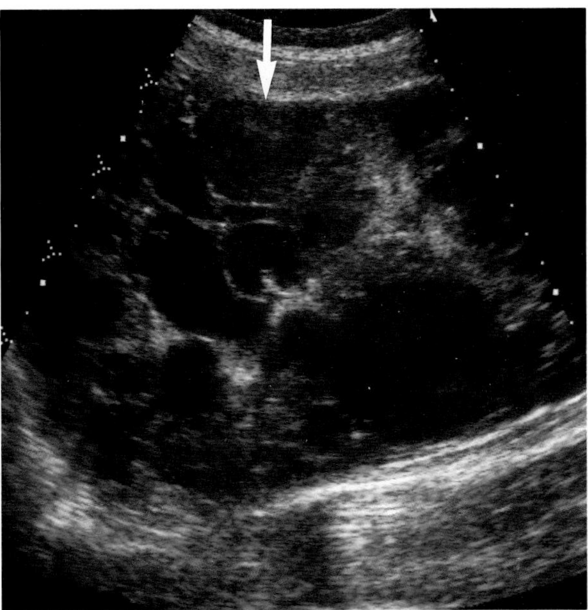

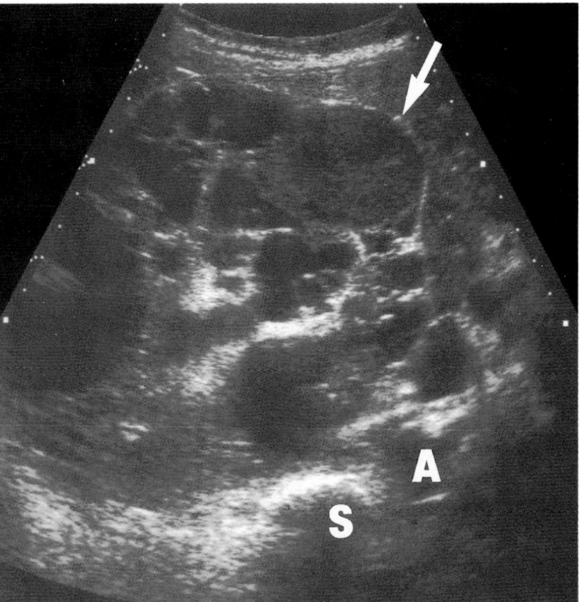

FIG. 5.50. Renal cystic disease, infected cyst. The longitudinal (**A**) and transverse (**B**) sonograms reveal extensive replacement of the kidney by cysts, many of which have irregular borders. Internal echoes are present in one cyst (*arrow*). Aspiration yielded pus. The patient was focally tender over the cyst, a finding that helped localize this as the symptomatic cyst. Often, several cysts have internal echoes. Sonographic localization of tenderness can indicate which cyst with internal echoes is responsible for the symptoms. S, spine; A, aorta.

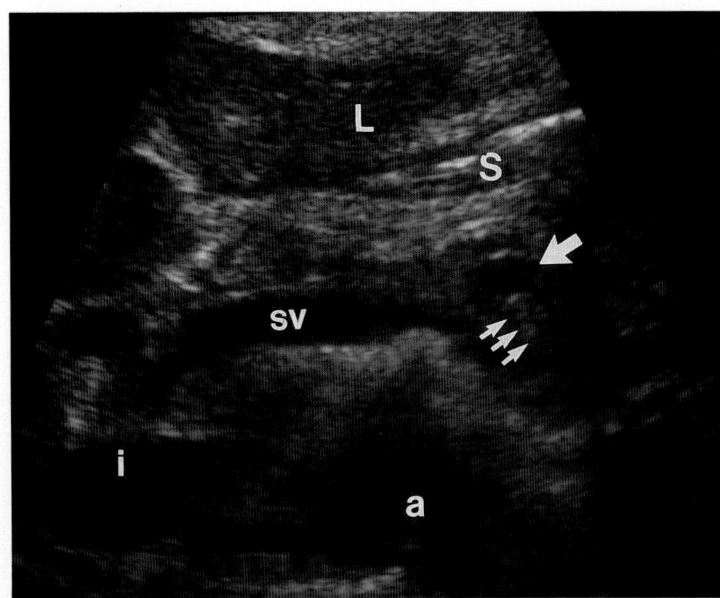

FIG. 5.51. Renal cystic disease, pancreatic cyst. Transverse sonogram of the pancreas reveals a small, 5-mm intrapancreatic cyst (*arrow*). Pancreatic cysts, reported to have a frequency of 5 to 10 percent in patients with renal polycystic disease, are actually quite rarely imaged. This is the only patient we have encountered with renal polycystic disease who had an imageable pancreatic cyst. a, aorta; i, inferior vena cava; sv, splenic vein; L, liver; S, stomach.

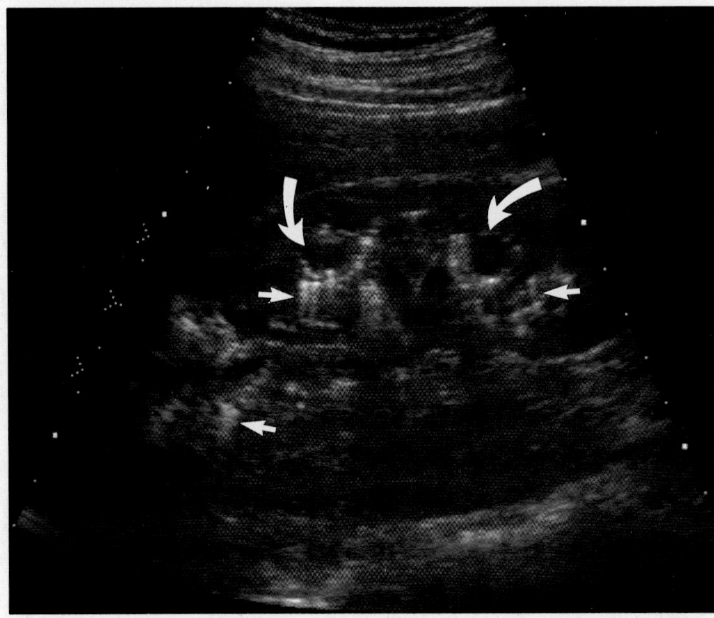

FIG. 5.52. Medullary sponge kidney. Longitudinal sonogram of the left kidney. Longitudinal coronal sonogram of the left kidney reveals multiple echogenic foci scattered about the renal pyramids (*curved arrows*). Note the comet-tail artifact (*small arrows*) associated with some of the small collecting tubule stones. The medullary calcifications and stones present in medullary sponge kidney can be detected sonographically but are more sensitively detected by CT and intravenous urography.

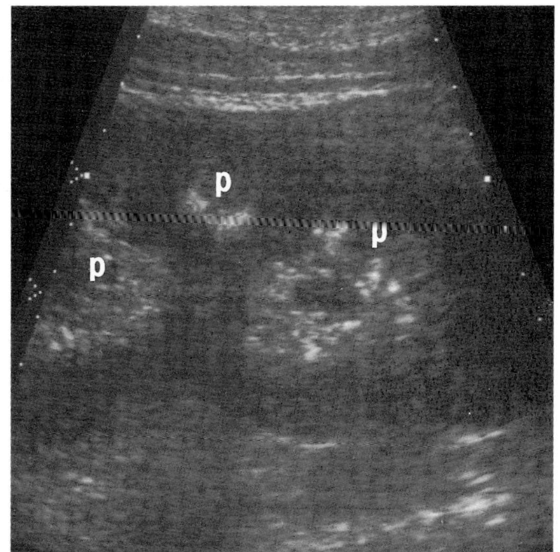

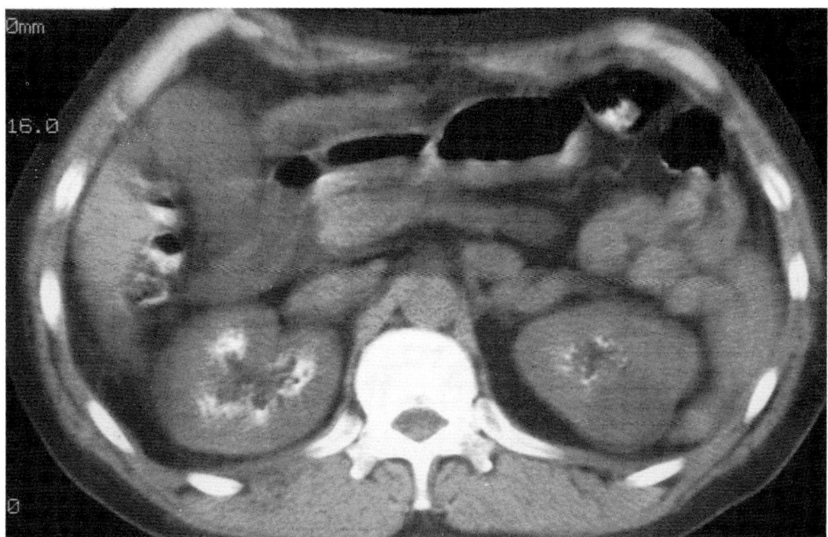

FIG. 5.53. Medullary sponge kidney. **A:** Longitudinal coronal sonogram of the right kidney reveals multiple echogenic foci scattered about the renal pyramids (p), essentially diagnostic of medullary sponge kidney. **B:** A CT scan also reveals these calcifications, located at the periphery of the medullary pyramids.

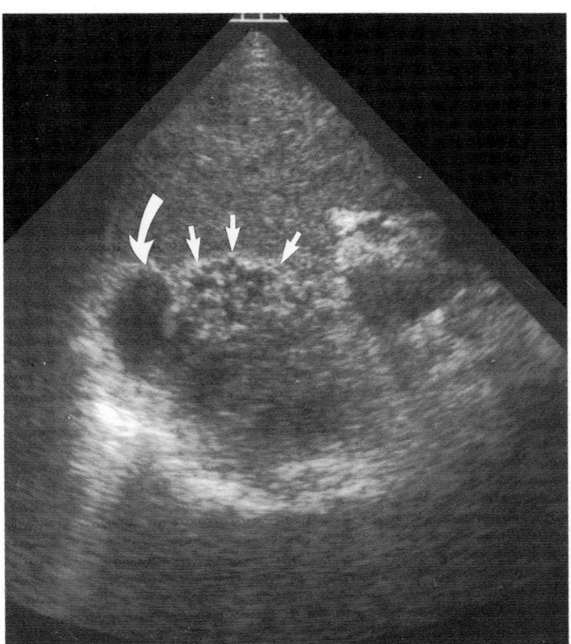

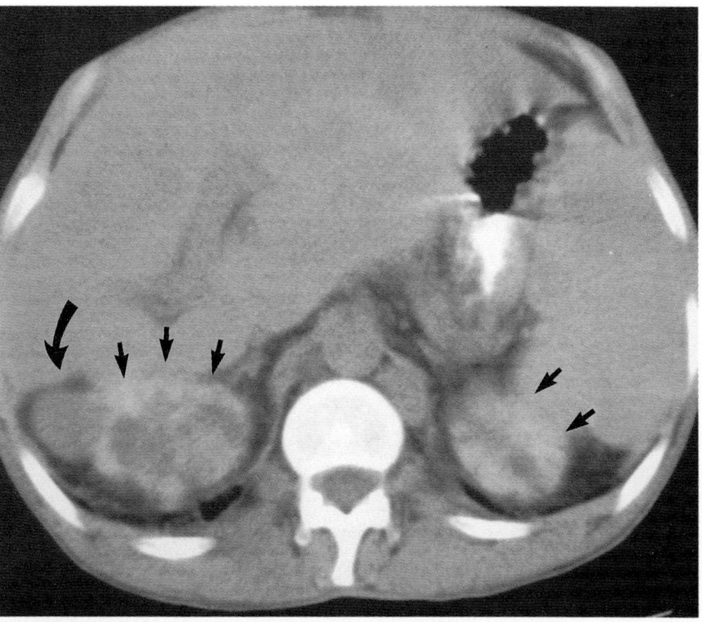

FIG. 5.54. Acquired cystic disease of the kidneys, dialysis related. The transverse sonogram (**A**) of the right kidney and noncontrast CT scan (**B**) reveal multiple small cysts (*small arrows*) that are high attenuation on CT because of intracystic hemorrhage. A larger, nonhemorrhagic cyst (*curved arrow*) is also noted. Intracystic hemorrhage is common in cysts caused by dialysis-related acquired cystic disease. Higher attenuation on CT is a more frequent finding in these cysts than is increased internal echogenicity on sonography. Enlarged azygos and hemiazygos veins are seen in the retrocrural region on CT. This patient had complete fibrous inferior vena caval occlusion of unknown etiology.

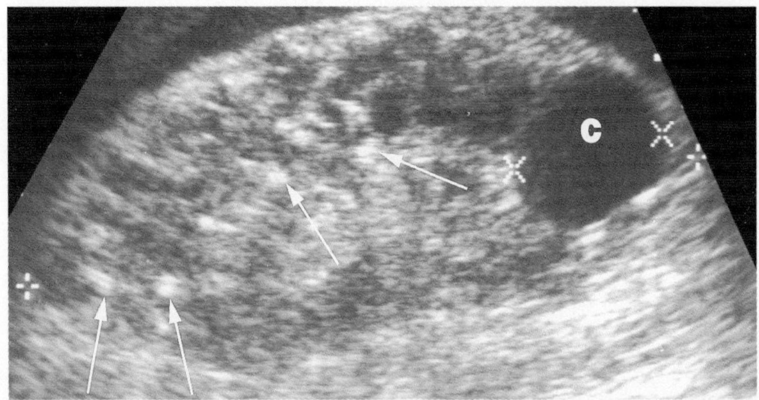

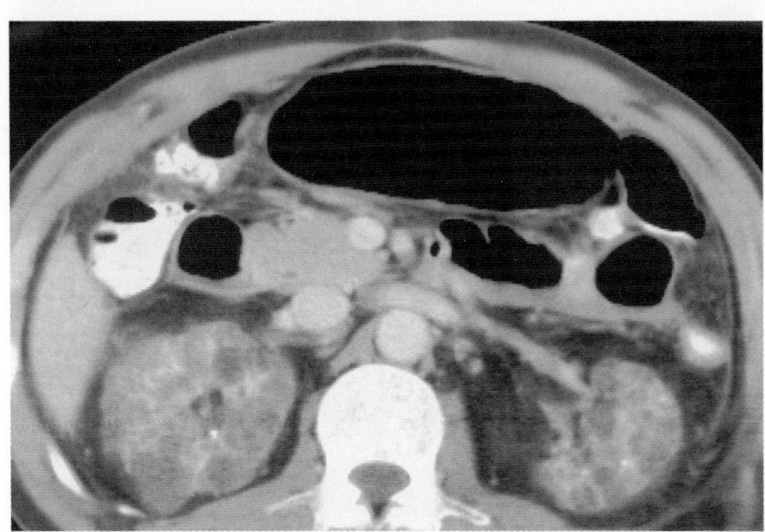

FIG. 5.55. Acquired cystic disease of the kidney (ACDK). **A:** Longitudinal sonogram of the right kidney reveals a large cyst (c) at the lower pole, multiple tiny cysts throughout the kidney, and many punctate areas of increased echogenicity representing calcification (*thin arrows*). **B:** A contrast-enhanced CT scan reveals areas of patchy enhancement coupled with multiple small cysts of varying sizes. In this patient with ACDK, fairly typical findings are present. As ACDK progresses, the kidneys enlarge and may eventually cause enlarged kidneys like those found in renal polycystic disease. Hemorrhagic cysts, tiny to large simple cysts, and punctate calcifications are typical findings in ACDK. These patients are at increased risk to develop renal cell carcinoma.

curs rarely in childhood and, occasionally, in young adults. RCC is more common in men and probably increases in prevalence with increasing age (47). While some feel that small benign renal adenomas are neoplasms distinct from RCC, most pathologists feel that adenomas are merely small RCCs (47,48). Patients with von Hippel–Lindau disease (34) and dialysis-related acquired cystic disease of the kidney (45) are at increased risk for renal cell carcinoma. Though controversial, some feel patients with renal (autosomal dominant) polycystic disease may also have slightly increased risk for developing RCC (35).

Sonographically, RCC is usually a heterogeneous hypoechoic to isoechoic solid mass (Figs. 5.56 and 5.57). Cystic areas (Fig. 5.58) and calcification (Fig. 5.59) may be present. Thicker and more irregular calcifications are suggestive of neoplasm, but any calcified cyst or mass should be evaluated with CT employing 5-mm sections before and after intravenous contrast enhancement to seek the presence of an RCC. Occasionally, predominantly cystic RCCs occur (Figs. 5.60 and 5.61) (49–51). RCCs of equal or greater echogenicity than the renal sinus fat (49) are much less frequent than hypoechoic or isoechoic lesions (Fig. 5.62). On occasion, RCC may cause only subtle sonographic abnormality (Fig. 5.63). Normal structures, such as renal cortical columns (Fig. 5.64), can simulate masses.

Tumor vascularity greater than that of normal renal parenchyma can be demonstrated in RCC by color flow sonography (Fig. 5.65), although flow may also be decreased or absent (Fig. 5.66). The frequency of increased flow in RCC on color flow sonography is unknown. As a general rule, abnormal vascularity in or at the periphery of a mass on color or spectral Doppler sonography should suggest the possibility of renal cell carcinoma. No correlation between RCC vascularity and tissue echogenicity has been demonstrated.

It has been reported that high-frequency shifts, related to small AV shunts, may be detected in RCC by spectral Doppler sonography, differentiating RCC from benign lesions (52–54). This technique may be time consuming, as in tissue characterization of liver tumors. Currently, diagnosis of RCC by spectral analysis is best considered investigational.

Sonography can be used to screen patients for RCC. More usually, intravenous urography is used for this purpose. If a mass suggestive of RCC is detected using intravenous urography (IVU), CT is used next to determine the stage and extent of the disease. When IVU reveals either a questionable or indeterminate mass (i.e., one that might represent a cyst), sonography is performed. CT is preferable to sonography in suspected RCC because it is more effective in detecting extracapsular invasion, lymph nodes, and distant metastasis. On occasion, sonography is superior to CT in determining whether a superior pole RCC invades or merely indents the liver (Fig. 5.67).

Color flow imaging is probably comparably accurate to CT, MRI, and venography in detecting tumor invasion of the renal vein and inferior vena cava (IVC). RCC is the commonest tumor that invades the IVC (Figs. 5.56, 5.68, and 5.69) (hepatocellular carcinoma is second) and may, on occasion, invade the heart. IVC invasion occurs in from 5 to 24 percent of RCCs (48). Metastasis from RCC occurs most often to (in order) lungs, mediastinum and other nodes, liver, bone, adrenal, and the opposite kidney. All other sites have a frequency of 5 percent or less (47).

Rarely, patients with RCC may present with perinephric or subcapsular hemorrhage. RCC is the most common cause of spontaneous perinephric or paranephric hemorrhage (55).

Urothelial Neoplasms of the Renal Pelvis and Ureter

Even though renal cell carcinoma (RCC) is relatively uncommon, it is four to five times more frequent than transitional cell carcinoma (TCC) of the upper collecting system. TCC is much more common in men, as is RCC. Urothelial tumors in the upper urinary tract are mainly (>90 percent) TCC. Most of the remainder are squamous cell and, rarely, undifferentiated carcinoma. Upper tract tumors occur much less often than those that arise in the bladder. The ratio of tumors occurring in the bladder, renal pelvis, and ureter has been reported as 50:3:1 (47). Fifty percent of patients with ureteral TCC and 32 percent of patients with renal TCC have or will eventually develop tumor in the bladder (56–58). If a mass suggestive of a urothelial tumor is detected, cystoscopy with retrograde pyelography is performed. Biopsy is done to determine histologic grade. CT is used next to determine the stage and extent of the disease.

Small and medium sized TCCs may be hard to detect with sonography or CT when the pelvicaliceal system is not dilated. Obstructing ureteral tumors may result in hydronephrosis or a dilated ureter (Figs. 5.70 and 5.71). Sonographically, TCC is typically a hypoechoic lesion in the collecting system. On occasion, a large sessile or pedunculated mass may be present (59). When a neoplasm invades both renal parenchyma and the renal sinus, it is essentially impossible to determine whether the tumor is RCC or TCC. In fact, RCC, rather than TCC, is the commonest tumor occurring in the renal sinus (Figs. 5.63 and 5.72).

Angiomyolipoma

Angiomyolipoma is a relatively uncommon neoplasm that consists of vessels, smooth muscle, and fat. These

(*text continues on page 323*)

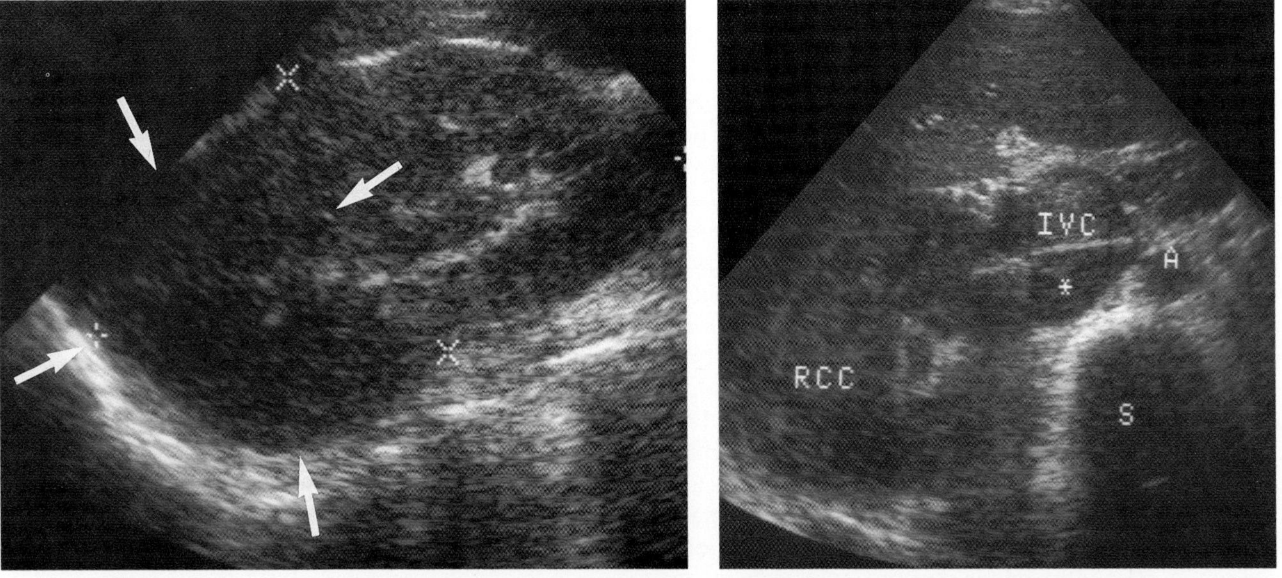

FIG. 5.56. Renal cell carcinoma with adenopathy and IVC invasion. **A:** Longitudinal sonogram of the right kidney reveals a large upper pole renal mass that is hypoechoic compared to the normal renal parenchyma. **B:** The transverse sonogram reveals retrocaval adenopathy (*) and tumor mass within the inferior vena cava (IVC). RCC, renal cell carcinoma; A, aorta; S, spine.

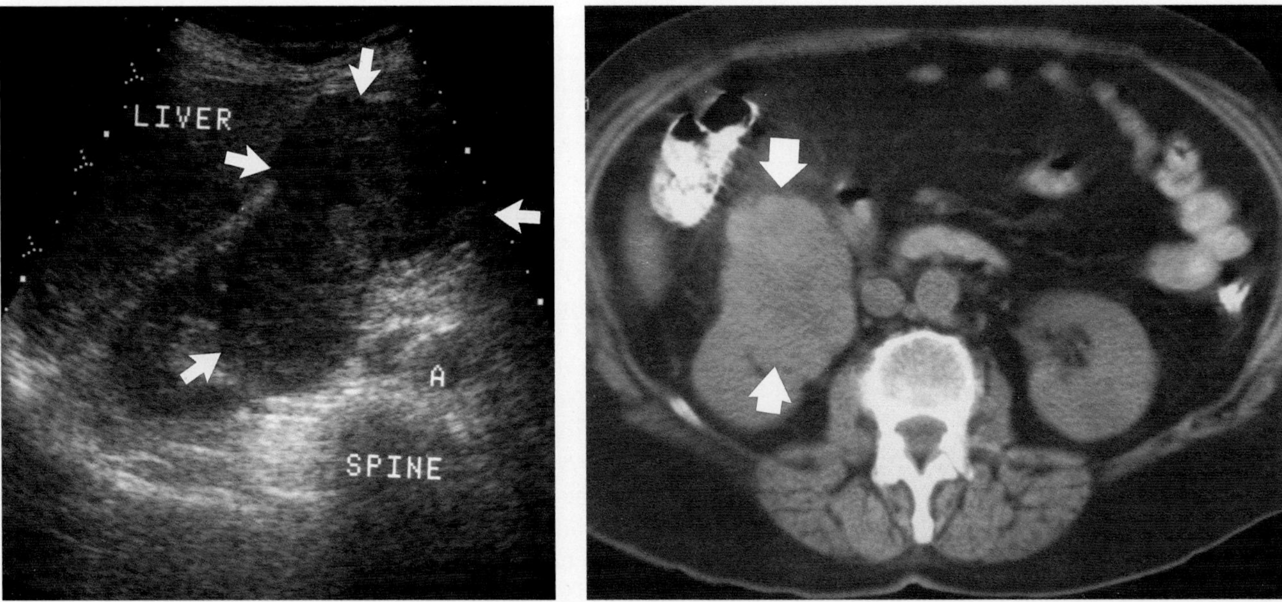

FIG. 5.57. Lobulated renal cell carcinoma. **A:** Transverse sonogram of the right kidney reveals a lobulated heterogeneous, predominantly isoechoic renal cell carcinoma (*arrows*). **B:** A noncontrast CT scan reveals similar morphology. Heterogeneous isoechoic masses such as this are a common sonographic pattern in renal cell carcinoma. A, aorta.

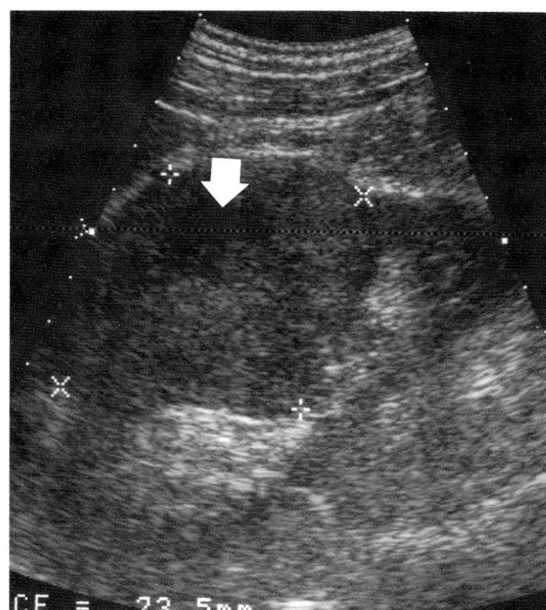

A

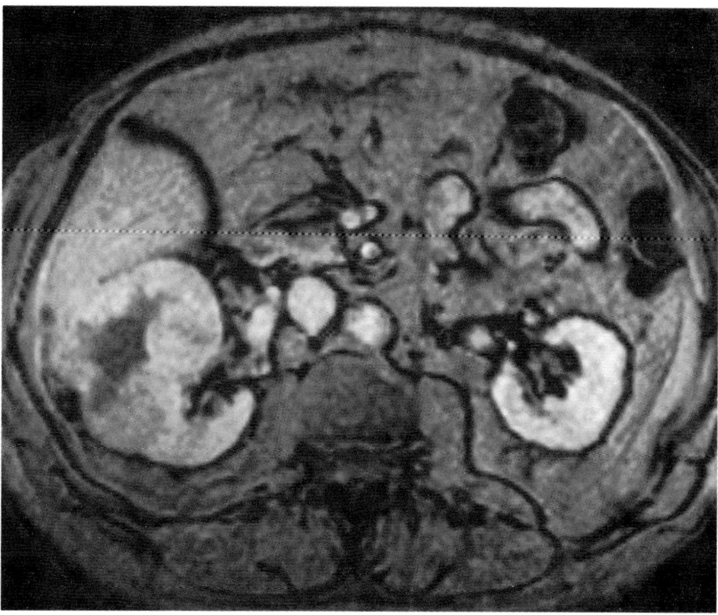

B

FIG. 5.58. Renal cell carcinoma. **A:** Longitudinal sonogram of the right kidney reveals a large mixed echogenicity renal cell carcinoma (calipers). There is an ill-defined hypoechoic area within this mass (*arrow*) that may represent an area of cystic necrosis. Note the enhanced through transmission of sound deep to the hypoechoic area. **B:** The gadolinium-enhanced MR study reveals similar morphologic features.

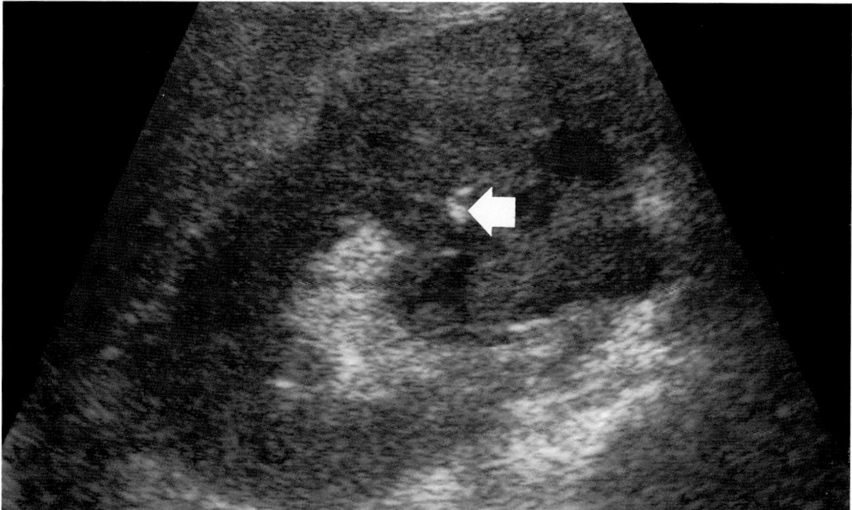

FIG. 5.59. Renal cell carcinoma with calcification. Longitudinal sonogram of the right kidney shows a large renal cell carcinoma of mixed echogenicity that invades the renal sinus. A prominent calcification with shadowing (*arrow*) is noted. This finding was confirmed on CT. Calcification within renal cell carcinoma is common. CT is a more sensitive detector of tumor calcification than sonography.

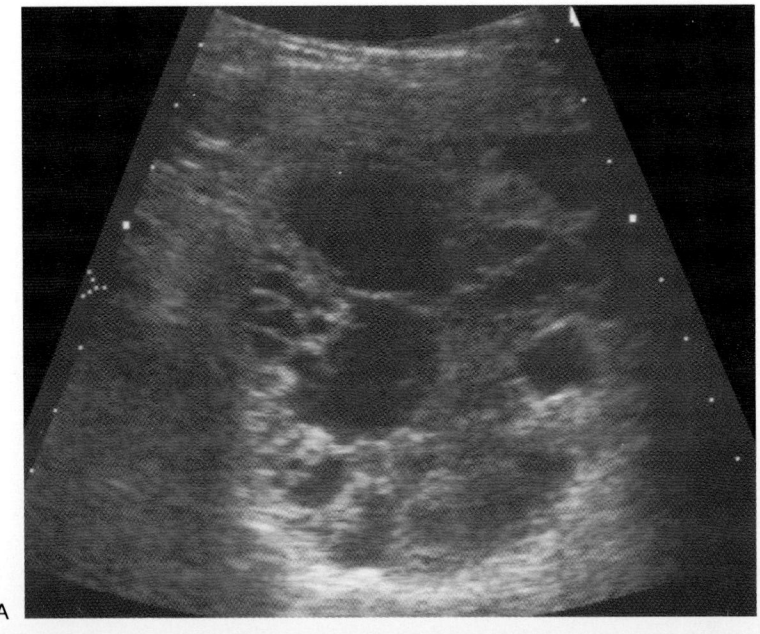

A

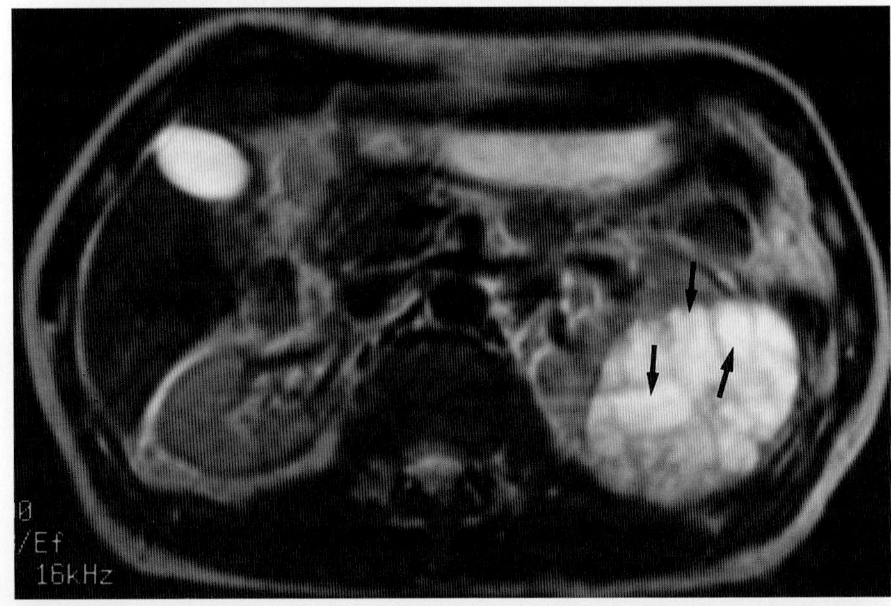

B

FIG. 5.60. Renal cell carcinoma with multiple cystic areas. **A:** Transverse sonogram of the left kidney reveals multiple cystic areas within the renal cell carcinoma. **B:** T2-weighted MR image also shows the fluid-containing areas as areas of high signal intensity (*arrows*). Cystic areas within renal cell carcinoma are encountered fairly frequently.

A

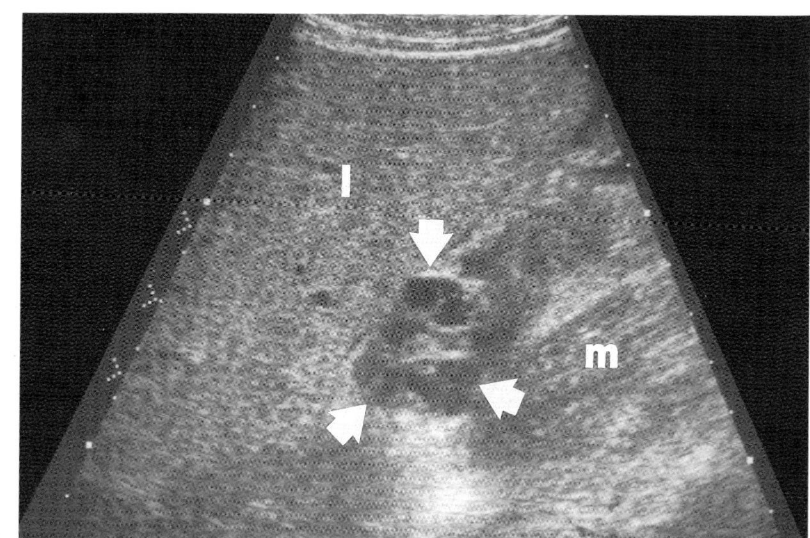

B

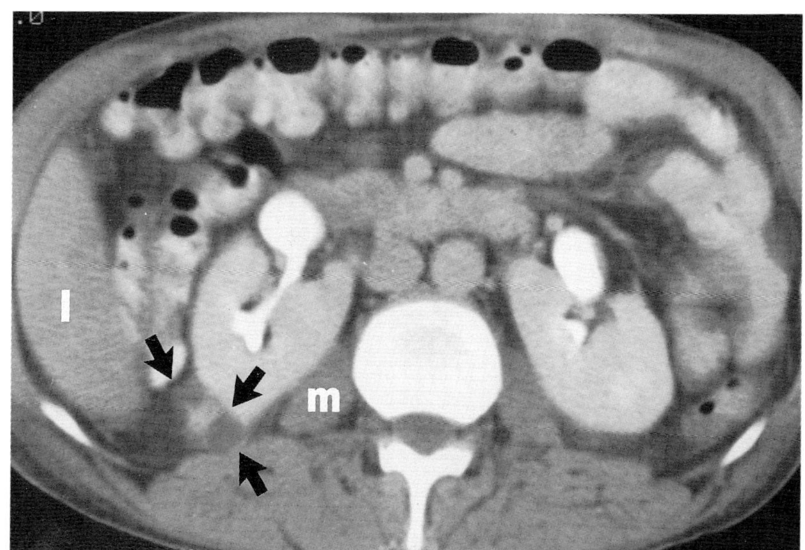

FIG. 5.61. Cystic renal cell carcinoma, horseshoe kidney. **A:** Longitudinal oblique sonogram of the right kidney reveals a cystic renal cell carcinoma (*arrows*) comprised of multiple small cysts with very little solid tissue. Note the through transmission deep to the lesion. **B:** A CT scan reveals similar findings. Although cystic change in renal cell carcinoma is not unusual, predominantly cystic renal cell carcinoma is rare. l, liver; m, psoas muscle.

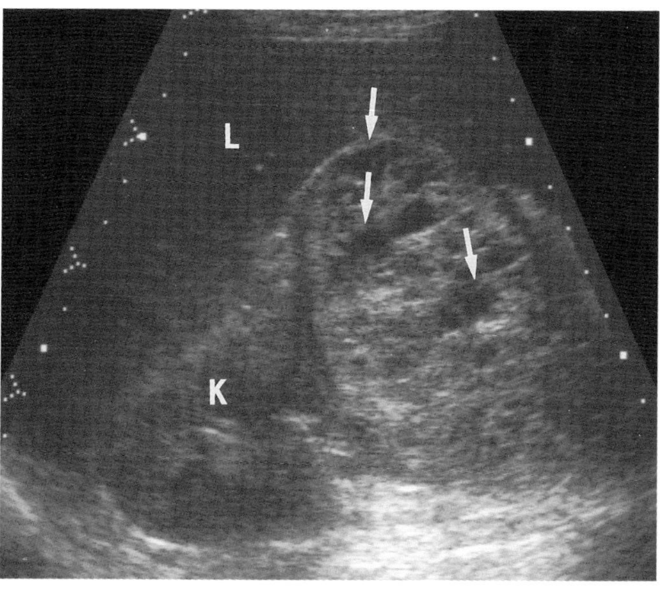

FIG. 5.62. Predominantly echogenic renal cell carcinoma. Longitudinal oblique sonogram of the right kidney. This large renal cell carcinoma has echogenicity greater than that of the renal sinus. Renal cell carcinoma of equal or greater echogenicity than renal sinus fat is unusual. In this instance, much of the increased echogenicity may be related to through transmission from the multiple small cystic areas within the tumor (*arrows*). K, normal upper pole; L, liver.

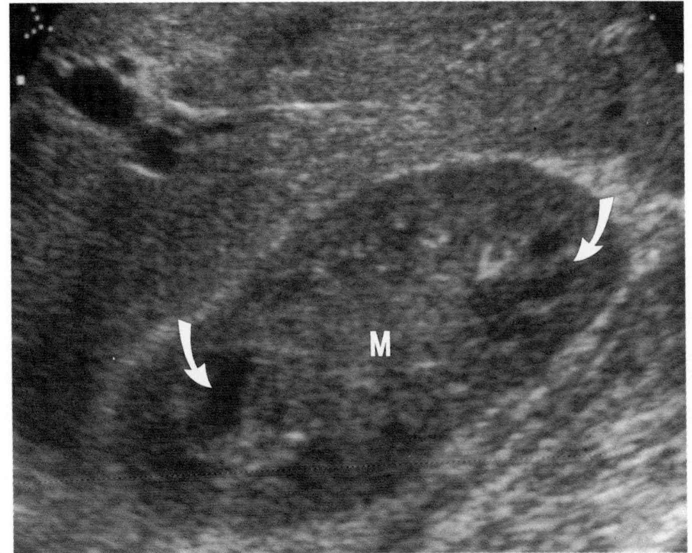

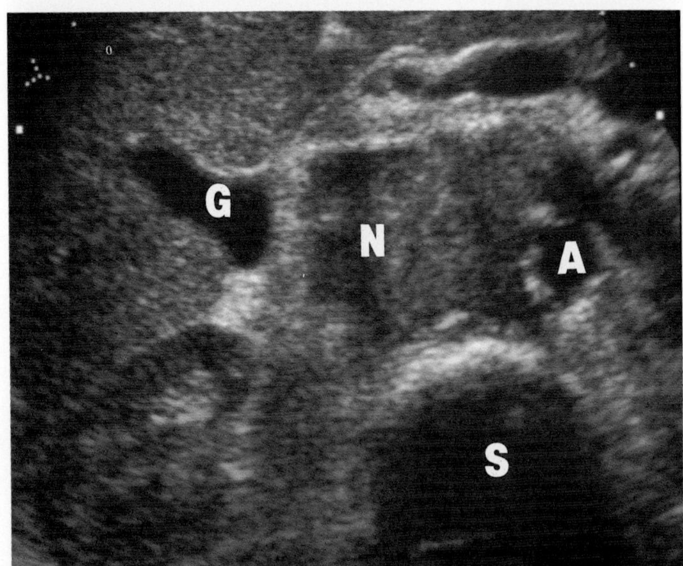

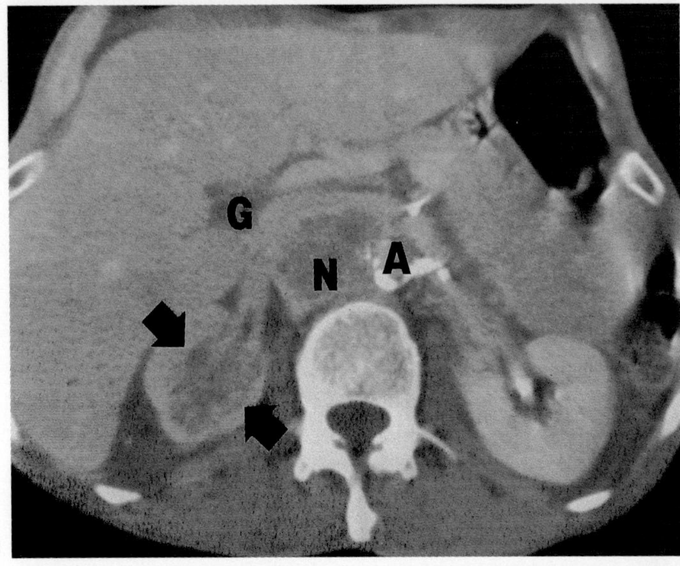

FIG. 5.63. Advanced renal cell carcinoma, subtle sonographically. **A:** Longitudinal sonogram of the right kidney reveals an ill-defined, slightly echogenic mass (M) in the middle portion of the renal sinus. The main abnormality is obliteration of the normal renal sinus structures (*curved arrows*) seen caudal and cephalad to the mass. **B:** This renal cell carcinoma was first discovered because of extensive adenopathy (nodes—N) in the periaortic region, visualized on the transverse sonogram. Note the displaced, calcified aorta (A). After the adenopathy had been discovered, the right kidney was carefully evaluated. The subtle architectural abnormality and renal sinus obliteration caused by the carcinoma were discovered. **C:** A contrast-enhanced CT scan demonstrates the mass (*arrows*) and the enlarged lymph node (N). S, spine; G, gallbladder.

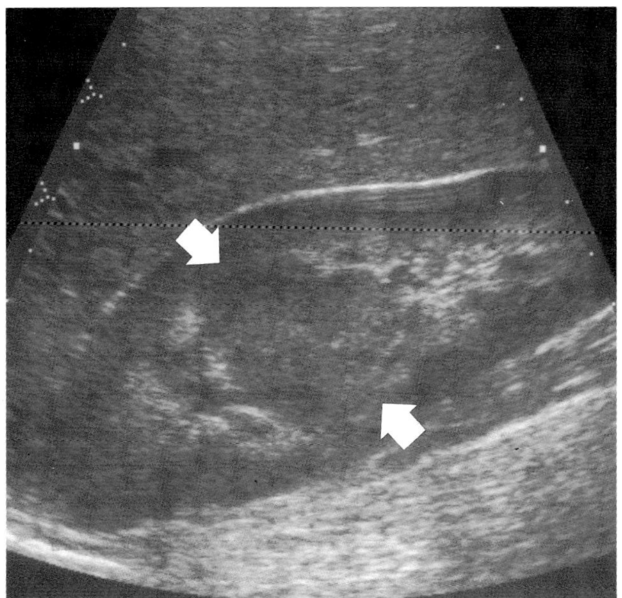

FIG. 5.64. Deceptive renal column simulates mass. Longitudinal sonogram of the right kidney. This deceptive renal column simulates a urothelial tumor or a renal cell carcinoma invading the renal sinus. The well-defined soft tissue mass (*arrows*) in the midst of the renal sinus was shown by subsequent studies to consist of normal renal parenchyma. It had normal flow on color flow sonography and was normal on a nuclear scan.

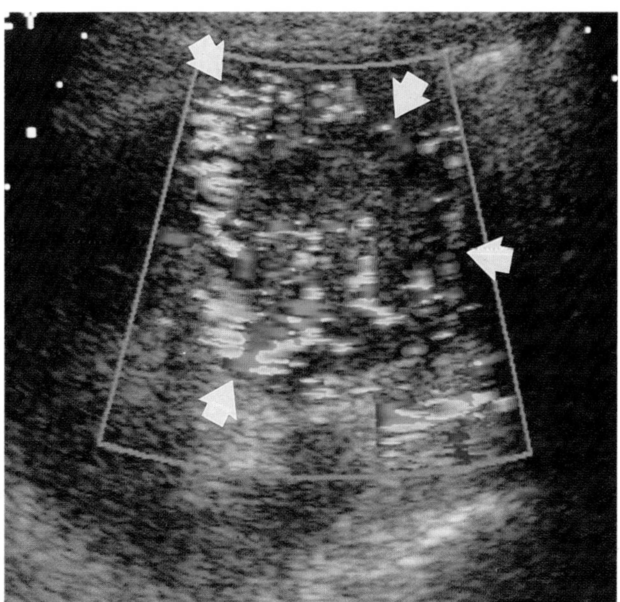

FIG. 5.65. Renal cell carcinoma, increased color flow. Transverse color Doppler sonogram of the right kidney reveals increased color flow within the renal cell carcinoma (*arrows*) compared to the normal parenchyma. Although renal cell carcinomas are hypervascular angiographically in three-fourths of patients, it is currently unknown what percentage have flow greater than renal parenchyma on color flow imaging.

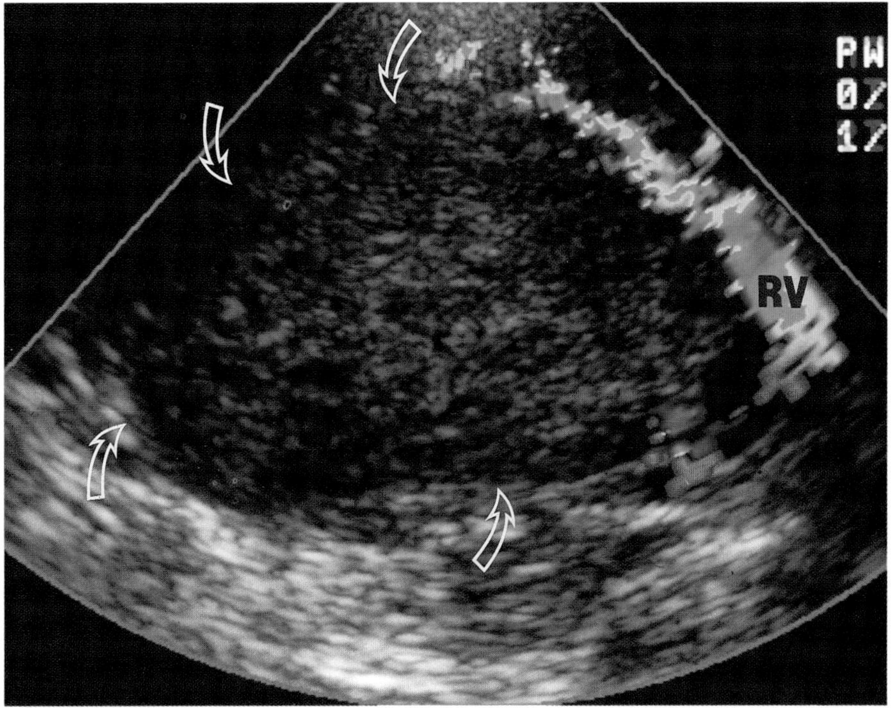

FIG. 5.66. Renal cell carcinoma, no internal color flow. Oblique longitudinal color Doppler sonogram of a large renal cell carcinoma (*curved open arrows*) reveals no flow within the tumor. The renal vein (RV) is displaced but not invaded by this tumor.

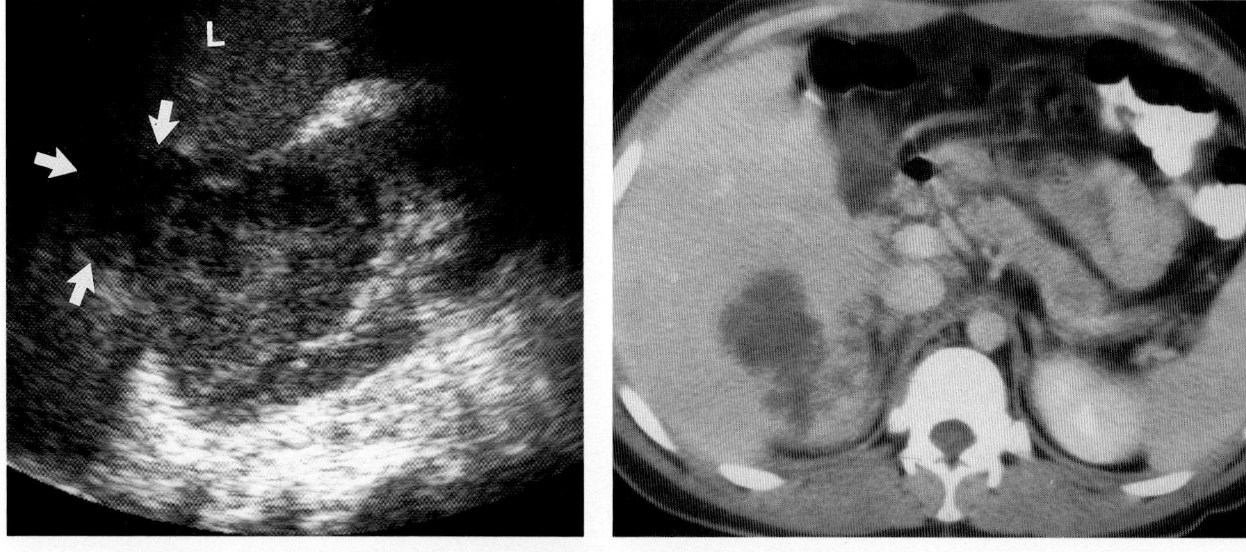

FIG. 5.67. Renal cell carcinoma invades the liver. **A:** Longitudinal sonogram of the right kidney and liver reveals a large renal mass that directly invades the liver (*arrows*). **B:** The CT scan showed the mass but could not definitively differentiate invasion from indentation caused by the tumor. Sonography's ability to scan in any plane is useful in making distinctions such as this. L, liver.

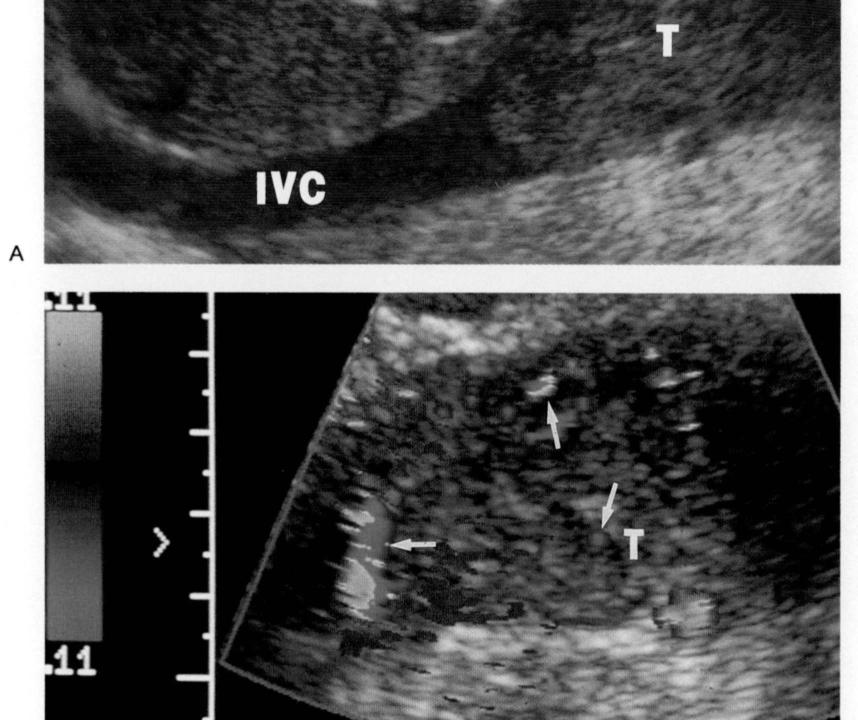

FIG. 5.68. Renal cell carcinoma invades the inferior vena cava. **A:** Longitudinal sonogram reveals a large tumor thrombus (T) within the inferior vena cava (IVC). **B:** Color flow sonogram reveals internal flow within the tumor thrombus (*arrows*). Renal cell carcinoma is the neoplasm that most frequently invades the IVC (hepatocellular carcinoma is second). Detection of color-coded flow within the thrombus documents the neoplastic nature of the thrombus. This is useful in distinguishing bland clot from tumor thrombus.

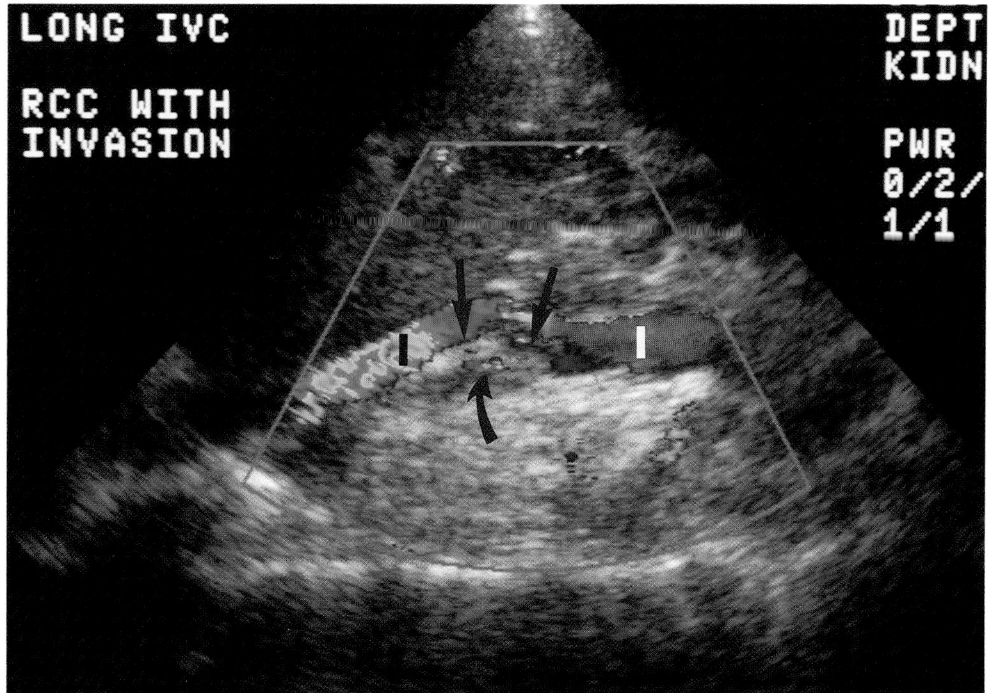

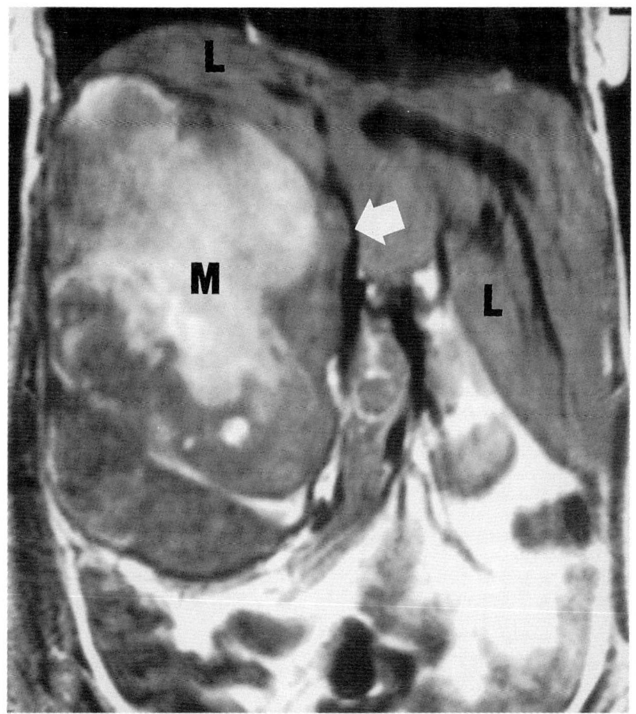

FIG. 5.69. Huge renal cell carcinoma invades inferior vena cava. **A:** Longitudinal color Doppler sonogram of the inferior vena cave reveals partial tumor thrombus within the inferior vena cava (*arrows*). The right renal artery (*curved arrow*) is noted dorsal to the tumor-containing inferior vena cava (I). **B:** A coronal MR image reveals a huge renal mass (M) representing the renal cell carcinoma. The inferior vena caval involvement (*arrow*) is also demonstrated by the MR study. L, liver.

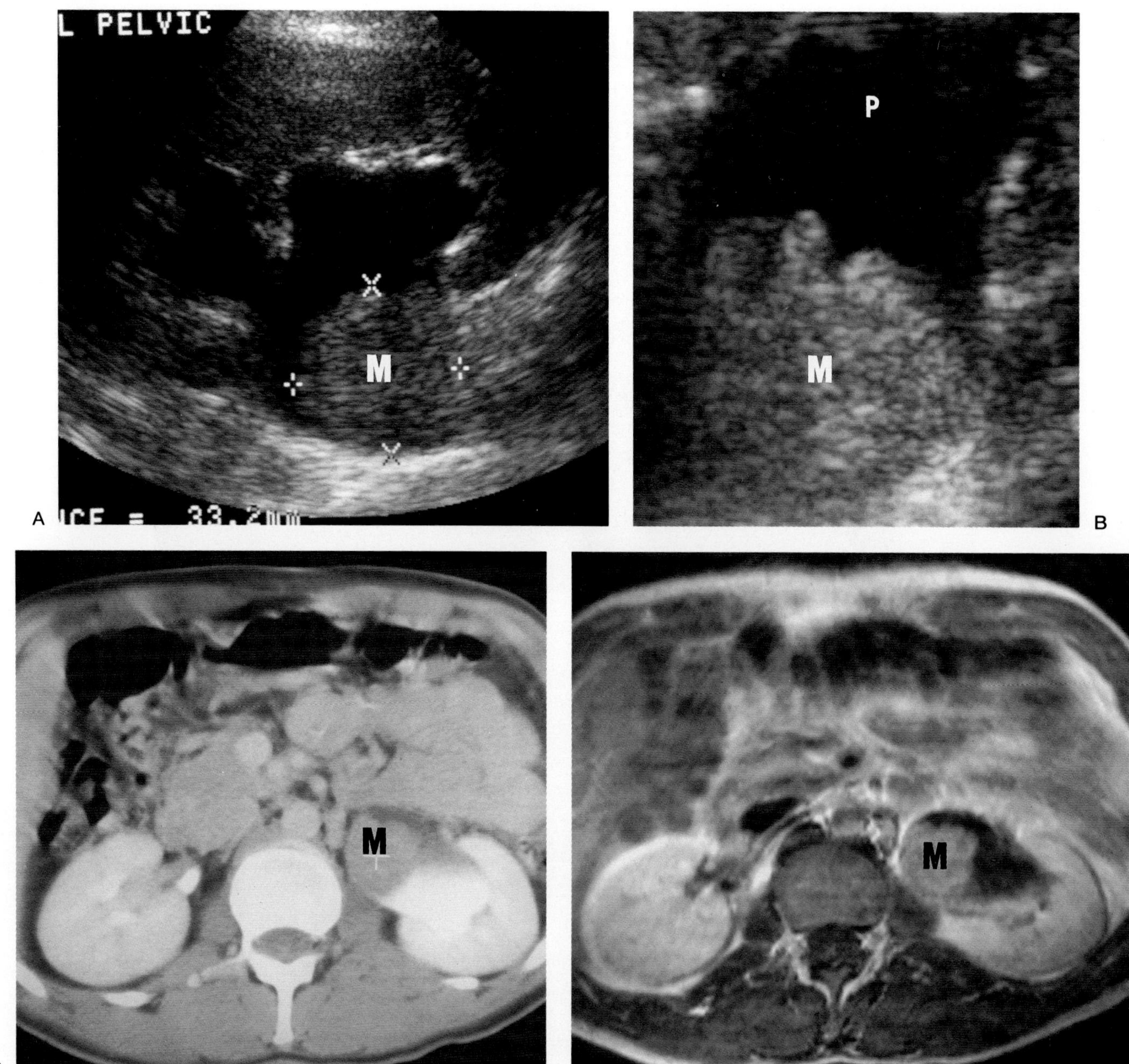

FIG. 5.70. Obstructing transitional cell carcinoma. Longitudinal coronal sonogram (**A**) of the left kidney reveals a 3- to 4-cm mass (M—outlined by calipers) that obstructs the ureteropelvic junction and causes hydronephrosis. The lobulated shape of this transitional cell carcinoma is shown on the magnified transverse sonogram through the renal pelvis (**B**). M, Transitional cell carcinoma; P, dilated renal pelvis. The transitional cell carcinoma mass (M) is also demonstrated on the CT scan (**C**) and the MR image (**D**). Although large transitional cell carcinomas such as this are relatively easy to image, small or medium sized nonobstructing tumors may be difficult to detect sonographically.

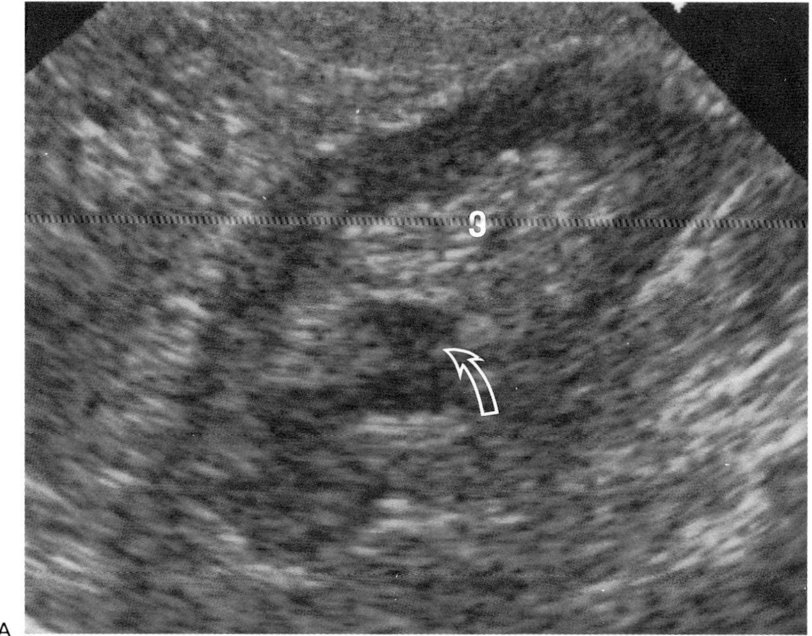

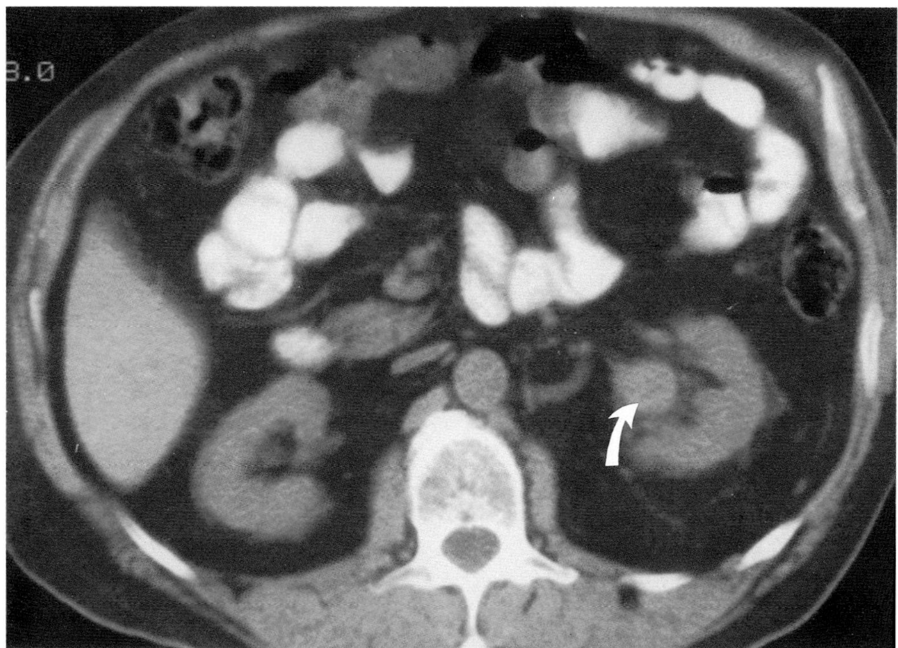

FIG. 5.71. Transitional cell carcinoma, left kidney. **A:** Longitudinal sonogram of the left kidney reveals a hypoechoic mass (*open curved arrow*) within the fat-containing renal sinus (S). **B:** A noncontrast CT reveals a renal pelvis mass (*curved arrow*) that is of higher attenuation than the unenhanced renal cortex. This is a small transitional cell carcinoma that was easily visualized on both sonography and CT. Small or moderate sized transitional cell carcinomas that do not cause hydronephrosis are often difficult to image. Sonographically, the differential diagnosis includes renal column (a normal variant) or a renal cell carcinoma involving the renal sinus.

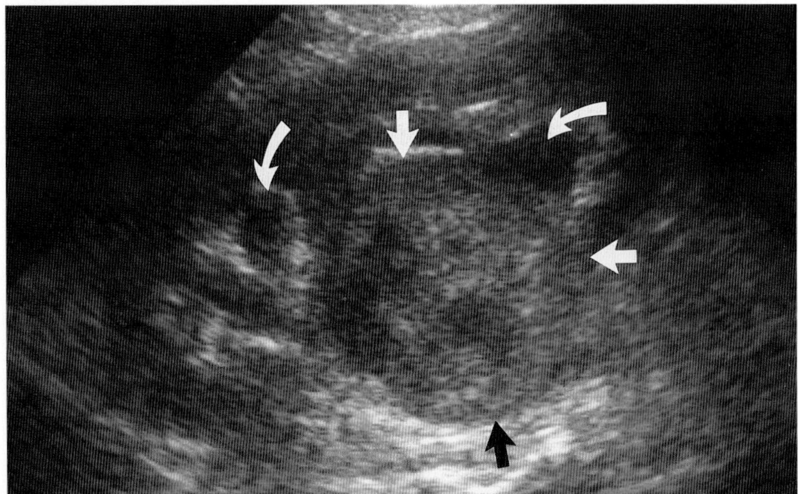

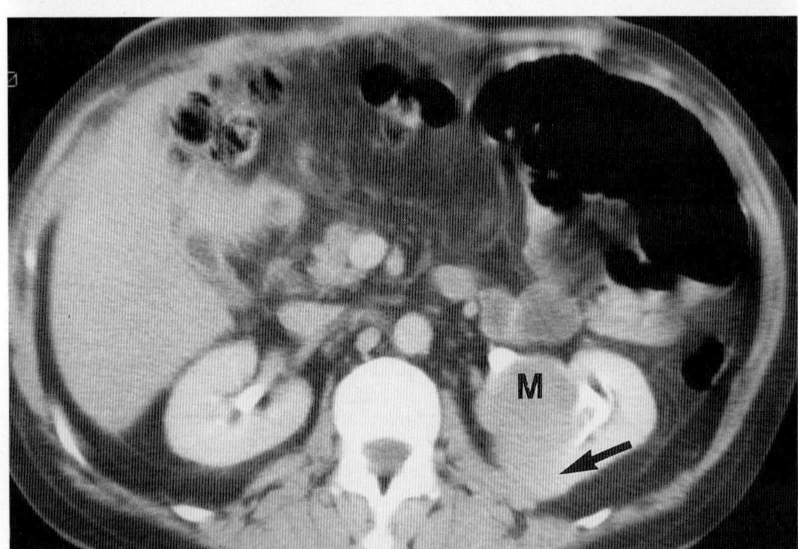

FIG. 5.72. Renal cell carcinoma simulates transitional cell carcinoma. Longitudinal coronal sonogram (**A**) of the left kidney reveals a mass within the renal pelvis similar to the transitional cell carcinoma depicted in Fig. 5.70. Note the heterogeneous mass (*arrows*) and the slightly dilated intrarenal collecting system (*curved arrows*). Other sonograms (not shown) and the CT scan (**B**) showed that the mass (M) originated from the renal cortex dorsally (*arrow*). Renal cell carcinoma is the commonest mass to involve the renal sinus. It is even more frequent than urothelial tumors such as transitional cell carcinoma.

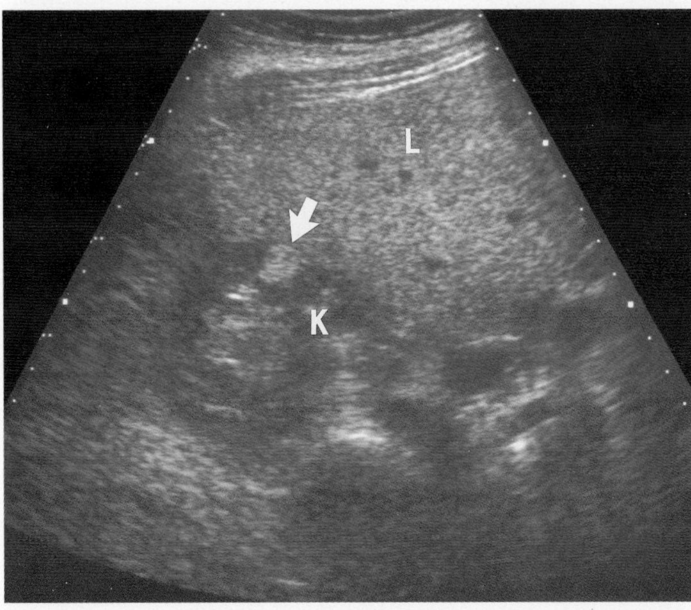

FIG. 5.73. Small angiomyolipoma. Transverse oblique sonogram of the right kidney reveals a small right renal angiomyolipoma (*arrow*). This less than 1-cm lesion was incidentally discovered during routine abdominal sonography requested because of vague abdominal pain. Finding a well-circumscribed echogenic mass such as this is highly suggestive of angiomyolipoma, but a CT scan is necessary to definitively demonstrate the intralesional fat and confirm the diagnosis. This patient had no evidence of tuberous sclerosis. L, liver; K, right kidney.

lesions are important as they may cause symptoms and have angiographic findings similar to those of RCC. About 80 percent of tuberous sclerosis patients have multiple bilateral angiomyolipomas. Approximately half of all patients with angiomyolipomas have tuberous sclerosis. In patients without tuberous sclerosis, angiomyolipomas are often incidental findings in asymptomatic patients (Fig. 5.73). Tumors of any size may occur in this group (Fig. 5.73). Almost 80 percent of these patients are middle-aged females (60,61).

The presence of fat in angiomyolipoma results in a sonographic appearance of a relatively homogeneous renal mass with echogenicity greater than or equal to the renal sinus fat. Mixed echogenicity is not unusual, especially when intralesional hemorrhage is present (Figs. 5.74 and 5.75) (60). Finding a well-defined echogenic renal lesion on sonography suggests the presence of an angiomyolipoma (Figs. 5.75 and 5.76). CT, which can demonstrate fat density within the lesion (Figs. 5.75 and 5.76), is required for definitive diagnosis.

Renal Metastases

Metastases are the most frequent renal tumor in autopsy series (62,63). Renal metastases are usually a relatively late manifestation of widespread metastatic disease; hence they are rarely clinically significant. Occasionally, a single renal metastasis from an unsuspected primary may be confused with a renal cell carcinoma. Typically, multiple masses are present, although a single metastasis can occur. Metastases are usually hypoechoic (Fig. 5.77), although renal enlargement without a discrete mass may occur. CT is more sensitive than sonography in detecting renal metastasis (62).

Renal Lymphoma

Primary renal lymphoma is rare. Renal involvement most often occurs as a manifestation of widespread lymphoma. Non-Hodgkin's lymphoma of the kidney is much more common than Hodgkin's lymphoma. It is estimated that 5 percent of patients have renal involvement at the time of diagnosis and 33 percent at autopsy (64).

Sonographic patterns of renal lymphoma are varied. Fifty percent of patients have a solitary renal mass, 30 percent multiple small masses (Fig. 5.78), and 20 percent have diffuse parenchymal infiltration (64,65). Renal masses are typically hypoechoic or even anechoic. On occasion, through transmission of sound may occur deep to lymphomatous masses (64–66). Diffuse involvement may be hypoechoic or echogenic (Figs. 5.79 and 5.80). Many patients have perinephric disease (Figs. 5.80 and 5.81) (64). On occasion, perirenal or subcapsular lymphomatous involvement may be confused with hematoma, extramedullary hematopoiesis (14,15), or infection.

RENAL STONES

Renal calculi are common and typically arise within the collecting system. Plain films and intravenous urography are the primary examinations used to diagnose renal calculi in patients with renal colic. In some studies, ultrasound has detected more than 90 percent of renal calculi (67–70). Because of this, some have suggested that patients with renal colic should be evaluated with the combination of sonography and plain radiography, rather than intravenous urography (70–72). Others still favor urography to screen patients with suspected renal colic that may be caused by renal stones (73).

Most renal calculi (about 80 percent) are calcified. Sonographically, stones usually appear as hyperechoic foci with distal acoustic shadowing (Fig. 5.82). Small stones may not engender shadowing deep to the stone (Fig. 5.83). When there is no shadowing, it may be difficult to distinguish small calculi from echogenic foci caused by fat or other echogenic reflectors within the renal sinus. Vascular or parenchymal calcification may mimic stones; false-positive studies may result. In addition, stones may be missed (false-negative) because of suboptimal studies in difficult or uncooperative patients.

Sonographically, staghorn calculi often appear as multiple, disconnected calculi within the collecting system (Fig. 5.84). Careful real-time scanning can reveal the true diagnosis, though sonography generally underestimates the extent and size of stones in patients with staghorn and other large calculi. The presence of a staghorn calculus may make it difficult to diagnose underlying caliceal and pelvicaliceal dilatation. Renal calcifications also occur in patients with medullary sponge kidney (Figs. 5.52 and 5.53) and in patients with nephrocalcinosis (Fig. 5.85).

HYDRONEPHROSIS AND OBSTRUCTION

Hydronephrosis refers to pelvicaliceal dilatation often, but not always, resulting from urinary tract obstruction (Figs. 5.86 to 5.88). Urinary obstruction, usually bilateral, causes less than 5 percent of all renal failure. Sonography can sensitively detect dilatation of the renal pelvis and calices. Unfortunately, dilatation is not always indicative of obstruction. Hydronephrosis may occur without obstruction and, less commonly, obstruction may occur without dilatation.

Reflux is a major cause of hydronephrosis without obstruction (Figs. 5.89 to 5.91). Other causes of pelvicaliceal dilatation without obstruction (false-positive for ob-

(*text continues on page 334*)

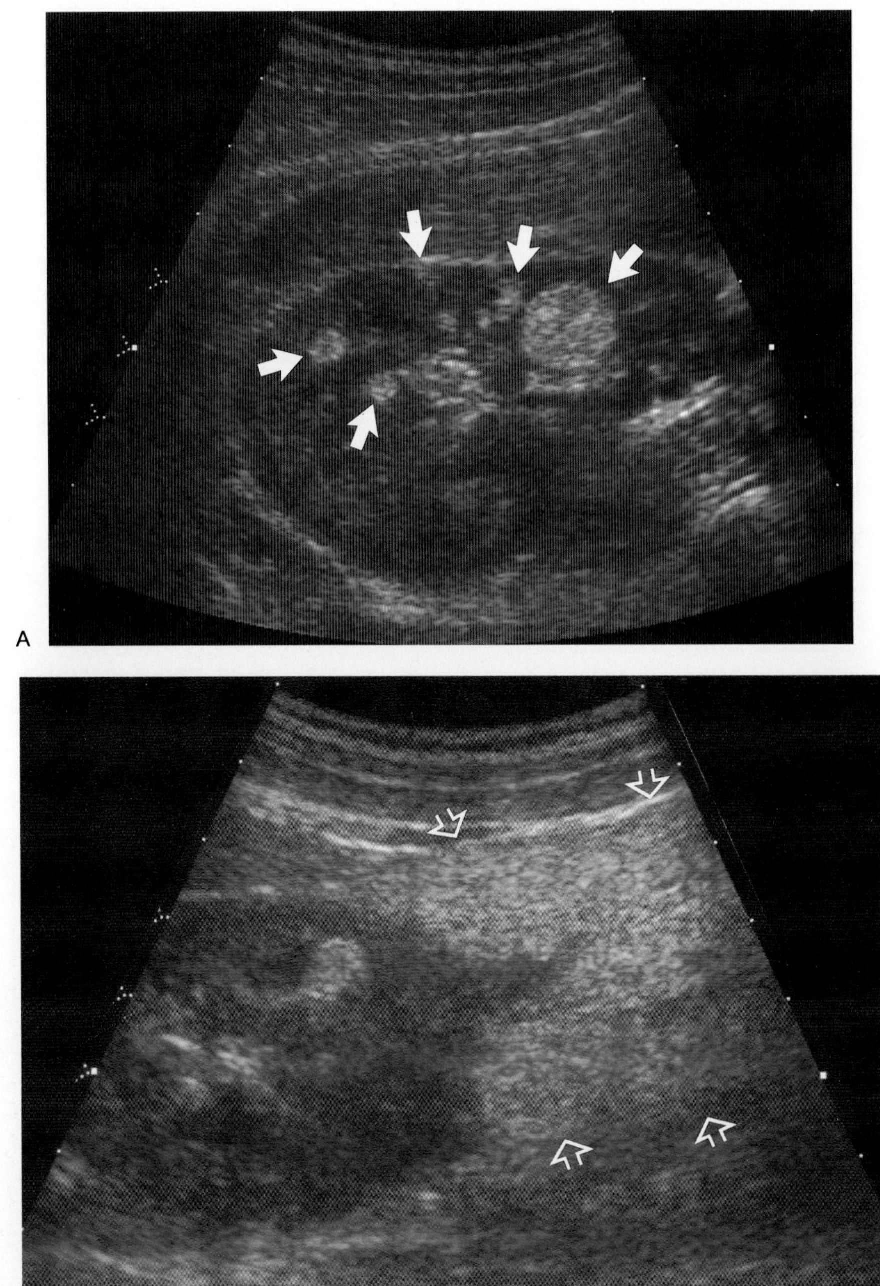

FIG. 5.74. Multiple angiomyolipomas, varying sizes. Transverse (**A**) and longitudinal (**B**) sonograms of the right kidney reveal multiple angiomyolipomas of varying sizes. This patient does not have tuberous sclerosis. Multiple intrarenal lesions varying in size from less than 1 to 1.5 cm (*arrows*) are noted on the transverse image. The sagittal image reveals a large exophytic angiomyolipoma (*open arrows*).

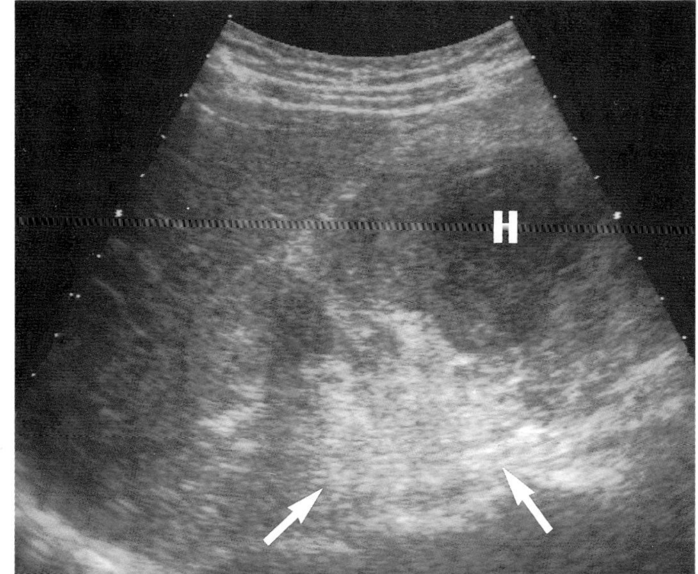

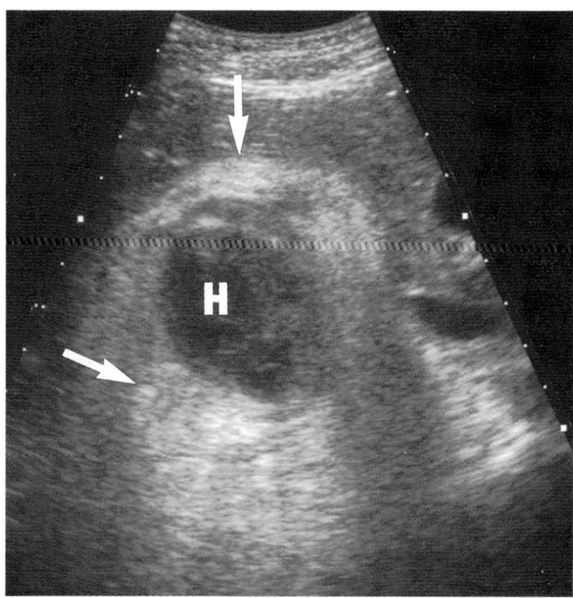

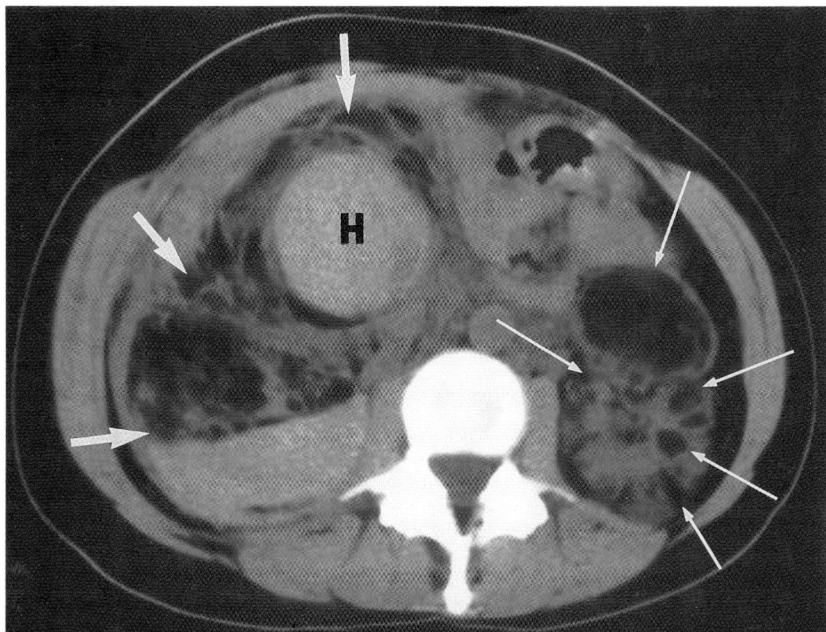

FIG. 5.75. Angiomyolipoma with hemorrhage. Longitudinal (**A**) and transverse (**B**) sonograms of the right kidney reveal heterogeneous echogenicity within the right kidney. Although areas of increased echogenicity (*arrows*) are present, angiomyolipoma cannot be definitively diagnosed. The hypoechoic region is an intralesional hematoma (H). The presence of fat (*arrows*) within the lesion on the CT scan (**C**) makes definitive diagnosis of angiomyolipoma possible. The CT scan reveals high-attenuation hemorrhage in the intralesional hematoma (H) that is hypoechoic sonographically. This patient has tuberous sclerosis. Left renal angiomyolipomas (*thin arrows*) are demonstrated on the CT scan.

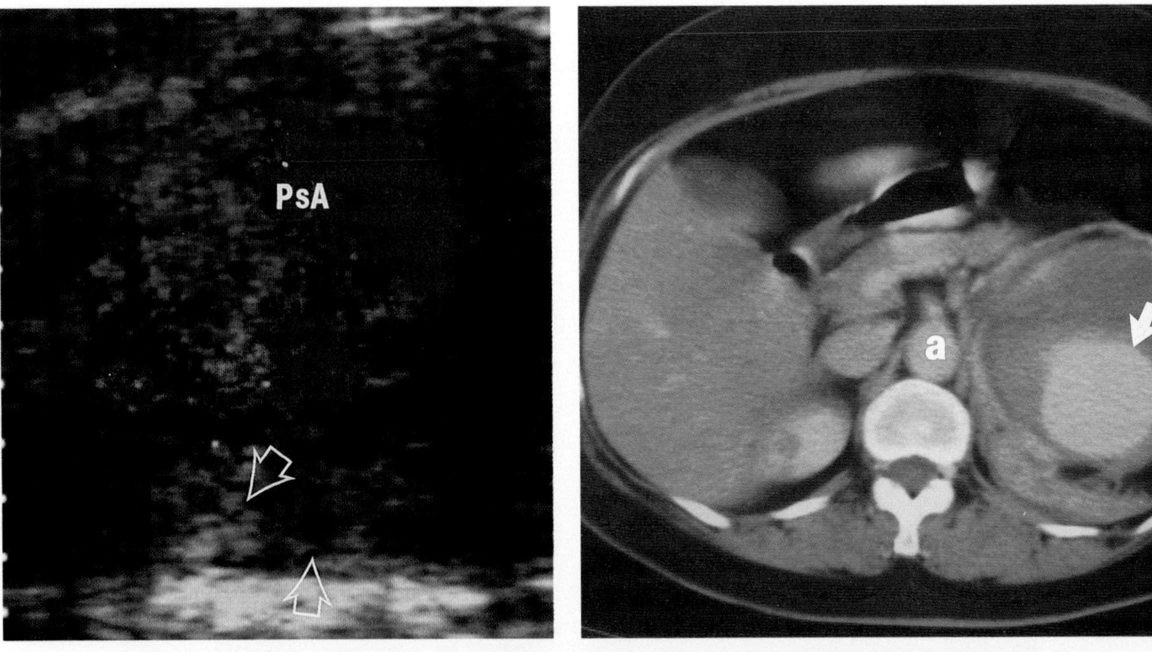

FIG. 5.76. Angiomyolipoma with large pseudoaneurysm. **A:** Longitudinal color Doppler sonogram reveals a large, 6-cm pseudoaneurysm with swirling, alternating red- and blue-coded flow (PsA). A mixed echogenicity mass, related to hemorrhage, is noted around the pseudoaneurysm. Note the feeding vessel (*open arrows*). **B:** A CT scan reveals vascular type contrast enhancement within the pseudoaneurysm (*arrow*). The surrounding hematoma is of lower attenuation. Note that the CT scan allows definitive diagnosis, since it demonstrates the presence of fat (*open curved arrow*). a, aorta. (From ref. 7a, with permission.)

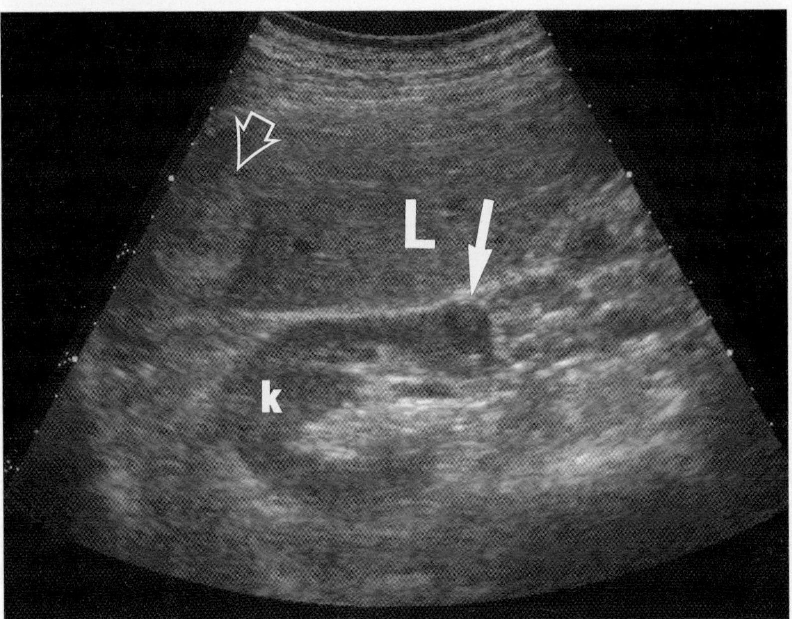

FIG. 5.77. Lung carcinoma metastasis to the kidney. Transverse sonogram through the right kidney reveals a small, approximately 1.5-cm hypoechoic metastasis from lung carcinoma (*arrow*). Metastases can be large or small or even have an infiltrative pattern. Typically, renal metastases are a late manifestation of metastatic disease. They are rarely clinically significant. Note the incidental hepatic hemangioma (*open arrow*). L, liver; K, right kidney.

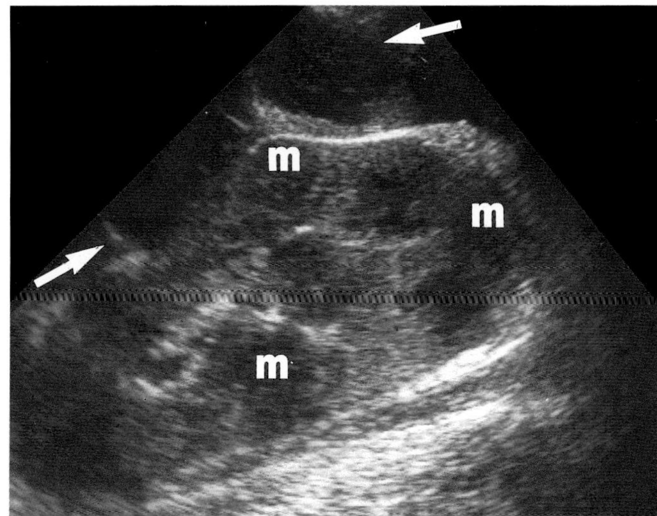

FIG. 5.78. Multifocal non-Hodgkin's lymphoma. Longitudinal sonogram of the right kidney reveals multiple focal masses (some indicated—m). Renal masses from lymphoma are typically hypoechoic, as in this case. This patient has AIDS-related lymphoma. Hypoechoic liver masses (*arrows*) are present, adjacent to the abnormal kidney.

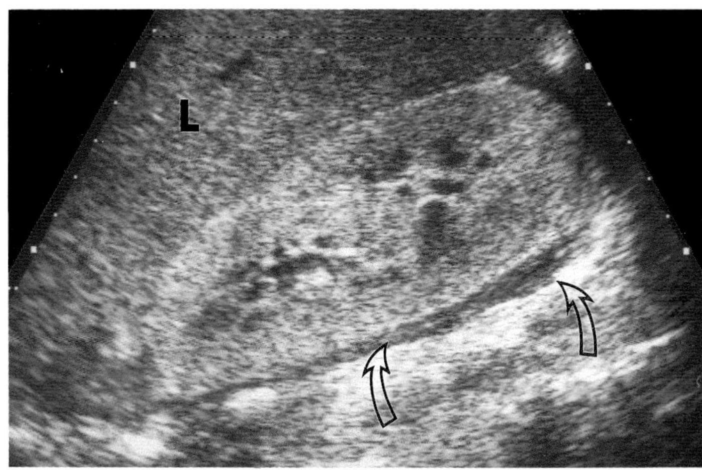

FIG. 5.79. Diffuse Hodgkin's lymphoma. Longitudinal sonogram of the right kidney reveals diffuse increased echogenicity in this patient with bilateral diffuse Hodgkin's lymphoma of the kidneys. Diffuse renal involvement with lymphoma may be echogenic, as in this patient, or hypoechoic. L, liver; *curved open arrows,* quadratus lumborum muscle.

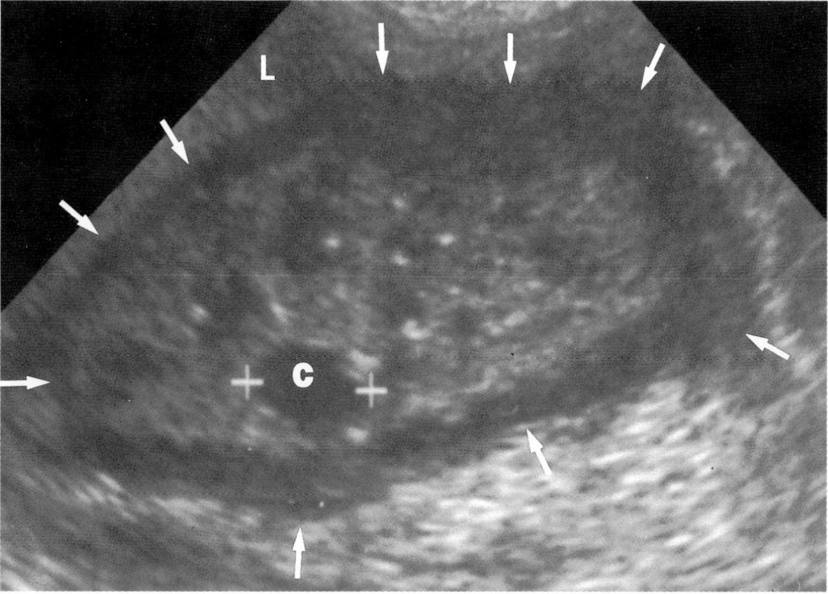

FIG. 5.80. Diffuse renal and perinephric non-Hodgkin's lymphoma. Longitudinal sonogram through the right kidney reveals diffuse increased renal echogenicity in this patient with diffuse renal non-Hodgkin's lymphoma. A small simple cyst (c) is noted. Note the extrarenal hypoechoic perinephric lymphomatous involvement (*arrows*). L, liver.

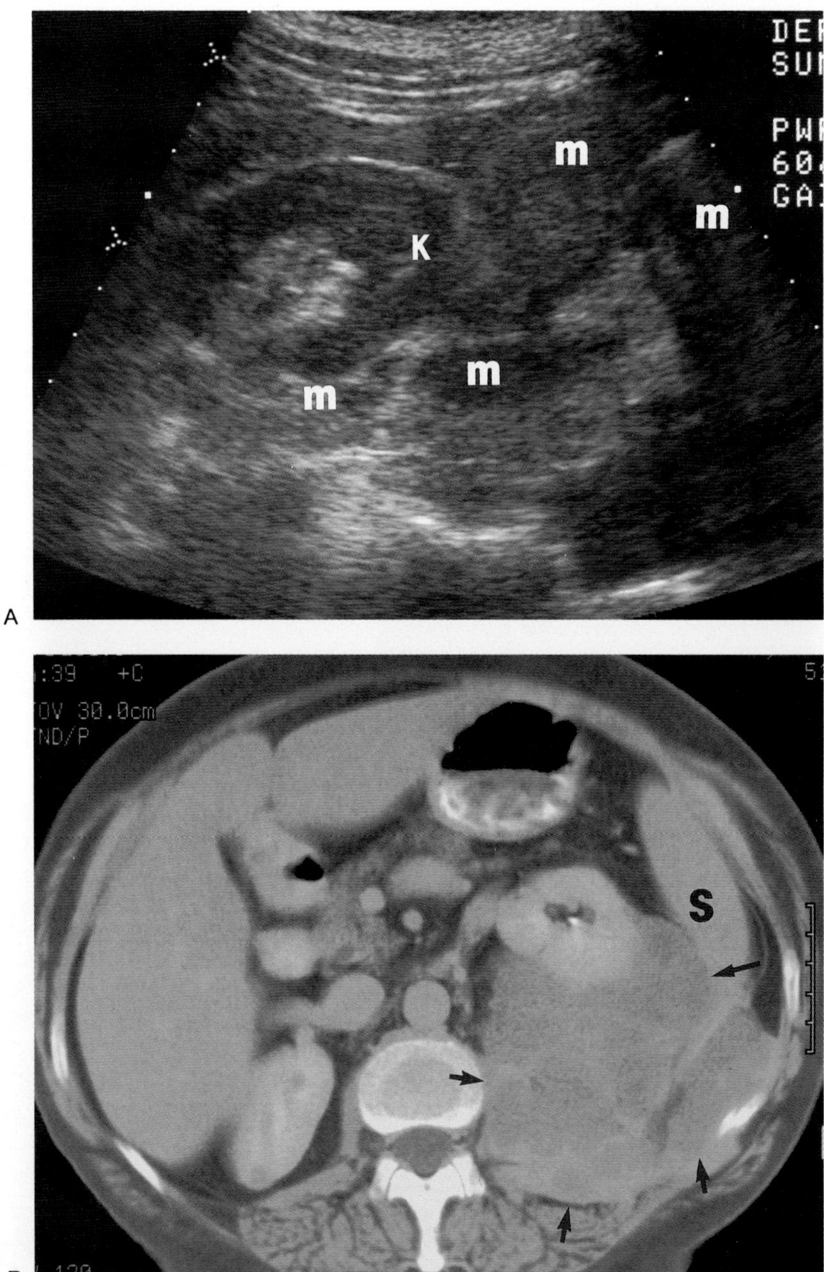

FIG. 5.81. Perirenal non-Hodgkin's lymphoma. **A:** Longitudinal sonogram of the left kidney (K) reveals multiple perinephric masses (m) that displace the kidney. **B:** The CT scan delineates massive involvement (*arrows*) dorsal to the kidney and adjacent to the spleen (S).

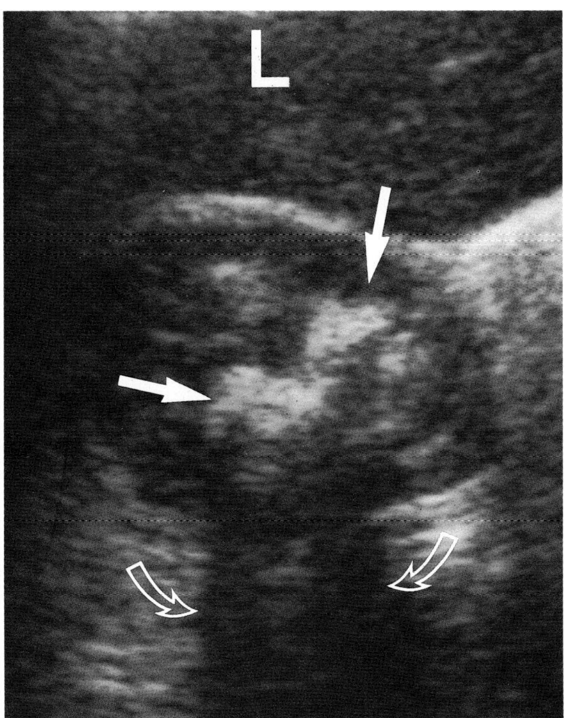

FIG. 5.82. Large renal calculi. Transverse sonogram through the lower pole of the right kidney reveals multiple echogenic renal calculi (*arrows*) that exhibit prominent distal sonic shadowing (*curved open arrows*). This is an example of classic sonographic findings for renal stones. On occasion, it may be difficult to distinguish stones from echogenic foci caused by gas or fat within the renal sinus. L, liver.

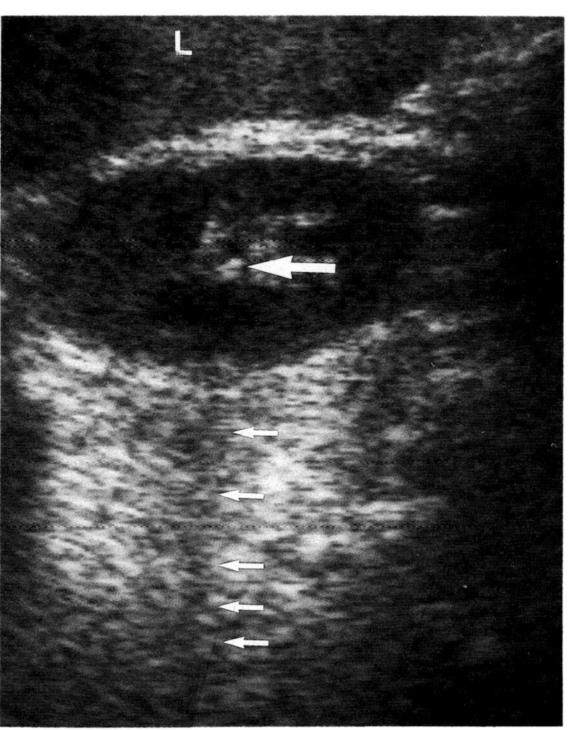

FIG. 5.83. Small stone with faint shadowing. Transverse sonogram through the region of the right kidney reveals a small echogenic focus (*arrow*) with subtle acoustic shadowing (*small arrows*). Small stones such as this often do not exhibit distal acoustic shadowing. When there is no shadowing, it is difficult, if not impossible, to distinguish small stones from normal echogenic structures within the renal sinus. L, liver.

A

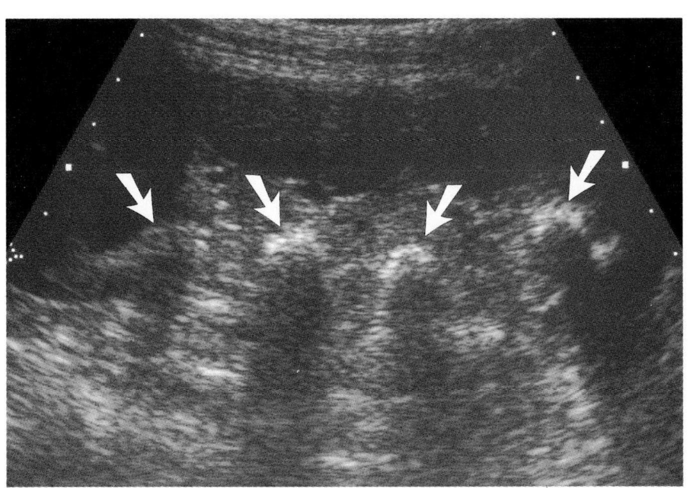

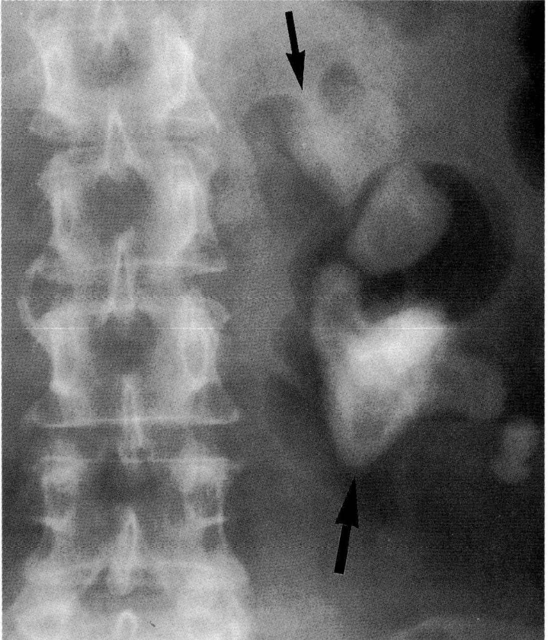

B

FIG. 5.84. Staghorn calculus. **A:** Longitudinal sonogram of the left kidney shows multiple, apparently discrete, shadowing calcifications (*slanted arrows*) through most of the renal sinus. **B:** The plain film of the left upper abdomen reveals the staghorn calculus (*arrows*) in the left kidney. Often, sonography underestimates the size of the calculus in patients with staghorn and other large calculi. Careful real-time survey will reveal the true diagnosis.

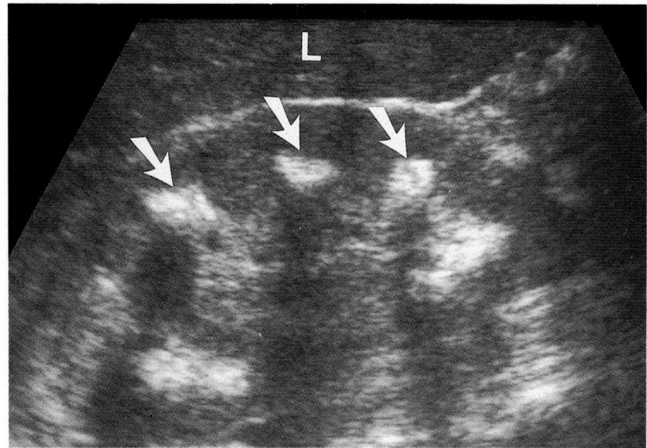

FIG. 5.85. Nephrocalcinosis related to primary hyperparathyroidism. Longitudinal sonogram of the right kidney reveals multiple fine medullary calcifications (*arrows*), which, in aggregate, engender acoustic shadowing. This patient had a large parathyroid adenoma and severe hypercalcemia. Nephrocalcinosis may occur in many abnormal metabolic states, especially those leading to hypercalcemia. L, liver.

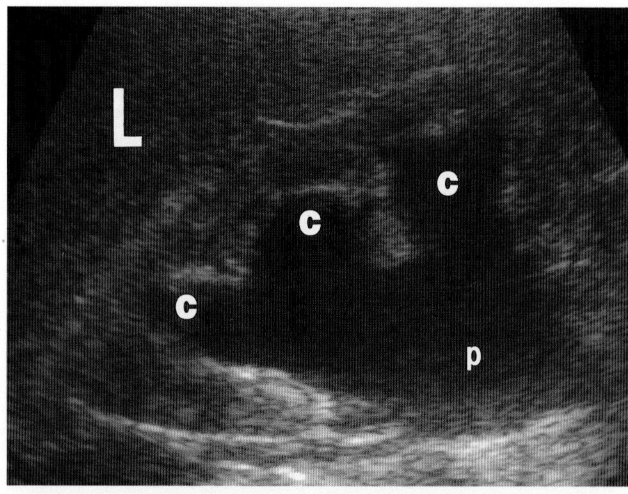

FIG. 5.86. Hydronephrosis, obstruction from cervical carcinoma. Longitudinal sonogram of the right kidney reveals marked pelvicaliceal dilatation. p, pelvis; c, calices. Hydronephrosis (pelvicaliceal dilatation) often, but not always, results from urinary tract obstruction. L, liver.

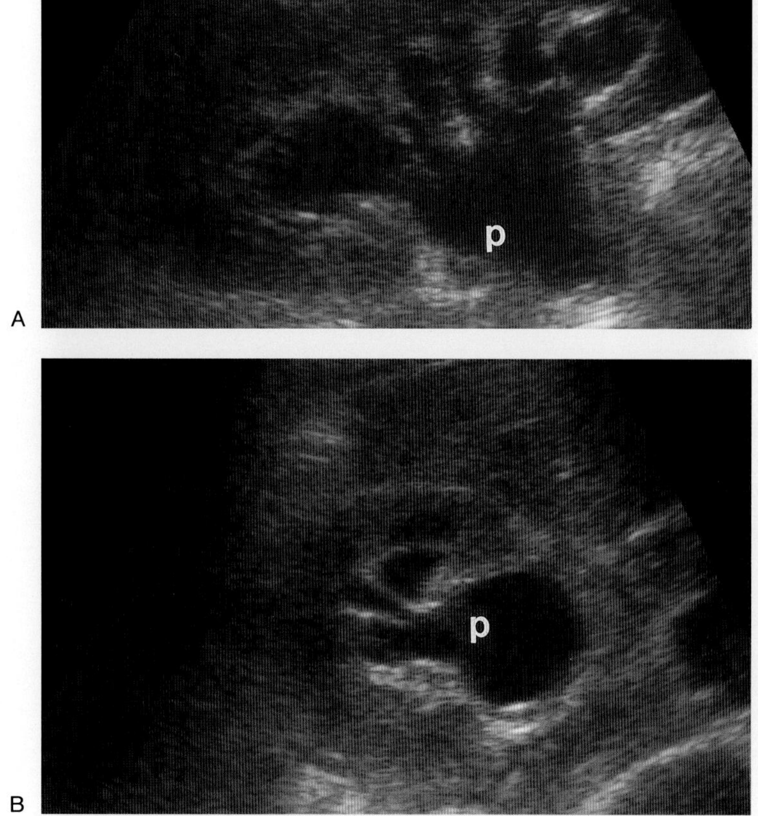

FIG. 5.87. Hydronephrosis, cervical carcinoma. **A:** Longitudinal oblique coronal sonogram of the right kidney reveals moderate to marked hydronephrosis with dilatation of the calices and renal pelvis (p). **B:** The transverse sonogram confirms the dilatation, especially of the extrarenal portion of the renal pelvis (p).

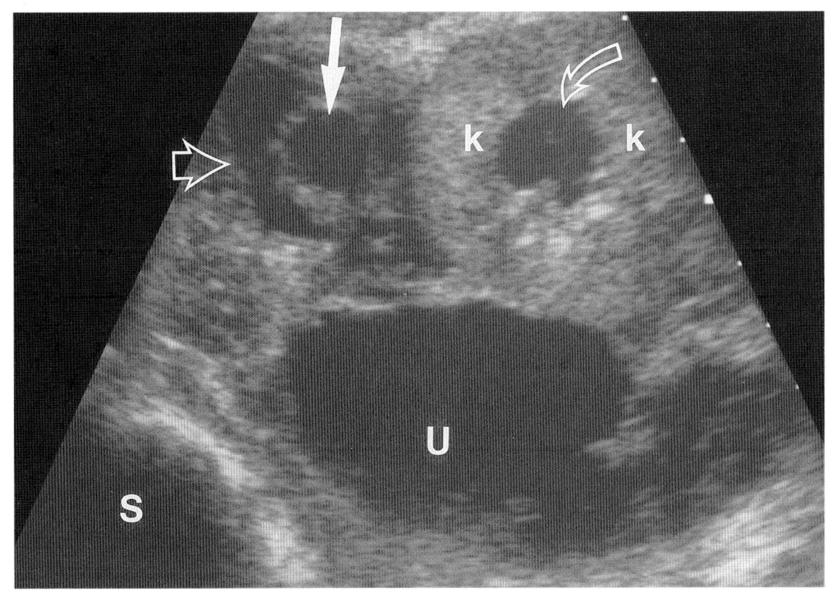

FIG. 5.88. Hydronephrosis, periureteral and perinephric urinomas. This transverse sonogram of the region of the left kidney (k) reveals a large dorsal perinephric urinoma (U). A small periureteral urinoma (*open arrow*) is seen surrounding the dilated ureter (*arrow*). Note the dilated lower pole calyx (*open curved arrow*). Ureteral obstruction from recurrent colon carcinoma resulted in forniceal rupture and the urinomas illustrated. A forniceal disruption may result in a nondilated pelvicalyceal system, even when the ureter is obstructed. There is often persistent dilatation as noted here. S, spine.

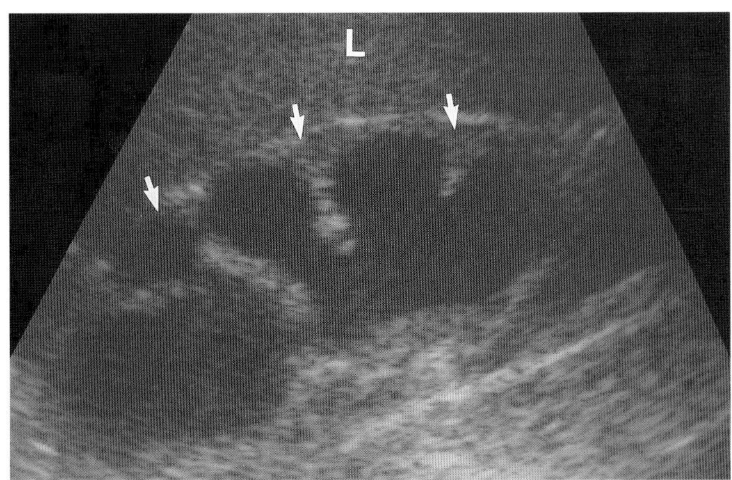

FIG. 5.89. Reflux-related hydronephrosis. Longitudinal sonogram of the right kidney reveals marked pelvicaliceal dilatation caused by reflux in a patient with a neurogenic bladder. Note that there is little residual cortex (*arrows*). This patient presented with renal failure caused by reflux-related cortical loss. It may be difficult to differentiate bilateral obstruction from the changes associated with reflux. Elevated peripheral resistance, diagnosed by abnormally increased resistive index using spectral Doppler sonography, suggests obstruction, rather than reflux-related hydronephrosis. Unfortunately, peripheral resistance may be normal in obstruction and elevated in other conditions. L, liver.

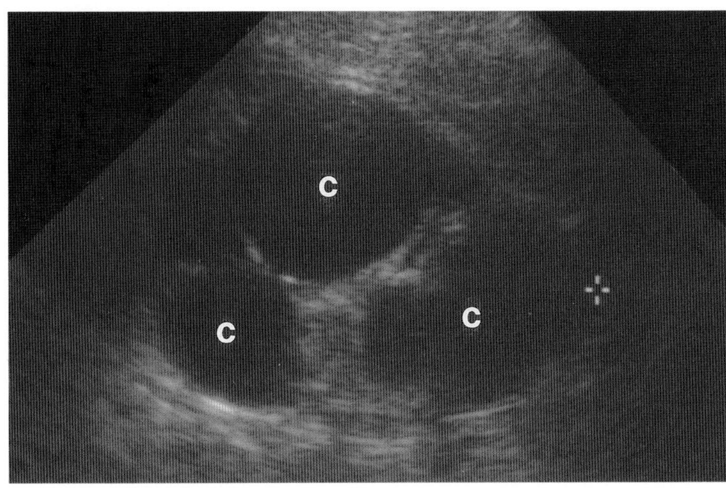

FIG. 5.90. Massive hydronephrosis related to reflux. Longitudinal sonogram of the left kidney reveals complete destruction of all of the renal cortex and a massively dilated pelvicaliceal system related to reflux. Multiple dilated calices (c) are noted.

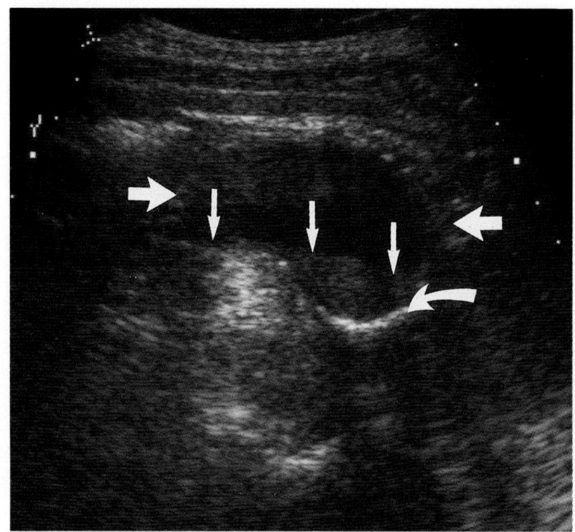

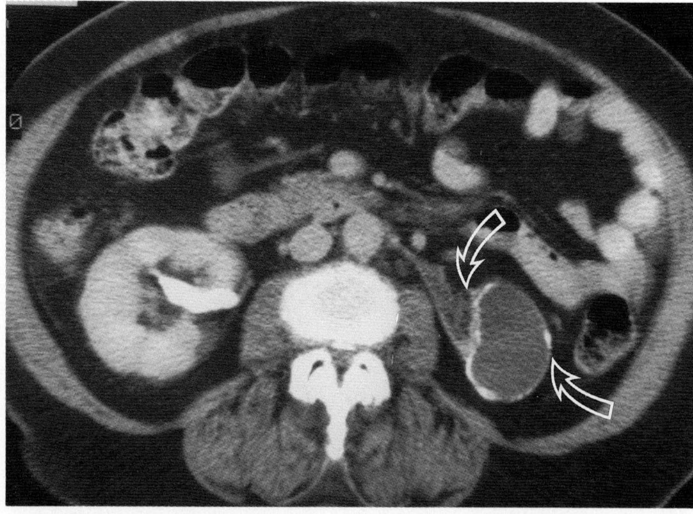

FIG. 5.91. Calcified cystic remnant, reflux nephropathy. **A:** Longitudinal coronal sonogram of the region of the left kidney reveals a small cystic structure (*arrows*) that has rim calcifications (*curved arrow*) and some internal dependent debris (*small arrows*). This patient had long-standing reflux and recurrent infection that resulted in total destruction of the left kidney, leaving a shrunken, calcified remnant of the pelvicaliceal system. No normal renal tissue is evident. **B:** The CT scan confirms the sonographic findings. Note the rim calcifications (*curved open arrows*).

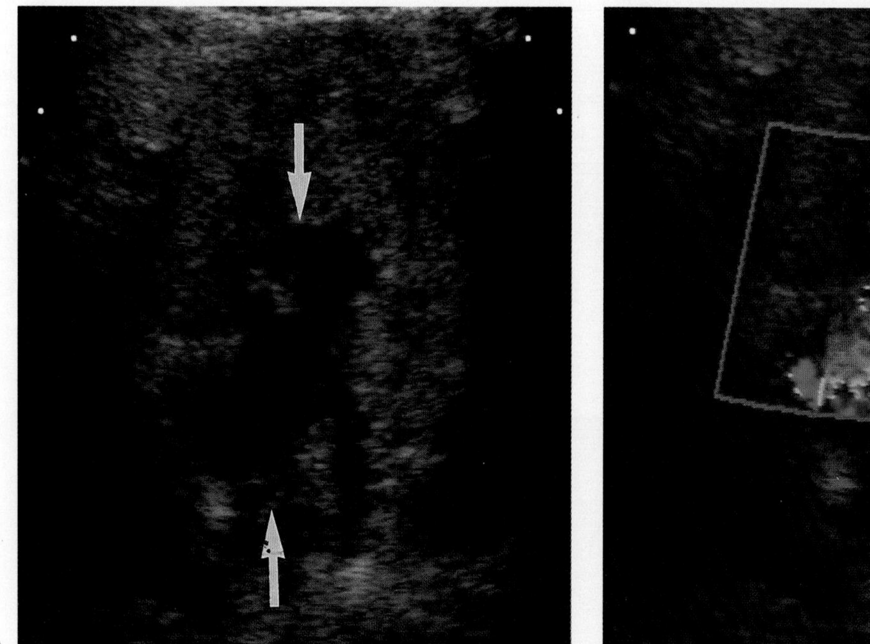

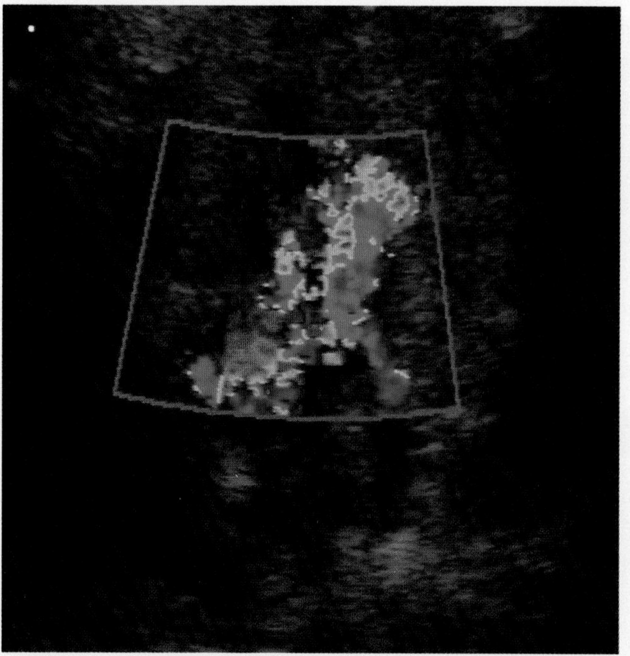

FIG. 5.92. Dilated renal veins simulate hydronephrosis. **A:** Transverse coronal sonogram of the left kidney shows a dilated anechoic structure (*arrows*) in the renal sinus. **B:** Color Doppler sonography reveals that this is an enlarged renal vein, rather than dilated pelvicaliceal structures. Patients with heart failure and tricuspid insufficiency may have findings that simulate collecting system dilatation. Color Doppler is useful in distinguishing between these two conditions.

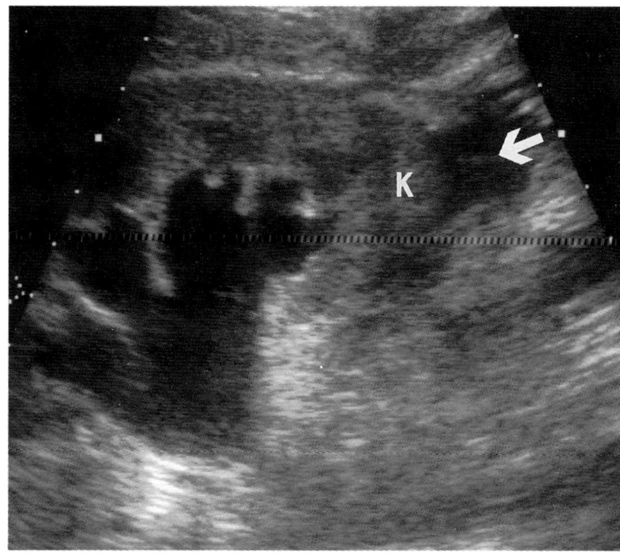

A

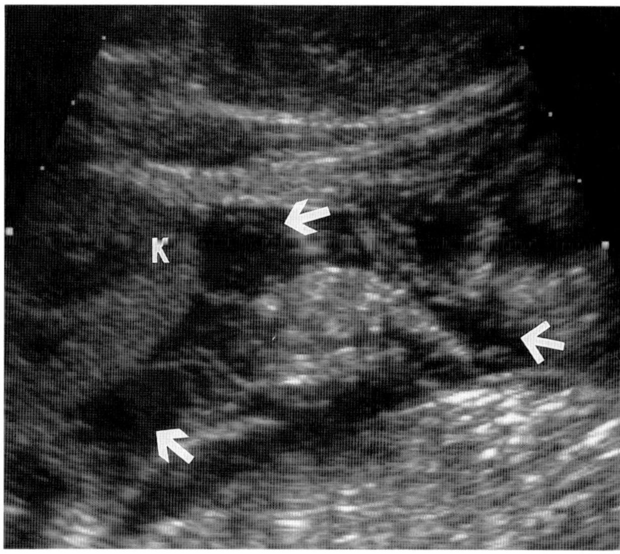

B

FIG. 5.93. Forniceal rupture from distal ureteral stone. **A:** Longitudinal coronal sonogram of the left kidney reveals moderate hydronephrosis. Part of the urinoma (*arrow*) is seen adjacent to the lower pole. **B:** A more caudal longitudinal scan reveals the hypoechoic perinephric urinoma (*arrows*). Forniceal rupture related to obstruction often leads to perinephric and periureteric urinomas, as seen here. On occasion, with forniceal rupture, the pelvicaliceal system may collapse, leading to a false-negative diagnosis for obstruction. In other situations, as in this case, residual hydronephrosis is present. *Arrows,* perinephric urinoma; K, left kidney.

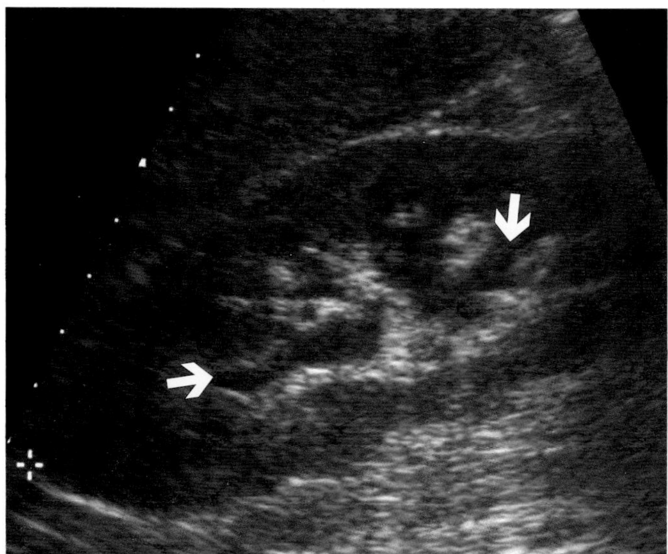

A

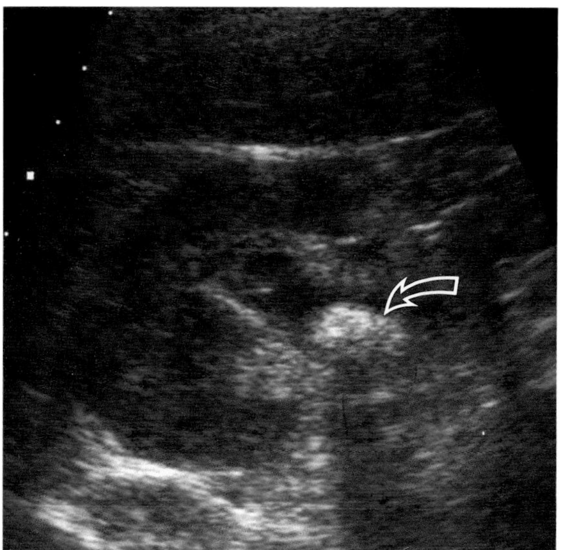

B

FIG. 5.94. Minimal hydronephrosis, UPJ Stone. **A:** Longitudinal sonogram of the right kidney reveals minimal dilatation of the pelvicaliceal system (*arrows*). **B:** A transverse sonogram reveals an obstructing ureteropelvic junction stone (*curved open arrow*). An obstructing ureteral calculus may cause varying degrees of hydronephrosis. When only minimal pelvicaliceal dilatation is present, it may be difficult to diagnose obstruction. The likelihood of mild pelvicaliceal dilatation being related to obstruction depends on whether the patient has high-risk or low-risk symptoms. Minimal pelvicaliceal dilatation is associated with a 5 percent chance of obstruction in a low-risk situation; 45 percent of patients in high-risk clinical situations are obstructed.

struction) occur in normal variants such as overly distensible collecting system (external pelvis, overly full bladder), increased urine production (overhydration, diuretics, diabetes insipidus), postobstructive dilatation, papillary necrosis, and congenital megacalices (73). Distended renal sinus blood vessels (Fig. 5.92) and parapelvic cysts (Fig. 5.45) in the renal sinus may falsely simulate hydronephrosis. Obstruction without hydronephrosis (false-negative results) occurs in congenitally small renal pelves and in encasement of the collecting system by tumor or fibrosis. Forniceal rupture may result in collapse of the collecting system, but in many instances some dilatation may persist (Figs. 5.88 and 5.93) (74–79).

Minimal (grade I) hydronephrosis may be hard to detect and interpret (Fig. 5.94). The clinical probability for obstruction significantly affects the predictive value of grade I hydronephrosis. Cronan and colleagues found that when the clinical probability for obstruction was judged as high, obstruction was present in 45 percent of patients with grade I hydronephrosis. In patients with low probability for obstruction, only 5 percent were obstructed (73,80).

Color and spectral Doppler sonography can help minimize errors. Color Doppler sonography allows confident differentiation of prominent renal sinus vessels that might otherwise simulate hydronephrosis (Fig. 5.92) (81). In addition, an absent or abnormal ureteral jet may indicate obstruction on that side (Fig. 5.95) (82,83).

Ureteral jets occur intermittently when a stripping peristaltic contraction wave passes through the ureteropelvic junction and ejects urine into the bladder. Ureteral jets are detected with color Doppler sonography only when the specific gravity of the urine ejected from the ureteral orifice is different from that of the urine already in the bladder (84,85). One should not expect to visualize ureteral jets soon after a patient has voided because the specific gravity of the urine in the bladder will be the same as that entering from the ureters. Jets occur with similar frequency bilaterally, but only occasionally simultaneously. Normal jets are typically oriented anteromedially and are flame-shaped (Fig. 5.95). When simultaneous, jets generally cross in the midline. Jet velocity and duration vary significantly in normals. Streaming flow (constant long-duration, low-velocity jets) may occur in some normals (86), although some feel that it is evidence for obstruction (83).

Evaluation of peripheral resistance in segmental and more distal renal parenchymal arteries, while nonspecific, may help determine whether or not acute obstruction is present. Increased peripheral resistance on spectral Doppler (resistive index greater than or equal to 0.75), supports the presumption that pyelocaliectasis is caused by acute obstruction (Figs. 5.96 and 5.97) (87). Potential pitfalls include increased peripheral resistance related to acute tubular necrosis (ATN) or other diffuse renal parenchymal diseases and persistent elevated peripheral resistance after obstruction has been relieved. Resistive index may be normal the first few hours after the onset of obstruction, and normal in obstructed patients with chronic renal failure who have significant cortical loss (88). Peripheral resistance may also be normal in obstructed patients for unexplained reasons (Fig. 5.98).

Antegrade pyelography, which is best performed with sonographic and fluoroscopic guidance, is a definitive test for complete urinary tract obstruction. The Whitaker test can be performed during antegrade pyelography when chronic low-grade or incomplete obstruction is suspected. During the Whitaker test, pressure in the renal pelvis is compared with that in the bladder as saline is infused at a rate of 10 ml/min. If renal pelvis pressure exceeds that in the bladder by 15 cm of water or more, then obstruction is present.

RENAL FAILURE/RENAL PARENCHYMAL DISEASE

Sonography evolved as a technique to evaluate patients with renal failure because it could noninvasively detect hydronephrosis related to obstruction, even though obstruction is an uncommon cause of renal failure. Subsequent attempts to stage or characterize renal parenchymal disease based on parenchymal echogenicity or other morphologic features have not proved useful or reliable. Both acute and chronic renal parenchymal diseases cause increased renal cortical echogenicity (Figs. 5.99 and 5.100). Thus abnormal cortical echogenicity cannot be used to differentiate acute from chronic renal parenchymal disease, much less distinguish among different renal diseases.

Renal size is often the most important information provided by ultrasound in patients with renal failure. The average adult kidney is about 10 to 10.5 cm in length with a standard deviation of slightly more than 1 cm (89). In a patient with renal failure, a kidney that is 9.0 cm or less in length usually indicates end-stage renal disease (Fig. 5.101). In these patients, biopsy is generally not indicated as the underlying renal disease is probably irreversible. Dialysis or transplant are the only viable therapeutic options. Biopsy is indicated when renal size is normal and a treatable course of renal failure is possible. All renal biopsies should be performed using sonographic guidance. Even so, complications, usually hematoma (Fig. 5.102), may occur occasionally.

Replacement of lost renal parenchyma by renal sinus fat (renal sinus lipomatosis) may occur in patients with renal failure (Figs. 5.103 and 5.104). Renal length may be normal when this occurs.

Most sonographic findings in acute and chronic renal parenchymal disease are nonspecific. In some patients

(*text continues on page 341*)

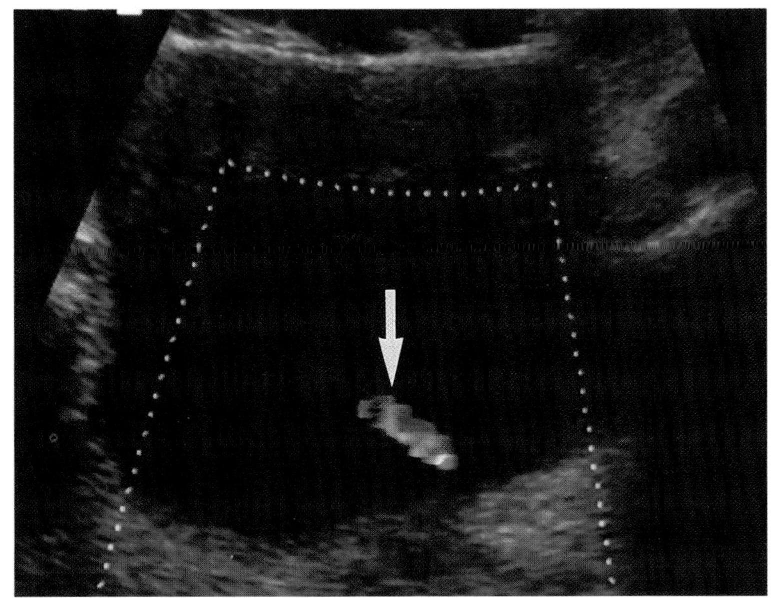

FIG. 5.95. Left ureteral jet, absent right ureteral jet. Transverse color Doppler sonogram of the urinary bladder reveals a left-sided ureteral jet (*arrow*). Fifteen minutes of observation revealed no right ureteral jet. A proximal obstructing calculus was present on the right. The absence of a ureteral jet on one side supports the diagnosis of obstruction. An absent jet suggests that pelvicalyceal dilatation is related to obstruction, rather than nonobstructive causes.

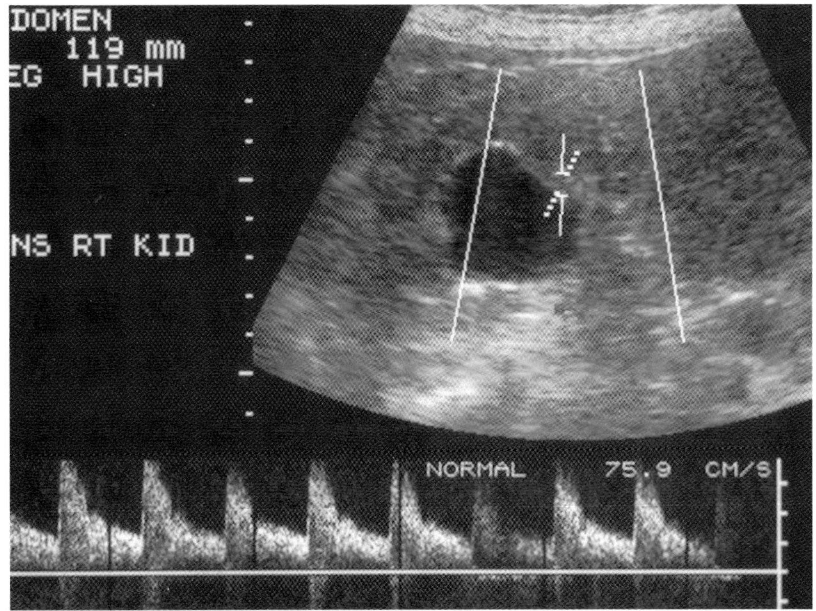

FIG. 5.96. Acute obstructive hydronephrosis, increased peripheral resistance. Transverse spectral Doppler sonogram of the right kidney reveals a high peripheral resistance waveform (RI = 0.80). This patient had acute obstruction related to squamous cell carcinoma of the cervix. Elevated peripheral resistance (RI > 0.75) supports an obstructive cause of pelvicaliceal dilatation. Unfortunately, increased peripheral resistance is not universally present in obstructive hydronephrosis, nor is it a specific indicator of obstruction.

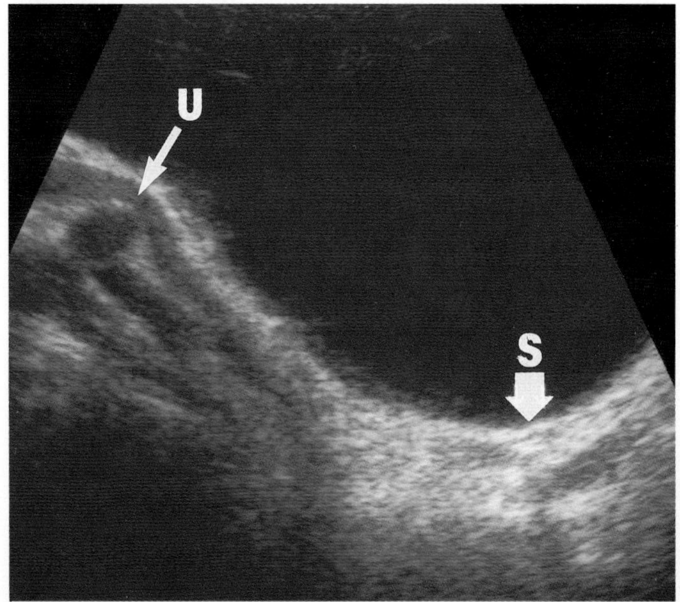

A

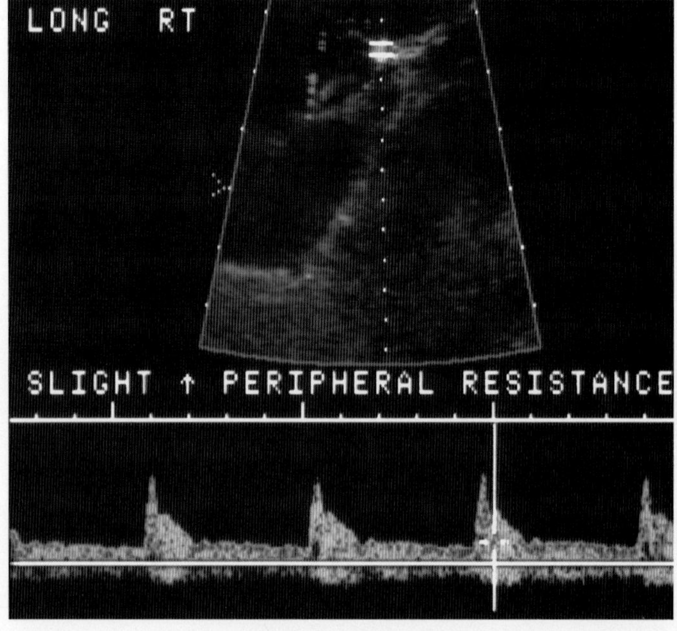

B

FIG. 5.97. Obstructing distal ureteral calculus, increased peripheral resistance. **A:** Longitudinal oblique sonogram shows the distal right ureter (U), where it crosses the iliac vessels. An obstructing distal ureteral stone (S) is noted near the ureterovesicle junction. **B:** A spectral Doppler sonogram of the right kidney reveals increased peripheral resistance (RI = 0.79). Moderate hydronephrosis is present. Although not a specific indicator of obstruction, an elevated peripheral resistance in a patient with pelvicaliceal dilatation suggests an obstructive cause of dilatation.

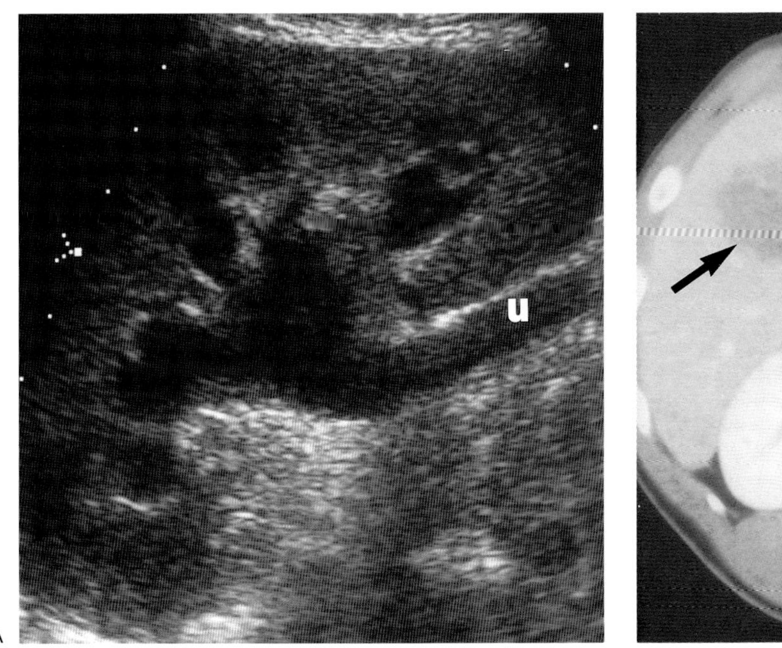

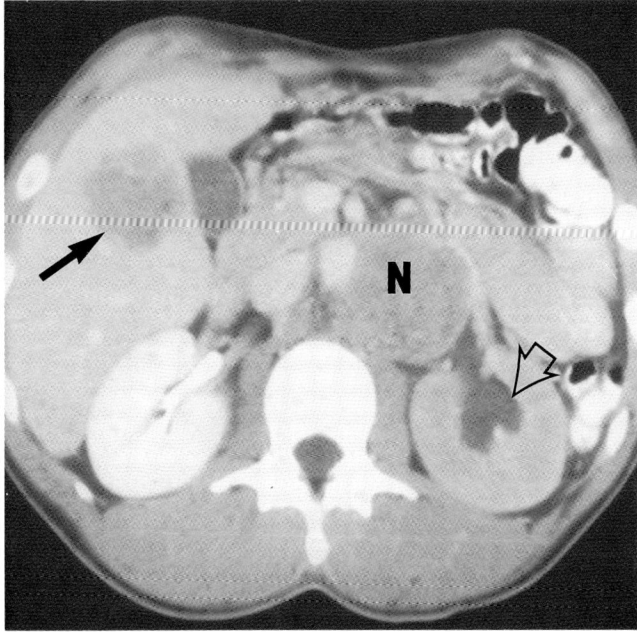

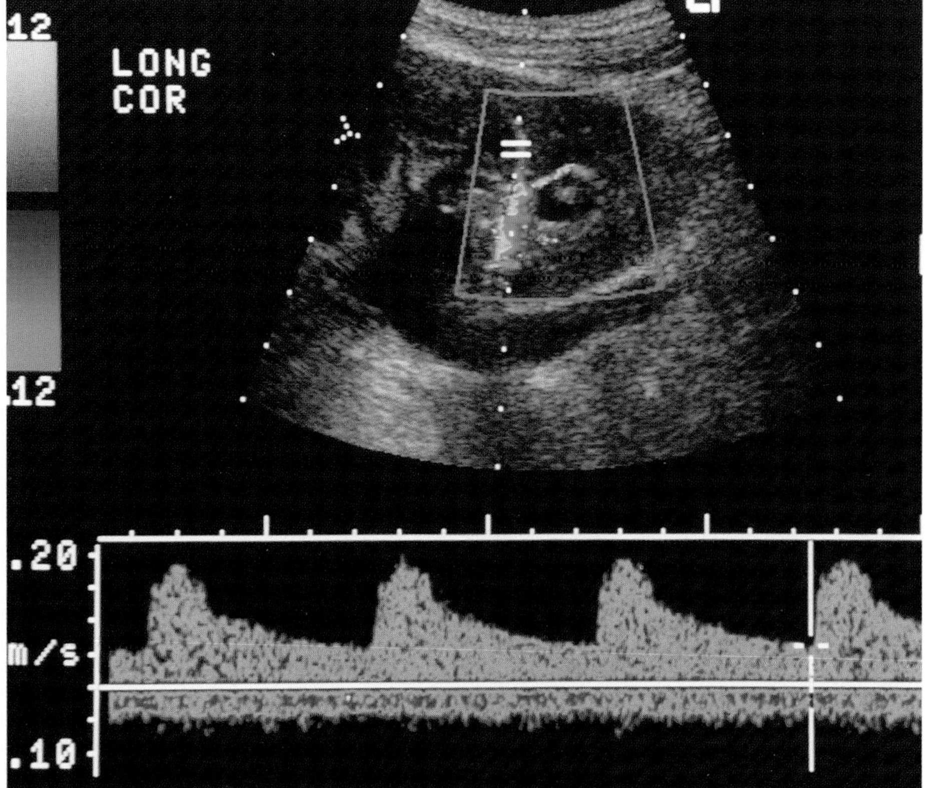

FIG. 5.98. Obstructive hydronephrosis with normal peripheral resistance. **A:** Longitudinal sonogram of the left kidney reveals moderate hydronephrosis and dilatation of the proximal ureter (u). This obstruction is caused by adenopathy from metastatic testicular carcinoma. **B:** The CT scan reveals left-sided hydronephrosis (*open arrow*) and a nodal mass (node—N) that caused the obstruction. Note the hepatic metastasis (*black arrow*). **C:** Color and spectral Doppler sonography revealed normal flow and normal intrarenal arterial peripheral resistance (RI = 0.68). While elevated peripheral resistance supports an obstructive cause for pelvicaliceal dilatation, there are some instances in which obstruction is present and the peripheral resistance is normal.

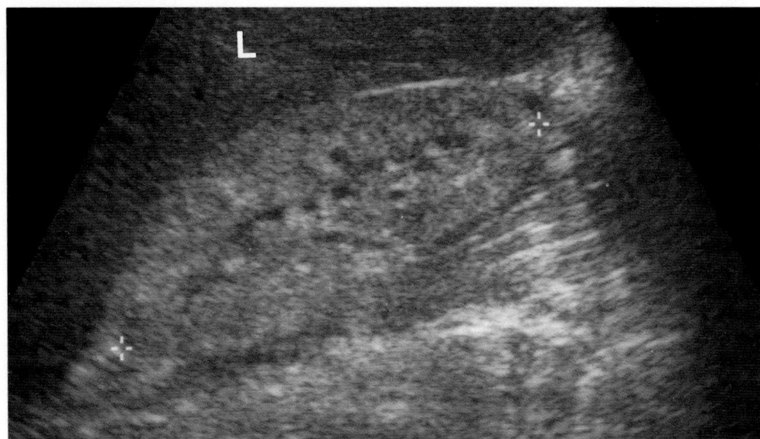

FIG. 5.99. Acute renal failure with increased cortical echogenicity. Longitudinal sonogram of the right kidney reveals an echogenic kidney that is normal in size. This patient had acute renal failure related to systemic lupus erythematosus. Increased cortical echogenicity is an indicator of diffuse renal parenchymal disease but is not useful in distinguishing acute from chronic causes of renal disease. L, liver.

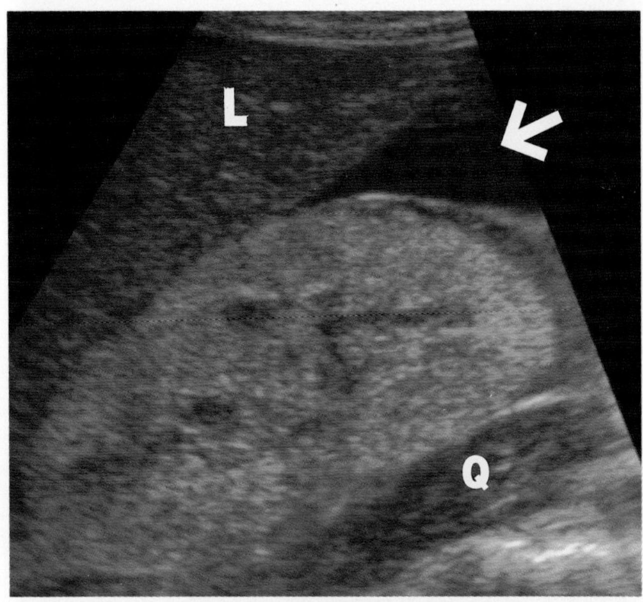

FIG. 5.100. Echogenic kidney, chronic renal failure. Longitudinal sonogram of the right kidney reveals a normal size echogenic kidney. This patient had chronic renal failure related to amyloid deposition. L, liver; *arrow,* ascites; Q, quadratus lumborum muscle.

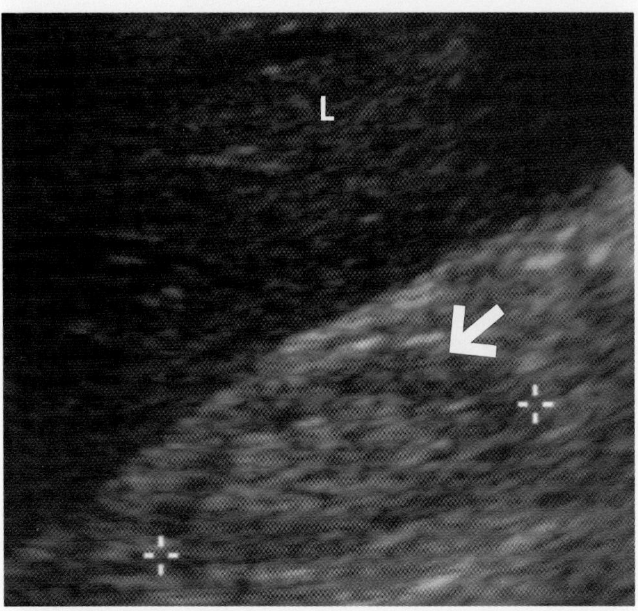

FIG. 5.101. Small kidney, end-stage renal parenchymal disease. Longitudinal sonogram of the right kidney reveals a 5.5-cm echogenic kidney. Note that the renal cortex (*arrow*) is more echogenic than the liver parenchyma (L). Renal cortical echogenicity is normally less than or equal to the echogenicity of normal liver parenchyma. In patients with small kidneys and renal failure, there is no need to perform renal biopsy; irreversible renal parenchymal disease is present. Dialysis and/or transplant are the only therapeutic options.

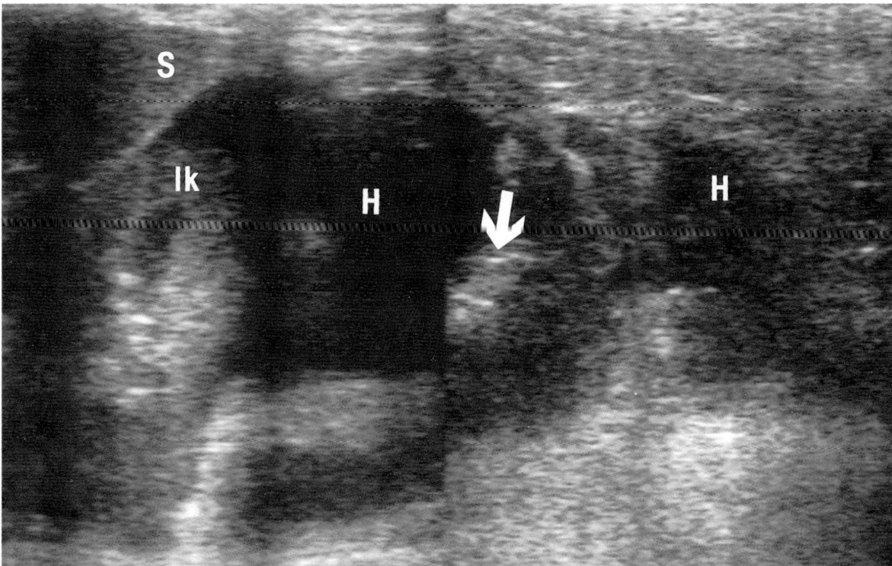

FIG. 5.102. Renal biopsy-related hematoma. Composite longitudinal coronal sonogram through the left flank. A large renal biopsy-related hematoma, anechoic portions of which are marked H, is seen extending caudally from the left kidney (lk). While small hematomas occur often after almost all renal biopsies, large hematomas are unusual. A higher echogenicity area (*arrow*) of the hematoma is indicated. S, spleen; lk, left kidney.

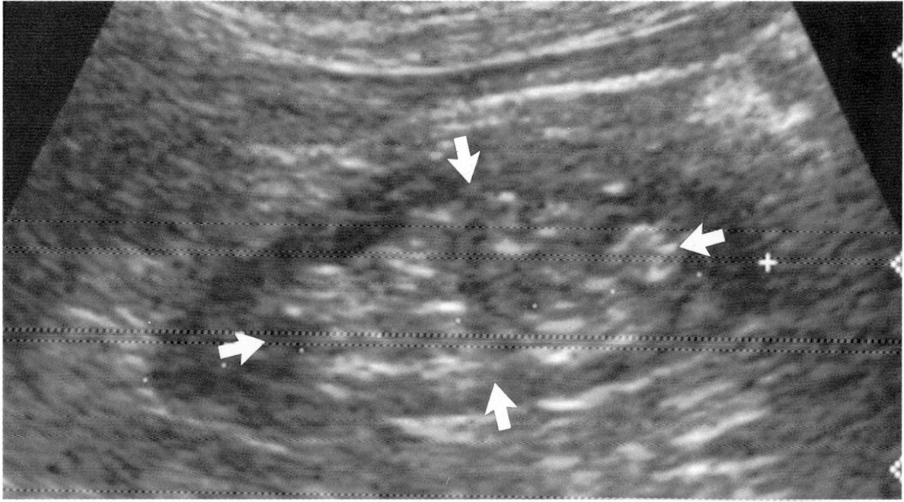

FIG. 5.103. Chronic renal failure, renal sinus lipomatosis. Longitudinal sonogram of the right kidney reveals an abnormally small, 8-cm kidney with an enlarged fatty renal sinus (renal sinus lipomatosis). In this patient with chronic renal disease, renal parenchymal loss has resulted not only in decreased length but also in enlargement of the renal sinus (*arrows*).

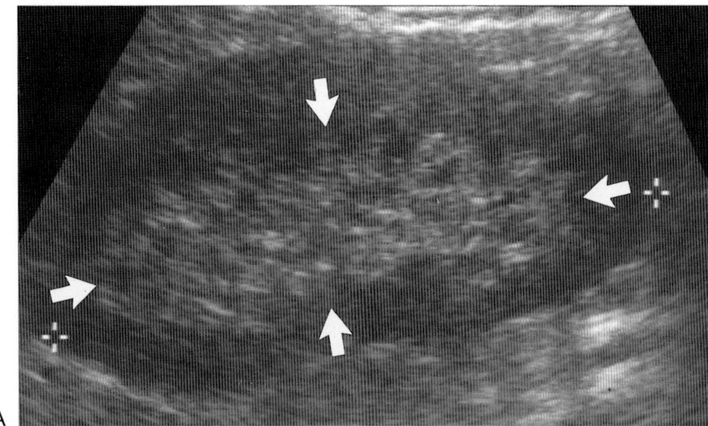

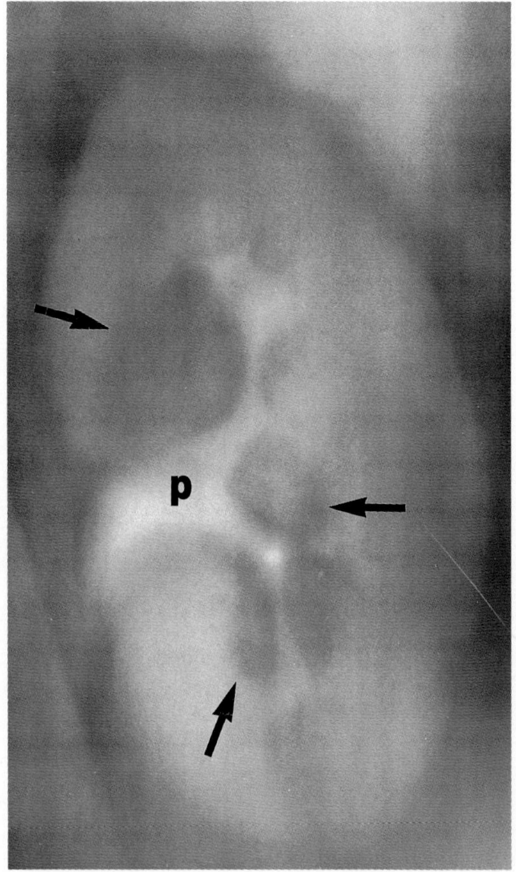

FIG. 5.104. Renal sinus lipomatosis, normal renal function. **A:** Longitudinal sonogram of the left kidney reveals enlargement of the renal sinus (*arrows*). Renal length and cortical thickness are normal. **B:** A nephrotomogram of the left kidney reveals renal sinus fat (*arrows*) adjacent to the pelvicaliceal system (p). Renal sinus lipomatosis may occur in individuals with normal renal function or, occasionally, in patients who have excess fat deposition.

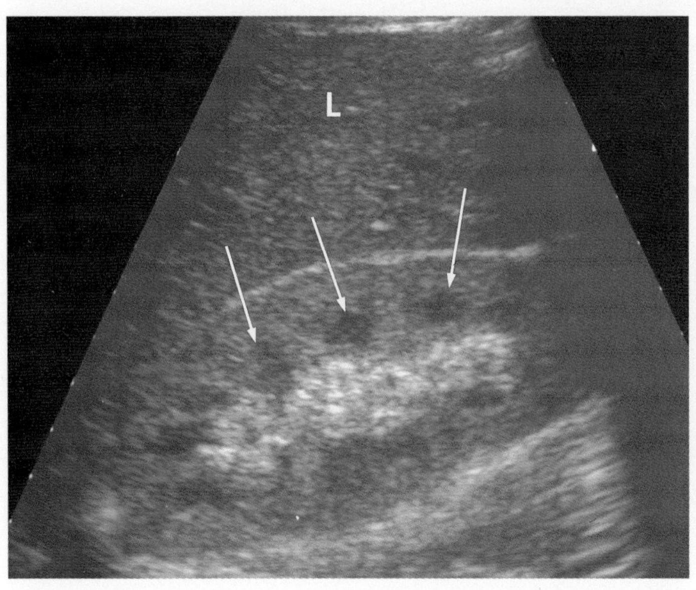

FIG. 5.105. Rhabdomyolysis—acute renal failure with increased peripheral resistance. Longitudinal sonogram of the right kidney reveals increased cortical echogenicity and prominent medullary pyramids (*thin arrows*). The increased cortical echogenicity is caused by post-traumatic rhabdomyolysis. Note the increased parenchymal echogenicity compared to the liver (L). Peripheral resistance is increased (RI = 0.90) in this patient with acute renal failure (creatinine of 4.6). Some, but not all, patients with acute renal parenchymal disease have increased peripheral resistance. Increased peripheral resistance is a nonspecific abnormality, present in many kinds of renal disease.

with acute renal failure, the kidney may actually enlarge due to acute edema. Other common but nonspecific findings include diffuse increased renal cortical parenchymal echogenicity (greater than the liver or spleen) and prominent pyramids (accentuated corticomedullary definition).

Spectral Doppler sonography can be used to evaluate peripheral intrarenal arterial resistance. Peripheral arterial resistance is usually measured by resistive index (RI):

$$RI = \frac{\text{peak systolic velocity} - \text{lowest diastolic velocity}}{\text{peak systolic velocity}}$$

There is debate whether increased peripheral resistance is merely a nonspecific indicator of disease (Fig. 5.105) or a parameter that is useful to distinguish different causes of renal pathology. Some studies have suggested that increased peripheral resistance ($RI > 0.7$) is characteristic of diseases with vasculitis or tubulointerstitial abnormalities (e.g., ATN, interstitial nephritis–SLE, and Wagner's granulomatosis) and does not occur in glomerular disease (glomerulonephritis, etc.) (90). Platt et al. (90) feel that prerenal causes of renal failure do not result in elevated peripheral resistance (with the exception of hepatorenal syndrome) and thus can be differentiated from renal causes of renal failure.

Unfortunately, there are many instances when peripheral resistance is normal in patients with renal parenchymal disease. In addition, elevated peripheral resistance can occur in many other conditions. Among these are extrinsic compression by perinephric collections (Fig. 5.106), pyelonephritis, renal obstruction (Figs. 5.96 and 5.107), and renal vein thrombosis (Fig. 5.108).

Despite the problems and pitfalls, Doppler appraisal of peripheral resistance may be helpful in renal parenchymal disease. Elevated peripheral resistance may be the only indication of renal disease when no other sonographic abnormality is present. Elevated peripheral resistance suggests that obstructive hydronephrosis is present, rather than pelvicaliceal dilatation related to other problems, such as reflux. The level of increased peripheral resistance may be predictive of eventual chronic renal function impairment in patients with acute renal failure (91).

RENAL TRANSPLANTATION

The kidney is the organ most frequently transplanted. Transplantation is recommended for most patients with irreversible renal failure. It is performed routinely in most major medical centers and in many community hospitals. Sonography, along with nuclear medicine techniques, plays an integral role in evaluating and managing renal transplant patients. Doppler technology has only enhanced sonography's value as a means to evaluate renal transplants. Sonography is useful in evaluating perinephric fluid collections and urinary obstruction and assessing major vascular complications. It plays a role in evaluating suspected renal transplant rejection.

Transplant-Associated Fluid Collections

Perinephric fluid collections are quite frequent. They include lymphoceles, hematomas, urinomas, seromas, and abscess (92). Hematomas and seromas often occur soon after transplantation or renal transplant biopsy. These collections are usually self-limited and do not require therapy (93). Hematomas have a variable appearance depending on their age. Early on, they may appear as complex, mainly echogenic masses (Fig. 5.109). With breakdown, fibrin strands and fluid collections may be seen. Seromas are often anechoic and may conform to adjacent tissue planes. Aspiration need not be performed unless there is suspicion of an abscess.

Lymphoceles, probably the most common posttransplant fluid collections, are not usually seen immediately subsequent to transplant but arise several weeks to as long as a year after surgery. Sonographically, lymphoceles are usually rounded or lobulated and contain septations. They may be totally echo-free or contain debris of varying echogenicity. On CT, lymphoceles may have lower attenuation than water. Drainage is indicated when there are complications: compression of the transplant, compromise of the major renal vessels or collecting system, or occurrence of infection. Percutaneous drainage of lymphoceles is usually effective, though some lesions may require surgery.

Urinomas may occur quite early after transplant owing to anastomotic leaks or disruption of the renal collecting system. If the parietal peritoneum is not intact (transplantation is usually done extraperitoneally), urinary ascites may occur. Some urinomas resolve spontaneously, but others require surgery. Percutaneous drainage is generally not useful.

Renal transplant-associated abscesses generally result from infection of one of the previously described fluid collections. Clinical suspicion, coupled with percutaneous aspiration and drainage, may serve to diagnose and manage peritransplant abscesses effectively.

Transplant Urinary Tract Obstruction

Mild hydronephrosis from edema is common in the first week after transplantation and is occasionally identified later in unobstructed transplants. Urinary obstruction is likely when there is more pronounced hydronephrosis. There may be increased peripheral resistance on Doppler, though other problems (transplant rejection, ATN) may also cause this finding. Nuclear medicine techniques may be useful. Antegrade pyelograms may be performed in problematic cases.

(text continues on page 345)

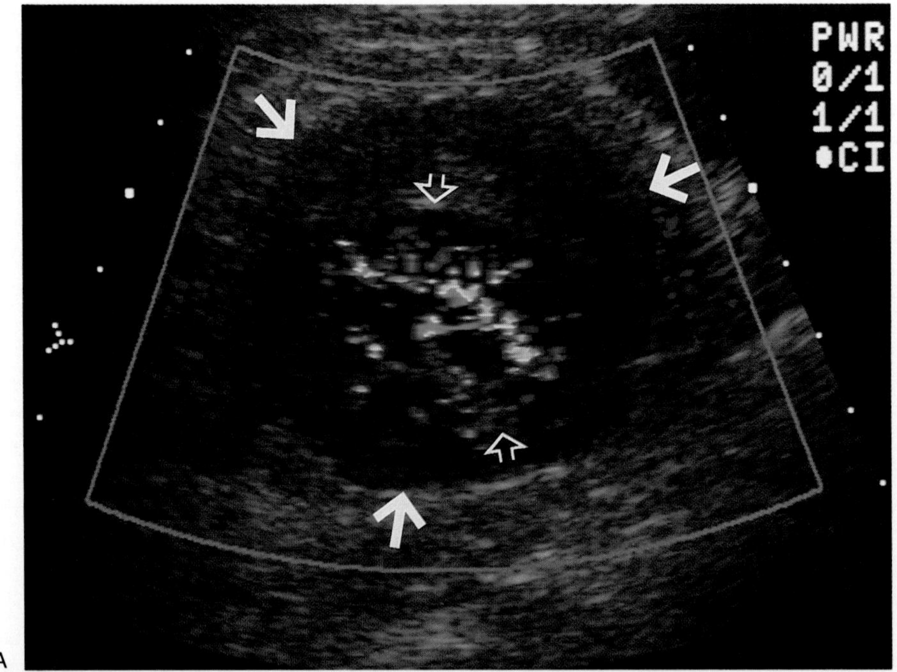

A

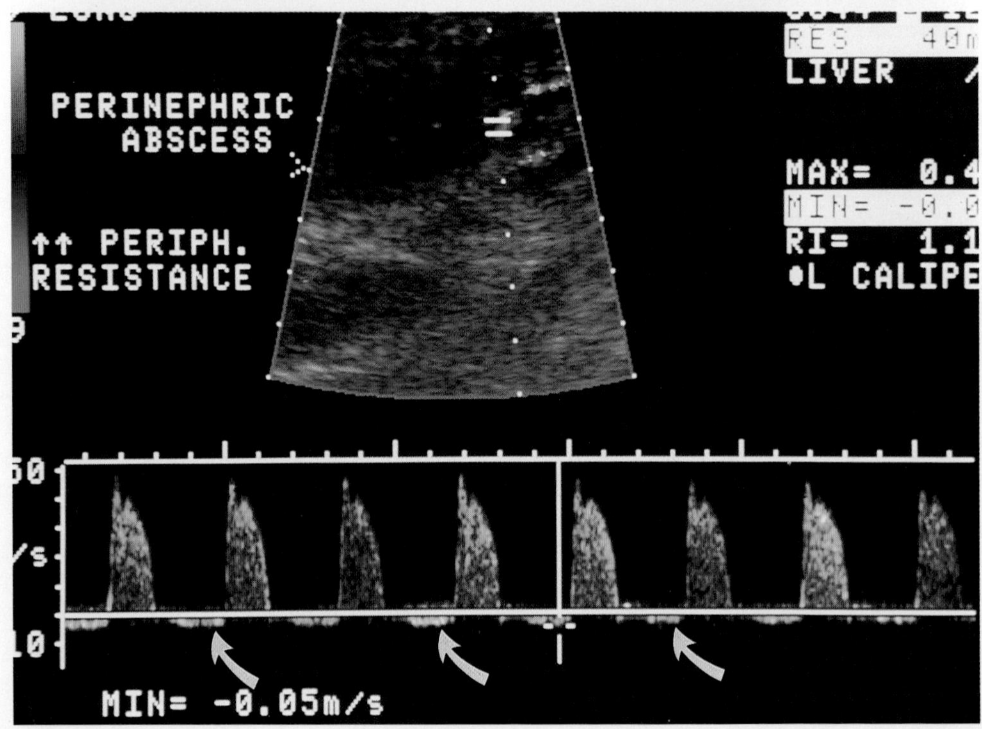

B

FIG. 5.106. Peripnephric abscess, increased peripheral resistance. **A:** Transverse color Doppler sonogram shows flow within the lower pole of the kidney (*open arrows*). There is a circumferential perinephric abscess (*arrows*) that is surrounding and compressing the kidney. **B:** Spectral Doppler analysis reveals markedly increased peripheral resistance with flow reversal (*curved arrows*). Resistive index was 1.1 (normal is less than 0.70).

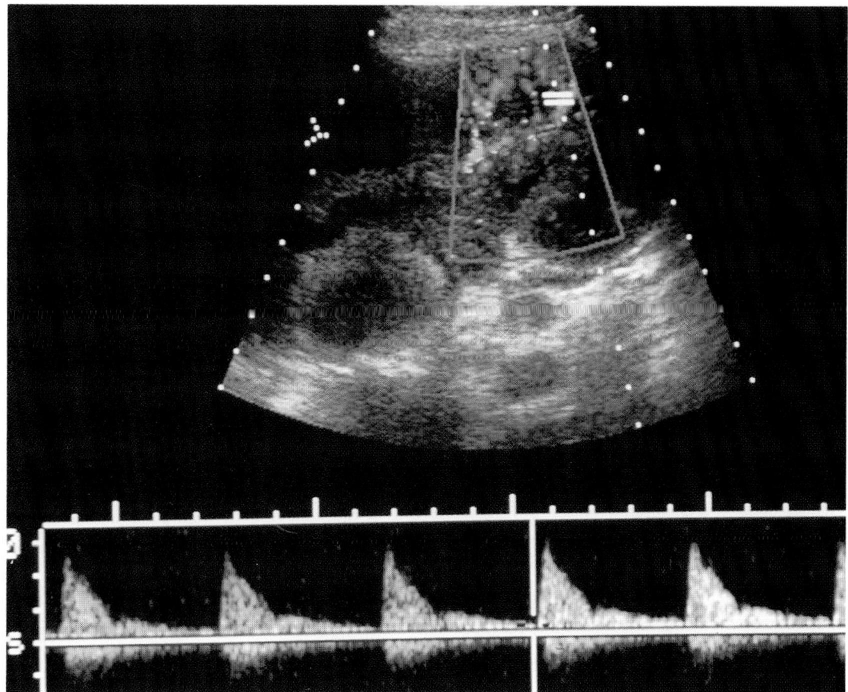

FIG. 5.107. Renal tuberculosis with elevated peripheral resistance. Longitudinal color Doppler and spectral sonogram reveals increased peripheral resistance (RI = 0.92) in a patient with renal tuberculosis. It is uncertain whether the elevated peripheral resistance is related to increased intracapsular pressure from the inflammatory process or from obstruction of the collecting system. Both renal infection and pelvicaliceal obstruction can cause increased peripheral resistance.

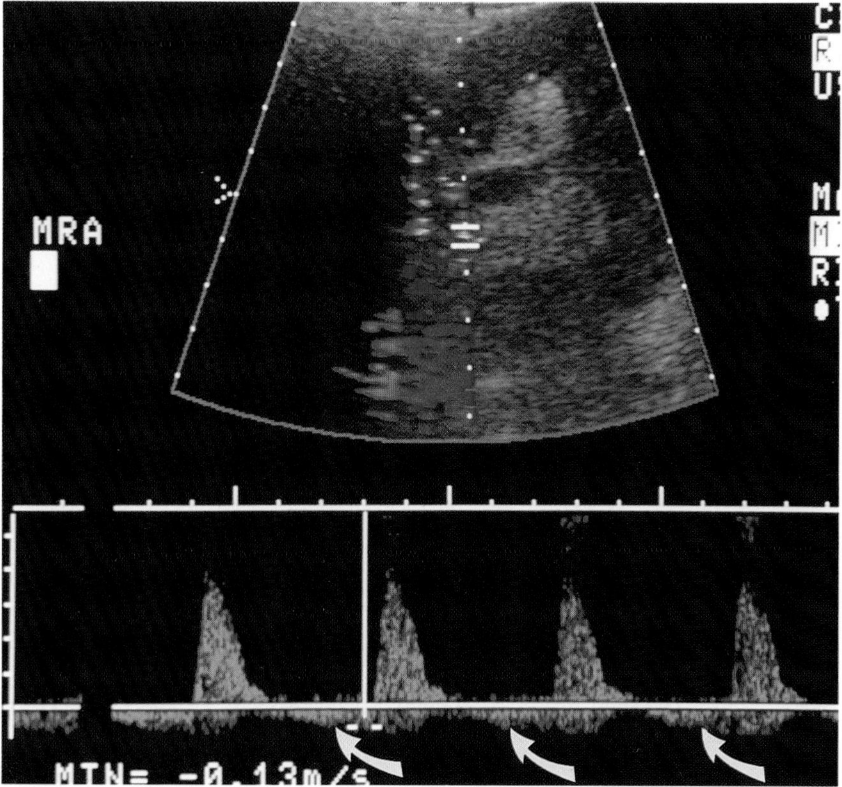

FIG. 5.108. Renal vein thrombosis with increased peripheral resistance. Transverse sonogram of the left kidney reveals increased peripheral resistance in a patient with renal vein thrombosis related to dehydration. The resistive index in this patient is 1.17. Note the diastolic flow reversal (*curved arrows*). Renal vein thrombosis is another cause of increased peripheral resistance.

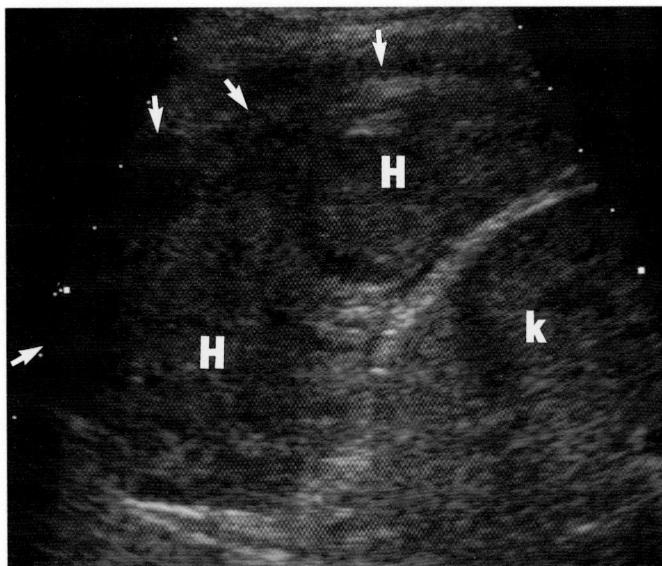

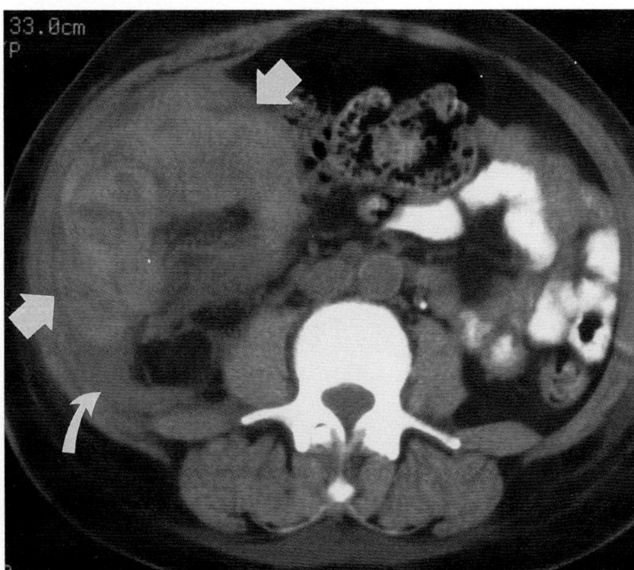

FIG. 5.109. Post-renal-transplant hematoma. **A:** Longitudinal sonogram through the right flank reveals a complex appearing hematoma (H—*arrows*) adjacent to the upper pole of the transplanted kidney (k). **B:** A CT scan reveals a predominantly increased attenuation area (*arrows*) diagnostic of hematoma. Some lower attenuation fluid is noted more dorsally (*curved arrow*). Large post-transplant hematomas such as this are unusual. It is not unusual to detect small hematomas or seromas in the immediate post-transplantation period.

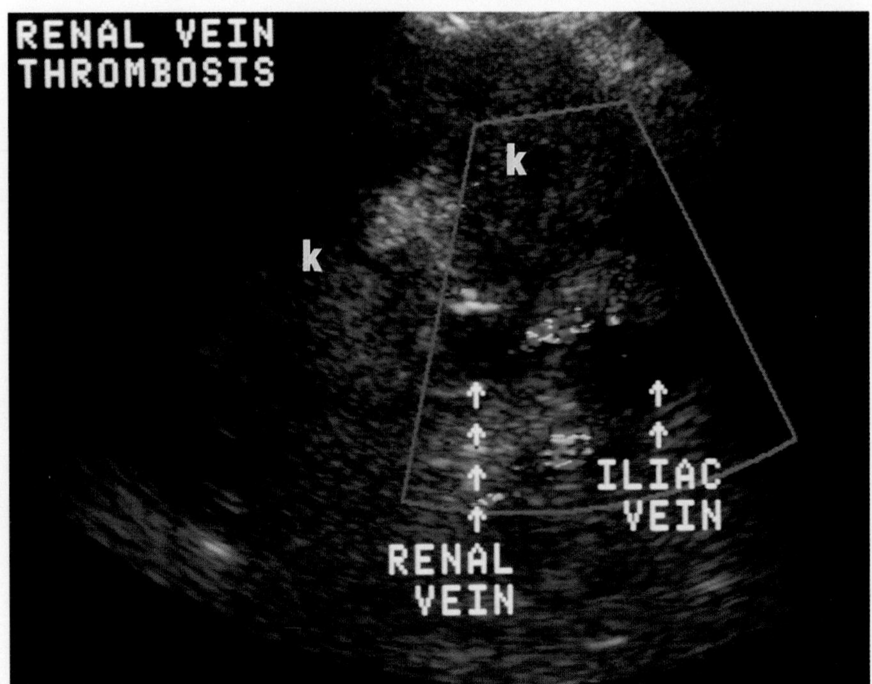

FIG. 5.110. Renal vein thrombosis, renal transplant. Oblique longitudinal color Doppler sonogram of the renal transplant kidney (k) reveals thrombosis of the renal vein and the iliac vein. Color Doppler sonography is an invaluable tool in assessing major vessels in renal transplants.

Major Vascular Obstruction

Color Doppler sonography can often delineate the anastomoses of the renal artery and vein, even when they are totally invisible on grayscale images. Complete and partial renal vein thrombosis can be effectively evaluated using color Doppler sonography (Figs. 5.110 and 5.111). Segmental intrarenal perfusion defects may also be detected with color Doppler techniques. Color Doppler sonography can easily diagnose renal artery occlusion and, with less certainty, renal artery stenosis. Renal artery stenosis is generally present when peak velocity greater than 190 cm/sec is detected. Color Doppler sonography is also successful in demonstrating segmental infarcts, AV fistulas, and pseudoaneurysms (Fig. 5.112) (94).

Renal Transplant Dysfunction

Renal transplant dysfunction is a difficult diagnostic problem, often prompting renal transplant biopsy. Increased peripheral resistance, defined as a resistive index greater than 0.75 (or, more strictly, greater than 0.9), may be present in many patients with acute transplant rejection (Figs. 5.113 and 5.114). Unfortunately, other conditions such as acute obstruction and, more notably, acute tubular necrosis (ATN) may also result in elevated peripheral resistance. In addition, later in the course of renal transplant patients, cyclosporine toxicity may cause increased resistive indices, although rarely greater than 0.8 (95). Other causes of increased peripheral resistance include renal vein thrombosis, pyelonephritis, and extrarenal compression by the ultrasound transducer (96,97). Most feel that the presence of flow reversal at end diastole (RI > 1.0) is a bad prognostic sign (98). While many have suggested that increased peripheral resistance indicates the presence of transplant rejection (99–102), others have pointed out that sensitivity and specificity are suboptimal (103,104).

Perhaps the most reasonable approach to sonographic evaluation of patients with renal transplant rejection is the combined use of morphologic and Doppler findings, as suggested by Townsend and the UC San Francisco group (105). The presence of four morphologic criteria for rejection (decreased renal sinus fat, renal edema, pelvic infundibular thickening [Fig. 5.115], and conspicuous pyramids) had 100 percent positive predictive value for rejection. Unfortunately, all four findings were found in only 21 percent of patients with rejection (21 percent sensitivity). In the first 3 weeks after transplant, increased peripheral resistance was not useful as it did not distinguish between acute tubular necrosis and acute transplant rejection. From 3 weeks to 6 months after transplant, increased peripheral resistance usually indicated rejection. After 6 months, Doppler sonography was again less useful as cyclosporine toxicity could also cause increased peripheral resistance.

Peripheral resistance may be normal in certain types of acute rejection and also in many patients with chronic rejection. Because of the problems mentioned above, evaluation of peripheral resistance with spectral Doppler techniques is generally no substitute for other imaging tests or biopsy.

RENAL TRAUMA

In the United States, sonography typically plays little role in the evaluation of renal injury (106–108). In some countries, however, ultrasound used in combination with IVU is the technique of choice in suspected renal injury (109,110). Ultrasound is able to detect some major renal injuries including laceration (Fig. 5.116) and hematoma. It can also detect some major arterial injuries. The reliability of sonography in renal trauma is, however, uncertain; it probably cannot be depended on to definitively guide management. Further investigation is needed to define its role in trauma patients.

RENAL SONOGRAPHY IN HUMAN IMMUNODEFICIENCY VIRUS (HIV) INFECTION AND ACQUIRED IMMUNODEFICIENCY SYNDROME (AIDS)

Patients with HIV infection and AIDS may suffer from renal infection, renal lymphoma, evidence of disseminated pneumocystic infection, and HIV nephropathy (which leads to rapidly progressive renal failure).

Renal abnormalities in AIDS-related lymphoma are more likely to be discrete single or multiple focal masses than renal lesions in other types of lymphoma. On sonography, these masses are typically hypoechoic and thus indistinguishable from other lymphomatous lesions or other focal renal tumors (Fig. 5.78). In disseminated pneumocystic infection, diffuse medullary and cortical calcification may lead to increased echogenicity of the kidneys (111). Focal calcifications also occur (Fig. 5.117). This pattern may also be caused by MAI infection (112). HIV-related nephropathy results in focal segmental glomerulosclerosis with renal failure and proteinuria. The tubular and interstitial abnormalities that accompany glomerulosclerosis produce striking ultrasound findings including renal enlargement and pronounced increased cortical echogenicity (Fig. 5.118). HIV nephropathy occurs most frequently in intravenous drug abusers but also occurs in other risk groups in the absence of intravenous drug abuse (113).

ADRENAL SONOGRAPHY

Sonography was the first modality to directly image the adrenal gland (114,115) and can, with meticulous

(text continues on page 350)

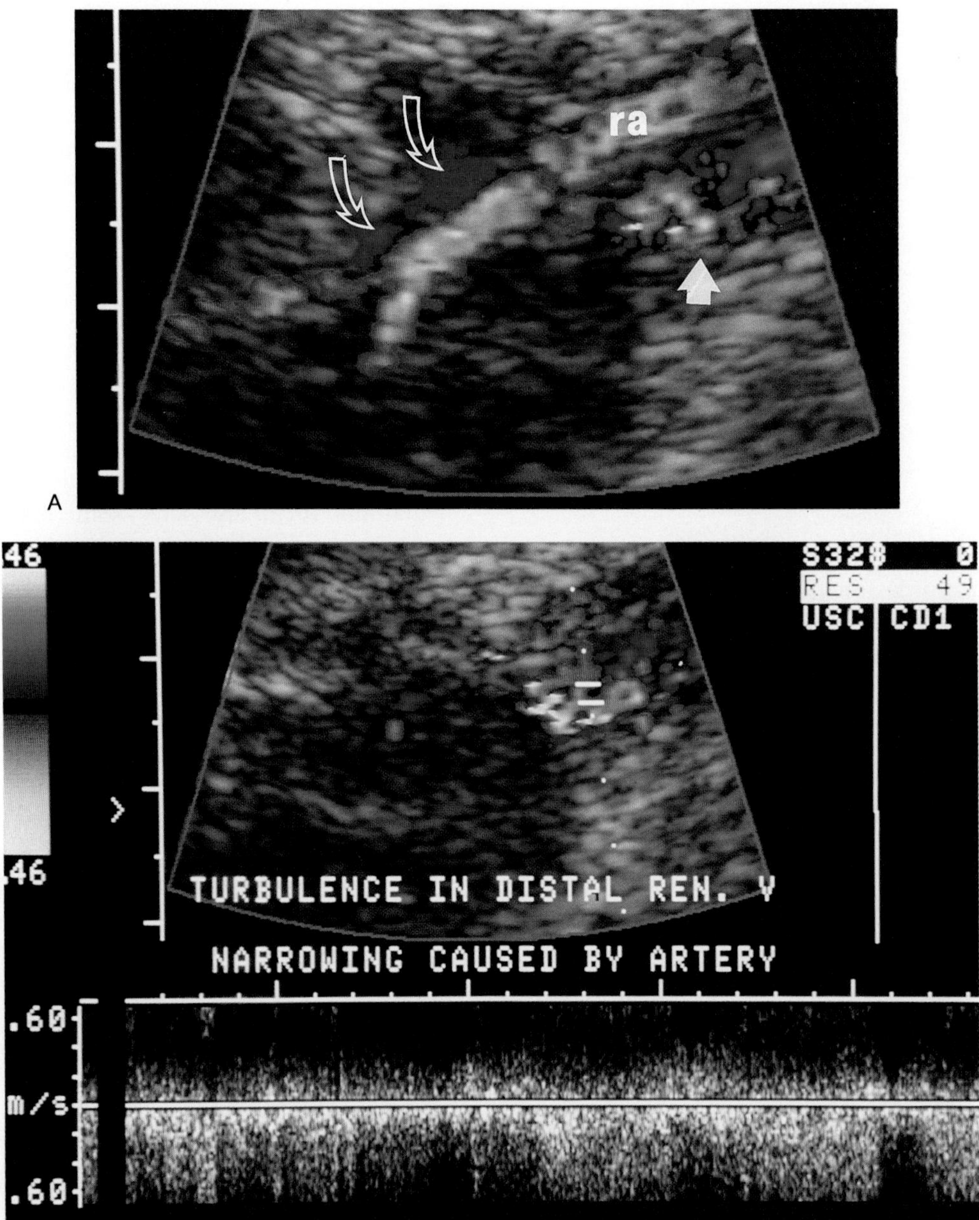

FIG. 5.111. Transplant renal vein stenosis. **A:** Oblique transverse sonogram reveals the renal artery (ra) crossing over the renal vein. The more peripheral renal vein (*curved open arrows*) has a lower velocity flow pattern. Turbulent flow (*arrow*) is noted in the more central renal vein. This turbulence was presumably caused by compression by the renal artery. **B:** The spectral Doppler sonogram reveals turbulent flow in the segment of the renal vein beyond the narrowing caused by the renal artery. In this patient, corrective surgery yielded good results. The general significance of similar stenoses in other patients is uncertain. We do not recommend intervention in all cases with findings like this.

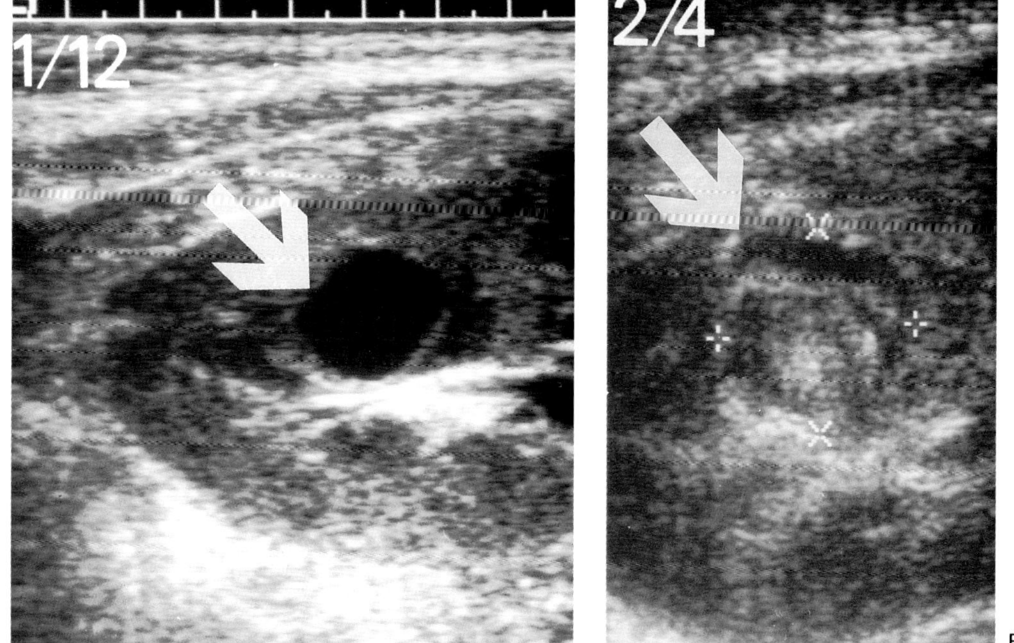

FIG. 5.112. Post-renal-transplant biopsy pseudoaneurysm. **A**: Oblique longitudinal sonogram of the transplant kidney reveals a pseudoaneurysm (*arrow*) at the biopsy site. Flow throughout the pseudoaneurysm was documented with color Doppler imaging (not shown). **B**: Three weeks later, the pseudoaneurysm had thrombosed spontaneously (*arrow*). (Case courtesy of E. Meredith James, MD.)

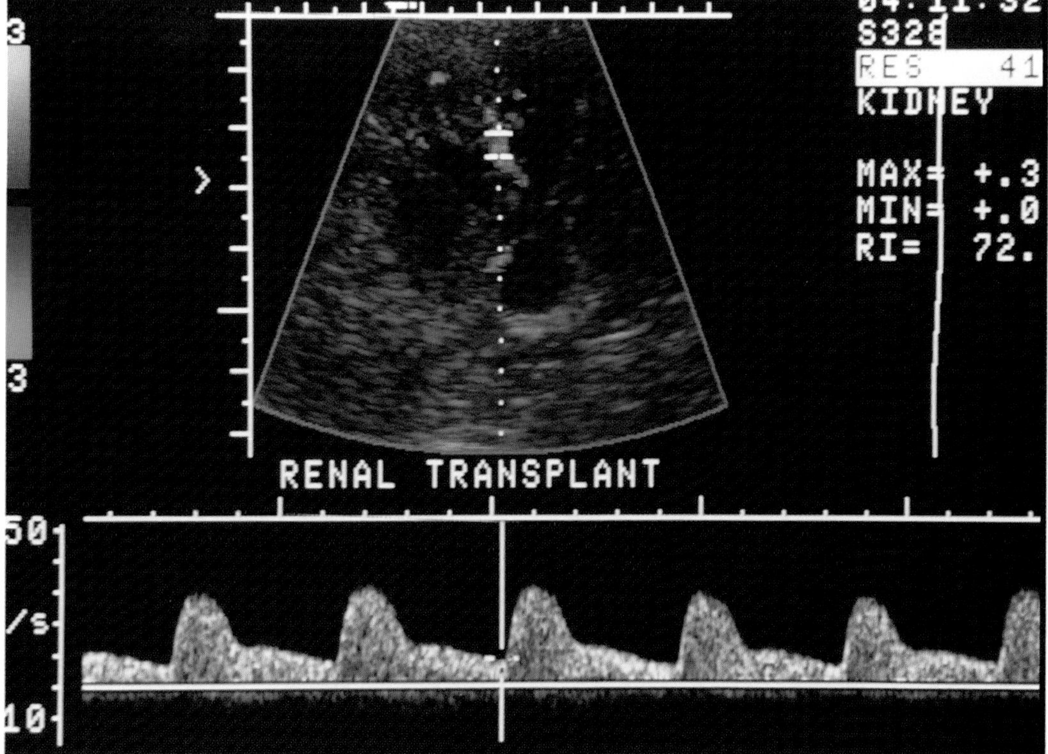

FIG. 5.113. Renal transplant, normal peripheral resistance. Longitudinal oblique spectral Doppler sonogram reveals a normal intrarenal arterial waveform with a resistive index of 0.72 (lower limit of normal in renal transplants is RI < 0.75). Many feel that values less than 0.90 should be considered normal. Color Doppler sonography can facilitate spectral analysis of renal transplant by guiding placement of the sample volume. Unfortunately, Doppler findings are often normal in patients with chronic rejection. Peripheral resistance is occasionally normal even in acute rejection.

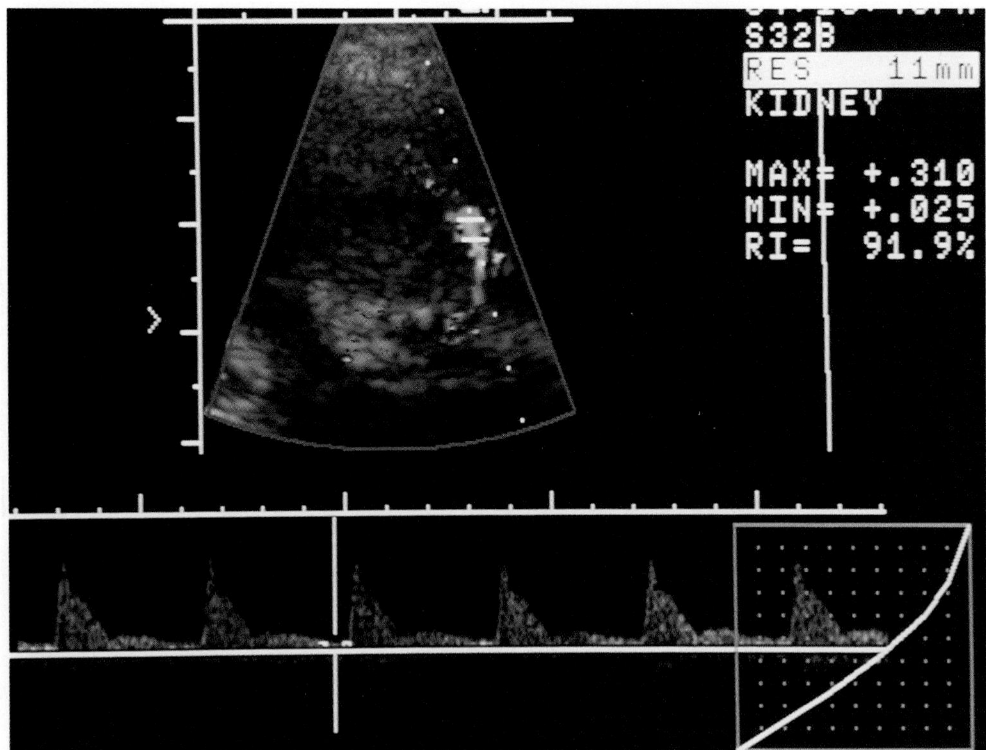

FIG. 5.114. Renal transplant rejection, increased peripheral resistance. Oblique longitudinal color Doppler and spectral Doppler sonogram reveals evidence of increased peripheral resistance (RI = 0.92). This patient had biopsy-proved transplant rejection. Unfortunately, increased peripheral resistance is nonspecific. Peripheral resistance may be elevated in other conditions commonly present in renal transplant patients, such as acute tubular necrosis and cyclosporine toxicity.

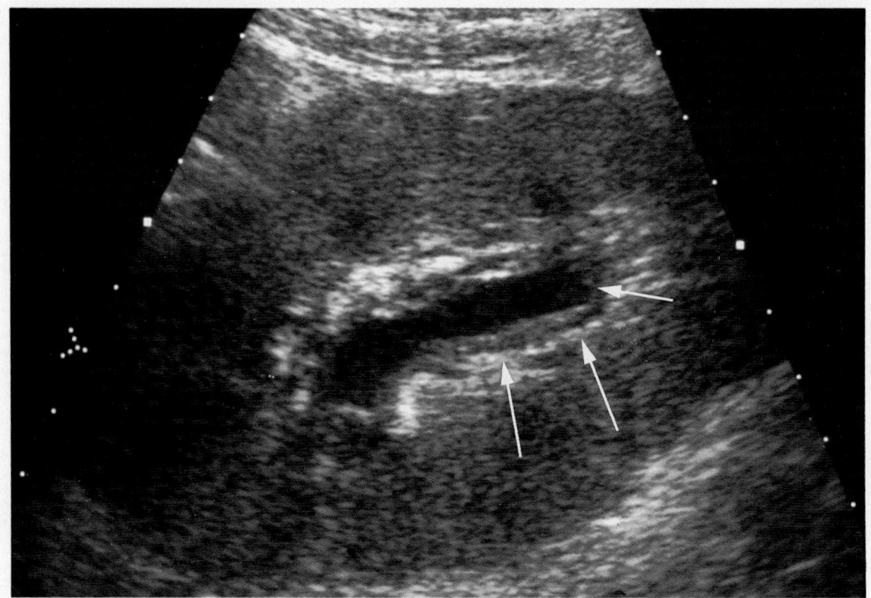

FIG. 5.115. Renal transplant rejection, thickening of collecting system walls. Transverse oblique sonogram through this transplant kidney reveals mild to moderate pelvicaliceal dilatation and thickened renal pelvis walls (*thin arrows*). Renal pelvic and infundibular wall thickening is one of the four morphologic criteria for rejection described by the UC San Francisco group. The others are decreased renal sinus fat, renal edema (also present here), and conspicuous pyramids. The presence of all four findings together had a 100 percent positive predictive value for rejection in their series. Unfortunately, all four findings were found in only 21 percent of patients with rejection (21 percent sensitivity).

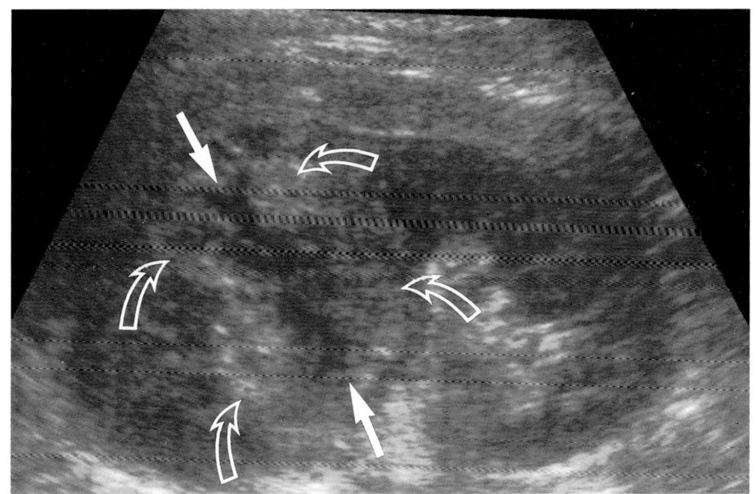

FIG. 5.116. Renal gunshot wound, upper pole laceration. Longitudinal coronal sonogram of the left kidney. A jagged laceration (*arrows*) surrounded by echogenic hemorrhage (*open curved arrows*) is seen where a bullet passed through the upper pole of the kidney. Sonography is able to detect major renal injuries including laceration and hematoma. Color flow sonography can detect some vascular injuries. The reliability of sonography in renal trauma is uncertain. Further investigation is needed to define its role in assessing trauma patients.

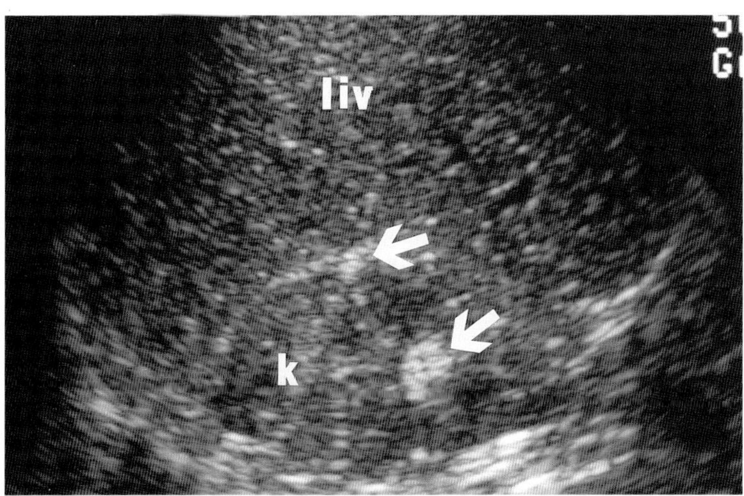

FIG. 5.117. Disseminated *Pneumocystis,* renal calcification. Transverse sonogram through the right kidney (k) shows many small calcifications within the kidney. Two larger calcifications (*arrows*) are also noted. Multiple tiny calcifications are present within the liver (liv), manifest as small punctate echogenic foci. Disseminated *Pneumocystis* can cause multiple parenchymal calcifications, as well as nodal calcifications, throughout the body. S, spleen.

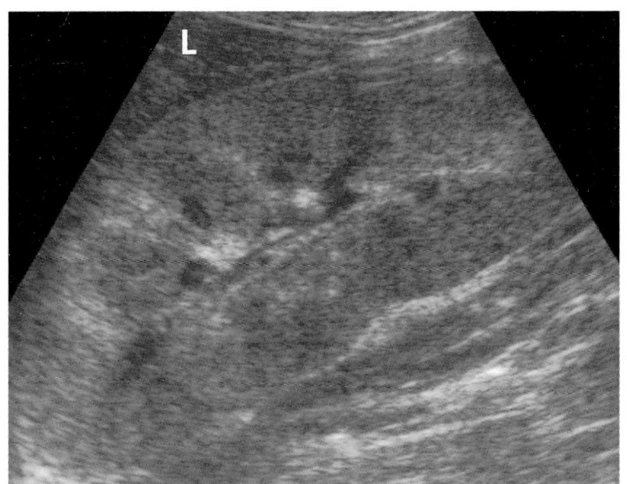

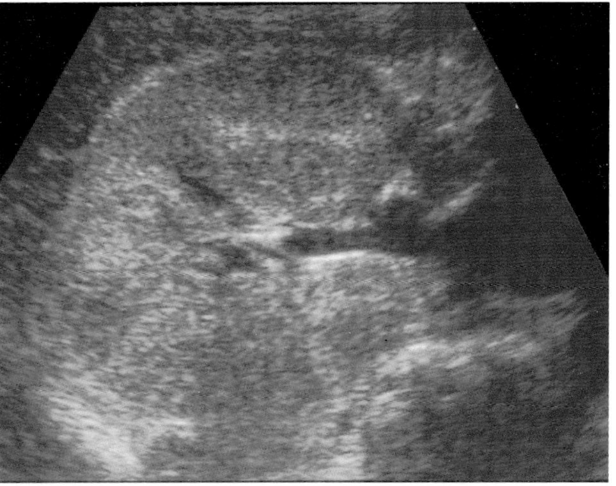

FIG. 5.118. HIV nephropathy. **A:** Longitudinal sonogram of the right kidney reveals increased echogenicity of the kidney compared to the parenchyma of the liver (L). The renal pyramids are indistinct and the renal sinus structures not well seen. **B:** A transverse sonogram shows a "plump" kidney caused by renal edema. HIV nephropathy is characterized by nephrosclerosis and rapidly progressive renal failure often ending in uremia. It occurs in HIV-infected patients from all risk groups and is not an AIDS-defining condition.

technique (116), reliably image the adrenal gland. Despite this, sonography is rarely used as a primary adrenal imaging modality. CT is generally considered best to assess adrenal masses and pathology.

On occasion, sonography may detect adrenal masses. These include metastases (Fig. 5.119), incidental adrenal adenomas (Figs. 5.120 and 5.121), pheochromocytomas (Fig. 5.122), adrenal carcinoma (Fig. 5.123), myelolipomas (Fig. 5.124), and other lesions such as abscess, hematoma (Fig. 5.125), and cyst.

Management and follow-up of adrenal masses should be the same whether detected sonographically, by CT, or in some other way. When a mass less than 5 cm in size is detected in a patient without malignancy, endocrine evaluation to rule out adrenal hyperfunction is indicated. All hyperfunctioning adrenal masses should be surgically resected. If the mass is not hyperfunctioning, follow-up imaging is indicated to ensure that the lesion is an insignificant nonhyperfunctioning adrenal adenoma. If the adrenal mass grows on follow-up examination, resection is appropriate. If there has been no change in size after 18 months, no further follow-up is needed.

Patients with adrenal masses larger than 5 cm should undergo CT for staging, as adrenal carcinoma is likely (Fig. 5.122). In patients with a known malignancy, biopsy is often needed to distinguish an adrenal metastasis from an incidental nonhyperfunctioning adenoma. If the presence of an adrenal metastasis would have no effect on the management of the patient, no biopsy is necessary.

REFERENCES

1. Taylor DC, Kettler MD, Moneta GL, et al. Duplex ultrasound scanning in the diagnosis of renal artery stenosis: a prospective evaluation. *J Vasc Surg* 1988;7:363–369.
2. Robertson R, Murphy A, Dubbins PA. Renal artery stenosis: the use of duplex ultrasound as a screening technique. *Br J Radiol* 1988;61:196–201.
3. Greene ER, Avasthi PS, Hodges JW. Noninvasive Doppler assessment of renal artery stenosis and hemodynamics. *J Clin Ultrasound* 1987;15:653–659.
4. Berland LL, Koslin DB, Routh WD, et al. Renal artery stenosis: prospective evaluation of diagnosis with color duplex US compared with angiography. *Radiology* 1990;174:421–423.
5. Handa N, Fukunaga R, Etani H, et al. Efficacy of echo-Doppler examination for the evaluation of renovascular disease. *Ultrasound Med Biol* 1988;14:1–5.
6. Stavros AT, Parker SH, Yakes WF, et al. Segmental stenosis of the renal artery: pattern recognition of tardus and parvus abnormalities with duplex sonography. *Radiology* 1992;184:487–492.
7. Patriquin HB, Lafortune M, Jequier JC, et al. Stenosis of the renal artery: assessment of slowed systole in the downstream circulation with Doppler sonography. *Radiology* 1992;184:479–485.

7a. Sullivan RR, et al. Color Doppler sonographic findings in renal vascular lesions. *J Ultrasound Med* 1991;10:161–165.

8. Hillman BJ. Imaging advances in the diagnosis of renovascular hypertension. *AJR* 1989;153:5–14.
9. Soulen MC, Fishman EK, Goldman SM, et al. Bacterial renal infection: role of CT. *Radiology* 1989;171:703–707.
10. Jeffrey RB, Federle MP. CT and ultrasonography of acute renal abnormalities. *Radiol Clin North Am* 1983;21:515–525.
11. Gold RP, McClennan BL. Bacterial renal infection: role of CT. *Radiology* 1990;174:283–284.
12. Rigsby CM, Rosenfield AT, Glickman MG, et al. Hemorrhagic focal bacterial nephritis: findings on gray-scale sonography and CT. *AJR* 1986;146:1173–1177.
13. Ralls PW, Barakos AJ, Kaptein EM, et al. Renal biopsy-related hemorrhage: frequency and comparison of CT and sonography. *J Comput Assist Tomogr* 1987;11:1031–1034.
14. Cadman PJ, Lindsell DRM, Golding SJ. An unusual appearance of renal lymphoma. *Clin Radiol* 1988;39:452–453.
15. Deuskar V, Martin LF, Leung W. Renal lymphoma: an unusual example. *J Can Assoc Radiol* 1987;38:133–135.
16. Murray KK, McLellan GL. Renal peripelvic lymphangiectasia: appearance at CT. *Radiology* 1991;180:455–456.
17. Brammer HM, Smith WS, Lubbers PR. Septated hypoechoic perirenal fat on sonograms: a pitfall in renal ultrasonography. *J Ultrasound Med* 1992;11:361–363.

17a. Jeffrey RB. Jr. *CT and sonography of the acute abdomen.* New York: Raven Press, 1989.

18. Hoddick W, Jeffrey RB, Goldberg HI, et al. CT and sonography of severe renal and perirenal infections. *AJR* 1983;140:517–520.
19. Deyoe LA, Cronan JJ, Lambiase RE, et al. Percutaneous drainage of renal and perirenal abscesses: results in 30 patients. *AJR* 1990;155:81–83.
20. Sacks D, Banner MP, Meranze SG, et al. Renal and related retroperitoneal abscesses: percutaneous drainage. *Radiology* 1988;167:447–451.
21. Jeffrey RB, Laing FC, Wing VW, et al. Sensitivity of sonography in pyonephrosis: a reevaluation. *AJR* 1985;144:71–73.
22. Keeney PJ. Imaging of chronic renal infections. *AJR* 1990;155: 485–494.
23. Subramanyam BR, Megibor AJ, Raghavendra BN, et al. Diffuse xanthogranulomatous pyelonephritis: analysis by computed tomography and sonography. *Urol Radiol* 1982;4:5–9.
24. Premkumar A, Lattimer J, Newhouse JH. CT and sonography of advanced urinary tract tuberculosis. *AJR* 1987;148:65–69.
25. Schaffer R, Becker JA, Goodman J. Sonography of tuberculous kidney. *Urology* 1983;22:209–211.
26. Das KM, Vaidyanathan S, Rajwanshi A, et al. Renal tuberculosis: diagnosis with sonographically guided aspiration cytology. *AJR* 1992;158:571–573.
27. Bosniak MA. The current radiological approach to renal cysts. *Radiology* 1986;158:1–10.
28. Hayden CK Jr, Swischuk LE, Smith TH, et al. Renal cystic disease in childhood. *Radiographics* 1986;6:97–116.
29. Ralls PW, Esensten ML, Boger D, et al. Severe hydronephrosis and severe renal cystic disease: ultrasonic differentiation. *AJR* 1980;134:473–475.
30. Grossman H, Rosenberg ER, Bowie JD, et al. Sonographic diagnosis of renal cystic diseases. *AJR* 1983;140:81–85.
31. Cronan JJ, Amis ES Jr, Yoder IC, et al. Peripelvic cysts: an imposter of sonographic hydronephrosis. *J Ultrasound Med* 1982;1: 229–236.
32. Hidalgo H, Dunnick NR, Rosenberg ER, et al. Parapelvic cysts: appearance on CT and sonography. *AJR* 1982;138:667–671.
33. Mellins HZ. Cystic dilatations of the upper urinary tract: a radiologist's developmental model. *Radiology* 1984;153:291–301.
34. Horton WA, Wong V, Eldridge R. Von Hippel–Lindau disease. *Arch Intern Med* 1976;136:769–777.
35. Bernstein J, Evan AP, Gardner KD Jr. Epithelial hyperplasia in human polycystic kidney diseases. *Am J Pathol* 1987;129:92–101.
36. Witzelben CL. In: Zakim D, Boyer TD, eds. *Hepatology: a textbook of liver diseases.* Philadelphia: Saunders; 1990:1395–1411.
37. Grossman H, Rosenberg ER, Bowie JD, et al. Sonographic diagnosis of renal cystic disease. *AJR* 1983;140:81–85.
38. Garel LA, Habib R, Pariente D, et al. Juvenile nephronophthiasis: sonographic appearance in children with severe uremia. *Radiology* 1984;151:93–95.
39. Rego JD Jr, Laing FC, Jeffrey RB. Ultrasonographic diagnosis of medullary cystic disease. *J Ultrasound Med* 1983;2:433–436.
40. Madewell JE, Goldman SM, Davis CJ Jr, et al. Multilocular cystic nephroma: a radiographic–pathologic correlation of 58 patients. *Radiology* 1983;146:309–321.

(*text continues on page 356*)

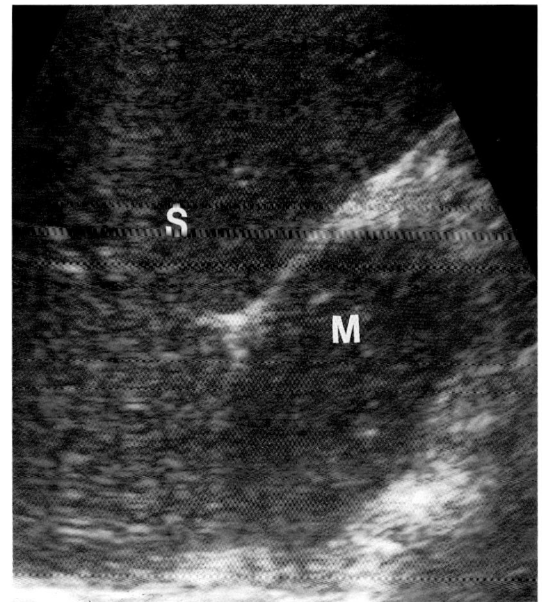

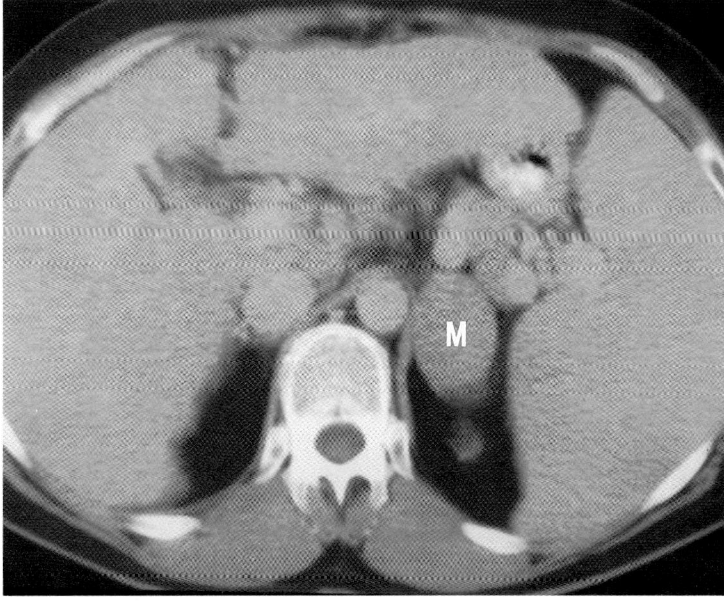

FIG. 5.119. Left adrenal metastasis, uterine leiomyosarcoma. **A:** Longitudinal sonogram through the region of the spleen and left kidney reveals a large ovoid adrenal metastasis (M). **B:** The CT scan shows a similar lesion. Adrenal metastasis is a common manifestation of metastatic disease. While adrenal metastases are generally discovered on CT scans, sonography may also identify them. Metastases may be unilateral or bilateral. Their internal morphology varies widely on CT and sonography. Any adrenal mass in a patient with malignancy must be considered a metastasis until proved otherwise.

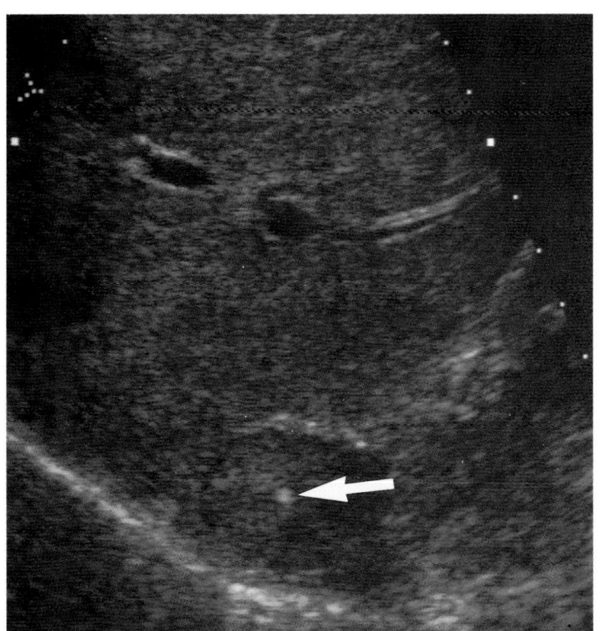

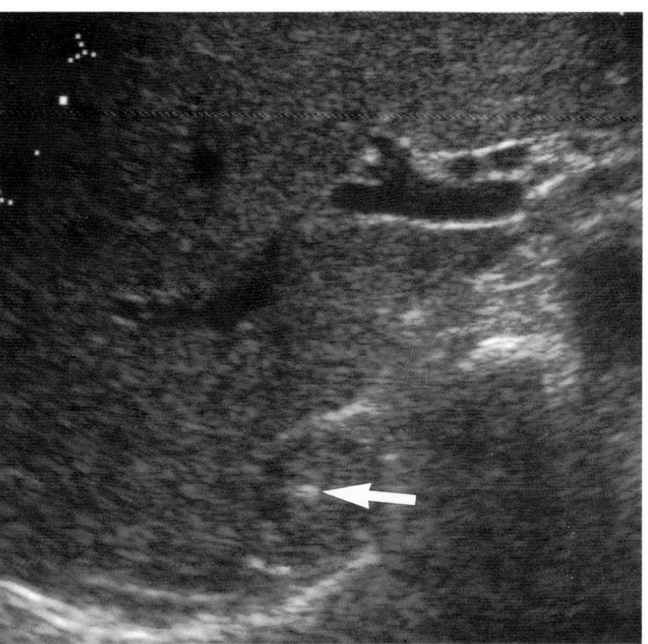

FIG. 5.120. Nonhyperfunctioning adrenal adenoma, central calcification. Longitudinal (**A**) and transverse (**B**) sonograms through the region of the right adrenal reveal a 2-cm spheroid adrenal mass that has a central, nonshadowing calcification (*arrow*). Nonhyperfunctioning adrenal adenomas are common lesions occurring in about 5 percent of the general population. Calcification, present in this patient, is not useful in distinguishing adenoma from carcinoma, or even from metastasis. Any patient with an incidentally discovered adrenal mass should have an endocrine evaluation to determine if adrenal hyperfunction is present. If no hyperfunction is present, follow-up images should be obtained at intervals, the first within 2 to 4 months. If there has been no change in size at 18 months, no further follow-up is necessary. Adrenal adenomas are rarely larger than 4 cm in diameter.

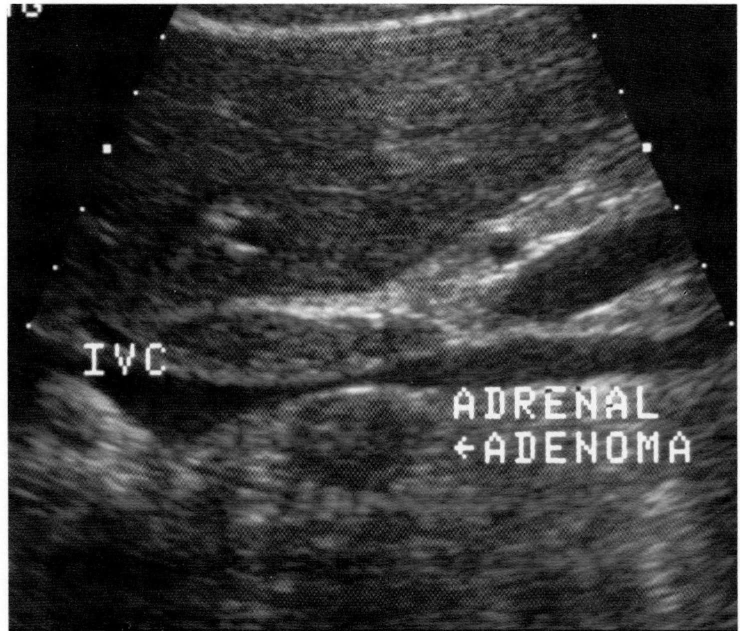

A

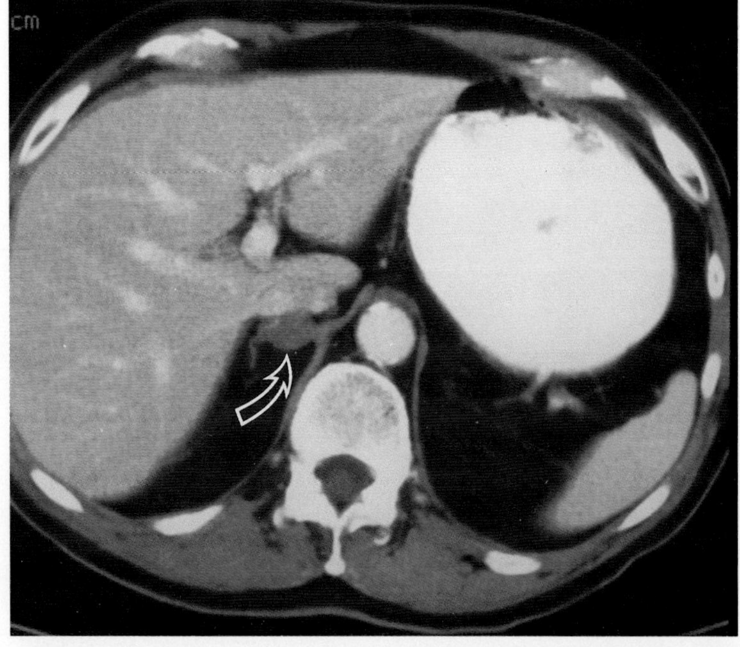

B

FIG. 5.121. A 1-cm nonhyperfunctioning adrenal adenoma. **A:** Longitudinal oblique sonogram reveals a small nonhyperfunctioning adrenal adenoma dorsal to the inferior vena cava. **B:** A contrast-enhanced CT scan reveals a relatively low-attenuation adenoma in the same location (*open curved arrow*). Small nonfunctioning adrenal adenomas such as this are common findings on routine abdominal CT scanning. If there is no evidence of endocrine hyperfunction, and follow-up imaging shows no change in size, no further evaluation is required. If an adrenal mass like this is discovered in a patient with malignancy, however, a biopsy may be needed to rule out metastasis. In a patient with malignancy, adrenal masses are biopsied only when the presence of metastasis would alter the therapy of the patient.

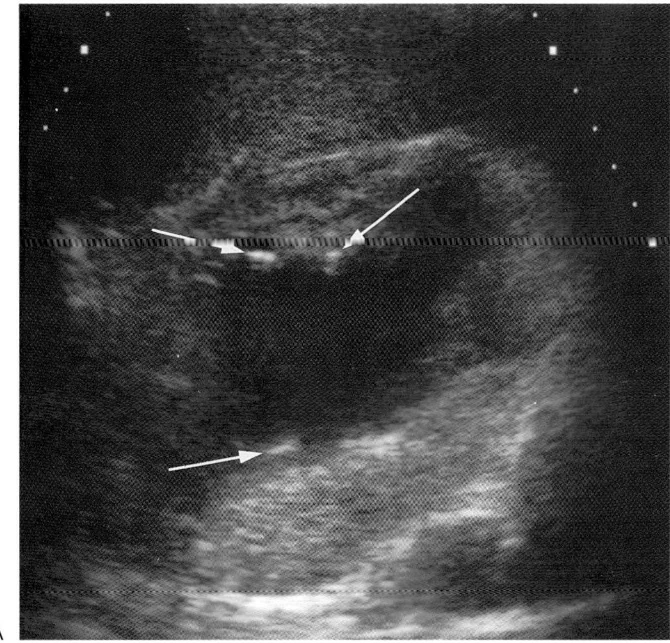

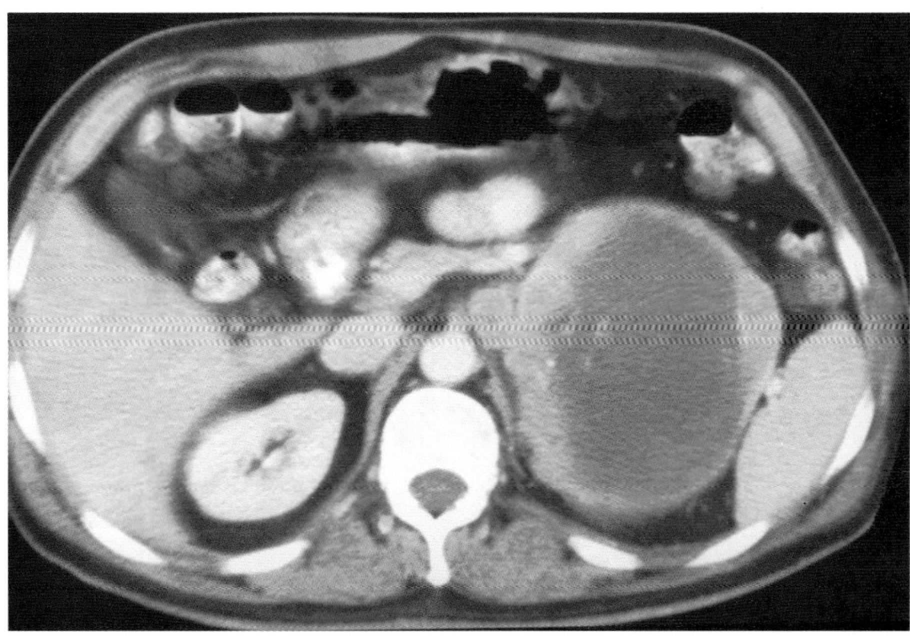

FIG. 5.122. Left adrenal pheochromocytoma, malignant. **A:** Longitudinal oblique sonogram through the region of the left adrenal reveals a large adrenal mass that has a central anechoic, presumably necrotic, central region. Note the small calcifications (*thin arrows*). **B:** The CT scan reveals similar findings with a low-attenuation, presumably necrotic, center. Calcifications are noted adjacent to the more solid-appearing peripheral portion of this large pheochromocytoma. This patient had hypertension and laboratory findings diagnostic of pheochromocytoma. Pheochromocytomas are usually large masses that have variable sized regions of internal decreased echogenicity. This is a malignant pheochromocytoma. Most pheochromocytomas are benign. Malignant pheochromocytomas may invade locally and metastasize. Other than by identifying local invasion or metastases, there is no way to distinguish benign from malignant pheochromocytomas on images.

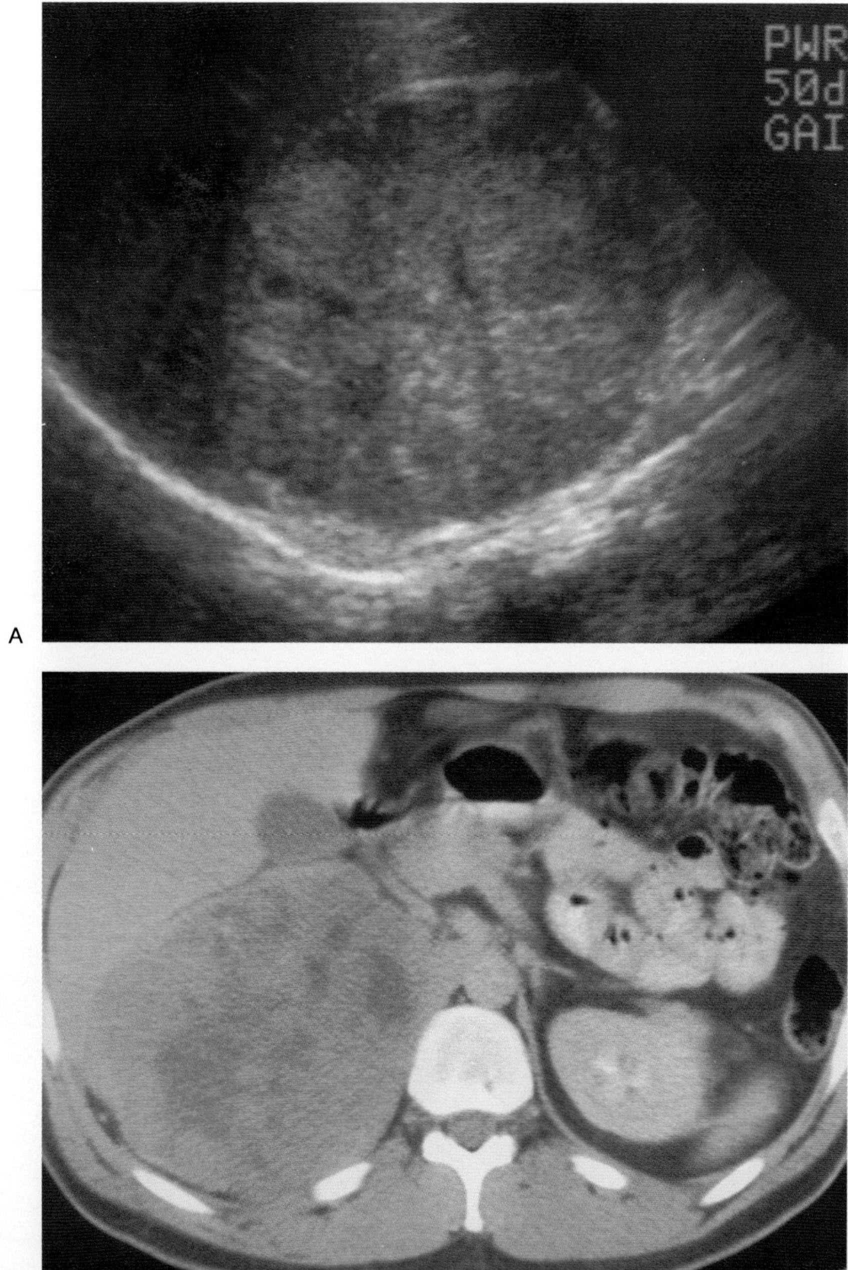

FIG. 5.123. Adrenal carcinoma. **A:** Longitudinal sonogram through the right suprarenal region reveals a large, solid, approximately 9-cm mixed echogenicity adrenal carcinoma. **B:** The CT scan reveals a similar mixed attenuation lesion, displacing the liver ventrally. Adrenal cell carcinomas are rarely less than 5 cm in size when detected. For this reason, all masses larger than 5 cm should be removed surgically regardless of the endocrine status of the patient. Adrenal carcinoma usually causes adrenal hyperfunction, but nonhyperfunctioning tumors may also be discovered. The only useful feature that allows discrimination between adrenal adenoma and carcinoma is size. When discovered, virtually all adrenal adenomas are less than 5 cm in size; virtually all adrenal carcinomas are larger than 5 cm. Although this lesion is uncalcified, adrenal carcinomas are frequently calcified.

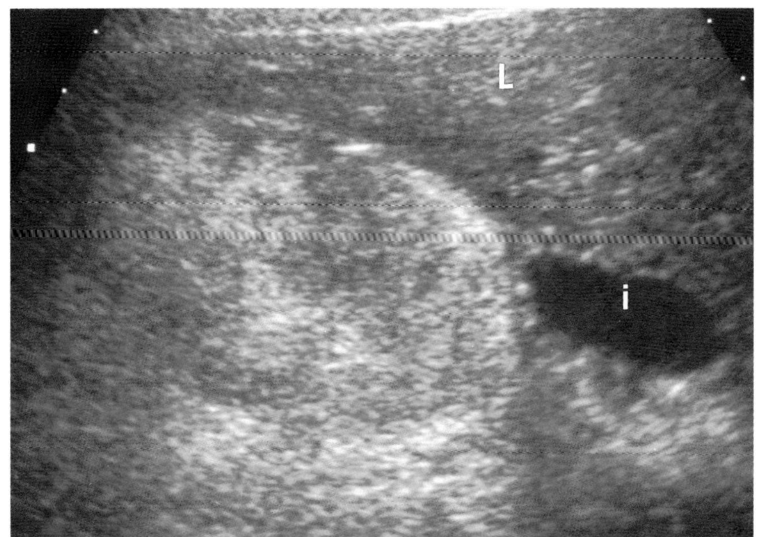

FIG. 5.124. Adrenal myelolipoma. Transverse sonogram through the region of the right adrenal gland reveals a large, predominantly echogenic, adrenal tumor. Increased echogenicity suggests the presence of fat, the hallmark of adrenal myelolipoma. Adrenal myelolipoma is an uncommon adrenal tumor comprised of bone marrow elements and fat. Fat, causing increased echogenicity on ultrasound and low attenuation on CT, allows a confident diagnosis from the images alone. Calcifications (not present here) are fairly frequent in this benign neoplasm. i, inferior vena cava; L, liver.

A

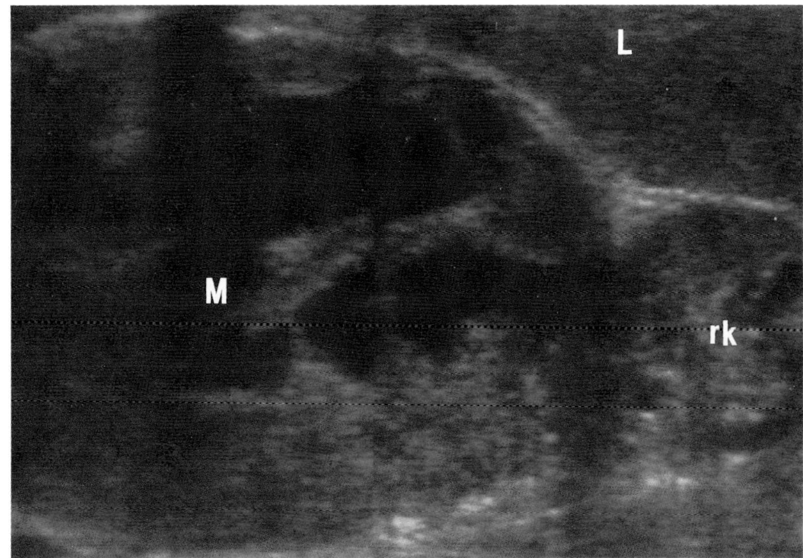

B

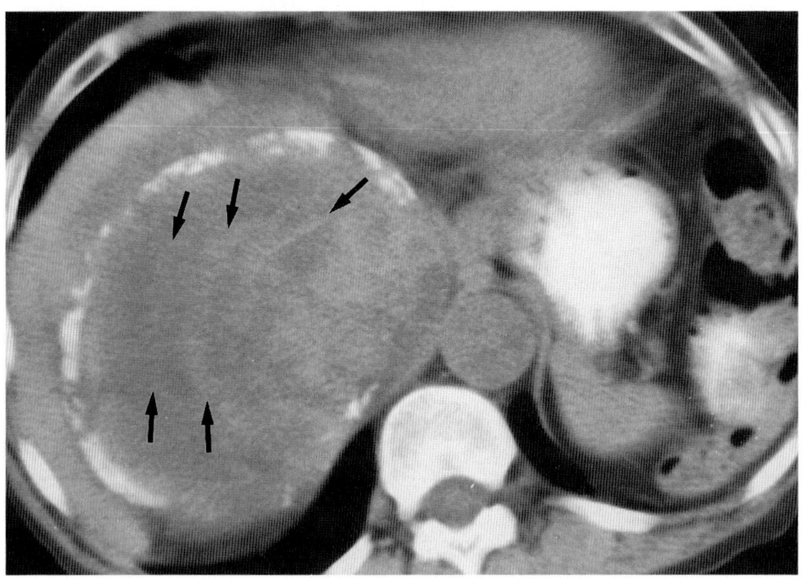

FIG. 5.125. Adrenal hematoma. **A:** A composite longitudinal sonogram through the region of the right kidney reveals a huge mixed echogenicity mass (M) that displaces the liver (L) and the right kidney (rk). **B:** A transverse CT scan shows calcification and a laminated appearance (note bands of higher attenuation—*thin arrows*). There is calcification around the periphery. Because of the size of the lesion and the presence of calcification, an adrenal carcinoma was suspected. At surgery, this lesion was easily resectable. Pathologically, it was a large adrenal hematoma. The cause of the hematoma was not determined, either pathologically or upon careful review of the patient's history. Adrenal hemorrhage is common in neonates and young children. Spontaneous hemorrhage in adults is rare.

41. Banner MP, Pollack HM, Chatten J, et al. Multilocular renal cysts: radiologic–pathologic correlation. *AJR* 1981;136:239–247.
42. Mindell HJ. Imaging studies for screening native kidneys in long-term dialysis patients. *AJR* 1989;153:768–769.
43. Jabour BA, Ralls PW, Tang WW, et al. Acquired cystic disease of the kidneys. Computed tomography and ultrasonography appraisal in patients on peritoneal dialysis and hemodialysis. *Invest Radiol* 1987;22:728–732.
44. Anderson BL, Curry NS, Gobien RP. Sonography of evolving renal cystic transformation associated with hemodialysis. *AJR* 1983;141:1003–1004.
45. Bretan PN Jr, Busch MP, Hricak H, et al. Chronic renal failure: a significant risk factor in the development of acquired renal cysts and renal cell carcinoma. *Cancer* 1986;57:1871–1879.
46. Boileau M, Foley R, Flechner S, et al. Renal adenocarcinoma and end stage kidney disease. *J Urol* 1986;138:603–606.
47. Bennington J, Beckwith JB. Tumors of the kidney, renal pelvis, and ureter. In: *Atlas of tumor pathology,* 2nd series, Fascicle 12. Washington DC: Armed Forces Institute of Pathology, 1975.
48. Curry NS, Schabel SI, Betsill WL Jr. Small renal neoplasms: diagnostic imaging, pathologic features, and clinical course. *Radiology* 1986;158:113–117.
49. Charboneau JW, Hattery RR, Ernst EC III, et al. Spectrum of sonographic findings in 125 renal masses other than benign simple cyst. *AJR* 1983;140:87–94.
50. Feldberg MAM, van Waes PFGM. Multilocular cystic renal cell carcinoma. *AJR* 1982;138:953–955.
51. Levine E, Huntrakoon M, Wetzel LH. Small renal neoplasms: clinical, pathologic, and imaging features. *AJR* 1989;153:69–73.
52. Taylor KJW, Ramos I, Carter D, et al. Correlation of Doppler US tumor signals with neovascular morphologic features. *Radiology* 1988;166:57–62.
53. Kuijpers D, Jaspers R. Renal masses: differential diagnosis with pulsed Doppler US. *Radiology* 1989;170:59–60.
54. Dubbins PA, Wells I. Renal carcinoma: duplex Doppler evaluation. *Br J Radiol* 1986;59:231–236.
55. Lafortune M, Breton G. Echographic demonstration of an oncocytoma. *J Can Assoc Radiol* 1983;34:144–146.
56. Grant DC, Dee GJ, Yoder IC, et al. Sonography in transitional cell carcinoma of the renal pelvis. *Urol Radiol* 1986;8:1–5.
57. Yousem DM, Gatewood OMB, Goldman SM, et al. Synchronous and metachronous transitional cell carcinoma of the urinary tract: prevalence, incidence, and radiographic detection. *Radiology* 1988;167:613–618.
58. Winalski CS, Lipman JC, Tumeh SS. Ureteral neoplasms. *Radiographics* 1990;10:271–283.
59. Subramanyam BR, Raghavendra BN, Madamba MR. Renal transitional cell carcinoma: sonographic and pathologic correlation. *J Clin Ultrasound* 1982;10:203–210.
60. Hartman DS, Goldman SM, Friedman AC, et al. Angiomyolipoma: ultrasonic–pathologic correlation. *Radiology* 1981;139:451–458.
61. Bret PM, Bretagnolle M, Gaillard D, et al. Small, asymptomatic angiomyolipomas of the kidney. *Radiology* 1985;154:7–10.
62. Choyke PL, White EM, Zeman RK, et al. Renal metastases: clinicopathologic and radiologic correlation. *Radiology* 1987;162:359–363.
63. Pagani JJ. Solid renal mass in the cancer patient: second primary renal cell carcinoma versus renal metastasis. *J Comput Assist Tomogr* 1983;7:444–448.
64. Hartman DS, Davis CJ Jr, Goldman SM, et al. Renal lymphoma: radiologic–pathologic correlation of 21 cases. *Radiology* 1982;144:759–766.
65. Charnsangavej C. Lymphoma of the genitourinary tract. *Radiol Clin North Am* 1990;28:865–877.
66. Richmond J, Sherman RS, Diamond HD, et al. Renal lesions associated with malignant lymphomas. *Am J Med* 1962;32:184–207.
67. Saita H, Matsukawa M, Fukushima H, et al. Ultrasound diagnosis of ureteral stones: its usefulness with subsequent excretory urography. *J Urol* 1986;140:28–31.
68. Middleton WD, Dodds WJ, Lawson TL, et al. Renal calculi: sensitivity for detection with US. *Radiology* 1988;167:239–244.
69. Haddad MC, Sharif HS, Shahed MS, et al. Renal coli: diagnosis and outcome. *Radiology* 1992;184:83–88.
70. Erwin BC, Carroll BA, Sommer FG. Renal colic: the role of ultrasound in initial evaluation. *Radiology* 1984;152:147–150.
71. Choyke PL. The urogram: are rumors of its death premature? *Radiology* 1992;184:33–36.
72. Laing FC, Jeffrey RB Jr, Wing VW. Ultrasound versus excretory urography in evaluating acuate flank pain. *Radiology* 1985;154:613–616.
73. Cronan JJ. Contemporary concepts in imaging urinary tract obstruction. *Radiol Clin North Am* 1991;29:527–542.
74. Wolfman MG, Thornberg JR, Barunstein EM. Nonobstructing radiopaque ureteral calculi. *Urol Radiol* 1979;1:97–104.
75. Maillet PJ, Pelle-Francoz D, Laville M, et al. Nondilated obstructive acute renal failure: diagnostic procedures and therapeutic management. *Radiology* 1986;160:659–662.
76. Harrison RB, Widner LA, Johnstone WH, et al. Subtle obstructive uropathy resulting from encasement of the ureters by tumor. *J Urol* 1979;122:835–836.
77. Rascoff JH, Golden RA, Spinowitz BS, et al. Nondilated obstructive nephropathy. *Arch Intern Med* 1983;143:696–698.
78. Naidich JB, Rackson ME, Mossey RT, et al. Nondilated obstructive uropathy: percutaneous nephrostomy performed to reverse renal failure. *Radiology* 1986;160:653–657.
79. Curry NS, Gobien RP, Schabel SI. Minimal-dilatation obstructive nephropathy. *Radiology* 1982;143:531–534.
80. Kamholtz RG, Cronan JJ, Dorfman GS. Obstruction and the minimally dilated renal collecting system: US evaluation. *Radiology* 1989;170:51–53.
81. Scola FH, Cronan JJ, Schepps B. Grade I hydronephrosis: pulsed Doppler US evaluation. *Radiology* 1989;171:519–520.
82. Baker SM, Middleton WD. Color Doppler sonography of ureteral jets in normal volunteers: importance of the relative specific gravity of urine in the ureter and bladder. *AJR* 1992;159:773–775.
83. Burge HJ, Middleton WD, McClennan BL, et al. Ureteral jets in healthy subjects and in patients with unilateral ureteral calculi: comparison with color Doppler US. *Radiology* 1991;180:437–442.
84. Price CI, Adler RS, Rubin JM. Ultrasound detection of differences in density explanation of the ureteric jet phenomenon and implications for new ultrasound applications. *Invest Radiol* 1989;24:876–883.
85. Dubbins PA, Kurtz AB, Darby J, et al. Ureteric jet effect: the echographic appearance of urine entering the bladder. *Radiology* 1981;140:513–515.
86. Cox IH, Erickson SJ, Foley WD, et al. Ureteric jets: evaluation of normal flow dynamics with color Doppler sonography. *AJR* 1992;158:1051–1055.
87. Platt JF, Rubin JM, Ellis JH, et al. Duplex Doppler US of the kidney: differentiation of obstructive from nonobstructive dilatation. *Radiology* 1989;171:515–517.
88. Platt JF. Duplex Doppler evaluation of native kidney dysfunction: obstructive and nonobstructive disease. *AJR* 1992;158:1035–1042.
89. Brandt TD, Neiman HL, Dragowski MJ, et al. Ultrasound assessment of normal renal dimensions. *J Ultrasound Med* 1982;1:49–52.
90. Platt JF, Rubin JM, Ellis JH. Acute renal failure: possible role of duplex Doppler US in distinction between acute prerenal failure and acute tubular necrosis. *Radiology* 1991;179:419–423.
91. Patriquin HB, O'Regan S, Robitaille P, et al. Hemolytic–uremic syndrome: intrarenal arterial Doppler patterns as a useful guide to therapy. *Radiology* 1989;172:625–628.
92. Letourneau JG, Day DL, Ascher NL, et al. Imaging of renal transplants. *AJR* 1988;150:833–838.
93. Pozniak MA, Dodd GD III, Kelcz F. Ultrasonographic evaluation of renal transplantation. *Radiol Clin North Am* 1992;30:1053–1066.
94. Grenier N, Douws C, Morel D, et al. Detection of vascular complications in renal allografts with color Doppler flow imaging. *Radiology* 1991;178:217–223.
95. Kelcz F, Pozniak MA, Pirsch JD, et al. Pyramidal appearance and resistive index: insensitive and nonspecific sonographic indicators of renal transplant rejection. *AJR* 1990;155:531–535.

96. Warshauer DM, Taylor KJW, Bia MJ, et al. Unusual causes of increased vascular impedance in renal transplants: duplex Doppler evaluation. *Radiology* 1988;169:367–370.
97. Allen KS, Jorasky DK, Arger PH, et al. Renal allografts: prospective analysis of Doppler sonography. *Radiology* 1988;169:371–376.
98. Keveggia LP, Perrella RR, Grant EG, et al. Duplex Doppler sonography in renal allografts: the significance of reversed flow in diastole. *AJR* 1990;155:293–298.
99. Saarinen O. Diagnostic value of resistive index of renal transplants in the early postoperative period. *Acta Radiol* 1991;32:166–169.
100. Fleischer AC, Hinton AA, Glick AD, et al. Duplex Doppler sonography of renal transplants. Correlation with histopathology. *J Ultrasound Med* 1989;8:89–94.
101. Rigsby CM, Burns PN, Weltin GG, et al. Doppler signal quantitation in renal allografts: comparison in normal and rejecting transplants, with pathologic correlation. *Radiology* 1987;162:39–42.
102. Buckley AR, Cooperberg PL, Reeve C, et al. The distinction between acute renal transplant rejection and cyclosporine nephrotoxicity: value of duplex sonography. *AJR* 1987;149:521–525.
103. Perchik JE, Baumgartner BR, Bernardino ME. Renal transplant rejection. Limited value of duplex Doppler sonography. *Invest Radiol* 1991;26:422–426.
104. Genkins SM, Sanfilippo FP, Carroll BA. Duplex Doppler sonography of renal transplants: lack of sensitivity and specificity in establishing pathologic diagnosis. *AJR* 1989;152:535–539.
105. Townsend RR, Tomlanovich SJ, Goldstein RB, et al. Combined Doppler and morphologic sonographic evaluation of renal transplant rejection. *J Ultrasound Med* 1990;9:199–206.
106. Mee SL, McAninch JW. Indications for radiographic assessment in suspected renal trauma. *Urol Clin North Am* 1989;16:187–192.
107. Carroll PR, McAninch JW. Staging of renal trauma. *Urol Clin North Am* 1989;16:193–201.
108. Cass AS. Renovascular injuries from external trauma. *Urol Clin North Am* 1989;16:213–220.
109. Pollack HM, Wein AJ. Imaging of renal trauma. *Radiology* 1989;172:297–308.
110. Furtschegger A, Egender G, Jakse G. The value of sonography in the diagnosis and follow-up of patients with blunt renal trauma. *Br J Urol* 1988;62:110–116.
111. Radin DR, Baker EL, Klatt EC, et al. Visceral and nodal calcification in patients with AIDS-related *Pneumocystis carinii* infection. *AJR* 1990;154:27–31.
112. Falkoff GE, Rigsby CM, Rosenfield AT. Partial, combined cortical and medullary nephrocalcinosis: US and CT patterns in AIDS-associated MAI infection. *Radiology* 1987;162:343–344.
113. Carbone L, D'Agati V, Cheng JT, et al. Course and prognosis of human immunodeficiency virus-associated nephropathy. *Am J Med* 1989;87:389–395.
114. Sample WF. A new technique for the evaluation of the adrenal gland with gray scale ultrasonography. *Radiology* 1977;124:463–469.
115. Sample WF. Adrenal ultrasonography. *Radiology* 1978;127:461–466.
116. Yeh HC. Ultrasonography of the adrenals. *Semin Roentgenol* 1988;23:250–258.

CHAPTER 6

The Spleen

TECHNIQUE

Splenic sonography is best performed with patients in a 45° right posterior oblique (RPO) position. Scans are obtained first parallel to the intercostal spaces and then coronally through the left flank. It is generally not possible to adequately image the spleen with patients in supine position due to lack of adequate acoustic access from overlying ribs. Occasionally, prone scans may be useful. It is important for patients to vary their depth of respiration in order to image the entire spleen. The upper pole of the spleen is often best demonstrated by scans obtained with deep inspiration. Either a 5-MHz curved linear array transducer or a sector scanner may be used for splenic imaging. Color Doppler sonography is invaluable for diagnosis of splenic and perisplenic vascular abnormalities such as aneurysms, varices, and splenic vein thrombosis.

Coronal images through the spleen provide an important acoustic window to evaluate the pancreatic tail. The splenic hilum and the tail of the pancreas are difficult to image from a standard anterior approach. Larger lesions in the region of the tail of the pancreas can often be visualized by scanning coronally through the spleen.

SPLENOMEGALY

Sonography is an excellent technique to quickly evaluate patients for splenomegaly. In the Western world the most common cause of splenomegaly is portal hypertension from cirrhosis. However, a broad spectrum of infectious, hematologic, neoplastic, and storage disorders may result in moderate to severe splenomegaly. In many patients with splenomegaly the underlying etiology cannot be determined by sonography alone. Identifiable causes include splenic vein thrombosis and neoplastic replacement by lymphoma or metastatic disease. In patients with obvious signs of cirrhosis (nodular liver surface, recanalized paraumbilical, veins and varices), portal hypertension is the most likely cause of splenomegaly.

The normal spleen in adults has a length less than 12 cm and a maximal transverse diameter of 5 cm (1). These measurements may be of value in borderline cases of splenomegaly. In most patients with splenomegaly, visual inspection sonographically of the enlarged spleen is all that is required to establish the diagnosis (Fig. 6.1).

SPLENIC NEOPLASMS

When macroscopic, benign and malignant splenic neoplasms may cause focal parenchymal abnormalities. Micrometastases and diffuse microscopic infiltration from lymphoma generally do not have any appreciable sonographic findings. Hemangiomas are the most common benign neoplasms of the spleen and have been identified in as many as 14 percent of patients at autopsy (2,3). In clinical practice, however, detection of splenic hemangiomas with sonography is considerably less common. Splenic hemangiomas are usually focal echogenic lesions similar in appearance to hepatic hemangiomas (Fig. 6.1). Rarely, splenic hemangiomas may either be calcified or contain cystic components (4,5). A "halo" sign or a hypoechoic rim around a splenic hemangioma is unusual and should suggest splenic metastases (6).

Niizawa et al. (7) recently reported the color Doppler findings in a patient with a splenic hemangioma. Arterial flow was noted within an echogenic mass. With compression from the ultrasound transducer, the arterial flow could be occluded, suggesting a soft and pliable vascular mass. With release of compression arterial flow was again demonstrated within the mass. Surgery confirmed a splenic hemangioma (7). Whether color Doppler with compression will actually be of use in further characterizing echogenic splenic lesions must await larger clinical trials. Splenic angiomas are benign vascular lesions that demonstrate arterial flow with color Doppler (Fig. 6.2). It may not be possible to distinguish an angioma from

(text continues on page 361)

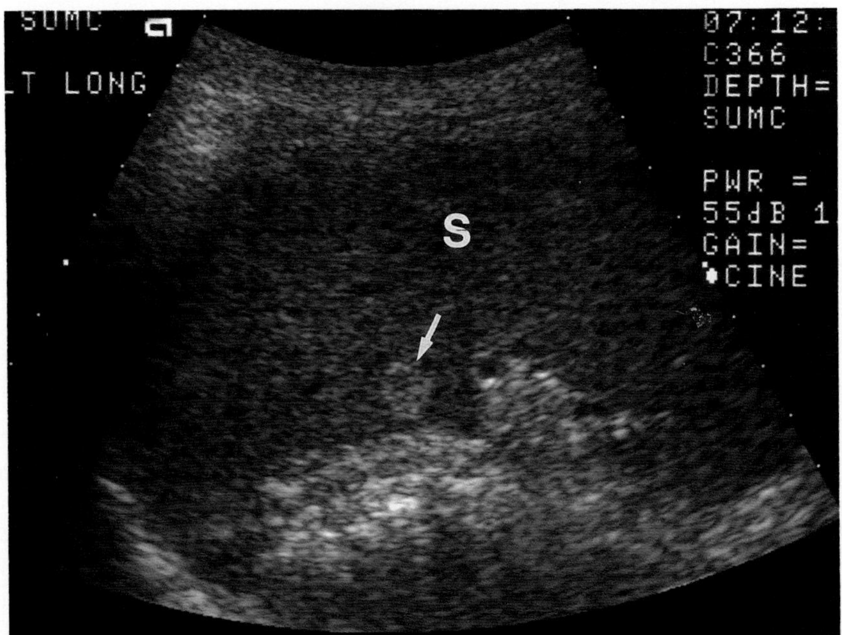

FIG. 6.1. Mild splenomegaly in a patient with splenic hemangioma. Sagittal scan demonstrates focal echogenic lesion (*arrow*) similar in appearance to hepatic hemangioma. Note mild splenic enlargement. S, spleen.

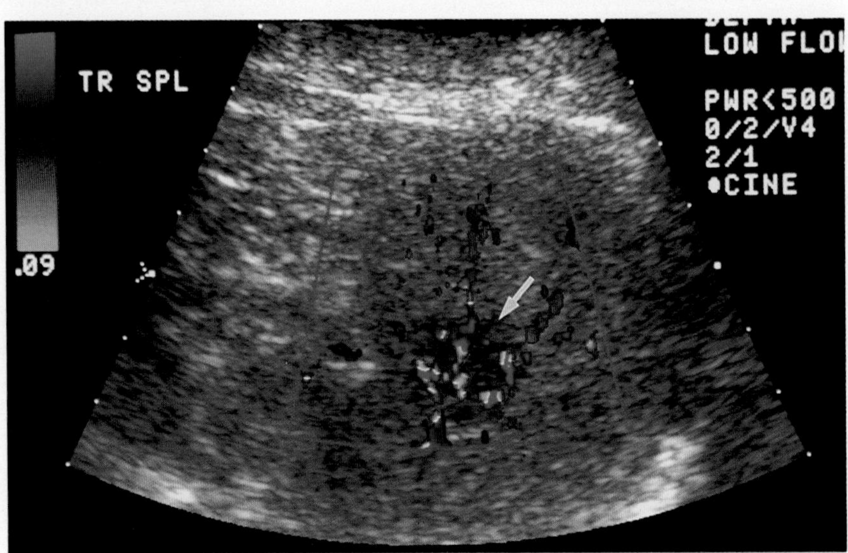

FIG. 6.2. Splenic angioma. Transverse color Doppler sonogram of spleen demonstrates small hypervascular lesion (*arrow*). Lesion was stable for several years.

other hypervascular lesions. Serial follow-up is recommended for small lesions.

Lymphoma and metastases are the most common malignant lesions of the spleen (8,9). Goerg et al. (8) noted that of 66 patients with splenic neoplasms identified by sonography, 55 had lymphoma and nine had metastases. Angiosarcoma, although an extremely rare lesion, is the most common primary splenic malignancy. Spontaneous rupture and hemoperitoneum may be the initial mode of clinical presentation (10).

Hypoechoic nodules are a characteristic sonographic finding in both splenic metastases and lymphoma (Fig. 6.3). A target sign or "bull's eye" appearance may occur with both types of neoplasms but is more common in metastatic disease. The overall sensitivity of sonography in the detection of splenic lymphoma is relatively poor. Siniluoto et al. (9) reported a sensitivity for sonography of only 54 percent in 61 patients with Hodgkin's disease involving the spleen. Of the 61 patients with splenic Hodgkin's disease, only 13 patients had splenomegaly (9). Thus it is important to recognize that splenomegaly is not a constant finding in lymphoma.

Splenic metastases are uncommon in clinical practice. Although autopsy series report splenic metastases in up to 10 percent of patients dying with cancer, many lesions are microscopic (11). The most common primary tumors to metastasize to the spleen are melanoma and carcinomas of the breast, lung, ovary, and stomach (Fig. 6.4). In a sonographic study of 31 patients with splenic metastases, Siniluoto et al. (11) noted that 16 had multifocal lesions, 12 had solitary lesions, and three had diffuse splenic infiltration. Splenic metastases were most often hypoechoic in appearance (11). Twenty-nine percent of lesions had mixed echogenicity (Fig. 6.5) and 14 percent were predominantly hyperechoic (Fig. 6.6). Three patients (11 percent) had target lesions with a hypoechoic halo surrounding an echogenic lesion (11). Goerg et al. (8) reported a halo sign in three of 13 patients with splenic metastases. Ovarian carcinoma and necrotic metastases may have a complex cystic appearance. Cystic metastases are characterized by thick irregular walls, mural nodules, and septations (Figs. 6.7 and 6.8).

Due to the nonspecific sonographic appearance of many splenic neoplasms, it may be necessary to perform guided fine-needle aspiration biopsy for definitive diagnosis. Percutaneous fine-needle aspiration biopsy of the spleen can generally be accomplished safely with little risk of bleeding (Fig. 6.9) (12). Larger cutting needles used to obtain core biopsies are not generally necessary to confirm the diagnosis of metastases. Histologic subtyping of Hodgkin's lymphoma, however, may not be possible with fine-needle aspiration cytology. In the past, most patients with lymphoma required splenectomy for definitive histologic subclassification. Suzuki et al. (13), however, reported that sonography may be helpful in guiding splenic biopsy with a 21-gauge core biopsy needle to classify non-Hodgkin's lymphoma. There were no complications in eight patients undergoing 21-gauge core biopsy. Two of the eight patients had histologic evidence of non-Hodgkin's lymphoma with a sonographically normal spleen (13).

SPLENIC VASCULAR ABNORMALITIES

Vascular abnormalities of the spleen are common and include infarction, splenic artery aneurysms, perisplenic varices, and splenic vein thrombosis. Color Doppler sonography is essential for establishing the diagnosis of many vascular disorders. Contrast-enhanced computed tomography (CT) and/or angiography may be required for confirmation in selected cases.

SPLENIC INFARCTION

In a review of 36 patients with splenic infarction, Goerg et al. (6) noted that the two most common etiologies were myeloproliferative disorders (15 patients) and endocarditis (17 patients). However, splenic infarction may be associated with many other diseases including hematologic disorders, lymphoma, lung cancer, and Whipple's disease. Splenomegaly was noted in 27 of the 36 patients with infarcts (6). Patients with splenic infarcts typically present with left upper quadrant pain (14). However, nine of 23 patients reported by Goerg and Schwerk (14) were asymptomatic.

Sonographically, segmental splenic infarcts are generally hypoechoic peripheral lesions with a wedge-shaped configuration (Figs. 6.10 and 6.11). On occasion, splenic infarction may have a rounded or nodular appearance that may mimic an abscess or a neoplasm. Global splenic infarction is rare due to its dual blood supply from the short gastric arteries and the splenic artery. Proximal occlusion of the splenic artery may rarely cause global splenic infarction (Fig. 6.12). The grayscale appearance of total splenic infarction may be deceptively normal and the diagnosis can only be established with confidence by color Doppler sonography or contrast CT.

In most patients, segmental splenic infarcts demonstrate a decrease in the size of the lesion over time. Chronic splenic infarcts may heal with areas of echogenic fibrosis. However, some patients with splenic infarcts develop complications such as superinfection, intralesional hemorrhage, and spontaneous splenic rupture (Fig. 6.13) (14). Hemoperitoneum and chronic intrasplenic pseudocysts may occur in a small percentage of patients (14).

Serial sonography may be helpful to document interval healing or delayed complications of splenic infarcts. In patients with septic emboli to the spleen, a wedged-shaped infarct may evolve into an abscess and become rounded or oval in configuration. Hemorrhage

(*text continues on page 371*)

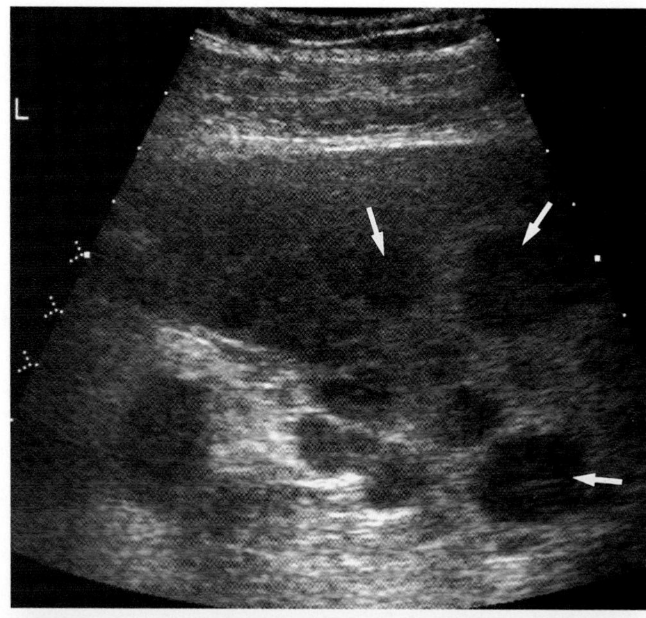

A

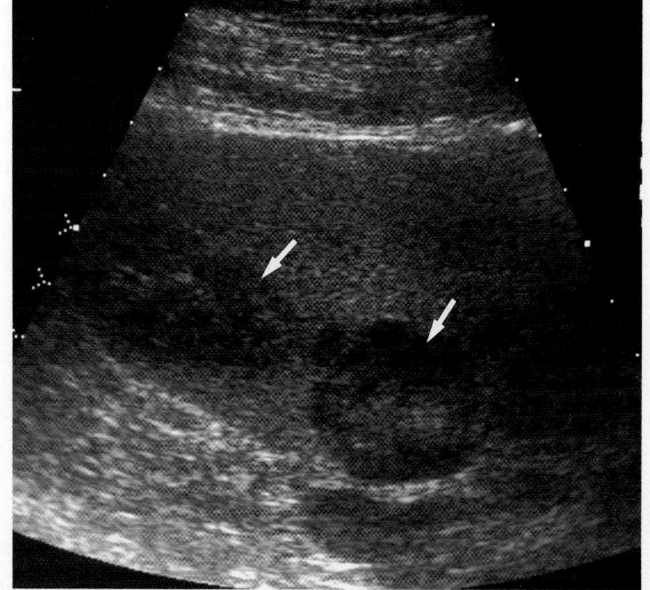

B

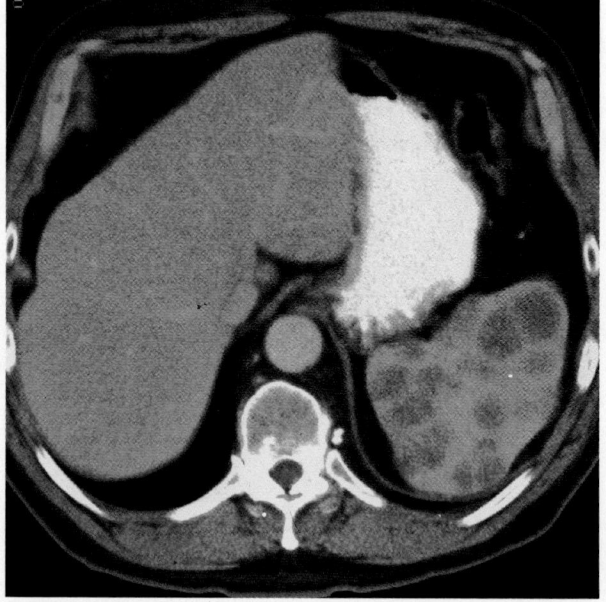

C

FIG. 6.3. Splenic lymphoma. **A, B:** Transverse scans of spleen demonstrate multiple hypoechoic nodules (*arrows*). **C:** CT scan confirms diffuse splenic lymphoma. Note lack of significant splenomegaly.

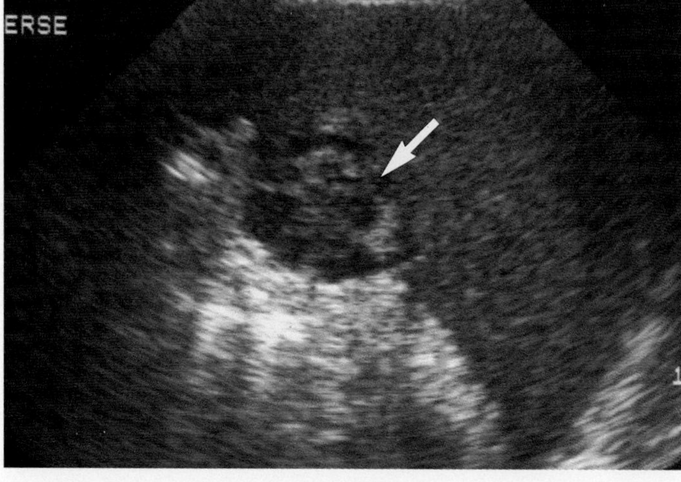

FIG. 6.4. Splenic metastasis from melanoma. Note lesion of mixed echogenicity (*arrow*) on transverse scan of spleen.

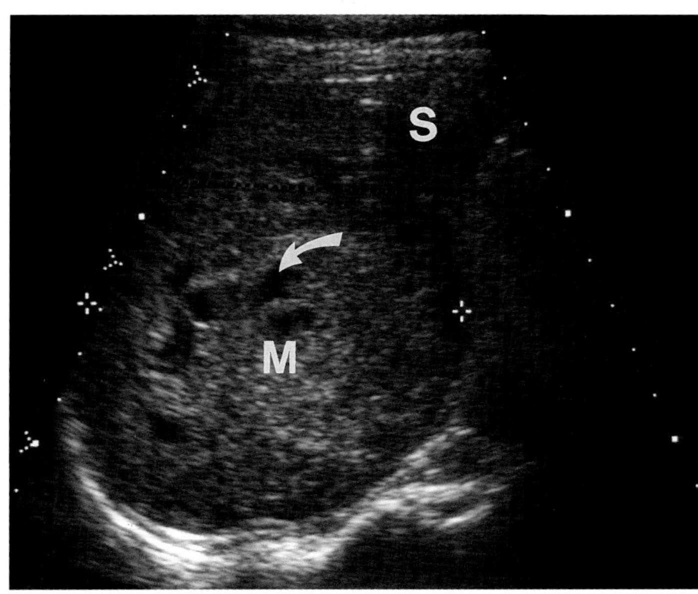

FIG. 6.5. Splenic metastasis from lung carcinoma. Sagittal scan of spleen (S) demonstrates large metastasis of mixed echogenicity. Note discrete hypoechoic areas probably representing necrosis (*arrow*).

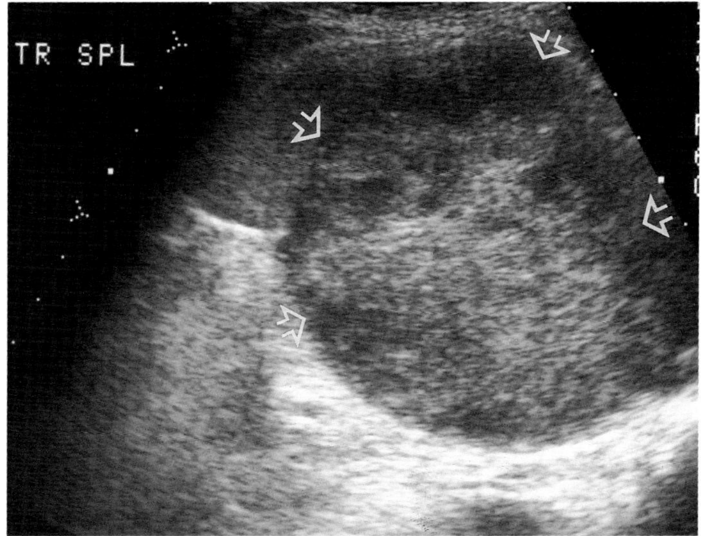

A

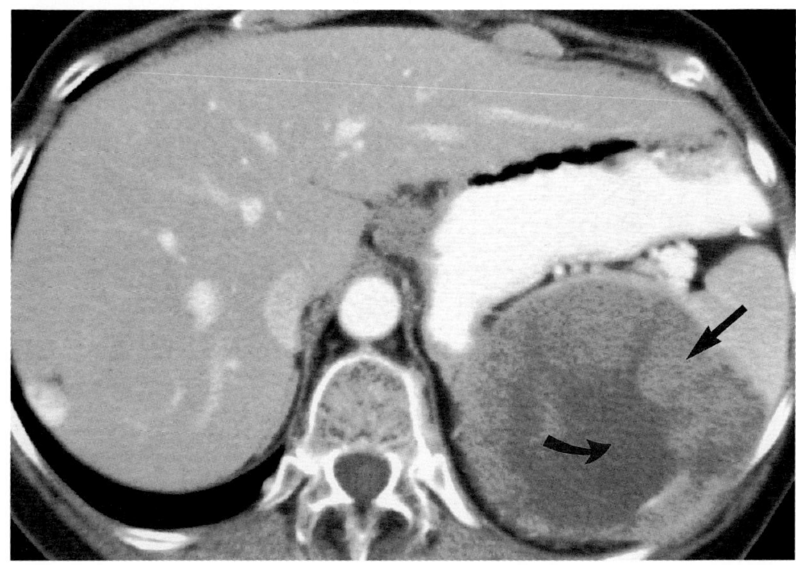

B

FIG. 6.6. Hyperechoic splenic metastasis from ovarian carcinoma. **A:** Transverse scan of spleen demonstrates echogenic ovarian metastasis (*arrows*). **B:** CT scan demonstrates solid peripheral component (*arrow*) and necrotic center (*curved arrow*).

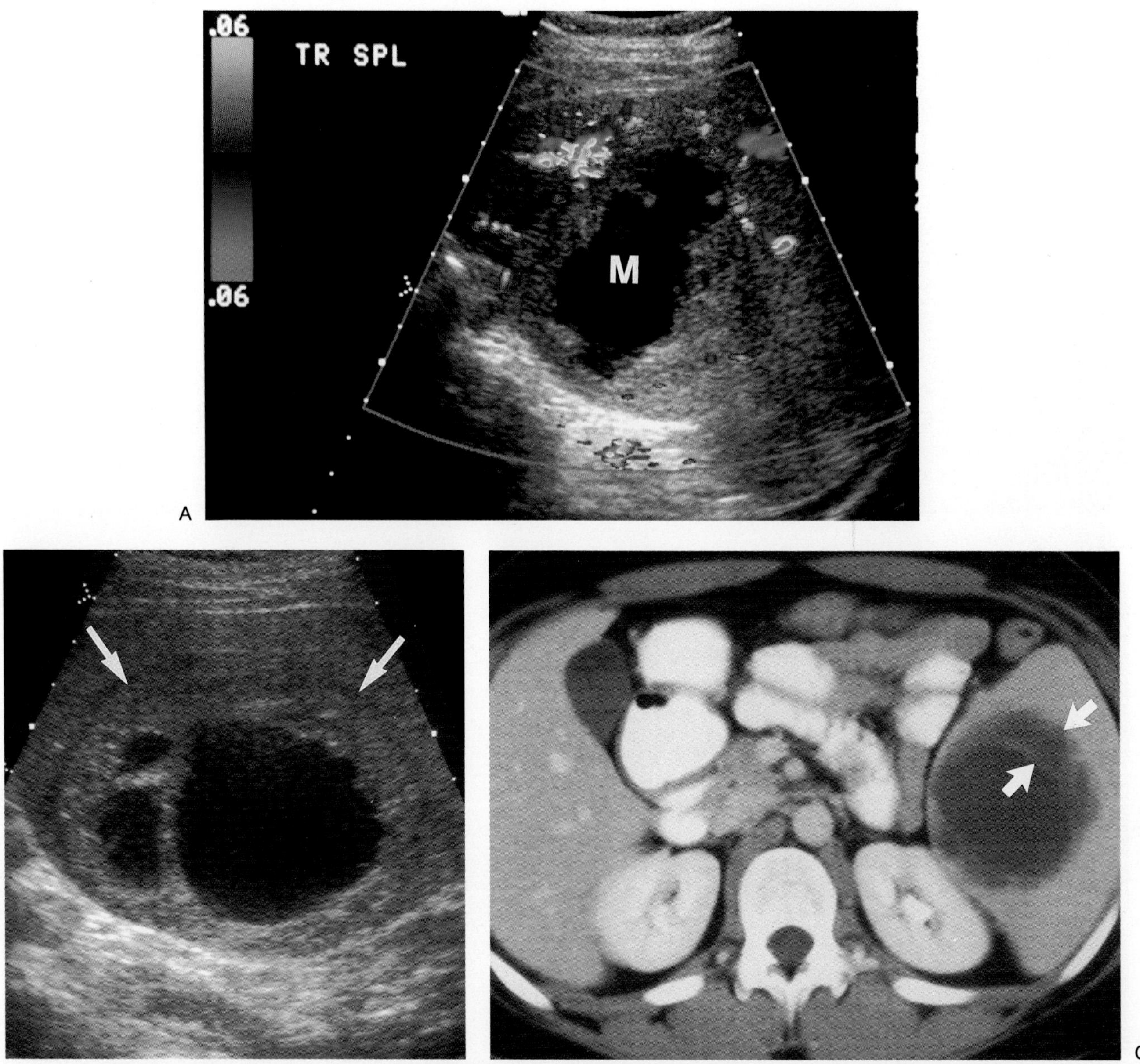

FIG. 6.7. Cystic splenic metastasis from nasopharyngeal carcinoma. **A:** Transverse color Doppler sonogram of spleen demonstrates necrotic center of metastasis (M). **B:** Sagittal grayscale image demonstrates cystic metastasis with thick capsule (*arrows*). **C:** CT scan confirms cystic metastasis. Note thick capsule (*arrows*).

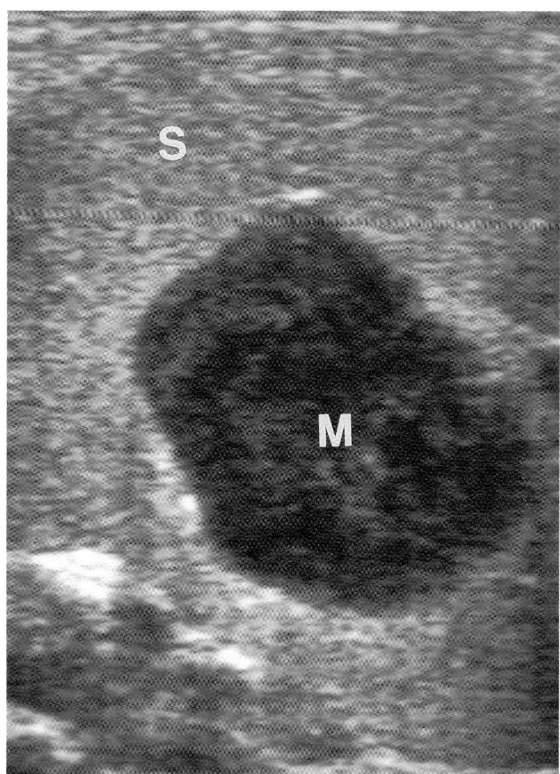

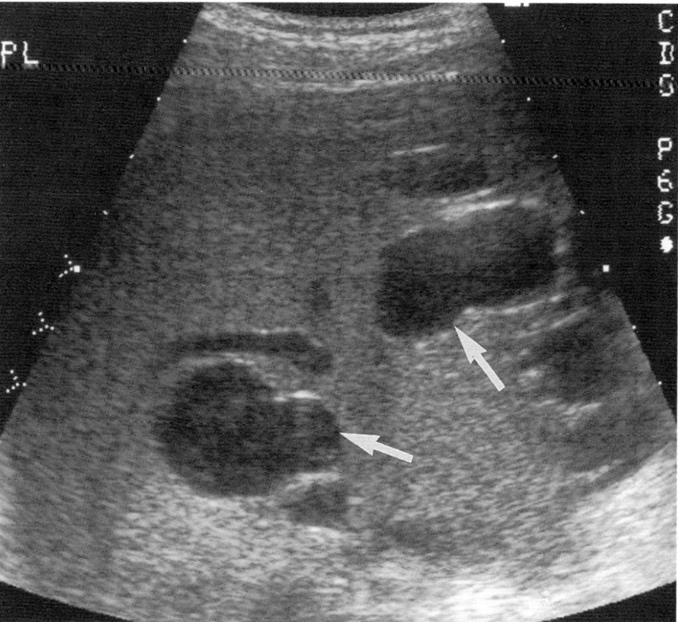

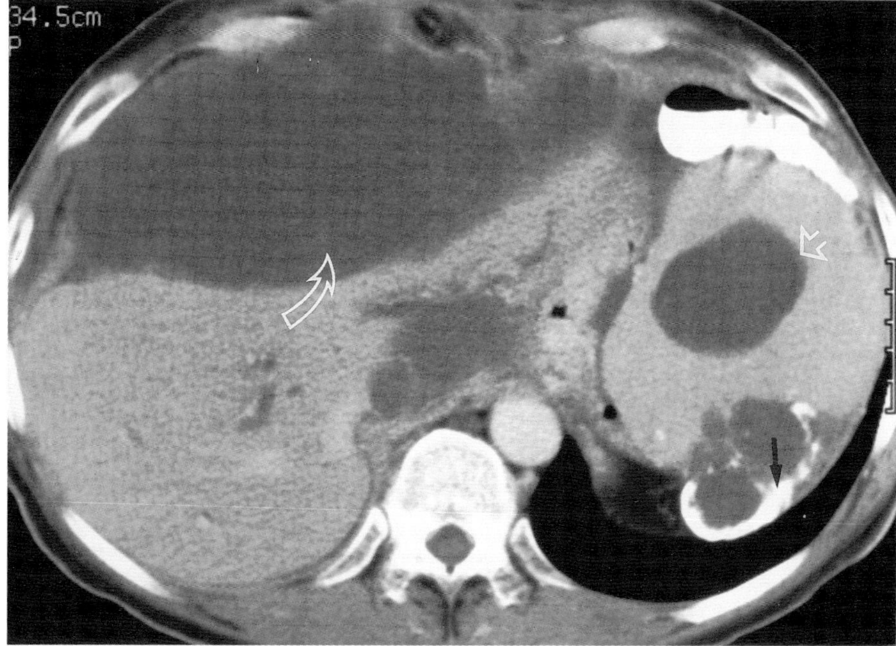

FIG. 6.8. Cystic splenic metastases in two patients. **A:** Transverse scan of spleen (S) demonstrates cystic metastasis (M) from ovarian carcinoma. **B:** In another patient, sagittal scan demonstrates multiple cystic metastases (*arrows*) from appendiceal carcinoma. **C:** CT scan confirms cystic metastases (*open arrow*) and areas of calcification (*black arrow*). Note peritoneal metastases adjacent to liver from pseudomyxoma peritonei (*curved arrow*).

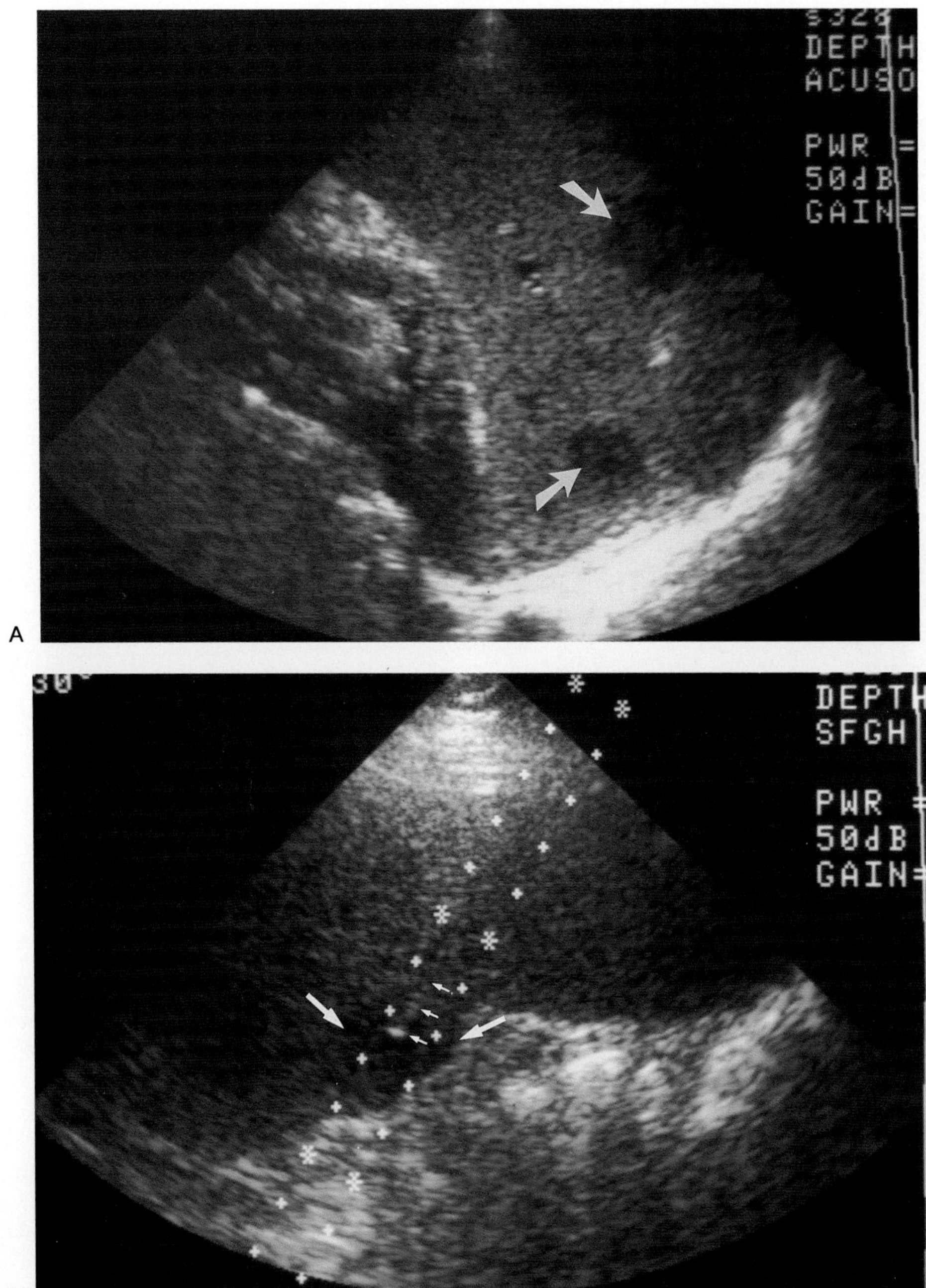

FIG. 6.9. Successful percutaneous biopsy of AIDS-related splenic lymphoma. **A:** Transverse scan of spleen demonstrates multiple hypoechoic nodules (*arrows*). **B:** Scan during biopsy with 22-gauge needle (*short arrows*). *Long arrows* indicate the lesion. Cytologic aspirate revealed immunoblastic lymphoma.

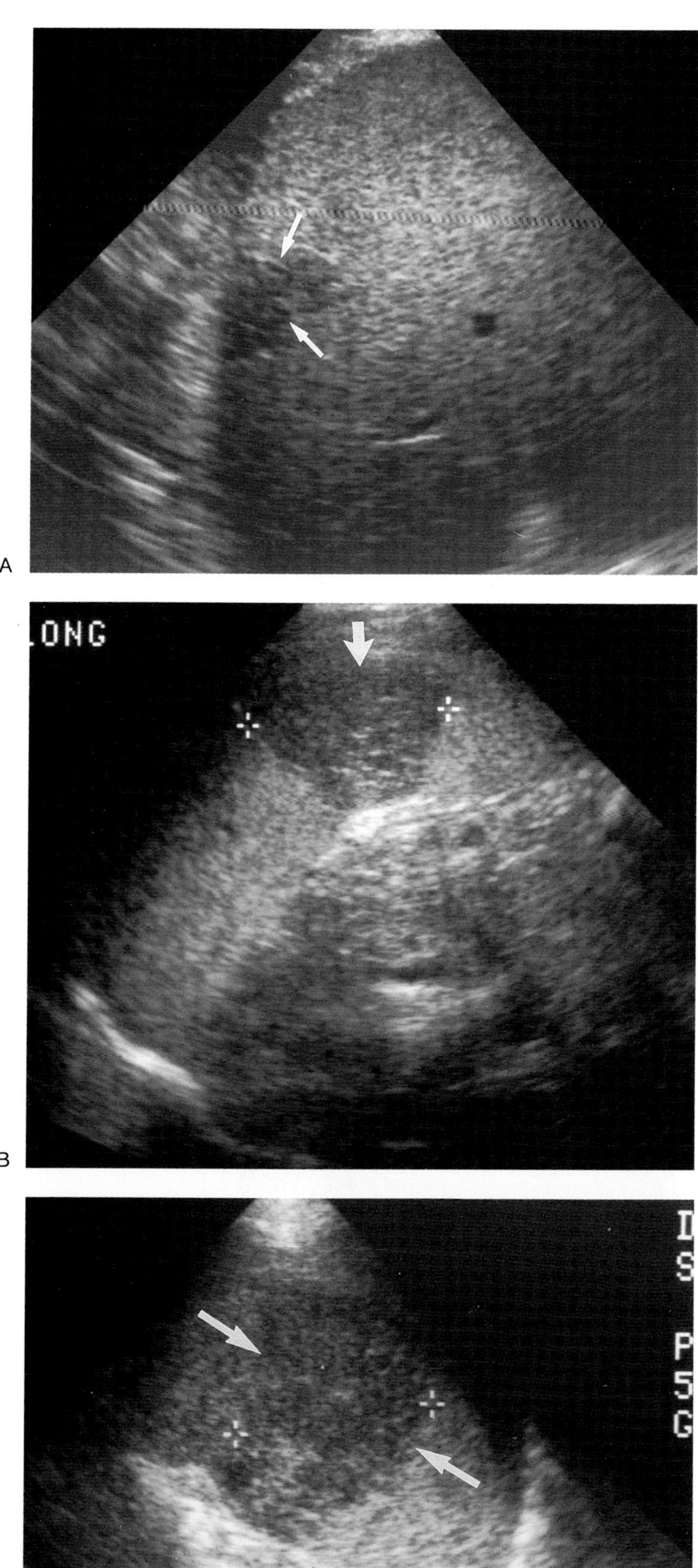

FIG. 6.10. Hypoechoic splenic infarcts in three patients. Note peripheral wedge-shaped infarcts (*arrows*) in all three patients.

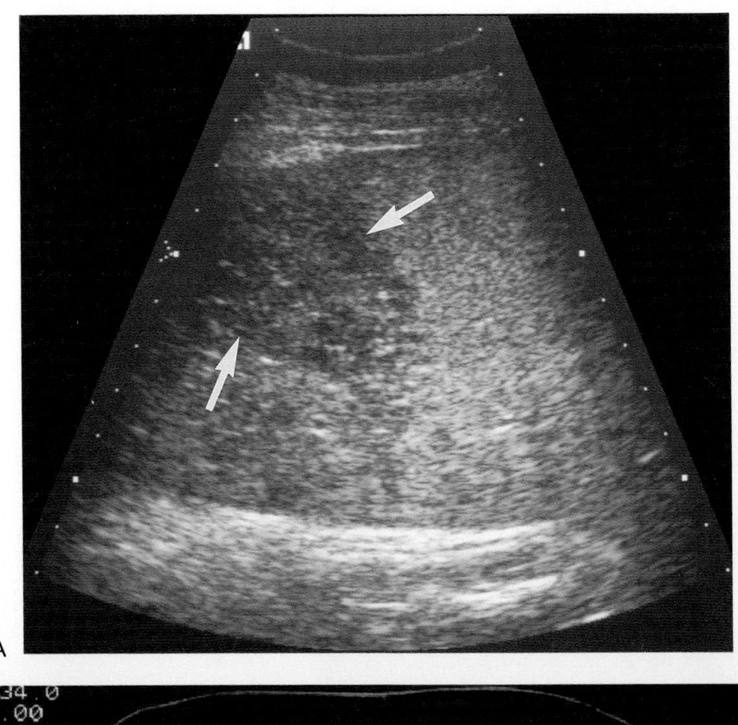

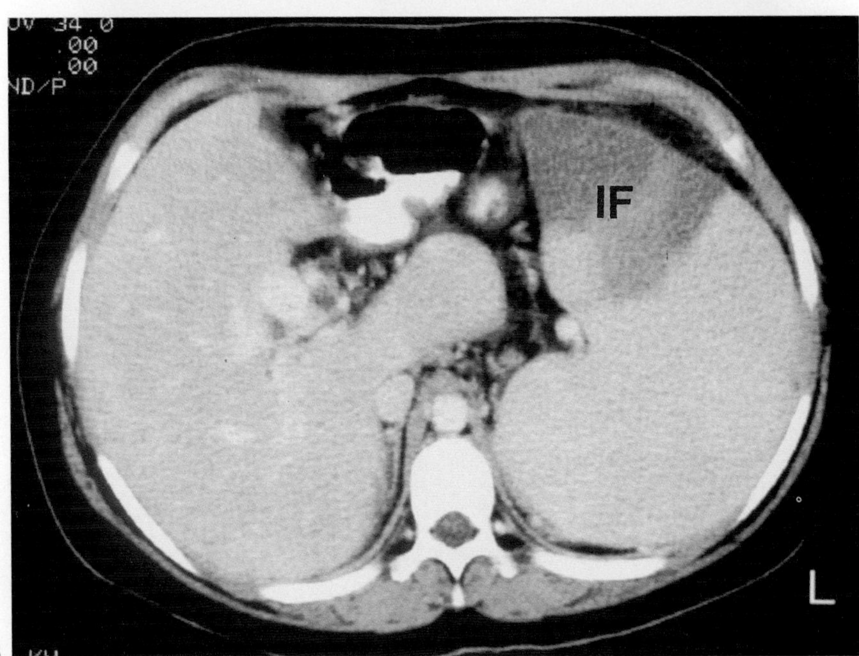

FIG. 6.11. Sonogram and CT scan of splenic infarction. **A:** Sagittal scan of spleen demonstrates typical hypoechoic infarct (*arrows*). **B:** CT scan confirms low-density infarct (IF).

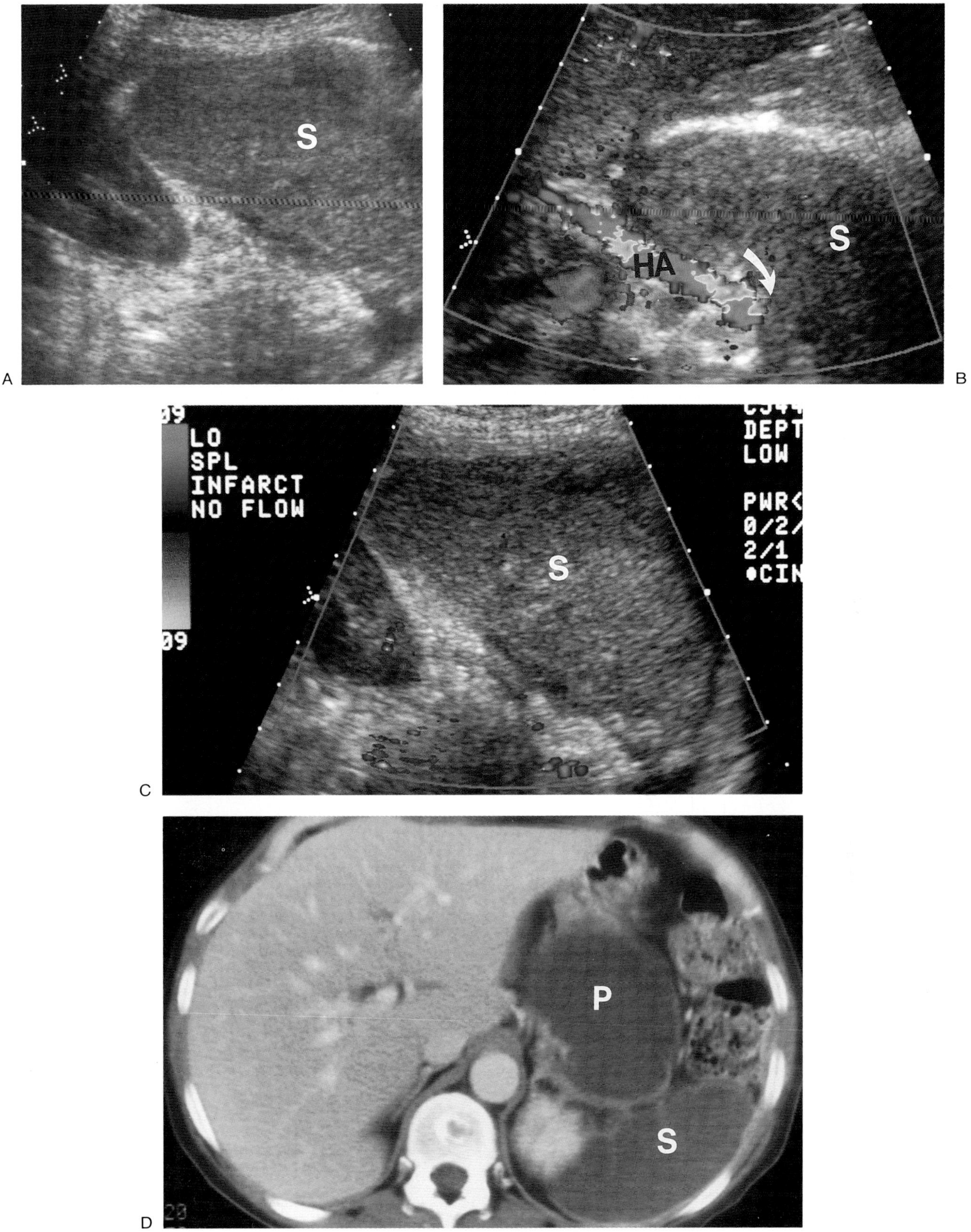

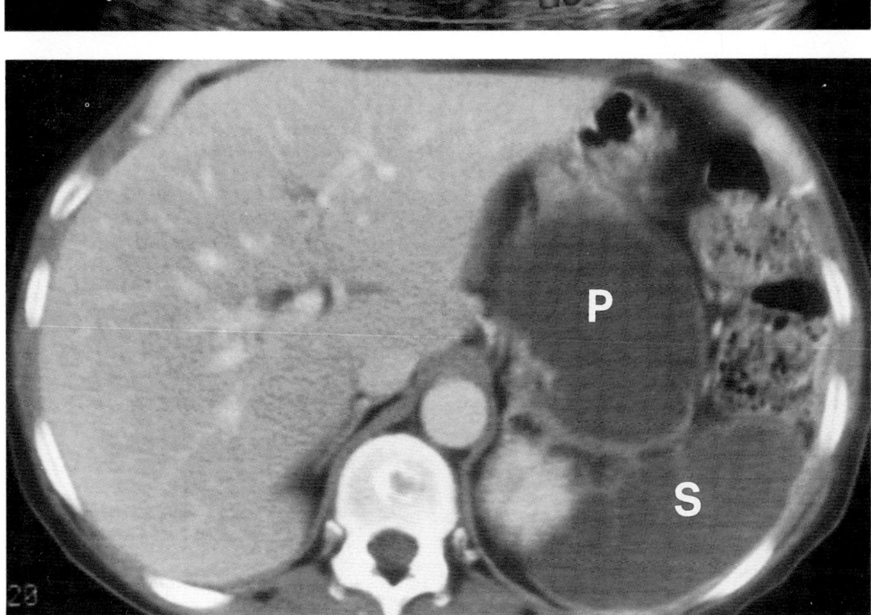

FIG. 6.12. Total splenic infarction in patient with pancreatitis and proximal splenic artery occlusion. **A:** Transverse scan of spleen (S) demonstrates relatively normal grayscale appearance. **B:** Color Doppler sonogram of celiac axis demonstrates patent hepatic artery (HA) and occlusion of splenic artery (*curved arrow*) at its origin. S, spleen. **C:** Color Doppler sonogram of spleen demonstrates complete lack of flow within spleen (S). **D:** Contrast CT scan confirms global splenic (S) infarction. Note extensive pancreatic (P) necrosis.

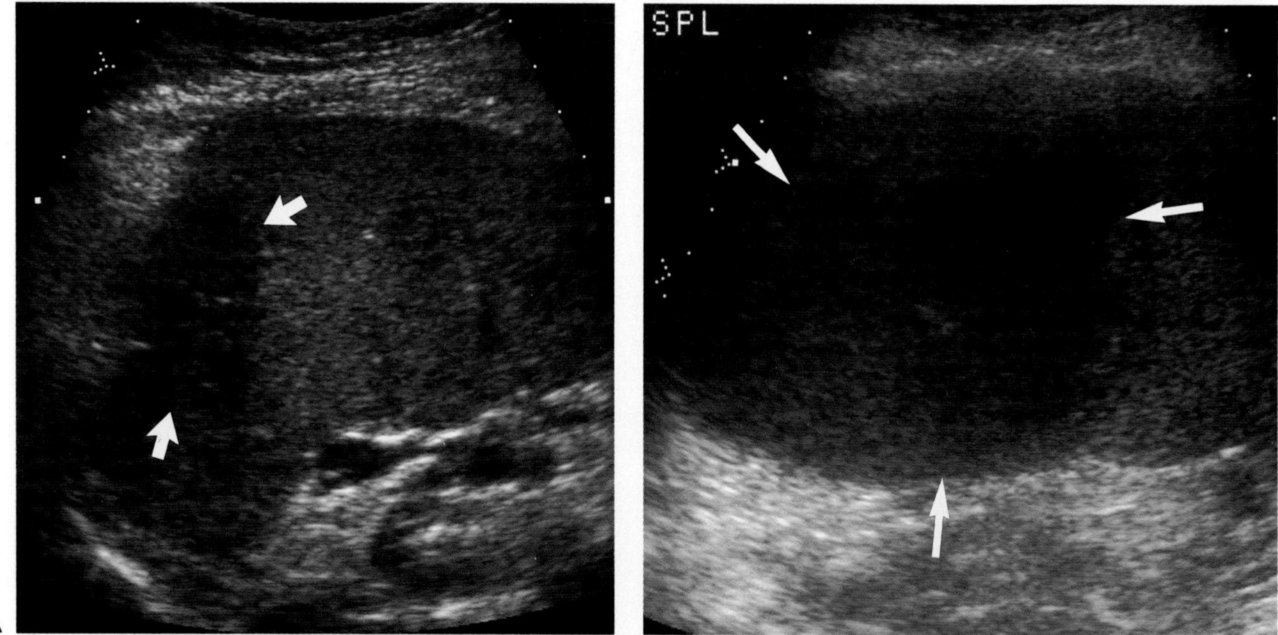

FIG. 6.13. Hemorrhage into splenic infarct. **A:** Note typical wedge-shaped hypoechoic infarct (*arrows*). **B:** One week later infarct is now much larger and rounded in configuration (*arrows*). Splenectomy revealed large hemorrhagic infarct.

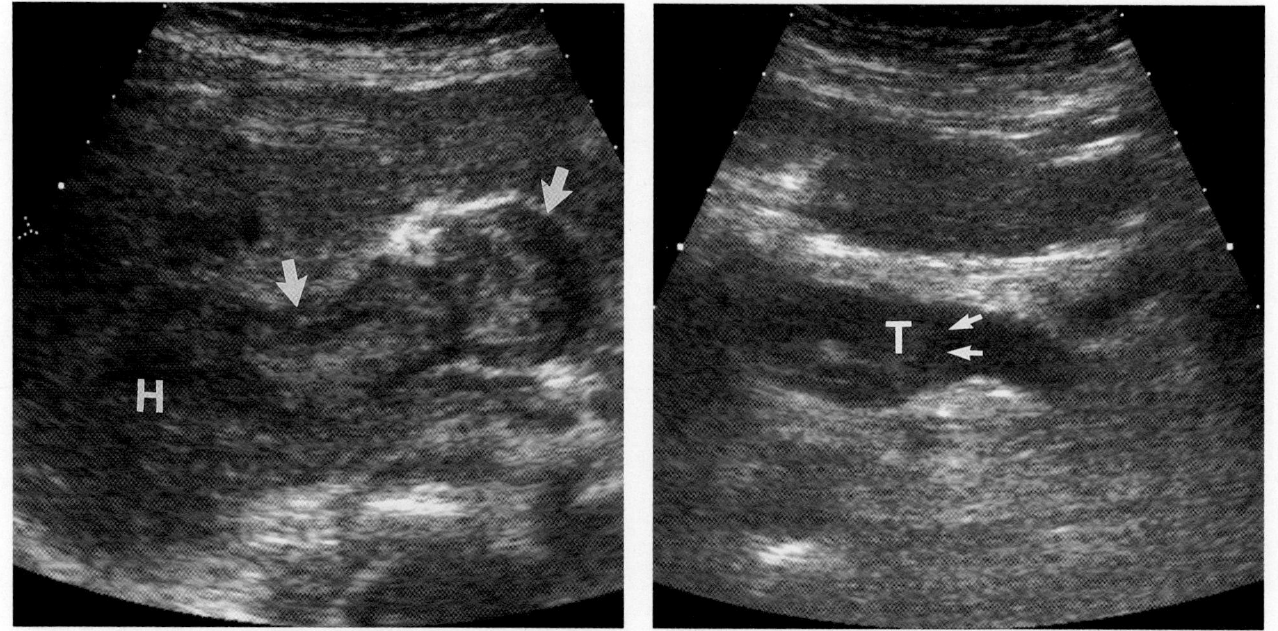

FIG. 6.14. Tumor thrombus from hepatocellular carcinoma extending into splenic vein. **A:** Transverse scan of right lobe of the liver demonstrates hepatoma (H) with tumor thrombus invading portal vein (*arrows*). **B:** Tumor thrombus (T) extends into splenic vein (*arrows*).

within a segmental infarction may at times mimic the appearance of an abscess. Either a noncontrast CT scan (to confirm a high-density hematoma) or fine needle aspiration may be required for definitive diagnosis.

SPLENIC VEIN THROMBOSIS

A broad spectrum of disorders may result in splenic vein thrombosis including pancreatitis and hypercoagulable states such a polycythemia vera or antithrombin-3 deficiency. Of 144 patients with splenic vein thrombosis reported by Moosa and Gadd (15), 56 percent were due to pancreatitis. Portal vein thrombus may occasionally extend into the splenic vein in patients with hepatocellular carcinoma (Fig. 6.14) or pyelophlebitis (Fig. 6.15).

Splenic vein thrombosis may cause no clinical symptoms. However, some patients with gastric varices present with acute gastrointestinal hemorrhage. Rarely, intramural hemorrhage may occur in the stomach from rupture of a gastric varix (Fig. 6.16). Splenomegaly is a common clinical finding in patients with isolated splenic vein occlusion but is not invariably present (16).

Contrast CT and color Doppler sonography have largely supplanted angiography in the diagnosis of splenic vein thrombosis (17). CT can more reliably demonstrate short gastric and gastroepiploic varices that are often important secondary clues to the presence of splenic vein occlusion (18). Acute splenic vein thrombus may be hypoechoic and difficult to detect without the use of color or spectral Doppler sonography (Fig. 6.17). Neoplastic invasion may result in marked distention of the splenic vein. Color Doppler sonography may reveal intrinsic neovascularity within the tumor thrombus (Fig. 6.18).

SPLENIC ARTERY ANEURYSMS AND PSEUDOANEURYSMS

Aneurysms of the splenic artery are the most common of all visceral aneurysms. The distal splenic artery near the splenic hilum is the most common anatomic site (19). Unless quite large (greater than 2 cm), splenic aneurysms are often an incidental finding of little clinical significance. Rarely, splenic aneurysms may rupture into the peritoneal cavity, pancreatic duct, or adjacent bowel (20,21). Splenic artery aneurysms are more prevalent in women and are most often due to atherosclerosis. Acoustic shadowing from calcification is common with atherosclerotic aneurysms. Sonographically, noncalcified splenic artery aneurysms may appear as rounded sonolucent "masses." Because of their cystic appearance, they can be mistaken for a pancreatic pseudocyst or other fluid collection (Fig. 6.19). As with all "cystic" abdominal masses, both color and spectral Doppler sonography are essential in order to avoid misdiagnosis of a pseudoaneurysm.

Splenic artery pseudoaneurysms may result in life-threatening hemorrhage and require either urgent angiographic embolization or splenectomy. Pancreatitis is the most common etiology. Enzymatic autolysis causes direct injury to the arterial wall. A splenic artery pseudoaneurysm should always be kept in mind in patients with pancreatitis and peripancreatic hemorrhagic fluid collections on CT scan or sonogram (22). Preliminary noncontrast CT is particularly helpful in confirming acute hemorrhage from rupture of a pseudoaneurysm. Attenuation values of an acute hematoma are generally greater than 30 HU. When technically feasible, angiographic embolization is the treatment of choice for splenic artery pseudoaneurysms (23).

SPLENIC ABSCESSES

Increasing numbers of immunosuppressed patients have altered the epidemiology and microbiology of splenic abscesses (24,25). In urban centers, fungal or mycobacterial splenic microabscesses are significantly more common than pyogenic abscesses. Pyogenic splenic abscesses are often due to hematogenous dissemination of septic emboli from endocarditis (24). Many causes of splenomegaly also predispose to pyogenic abscess formation including typhoid fever, sickle cell disease, and malaria. Post-traumatic splenic hematomas may also become secondarily infected in patients with bacteremia.

The clinical symptoms of splenic abscesses are generally nonspecific. Patients typically present with pleuritic and/or left upper quadrant abdominal pain. Most patients have systemic signs of infection with fever and leukocytosis (24,25). Although sonography and CT are sensitive for the detection of pyogenic splenic abscesses, the appearance is often nonspecific. Pyogenic abscesses are most often hypoechoic. The appearance may mimic a neoplasm such as lymphoma. Splenic abscesses may have relatively little enhanced through sound transmission and may mimic a "solid" lesion (Fig. 6.20). Gas within a splenic abscess is uncommon but may cause high-amplitude echoes with reverberation artifacts or diffuse shadowing.

Splenic microabscesses due to fungal infection typically have either a target or bull's eye appearance with an echogenic center surrounded by a hypoechoic rim (Fig. 6.21). Microabscesses may, however, appear sonographically as hypoechoic "nodules" indistinguishable from lymphoma (Fig. 6.21). Larger abscesses may demonstrate a more complex cystic appearance (Fig. 6.22).

Splenic calcifications are a common sequela of granulomatous infection, typically from histoplasmosis. In patients with acquired immunodeficiency syndrome (AIDS), punctate echogenic areas seen throughout the

(text continues on page 378)

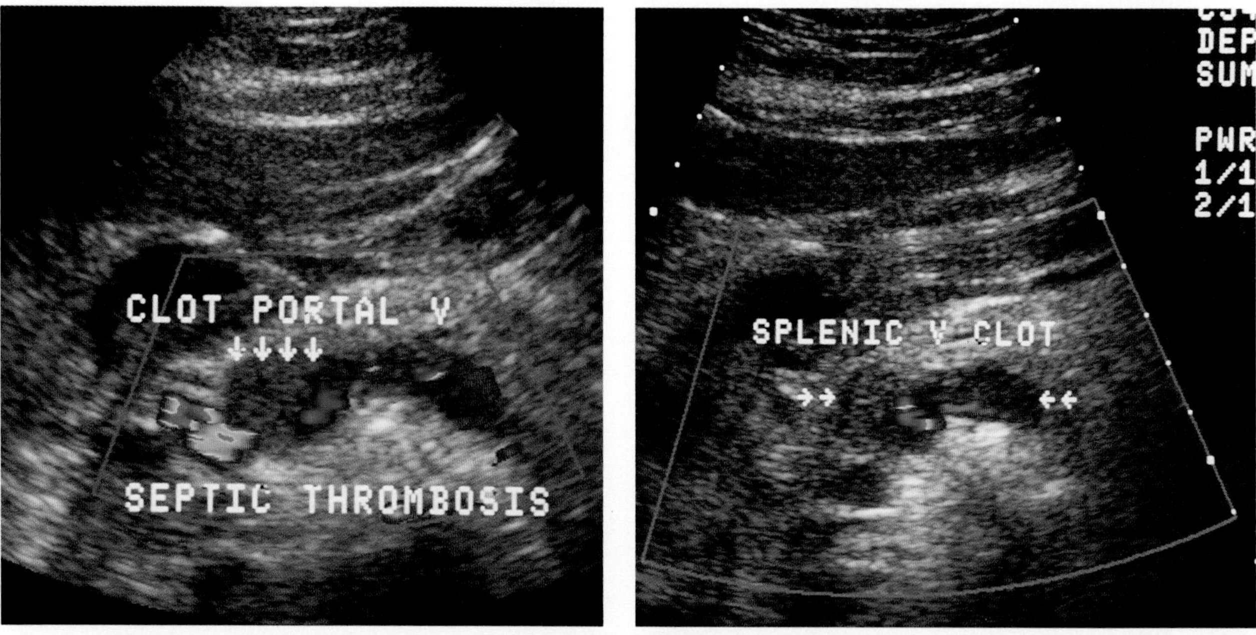

FIG. 6.15. Pyelophlebitis with septic thrombosis of splenic vein. Patient presented with bacteroides septicemia following laparoscopic cholecystectomy. **A:** Color Doppler sonogram demonstrates clot in portal vein (*arrows*). **B:** Note extension of thrombus into splenic vein (*arrows*).

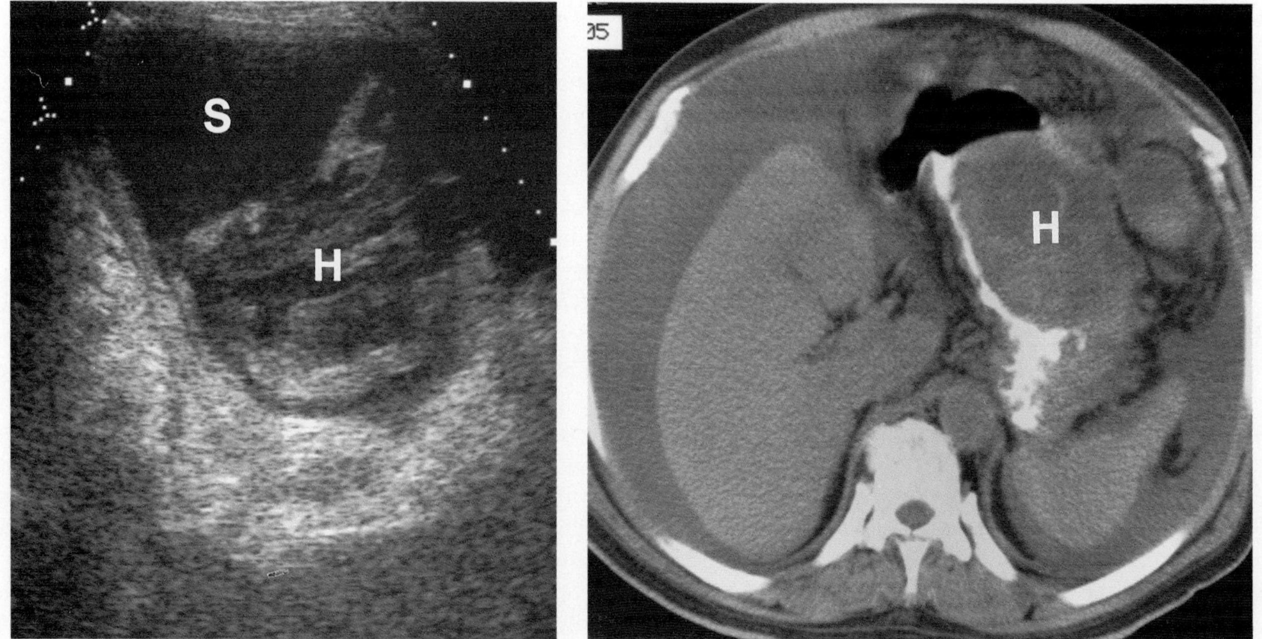

FIG. 6.16. Intramural hematoma of the stomach following rupture of gastric varix. Patient had pancreatic carcinoma with splenic vein occlusion and gastric varices. **A:** Transverse scan of the stomach (S) demonstrates echogenic intramural hematoma (H). **B:** CT scan confirms intramural hematoma of the stomach (H).

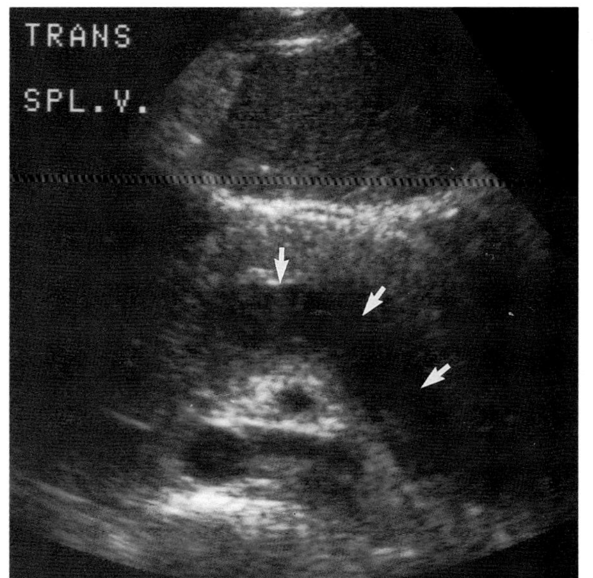

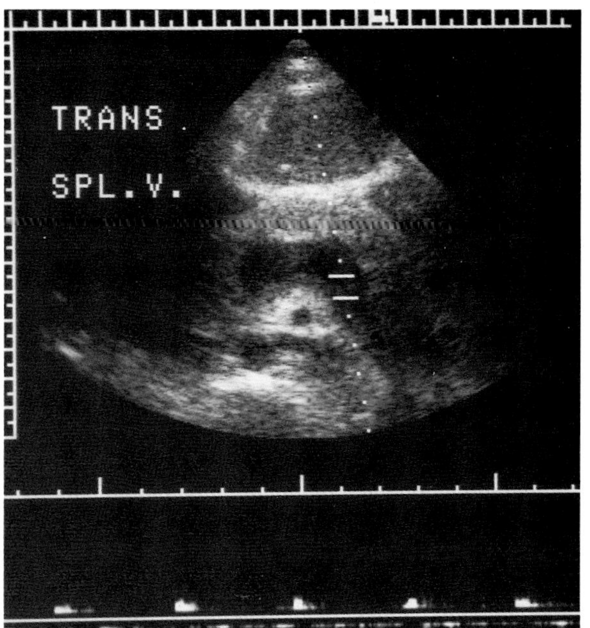

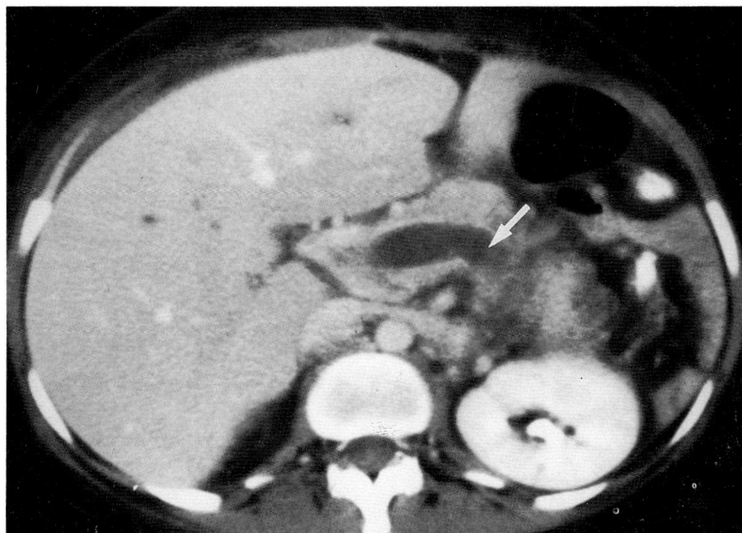

FIG. 6.17. Acute splenic vein thrombosis with anechoic thrombus. **A:** Transverse scan demonstrates anechoic splenic vein thrombus (*arrows*). **B:** Spectral Doppler sonogram confirms lack of flow within thrombosed splenic vein. **C:** Contrast CT scan reveals low-attenuation acute thrombus (*arrow*) within splenic vein. (Case courtesy of E. Meredith James, MD, Rochester, MN.)

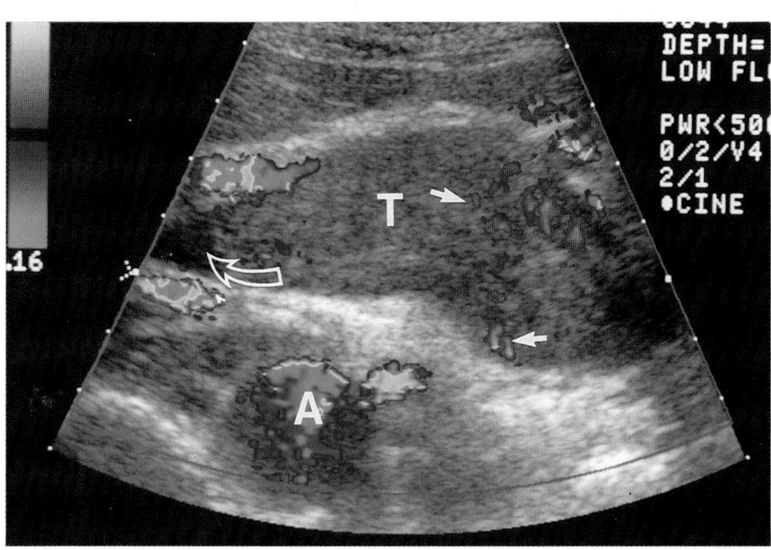

FIG. 6.18. Splenic vein tumor thrombus demonstrated by color Doppler sonography. Transverse scan reveals marked distention of splenic vein by tumor thrombus (T) from recurrent islet cell tumor of pancreas. Note neovascularity within tumor thrombus on color Doppler sonogram (*short arrows*). *Curved arrow,* portal vein; A, aorta.

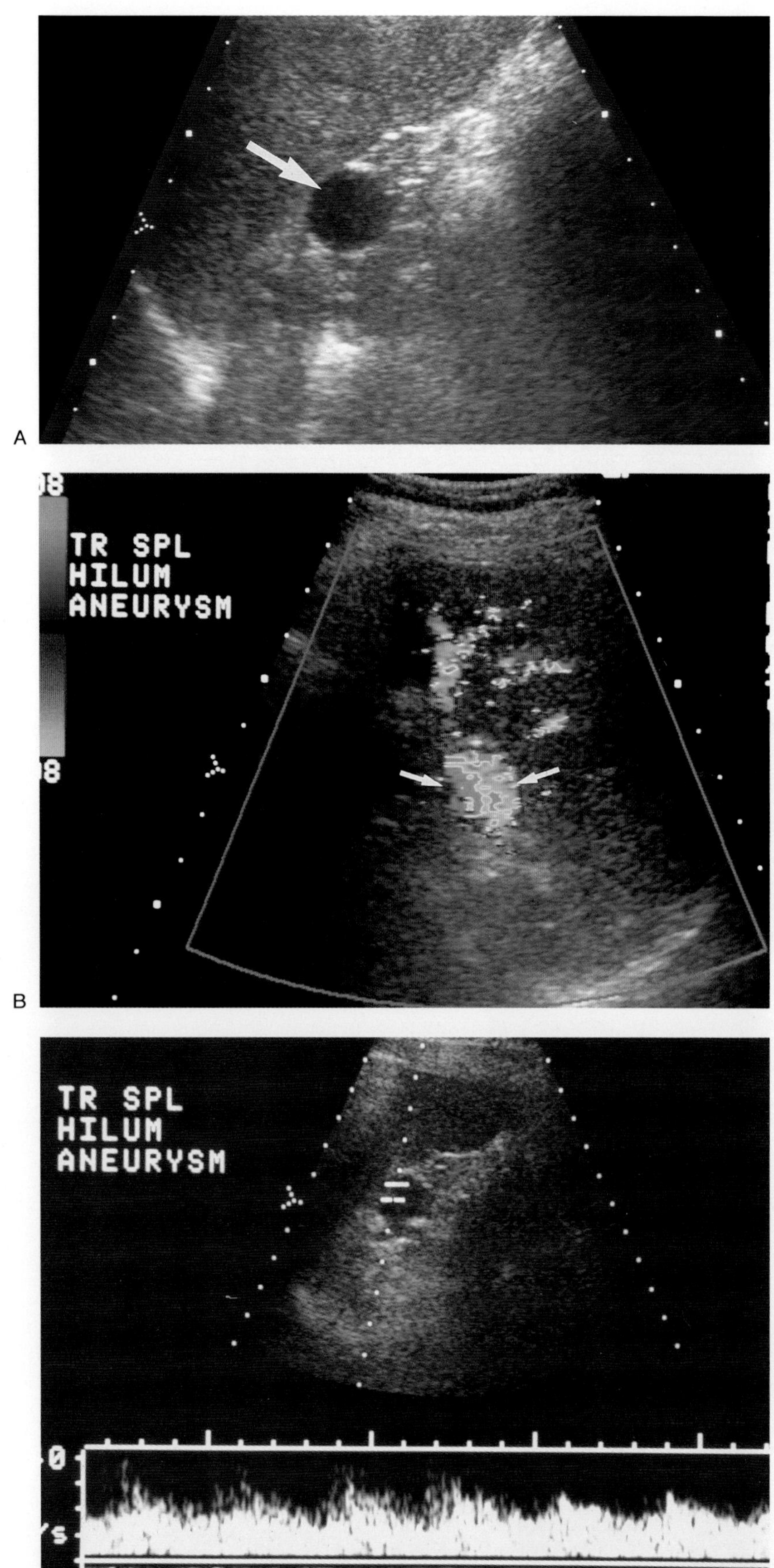

FIG. 6.19. Splenic artery aneurysm. **A:** Sagittal grayscale image of splenic hilum demonstrates "cystic" mass (*arrow*). **B:** Color Doppler sonogram confirms splenic artery aneurysm (*arrows*). **C:** Spectral tracing demonstrates arterial flow within aneurysm.

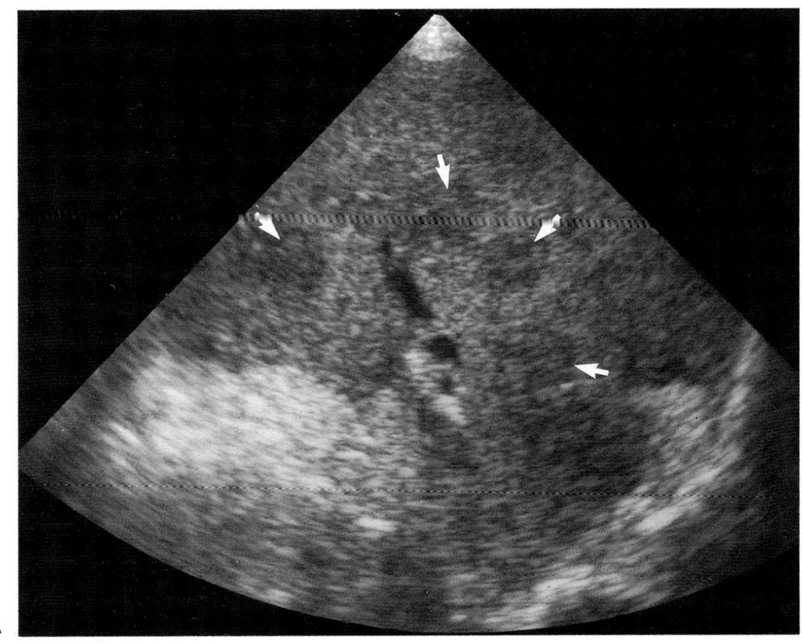
A

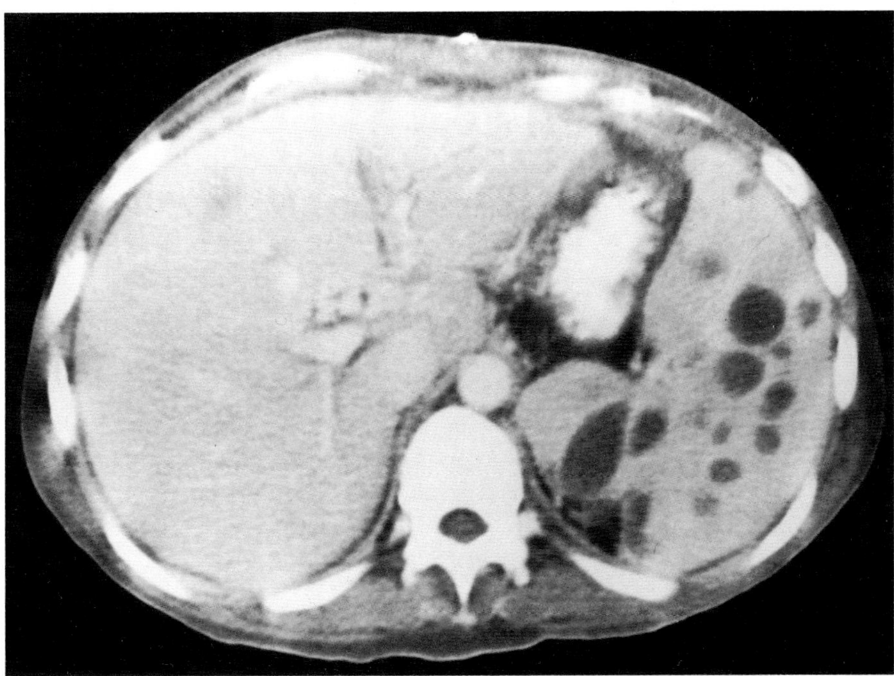
B

FIG. 6.20. Tuberculous microabscesses appearing as "solid" sonographic lesions. **A:** Transverse scan of the spleen demonstrates multiple, nearly isoechoic, splenic lesions (*arrows*). The appearance is similar to lymphoma or metastases. **B:** Contrast CT scan of spleen reveals multiple low-density tuberculous microabscesses.

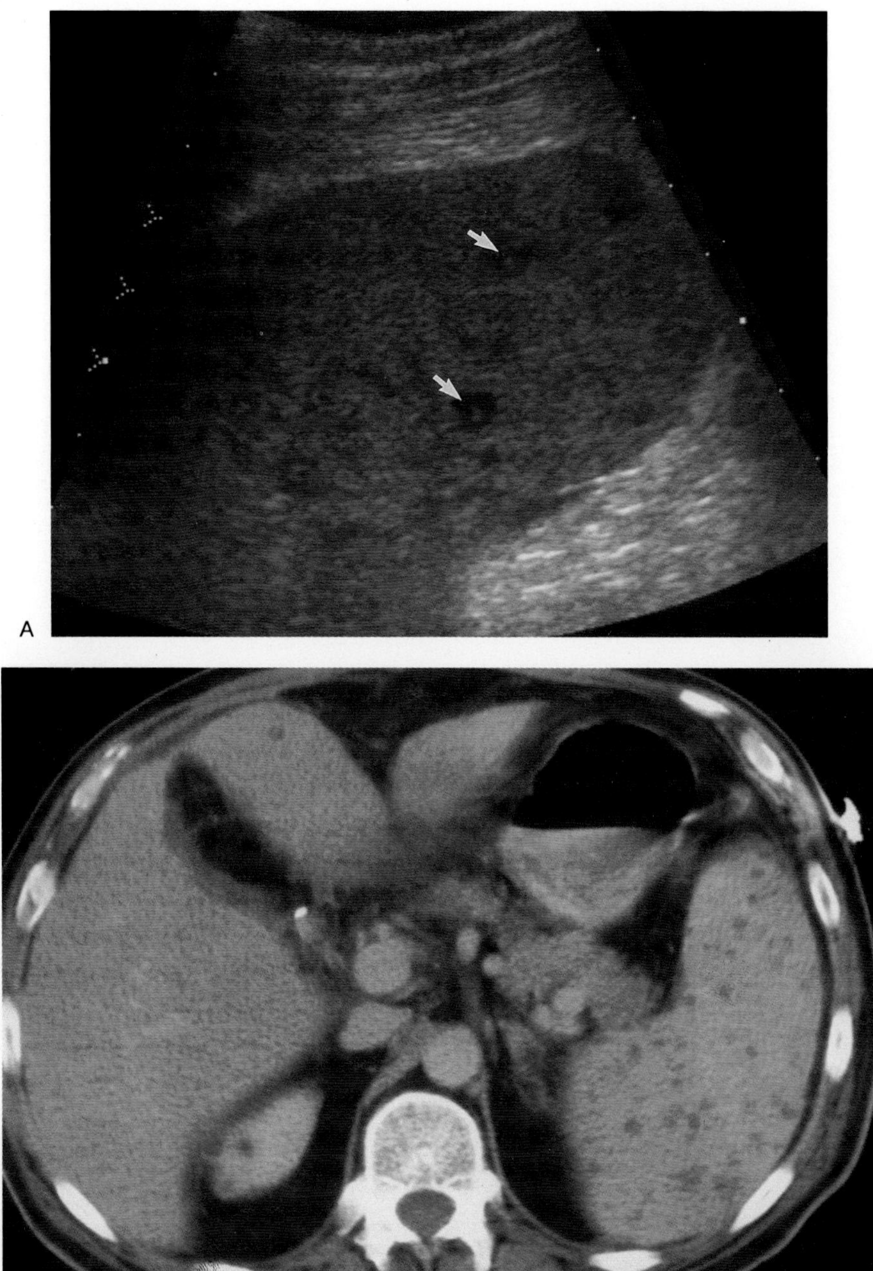

FIG. 6.21. Fungal microabscesses in leukemic patient. **A:** Sagittal scan of spleen demonstrates typical target lesions of fungal microabscesses. **B:** Contrast CT scan confirms multiple microabscesses.

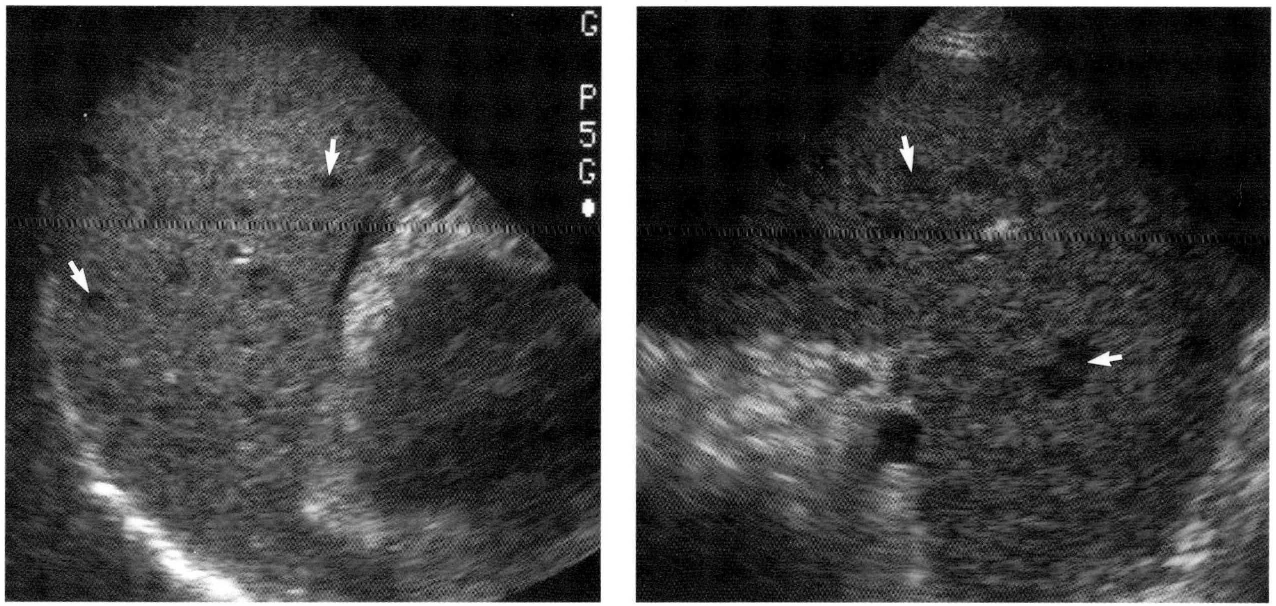

FIG. 6.22. Tuberculous microabscesses in patient with AIDS. **A, B:** Note numerous hypoechoic abscesses (*arrows*) throughout the spleen.

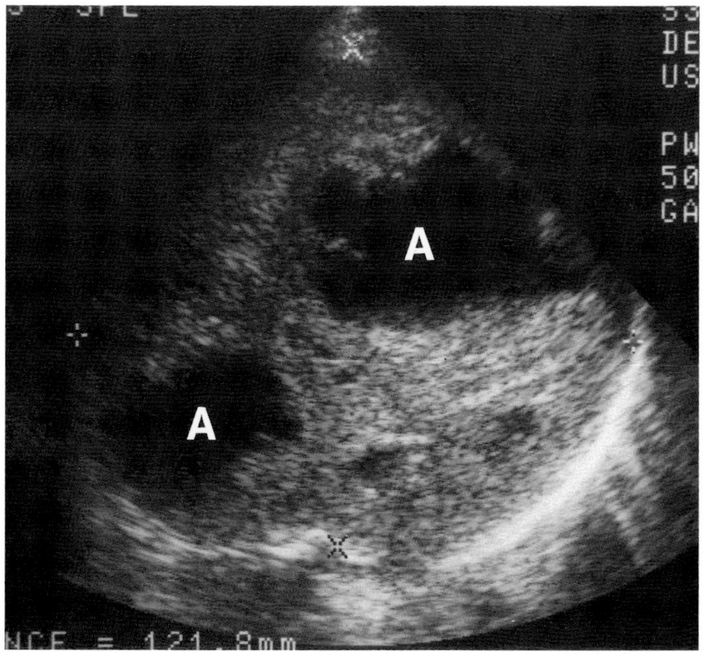

FIG. 6.23. Splenic abscesses due to *Pneumocystis carinii* in patient with AIDS. Note cystic appearances of abscesses (A).

spleen may also be due to calcifications from *Pneumocystis carinii* infection (Fig. 6.23) (26).

SPLENIC TRAUMA

CT is generally the imaging method of choice to evaluate patients with blunt abdominal trauma and possible splenic injury. Sonography, on occasion, may be helpful in patients who cannot undergo CT (27–29). Immediately after injury, acute intraparenchymal splenic lacerations are typically echogenic. Subacute hematomas are often hypoechoic. Residual areas of clot are echogenic (Fig. 6.24) (27). Subcapsular hematomas characteristically compress the lateral contour of the spleen (Fig. 6.25). With splenic capsular disruption, hemoperitoneum may be noted in the left paracolic gutter, pelvis, and/or upper abdomen. Intermittent hemorrhage may result in layers of echogenic clot adjacent to the spleen (Fig. 6.26). In patients treated nonoperatively, serial sonograms of the spleen may be useful to document interval resolution or to exclude ongoing hemorrhage. Following healing of splenic injuries, the spleen may appear sonographically normal or there may be an echogenic area of fibrosis. In some patients, focal post-traumatic pseudocysts persist for months or years (Fig. 6.27).

SPLENIC CYSTS

A variety of cystic lesions may involve the spleen. These include congenital or epidermoid cysts, post-traumatic cysts, cystic neoplasms, intrasplenic pancreatic pseudocysts, and parasitic cysts. Dachman et al. (30) reviewed 52 patients with splenic cysts including 24 congenital or epidermoid cysts and 28 post-traumatic cysts. Clinical symptoms were nonspecific, most often related to epigastric fullness or mass effect on adjacent organs (30). Acute pain was rare and was most often due to cyst rupture or superinfection (30).

Congenital cysts of the spleen are lined with epithelium. Sonographically, cysts are discrete sonolucent masses with enhanced through sound transmission. On occasion, low-level echoes may be noted in congenital cysts due to cholesterol crystals (Fig. 6.28). Although rare, congenital cysts may spontaneously rupture (31). Post-traumatic cysts do not have a true epithelial lining and most often represent areas of liquefied hematoma. Low-level echoes may be present due to breakdown of blood products within a hemorrhagic splenic cyst (Figs. 6.29 and 6.30). Patients with pancreatitis may develop intrasplenic pancreatic pseudocysts. Collections of pancreatic juice, proteolytic enzymes, and edema fluid extend from the tail of the pancreas directly into the splenic parenchyma via the splenorenal ligament.

Primary cystic neoplasms of the spleen are rare and include cystic hemangiomas and lymphangiomas. Cystic metastases to the spleen are more common than primary cystic tumors (Fig. 6.8). Unlike other cystic lesions that involve the spleen, cystic metastases often have a thick, irregular wall with mural nodules and septations. Ovarian carcinoma, melanoma, and sarcomas may cause cystic splenic metastases. Sonographically guided fine-needle aspiration biopsy of the periphery of the lesion is often the most effective way to establish the diagnosis of a cystic metastases.

Parasitic cysts may involve the spleen and are generally secondary to *Echinococcus granulosus* (32). Similar to hydatid cysts in the liver, there may be a dominant cyst with surrounding smaller daughter cysts as well as mural calcification. Other sonographic features include low-level echoes representing hydatid "sand" and multiple membranes (32). Origin from an edemic area and/or positive serologic tests for *Echinococcus* are essential clues for establishing the diagnosis.

PERISPLENIC NORMAL VARIANTS AND ABNORMALITIES

Masses in the splenic hilum may be due to perisplenic lymph nodes, metastases (Fig. 6.31), varices, or congenital variants, such as an accessory spleen (Fig. 6.32). In addition, aneurysms or pseudoaneurysms of the splenic artery are often located in the splenic hilum. Color Doppler sonography is essential for accurate characterization of splenic vascular abnormalities.

An accessory spleen or splenunculus has a typical sonographic appearance of a mass in the splenic hilus isoechoic to splenic parenchyma. These are extremely common and may occur in as many as 10 percent of the normal patients (33). On occasion, an accessory spleen may mimic a perisplenic nodal mass or a mass in the tail of the pancreas. Accessory spleens larger than 2 cm can be confirmed by sulfur colloid scintigraphy. Another normal variant that could be mistaken for a perisplenic "mass" is a left lobe of the liver that extends anteriorly over the dome of the spleen (Fig. 6.33). Perisplenic varices are common in patients with cirrhosis and portal hypertension. Color Doppler sonography with spectral tracings can readily establish the diagnosis of perisplenic varices (Fig. 6.34).

REFERENCES

1. Frank K, Linhart P, Kortsik C, et al. Sonographic determination of spleen size: normal dimensions in adults with a healthy spleen. *Ultraschall Med* 1986;7(3):134–137.
2. Manor A, Starinsky R, Gorfinkel D, et al. Ultrasound features of a symptomatic splenic hemangioma. *J Clin Ultrasound* 1984;12:94–97.
3. Pakter RL, Fishman EK, Nussbaum A, et al. Computed tomography findings in splenic hemangiomas in the Klippel–Trenaunay–Weber syndrome. *J Comput Assist Tomogr* 1987;11(1):88–91.
4. Moss CN, Van Dyke JA, Koehler RE, et al. Multiple cavernous hemangiomas of the spleen: computed tomography findings. *J Comput Assist Tomogr* 1986;10(2):338–340.

(*text continues on page 388*)

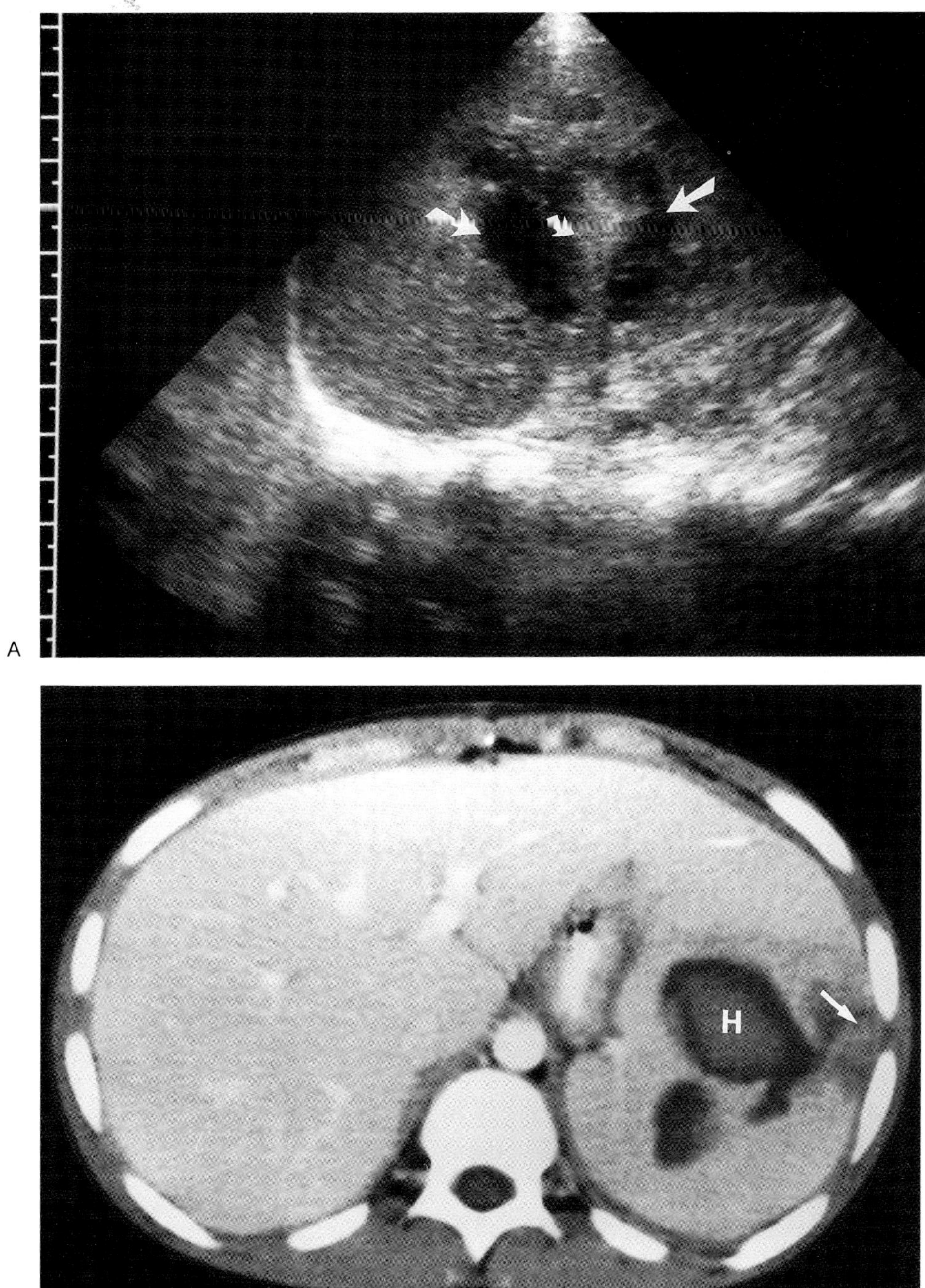

FIG. 6.24. Post-traumatic splenic hematoma. **A:** Patient was scanned 48 h postinjury. Patient underwent laparotomy and was felt to have only superficial laceration of spleen. This sagittal scan of spleen demonstrates intraparenchymal hematoma (*arrows*) with central echogenic clot (*curved arrow*). **B:** CT scan demonstrates central hematoma (H) with extension to splenic capsule (*arrow*).

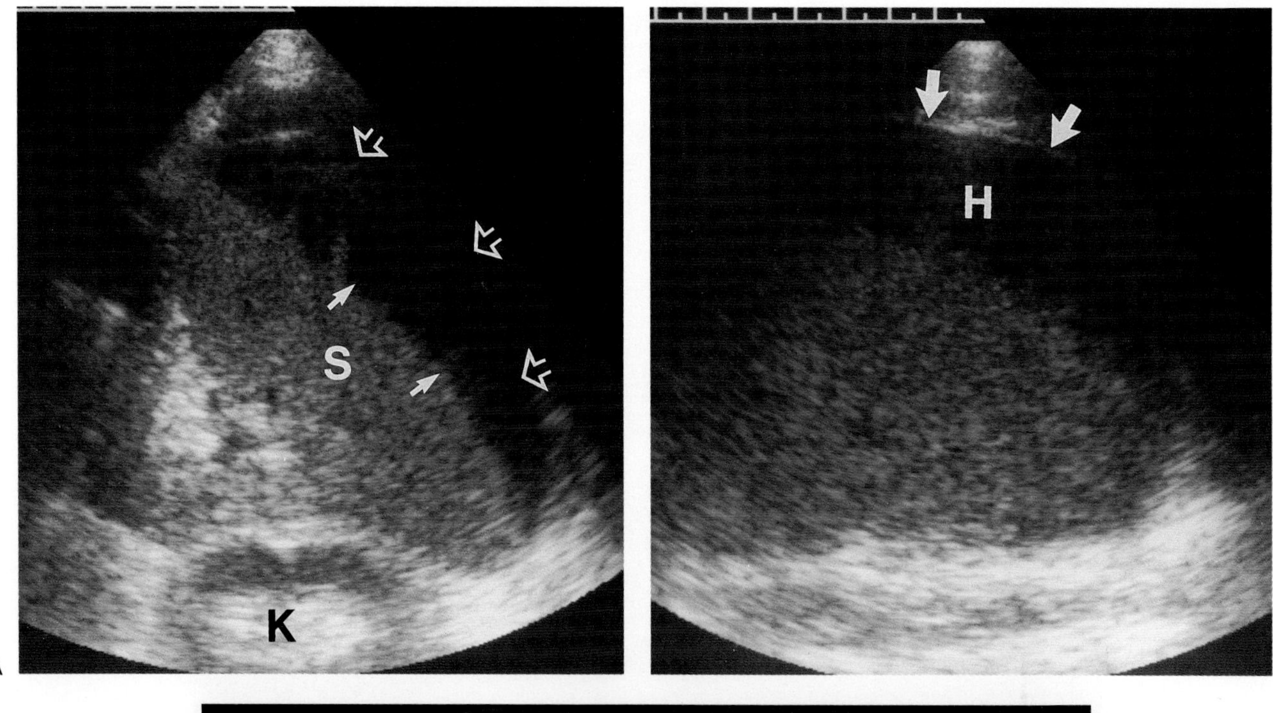

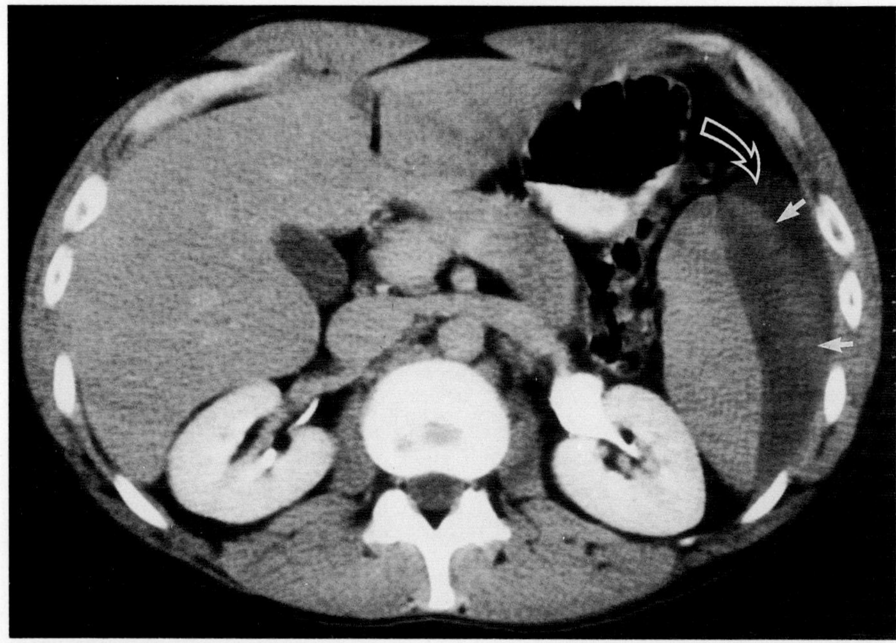

FIG. 6.25. Subcapsular hematoma of spleen. **A:** Note the characteristic flattening of lateral contour (*arrows*) of the spleen (S) by a subcapsular hematoma (*open arrows*). K, left kidney. **B:** Sagittal view of spleen demonstrates splenic capsule (*arrows*) displaced by hematoma (H). **C:** Corresponding contrast CT scan demonstrates subcapsular hematoma (*arrows*) and perisplenic hemoperitoneum (*curved arrow*).

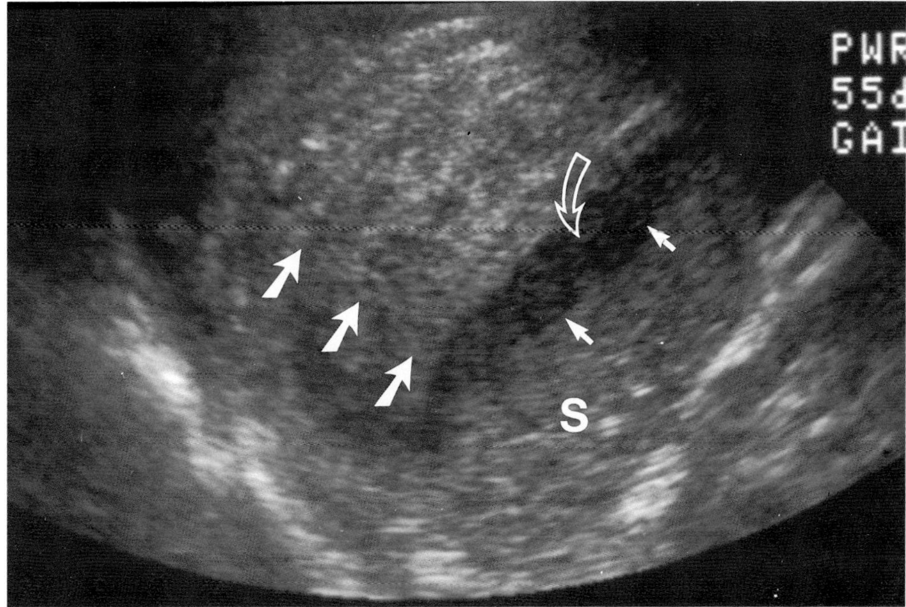

A

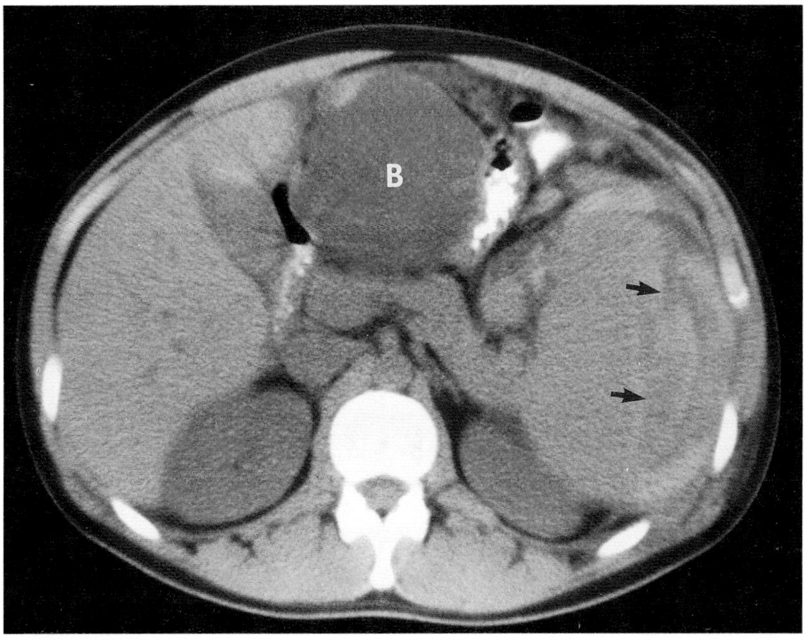

B

FIG. 6.26. Splenic trauma with layered perisplenic clot. **A:** Sagittal scan of spleen (S) demonstrates layers of echogenic clot (*long arrows*) from intermittent hemorrhage. Note hypoechoic subcapsular hematoma flattening contour of spleen (*short arrows*). **B:** Corresponding noncontrast CT scan demonstrates layered subcapsular and perisplenic clot (*arrows*). Note adjacent biloma (B) from hepatic injury.

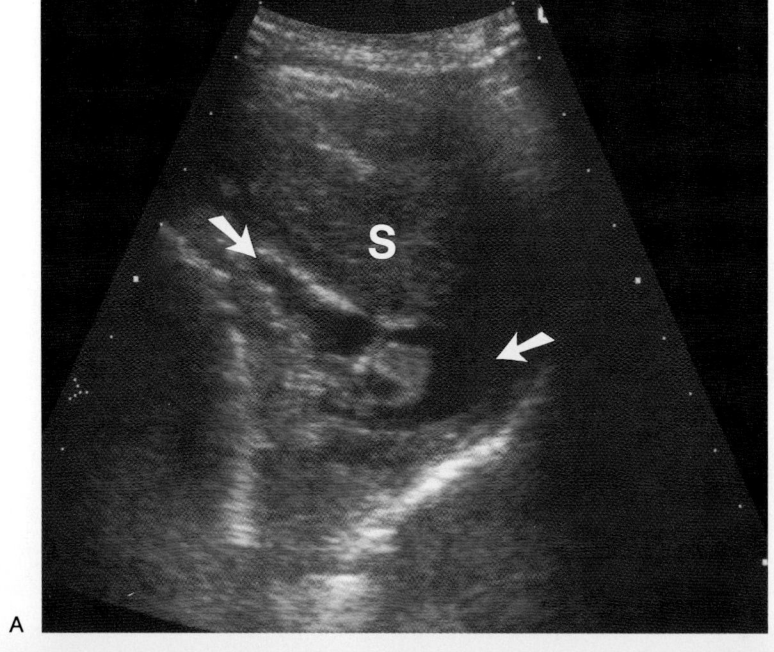

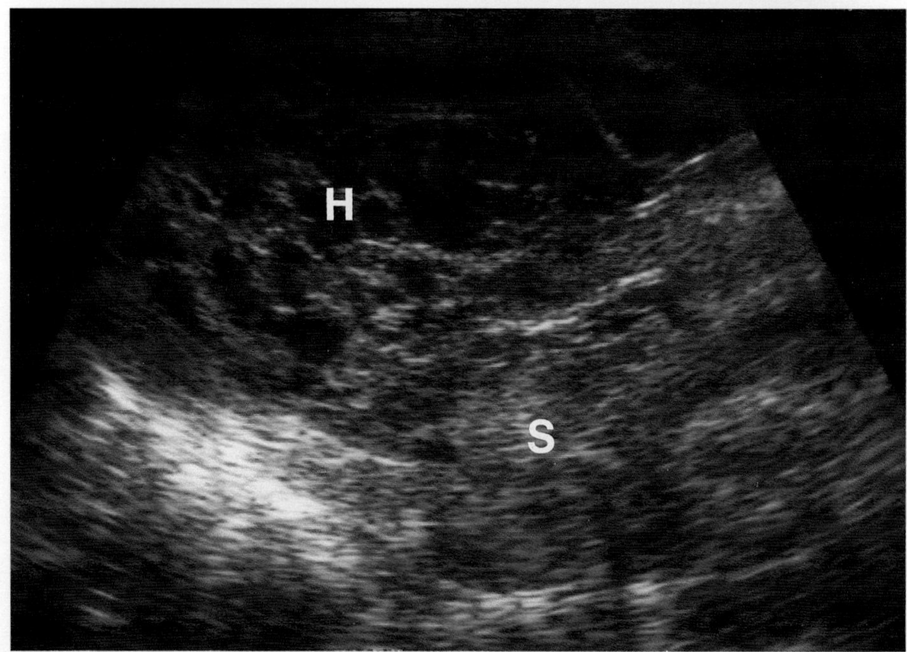

FIG. 6.27. Complications of splenic trauma in two patients. **A:** Note delayed healing of splenic hematoma (*arrows*) 1 month after injury. **B:** In second patient, perisplenic hematoma became infected. Note multisepted hematoma (H) from infection. S, spleen.

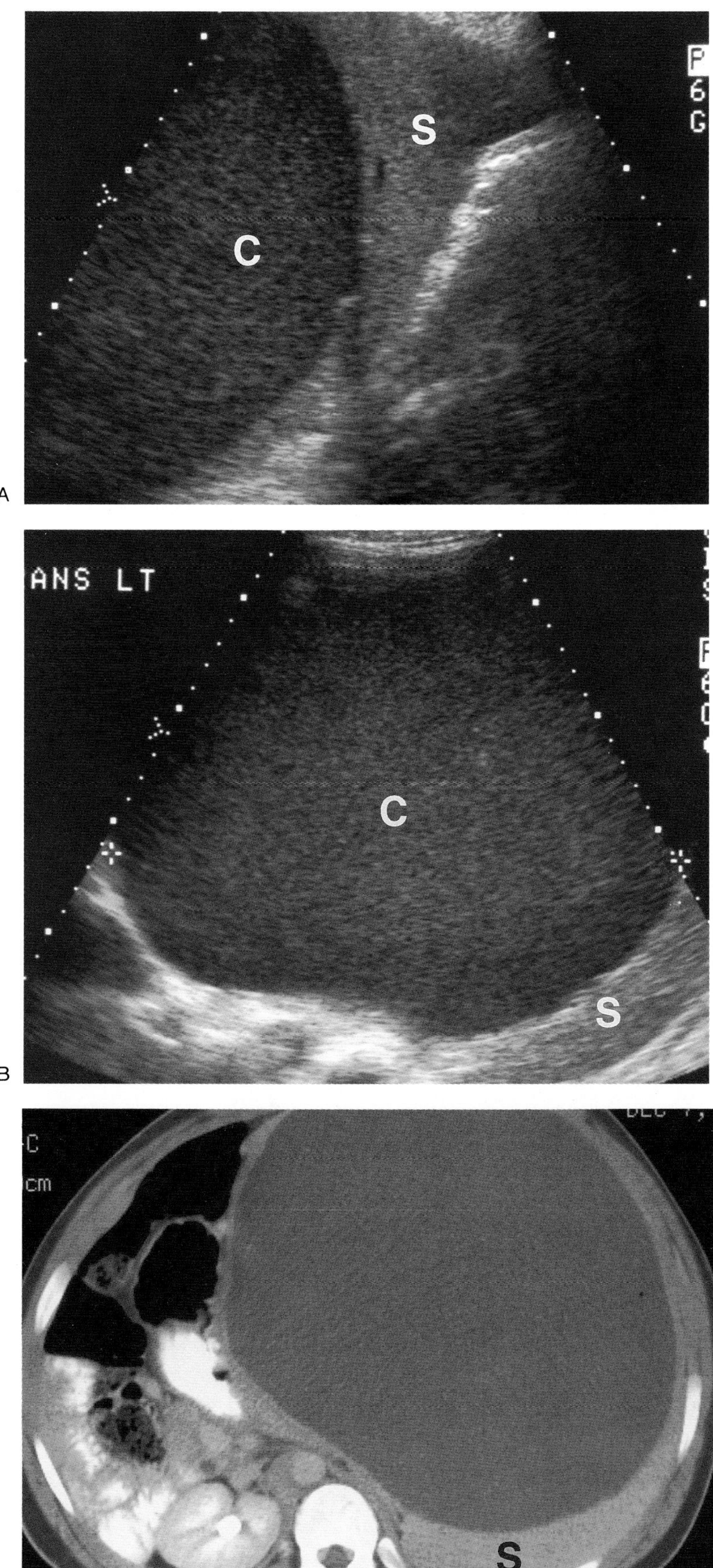

FIG. 6.28. Huge congenital cyst of the spleen. Sagittal (**A**) and transverse (**B**) scans of spleen (S) demonstrate large cystic (C) lesion with diffuse low-level echoes. CT scan (**C**) demonstrates large lesion crossing midline. S, spleen. Surgery revealed congenital cyst.

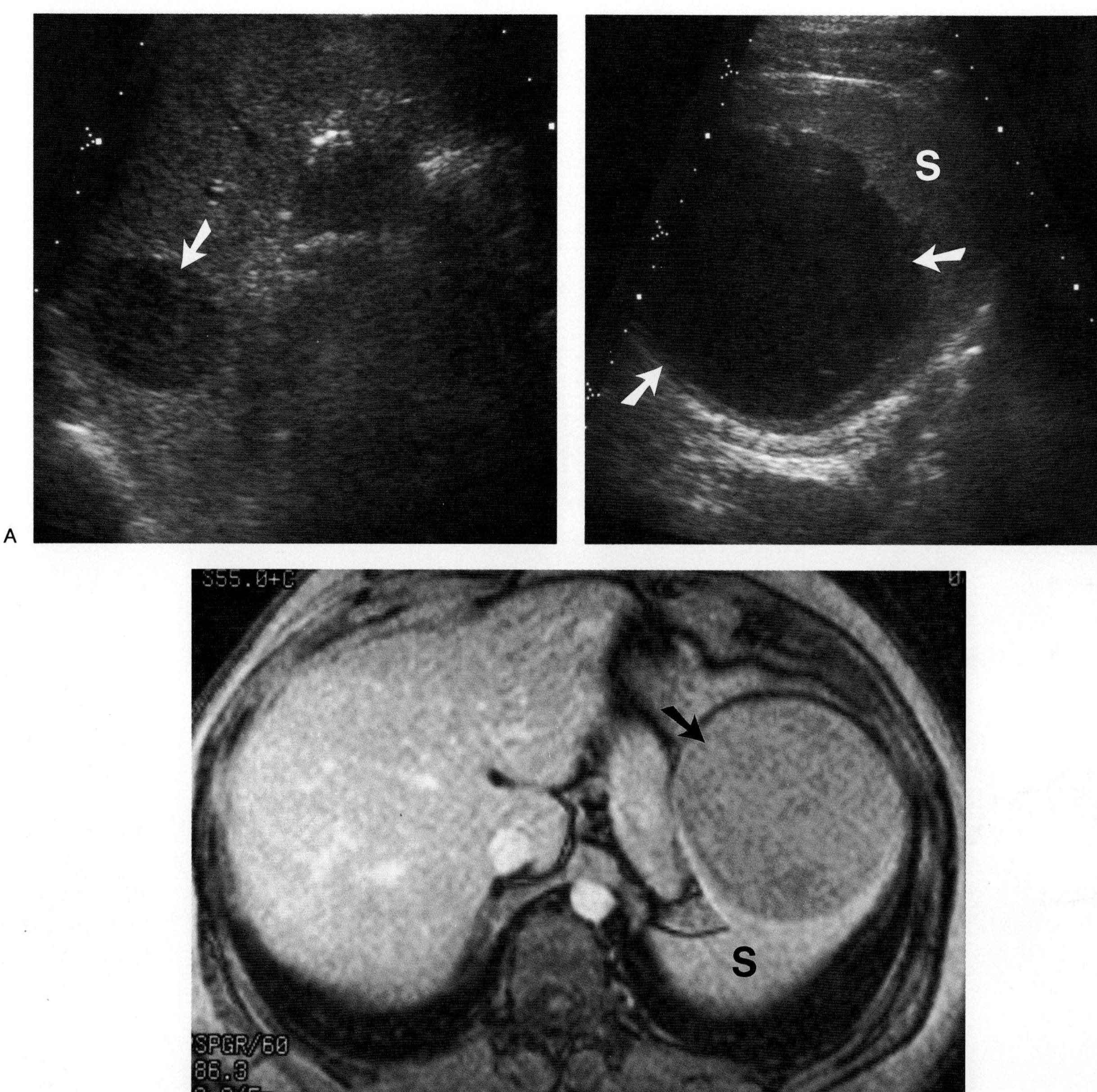

FIG. 6.29. Post-traumatic hemorrhagic splenic cysts in two patients. Sagittal scan (**A**) shows small hemorrhagic cyst with low-level echoes (*arrow*). In another patient, transverse sonogram (**B**) and MR image (**C**) reveal well-defined cystic lesion (*arrow*). S, spleen. Surgery revealed hemorrhagic cyst.

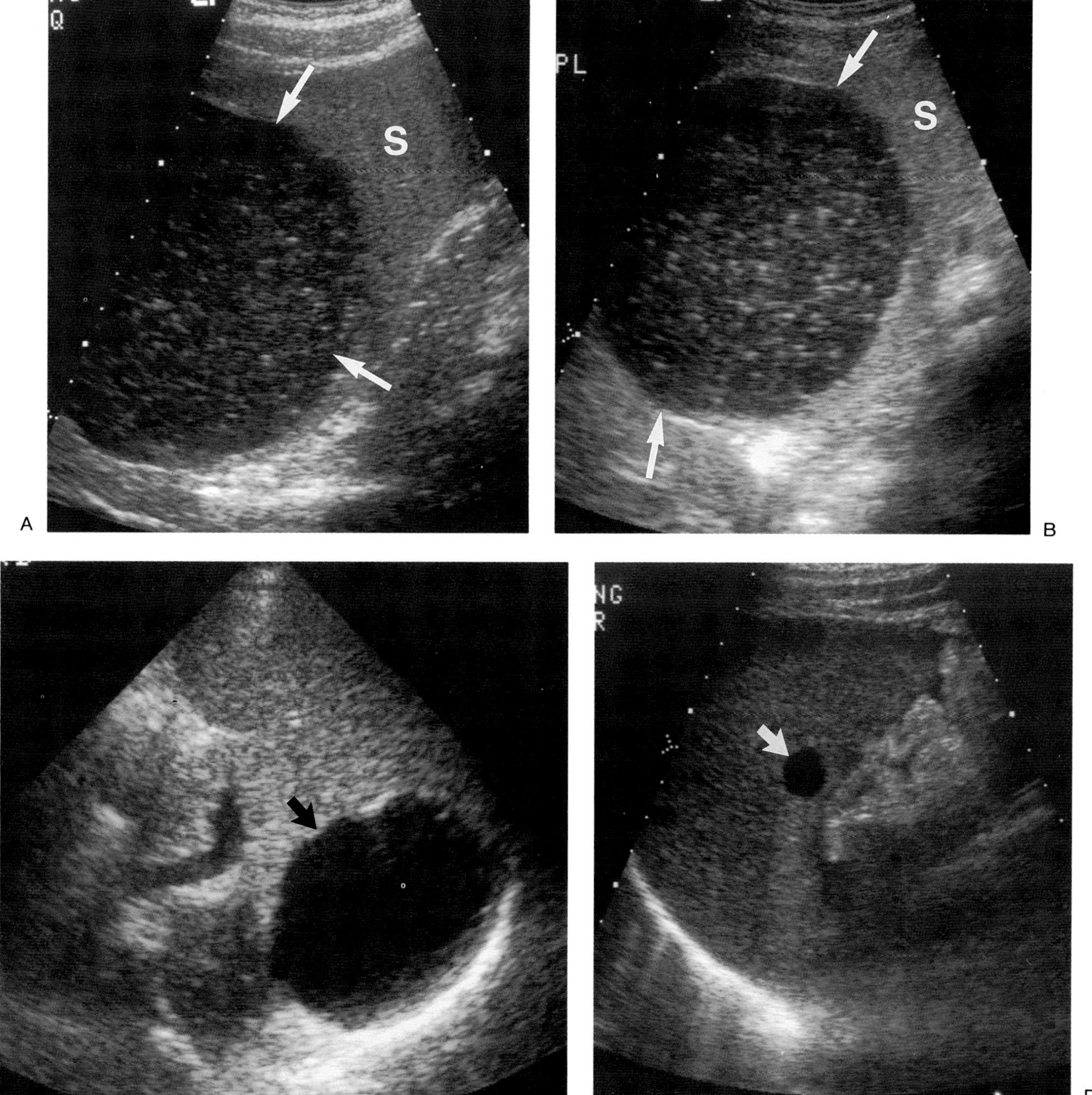

FIG. 6.30. Simple and hemorrhagic splenic cysts. **A, B:** Note large complex splenic cyst (*arrows*) with low-level echoes. S, spleen. Surgery revealed hemorrhagic cyst. **C, D:** Note anechoic simple splenic cysts (*arrows*).

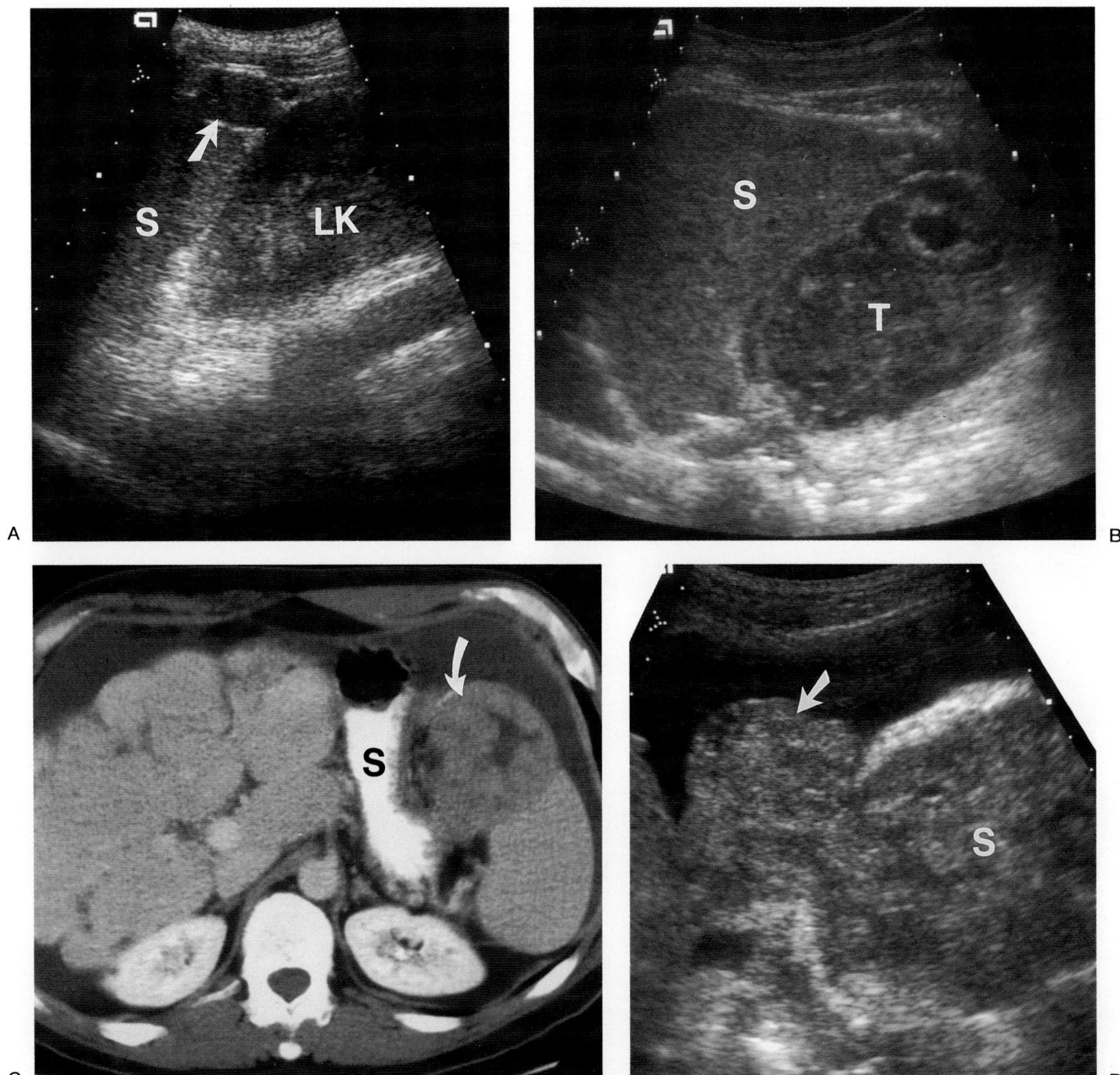

FIG. 6.31. Perisplenic metastases in three patients. **A:** Sagittal scan of lower pole of spleen (S). Note perisplenic metastasis (*arrow*) from ovarian carcinoma. LK, left kidney. **B:** In another patient with melanoma, sagittal sonogram demonstrates large metastatic tumor (T) in splenic hilum. S, spleen. **C:** CT scan demonstrates metastatic tumor (*curved arrow*) involving gastrosplenic ligament. S, stomach. Patient had metastatic sarcoma. **D:** In a third patient, note omental metastasis (*arrow*) adjacent to spleen (S).

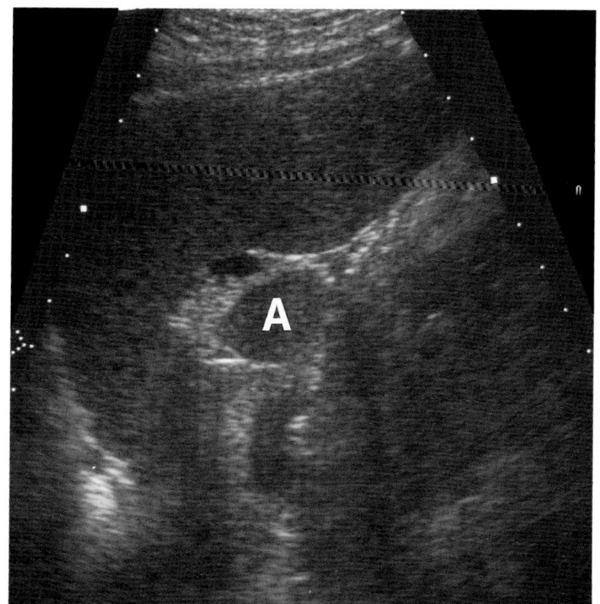

FIG. 6.32. Accessory spleen. Note isoechoic accessory spleen (A) in splenic hilum.

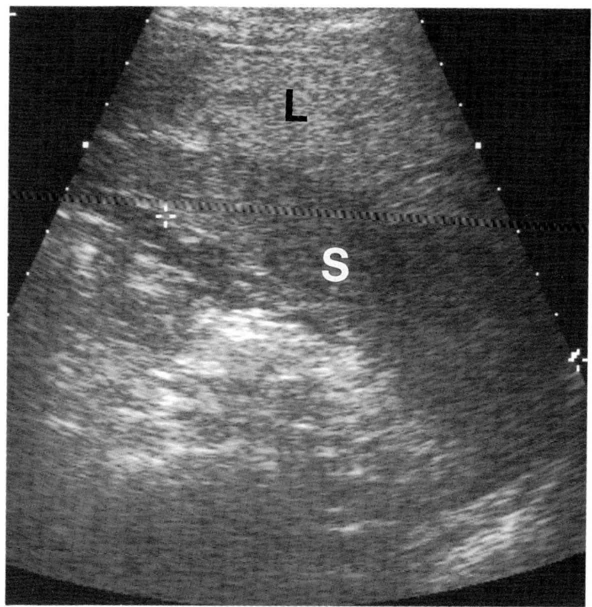

FIG. 6.33. Anatomic variant of lateral segment of left lobe of liver (L) located anterior to spleen (S). This could be misconstrued as perisplenic mass.

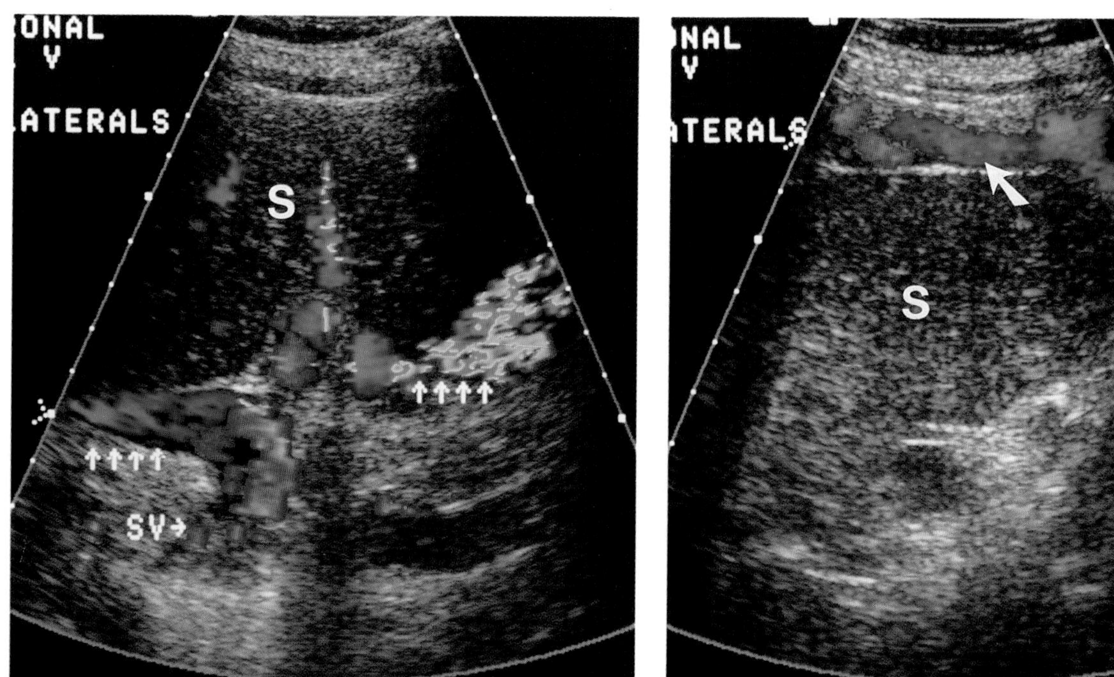

FIG. 6.34. Perisplenic varices. **A:** Coronal color Doppler sonogram of spleen demonstrates multiple perisplenic varices (*arrows*) in a patient with portal hypertension. S, spleen; SV, splenic vein. **B:** In another view of same patient, note varix (*arrow*) anterior to spleen (S).

5. Ros PR, Moser RP, Dachman AH, et al. Hemangioma of the spleen: radiologic–pathologic correlation in ten cases. *AJR* 1987;162:73–77.
6. Goerg C, Schwerk WB, Goerg K. Splenic lesions: sonographic patterns, follow-up, differential diagnosis. *Eur J Radiol* 1991;13:59–66.
7. Niizawa M, Ishida H, Morikawa P, et al. Color Doppler sonography in a case of splenic hemangioma: value of compressing the tumor. *AJR* 1991;157:965–966.
8. Goerg C, Schwerk WB, Goerg K. Sonography of focal lesions of the spleen. *AJR* 1990;156:949–953.
9. Siniluoto T, Päivänsalo M, Alavaikko M. Ultrasonography of spleen and liver in staging Hodgkin's disease. *Eur J Radiol* 1991;13:181–186.
10. Mahoney B, Jeffrey RB, Federle MP. Spontaneous rupture of hepatic and splenic angiosarcoma demonstrated by CT. *AJR* 1982;138:965–966.
11. Siniluoto T, Päivänsalo M, Lähde S. Ultrasonography of splenic metastases. *Acta Radiol* 1989;30:463.
12. Quinn SF, van Sonnenberg E, Casola G, et al. Interventional radiology in the spleen. *Radiology* 1986;161:289–291.
13. Suzuki T, Shibuya H, Yoshimatsu S, et al. Ultrasonically guided staging splenic tissue core biopsy in patients with non-Hodgkin's lymphoma. *Cancer* 1987;60:879–882.
14. Goerg C, Schwerk WB. Splenic infarction: sonographic pattern, diagnosis, follow-up, and complications. *Radiology* 1990;174:803–807.
15. Moosa AR, Gadd MA. Isolated splenic vein thrombosis. *World J Surg* 1985;9:384–390.
16. Itzchak Y, Glickman MG. Splenic vein thrombosis in patients with a normal size spleen. *Invest Radiol* 1977;12:158–163.
17. Weinberger G, Nitra SK, Yoeli G. Ultrasound diagnosis of splenic vein thrombosis. *JCU* 1982;10:345–346.
18. Marn CS, Glazer GM, Williams DM, et al. CT–angiographic correlation of collateral venous pathways in isolate splenic vein occlusion: new observations. *Radiology* 1990;175:375–380.
19. Jeffrey RB. *CT and sonography of the acute abdomen.* New York: Raven Press; 1989:105.
20. Harper PC, Garnelli RL, Kayle MD. Recurrent hemorrhage into the pancreatic duct from a splenic artery aneurysm. *Gastroenterology* 1984;87:417–420.
21. Bishop NL. Splenic artery aneurysm rupture into the colon diagnosed by angiography. *Br J Radiol* 1984;54:1149–1150.
22. Burke JW, Erickson SJ, Kellum CD, et al. Pseudoaneurysm complication pancreatitis: detection by CT. *Radiology* 1986;161:447–450.
23. Mandel SR, Jaques PF, Mauro MA, Sanofsky S. Nonoperative management of peripancreatic arterial aneurysm: a ten year experience. *Ann Surg* 1987;205:126–128.
24. Ralls PW, Quinn MF, Coletti P, et al. Sonography of pyogenic splenic abscess. *AJR* 1982;138:523–528.
25. Pawar S, Kay CJ, Gonzalez R, et al. Sonography of splenic abscess. *AJR* 1982;138:259–262.
26. Spouge AR, Wilson SR, Gopinath N, et al. Extrapulmonary *Pneumocystis carinii* in a patient with AIDS: sonographic findings. *AJR* 1990;155:76–78.
27. Lupien C, Sauerbrei EE. Healing in the traumatized spleen: sonographic investigation. *Radiology* 1984;151:181–185.
28. Filiatrault D, Longpŕe D, Patriquin H, et al. Investigation of childhood blunt abdominal trauma: a practical approach using ultrasound as the initial diagnostic modality. *Pediatr Radiol* 1987;17:373–379.
29. Weill F, Rohmer P, Didier D, et al. Ultrasound of the traumatized spleen: left butterfly sign in lesions masked by echogenic blood clots. *Gastrointest Radiol* 1988;13:169–172.
30. Dachman AH, Ros PR, Muirari PJ, et al. Nonparasitic splenic cysts: a report of 52 cases with radiologic–pathologic correlation. *AJR* 1986;147:537–542.
31. Rathaus V, Zissin R, Goldberg E. Spontaneous rupture of an epidermoid cyst of the spleen: preoperative ultrasonographic diagnosis. *JCU* 1991;19:235–237.
32. Franquet T, Montes M, Lecumberri FJ, et al. Hydatid disease of the spleen: imaging findings in nine patients. *AJR* 1990;154:525–528.
33. Subramanyam BR, Balthazar EJ, Harii SC. Sonography of the accessory spleen *AJR* 1984;143:47–49.

CHAPTER 7

Abdominal Aorta, Inferior Vena Cava, and Retroperitoneum

ABDOMINAL AORTA

Technique

Either a 5- or 3.5-MHz curved array transducer may be used for scanning the abdominal aorta. Linear array probes are also very helpful for graded-compression scans when overlying bowel gas obscures the aorta. In addition to sagittal and transverse views, coronal images are obtained in a steep oblique position to evaluate the aorta and periaortic retroperitoneum. The aorta is routinely imaged from the diaphragm to the aortic bifurcation. Sagittal views are best to identify the origins of the celiac and superior mesenteric arteries.

Color Doppler sonography may be of particular value in diagnosing abdominal aortic dissections and in demonstrating mural thrombus in patients with aortic aneurysms. Unlike smaller vessels in the abdomen with parabolic flow, the flow pattern in the abdominal aorta has been characterized as "plug flow" (1,2). In this flow state, red blood cells move at a uniform velocity throughout the entire volume of the aorta. In parabolic flow, red blood cells along the peripheral walls of vessels move slower than in the center of the vessel. Aortic aneurysms, however, have very chaotic flow patterns due to turbulence.

Abdominal Aortic Aneurysms

The diagnosis and surveillance of abdominal aortic aneurysms are the main indications for aortic sonography. The size of the aneurysm is directly related to the morbidity and risk of rupture (3). The incidence of rupture of abdominal aortic aneurysms increases substantially when the aneurysm exceeds 5 cm in maximal diameter (3–5). The rate of rupture of aortic aneurysms less than 5 cm in diameter varies between 1 and 5 percent (3–5). The risk of rupture dramatically increases with aneurysms 6 cm and greater. The 1-year mortality for a 6-cm aneurysm is approximately 50 percent (4).

Collin (5) noted that the prevalence of abdominal aortic aneurysms in men aged 65 to 75 is approximately 5.4 percent (5). In 2.3 percent of patients the aneurysm is 4 cm or greater in diameter (5). It has been estimated that abdominal aortic aneurysms 3 to 6 cm in diameter grow annually at 4 mm (3,4). However, in individual patients aortic aneurysms may grow quite rapidly; therefore continued surveillance at 6- to 12-month intervals is recommended for all abdominal aortic aneurysms greater than 3 cm. Russel (4) noted that because of the relatively low cost of sonography, screening for abdominal aortic aneurysm after the age of 60 is at least as effective as other radiologic screening techniques such as mammography.

Recent epidemiologic studies indicate that early surgery may be beneficial in improving survival in patients with aneurysms that are 4 cm in maximal diameter (6). Results of this study are somewhat controversial, as most centers do not generally perform elective surgery for aneurysms less than 5 cm. Nevertheless, continued surveillance with sonography is important as rapid increase in size is a clear indication for early surgery.

Pathologically, the vast majority of abdominal aortic aneurysms are due to atherosclerosis. Rarely, other etiologies such as Marfan's syndrome, cystic medial necrosis, or aortitis may cause abdominal aortic aneurysms. Mycotic aneurysms are generally pseudoaneurysms without all three layers of the arterial wall. In atherosclerotic aneurysms, there is degeneration of the elastic tissue within the media of the aortic wall, resulting in aortic dilatation. This results in decreasing wall thickness as well as increasing aortic wall tension. According to Laplace's law, wall tension is directly proportional to the product of intraluminal pressure and the radius of the vessel lumen. It is inversely proportional to the wall thickness (3). As the aorta dilates and has decreasing wall thickness, wall tension increases. Increasing wall tension is a major factor contributing to aortic rupture.

Computed tomography (CT), magnetic resonance imaging (MRI), and sonography can all reliably measure the dimensions of abdominal aortic aneurysms. The abdominal aorta should be measured in both true sagittal and transverse planes from outer wall to outer wall. Most abdominal aneurysms are fusiform, although saccular aneurysms may rarely occur (Figs. 7.1 and 7.2).

In addition to measuring the maximal diameter of the aneurysm, involvement of the suprarenal abdominal aorta and aortic bifurcation should be ascertained (Figs. 7.3 and 7.4). Although the vast majority of abdominal aortic aneurysms are infrarenal in location, sonography is often unable to define the relationship of the aneurysm to the renal arteries. MR angiography and three-dimensional CT angiography may obviate the need for conventional arteriograms in the near future.

Color Doppler sonography generally demonstrates markedly turbulent flow within abdominal aortic aneurysms (Fig. 7.5). Mural thrombus is a common finding in patients with larger aortic aneurysms (Fig. 7.6). Its echogenicity depends on the degree of organized or fresh thrombus. Color Doppler sonography excels at defining mural thrombus and the residual lumen.

Rupture of Abdominal Aortic Aneurysms

Rupture of an abdominal aortic aneurysm is a catastrophic event associated with 80 percent mortality if the patient becomes hypotensive (7). The classic clinical triad of rupture of an abdominal aortic aneurysm includes (a) severe abdominal pain, (b) hypotension, and (c) a pulsatile midabdominal mass. Imaging hypotensive patients with clinical signs of rupture may not be possible as immediate surgery is warranted. In patients who are hemodynamically stable, sonography in the emergency room may facilitate the diagnosis and occasionally prevent unnecessary surgery if an alternative abnormality is found. CT, however, is more reliable than sonography in defining small areas of retroperitoneal hemorrhage (8). Retroperitoneal hematomas from a ruptured aortic aneurysm are typically hypoechoic (Fig. 7.7). Hemorrhage may occur in multiple extraperitoneal compartments including the perirenal and posterior pararenal spaces and/or psoas compartment. These spaces are often difficult to appreciate accurately with sonography. However, the diagnosis of rupture is more important than localizing the exact site of retroperitoneal hematoma. CT can more accurately define a focal area of necrosis of the aneurysm wall (9).

Shuman et al. (10) performed sonography in the emergency department in 60 patients with suspected abdominal aortic aneurysm rupture. The purpose of the study was to determine the reliability of sonography in identifying aortic aneurysms in the clinical setting of suggested rupture. All studies were limited to 1 min of real-time examination in the emergency room. Sonography correctly identified 97 percent of aneurysms (10). However, the detection of periaortic hemorrhage was noted in only 4 percent of the patients (10).

Aortic Dissection

Contrast-enhanced CT and MRI are the imaging techniques of choice for evaluation of abdominal aortic dissections (11). Sonography can diagnose aortic dissection by demonstrating an intimal flap (Figs. 7.8 to 7.12). In many patients, demonstration of the intimal flap is facilitated by color Doppler sonography. Sonography is often limited, however, in determining the entire extent of the dissection as well as defining precisely which visceral vessels (celiac, superior mesenteric artery, and renal arteries) are supplied by the true or false lumen (12,13). On occasion, thrombus within a clotted false lumen can be identified with color Doppler sonography within branches of the aorta such as the superior mesenteric artery (Fig. 7.10) (13).

Isolated abdominal aortic dissections are uncommon. In well over 90 percent of cases, the dissection extends into the abdomen from the thoracic aorta. Color Doppler sonography and spectral waveforms may aid in the demonstration of differential flow patterns between the true and false lumen. There is often decreased flow or even reversal of flow within the false lumen. A "pseudodissection" may be noted with color Doppler sonography due to turbulent flow patterns within the aorta (Fig. 7.13). Therefore an intimal flap should always be identified prior to diagnosing a dissection.

Aortic Pseudoaneurysms

Pseudoaneurysms of the aorta are most often related to trauma or infection (Figs. 7.14 and 7.15). Life-threatening hemorrhage may occur unless the pseudoaneurysm is diagnosed and treated promptly. Color Doppler sonography is extremely valuable in suggesting the diagnosis and in defining the connection between the aorta and the pseudoaneurysm.

Perianeurysmal Fibrosis and Inflammation

Perianeurysmal fibrosis or inflammatory tissue may develop in some patients with abdominal aortic aneurysms (Fig. 7.16). Both abnormalities are important to detect preoperatively as they may affect surgical repair (14). Inflammatory reaction and fibrosis tissue appear sonographically as hypoechoic tissue surrounding the

(text continues on page 399)

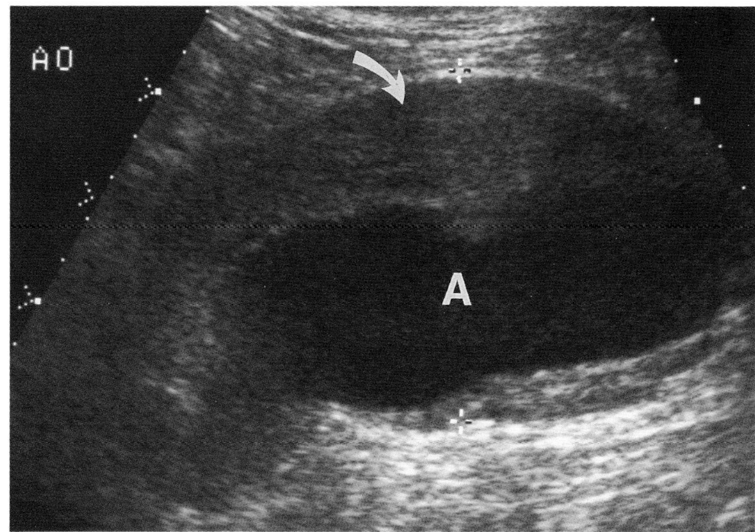

FIG. 7.1. Fusiform aneurysm of the abdominal aorta. Sagittal scan of the aorta (A) demonstrates 7-cm aneurysm (*cursors*) and extensive mural thrombosis (*curved arrow*). Note measurement taken from outer wall to outer wall of the aneurysm.

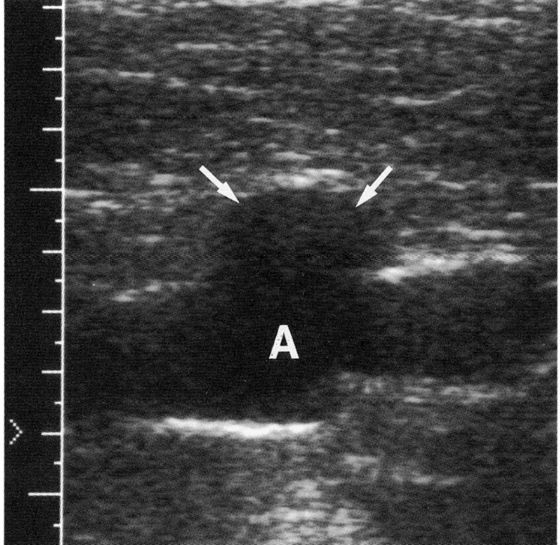

FIG. 7.2. Saccular aneurysm of the aorta. Sagittal scan of the aorta (A) demonstrates small saccular aneurysm (*arrows*).

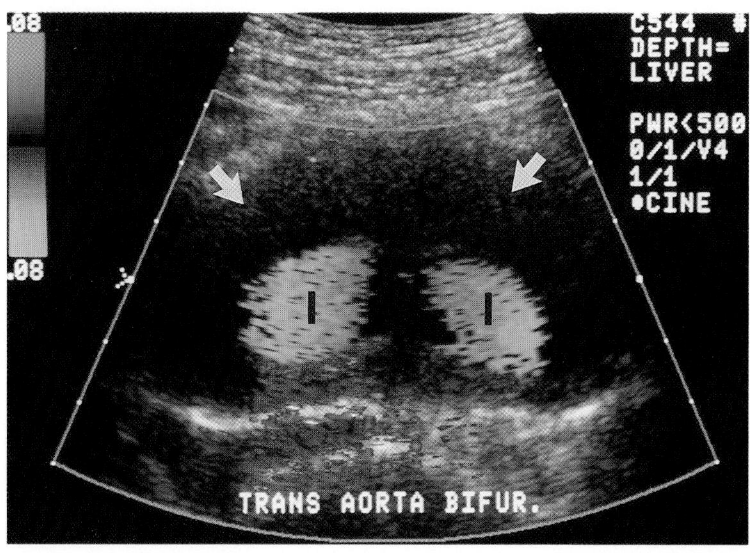

FIG. 7.3. Involvement of the aortic bifurcation with aortic aneurysm. Transverse color Doppler sonogram of the common iliac bifurcation demonstrates large aneurysm extending into the aortic bifurcation. Note extensive mural thrombus (*arrows*) surrounding common iliac (I) arteries.

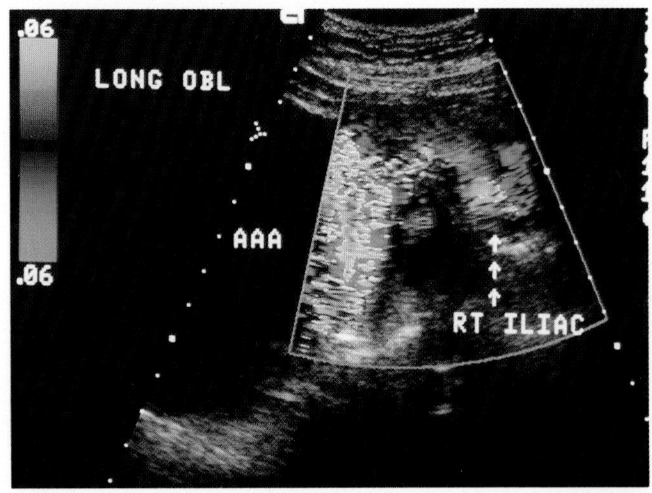

FIG. 7.4. Aortic aneurysm without extension into the common iliac artery. Oblique color Doppler scan of abdominal aortic aneurysm (AAA) demonstrates normal right common iliac artery (*arrows*).

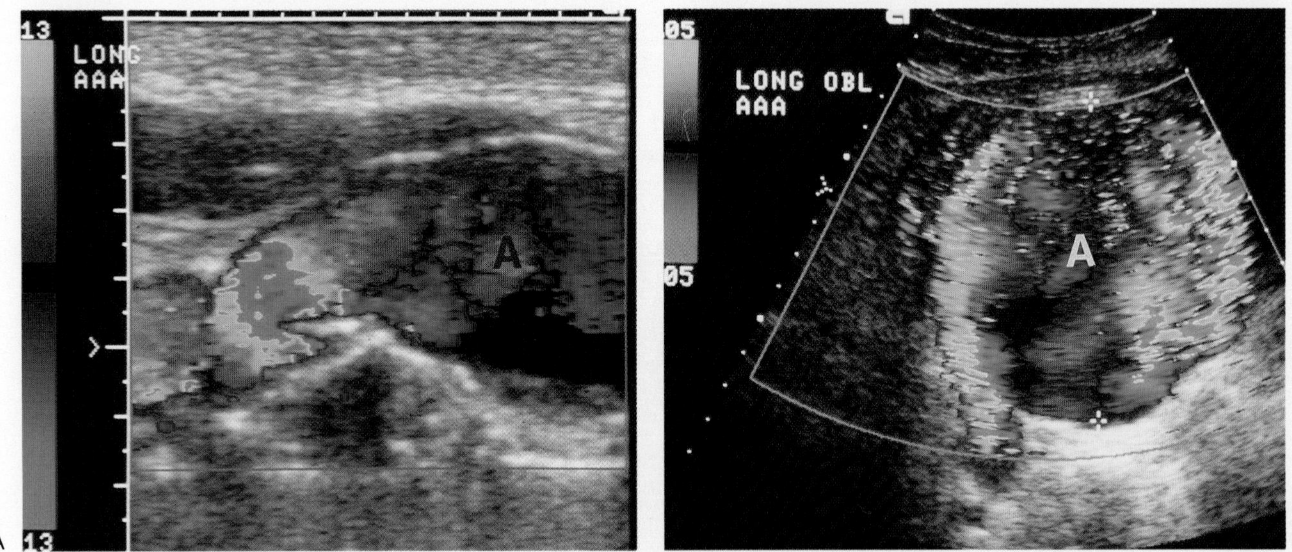

FIG. 7.5. Aortic aneurysms with turbulent flow in two patients. **A:** Sagittal scan of the aorta demonstrates a small aortic aneurysm (A) with turbulent flow. **B:** In another patient, a transverse scan demonstrates an 8.5-cm aneurysm (A) with markedly turbulent flow.

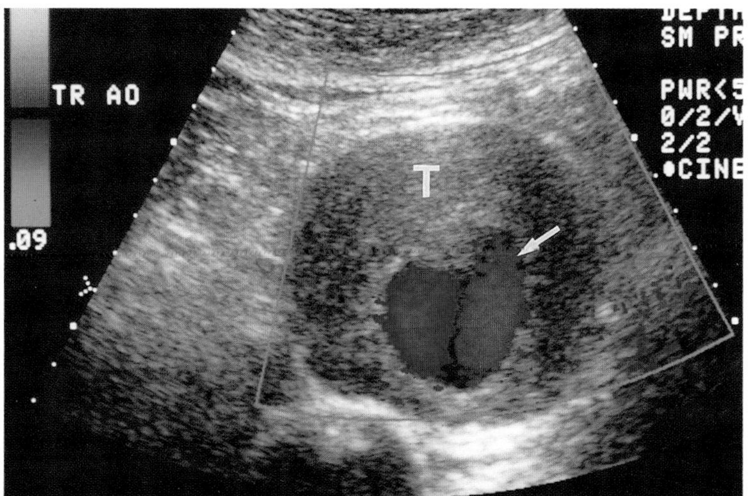

A

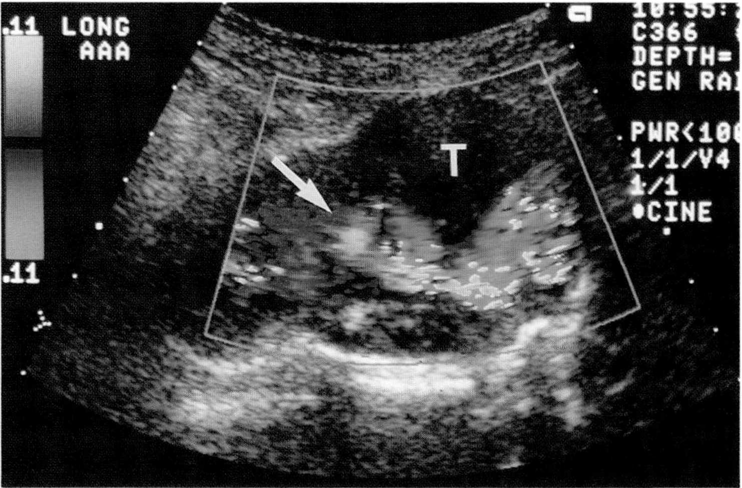

B

FIG. 7.6. Color Doppler scans of mural thrombus in abdominal aortic aneurysms in two patients. **A:** Transverse scan of the abdominal aorta demonstrates extensive circumferential thrombus (T) formation. Note relatively small residual lumen (*arrows*). **B:** In another patient, a longitudinal scan of the aorta demonstrates eccentric mural thrombus (T) and residual lumen (*arrow*).

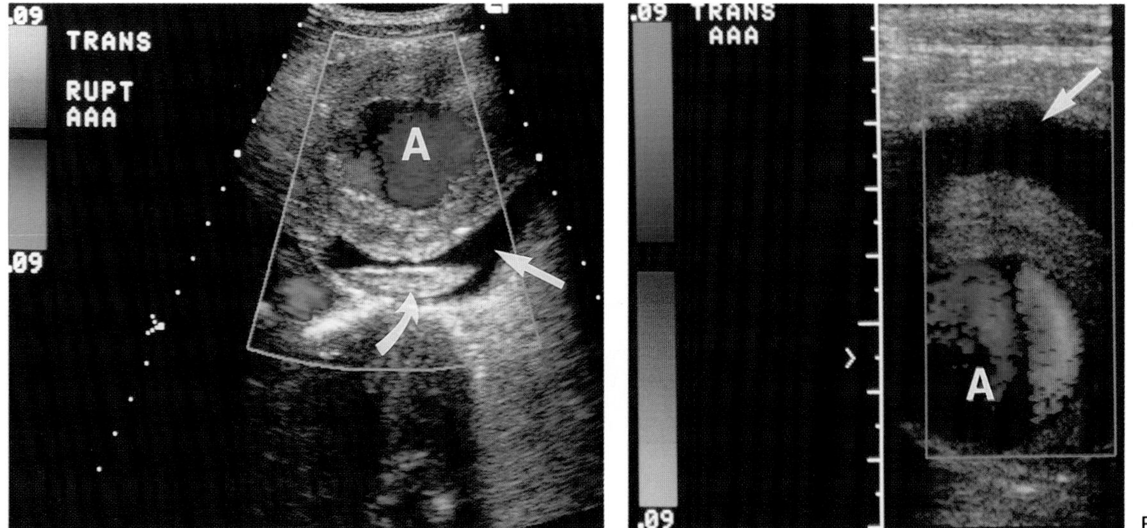

FIG. 7.7. Rupture of abdominal aortic aneurysm in two patients. **A:** Transverse color Doppler sonogram of the aorta demonstrates hypoechoic blood (*arrows*) posterior to aortic aneurysm (A) due to rupture. Note echogenic clot posteriorly (*curved arrow*). **B:** In another patient, note hypoechoic periaortic hemorrhage (*arrows*) anterior to the aneurysm (A). Both patients had ruptured aneurysms confirmed at surgery.

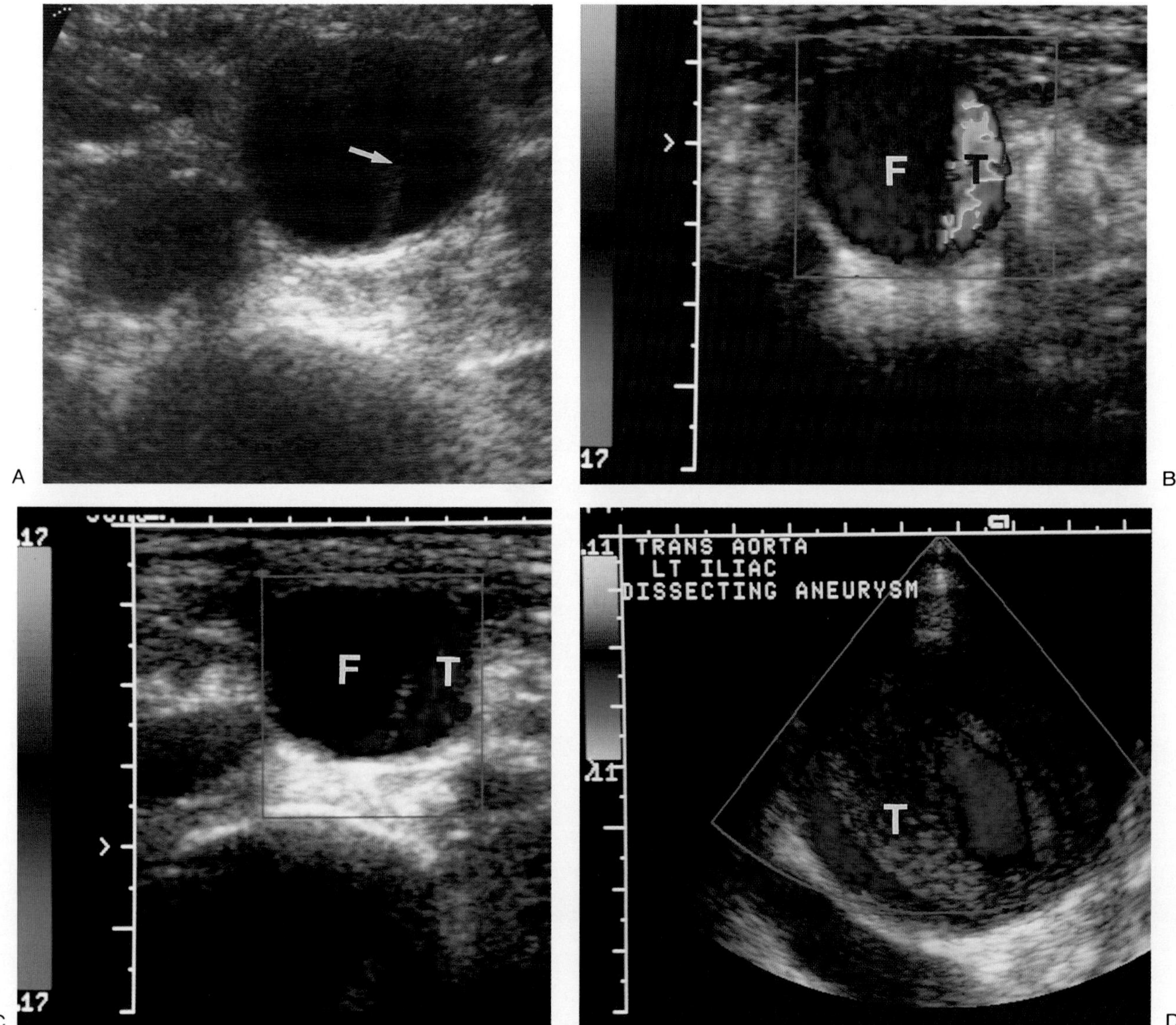

FIG. 7.8. Color Doppler sonography of aortic dissections in two patients. **A:** Transverse sonogram of an aortic dissection demonstrates a faintly visible intimal flap (*arrow*). **B:** Note differential flow pattern between the true (T) lumen and false (F) lumen. **C:** Note that in diastole there is no flow in the false (F) lumen. **D:** In another patient with a dissecting aortic aneurysm, note flow (*arrow*) posterior to large intramural thrombus (T).

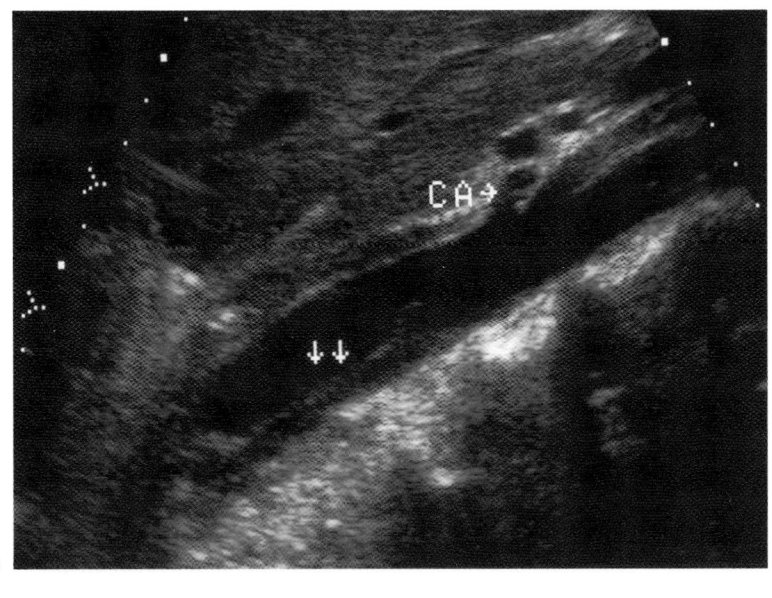

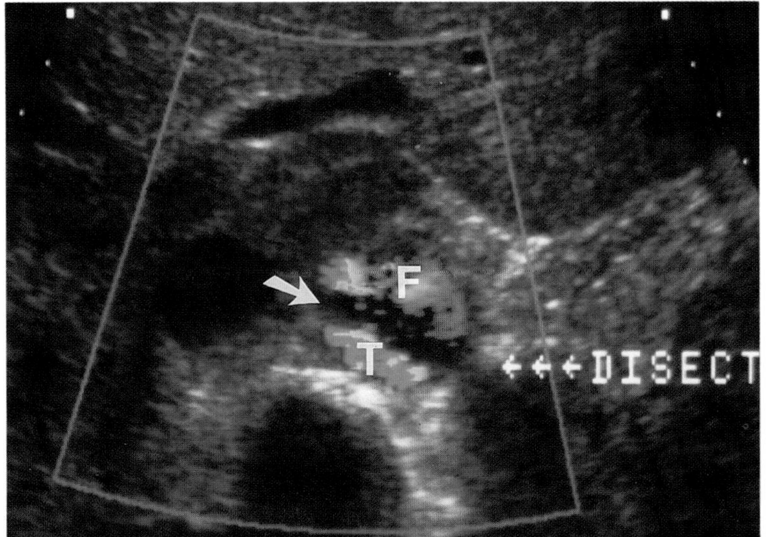

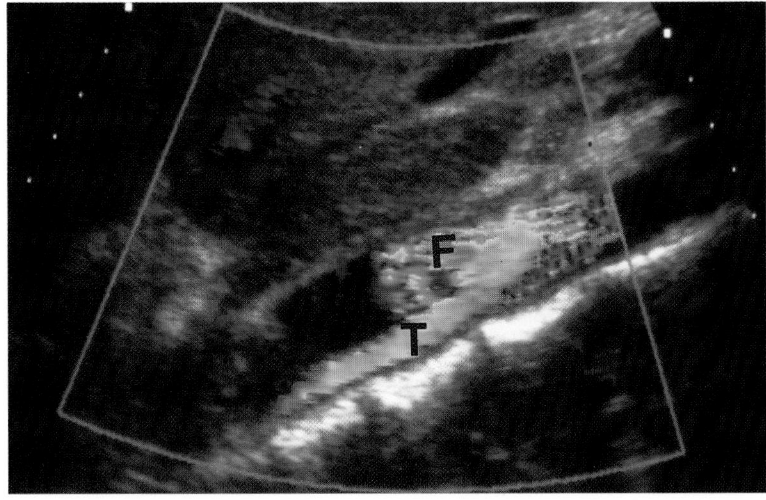

FIG. 7.9. Color Doppler sonography of aortic dissection. **A:** Sagittal sonogram of supraceliac dissection demonstrates intimal flap (*arrows*). CA, celiac artery. **B:** Transverse color Doppler scan demonstrates intimal flap (*arrow*) between true (T) lumen and false (F) lumen. **C:** Sagittal color Doppler image of dissection demonstrates true (T) and false (F) lumina.

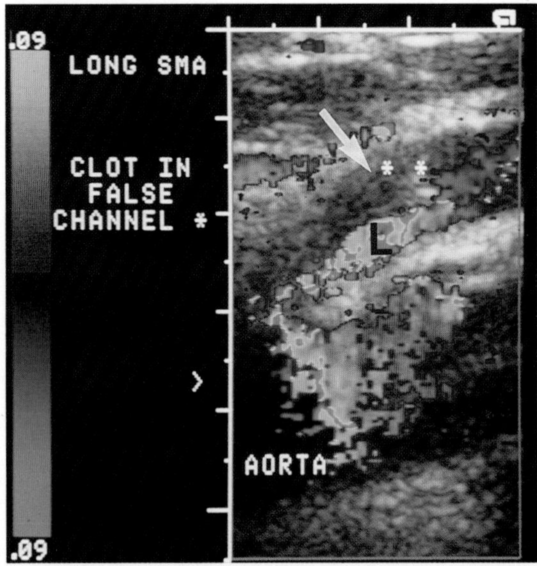

FIG. 7.10. Aortic dissection with clotted false lumen in the superior mesenteric aorta. Sagittal scan of the aorta demonstrates extensive thrombus (*arrow*) within the clotted false channel of dissection extending into the superior mesenteric artery. Note patent true lumen of superior mesenteric artery (L).

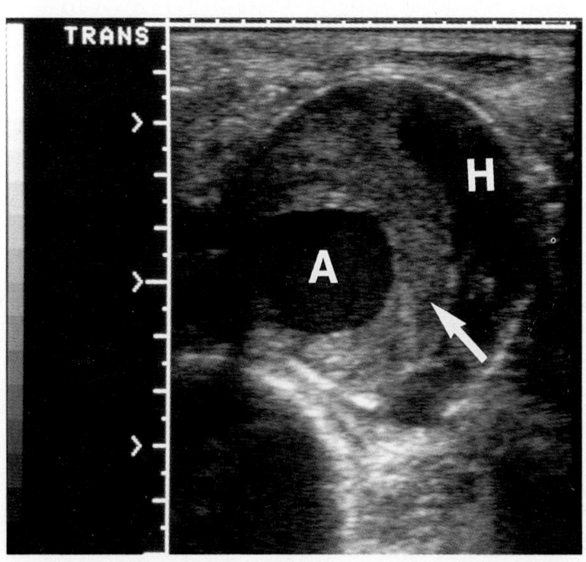

FIG. 7.11. Dissecting aneurysm with acute intramural hematoma. Transverse scan of the aorta (A) demonstrates acute intramural hematoma (H) displacing extensive mural thrombus (*arrow*) within the dissecting aneurysm.

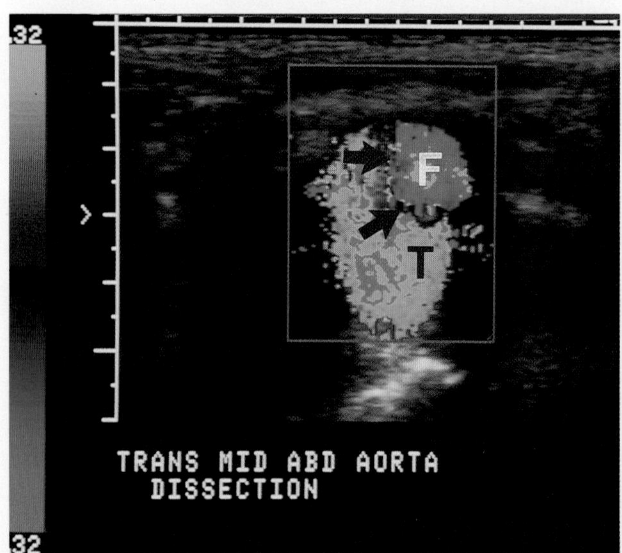

FIG. 7.12. Color Doppler sonography of localized aortic dissection. Transverse color Doppler sonogram of the aorta demonstrates a localized aortic dissection with intimal flap (*arrows*) between true (T) lumen and false (F) lumen.

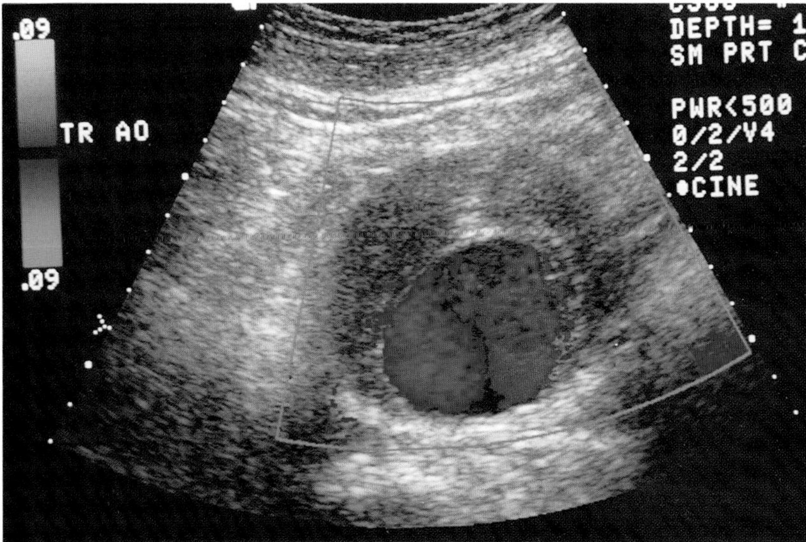

FIG. 7.13. "Pseudoaortic" dissection (same patient as in Fig. 7.5A). Transverse color Doppler of aortic aneurysm demonstrates turbulence creating the appearance of "pseudodissection." Intimal flap was not present.

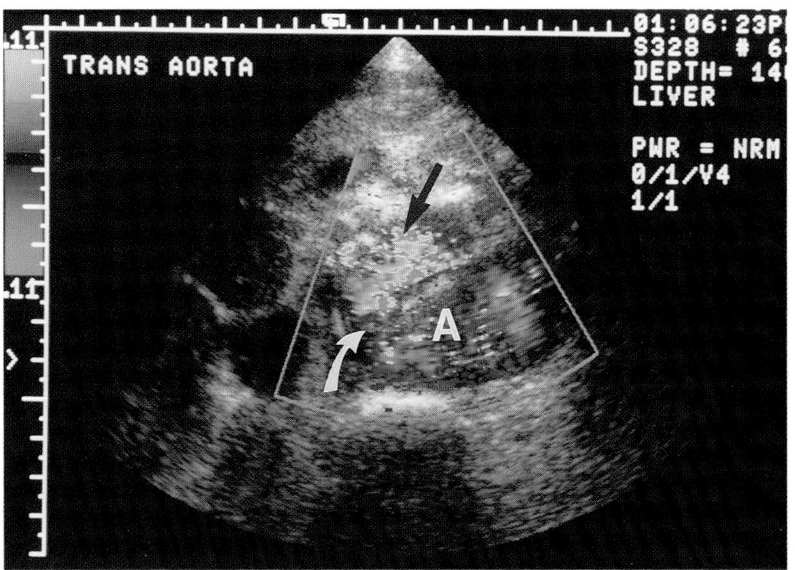

FIG. 7.14. Mycotic pseudoaneurysm of the aorta. Transverse color Doppler sonogram of the aorta demonstrates large mycotic pseudoaneurysm (*arrow*). Note connection (*curved arrow*) between aorta (A) and pseudoaneurysm.

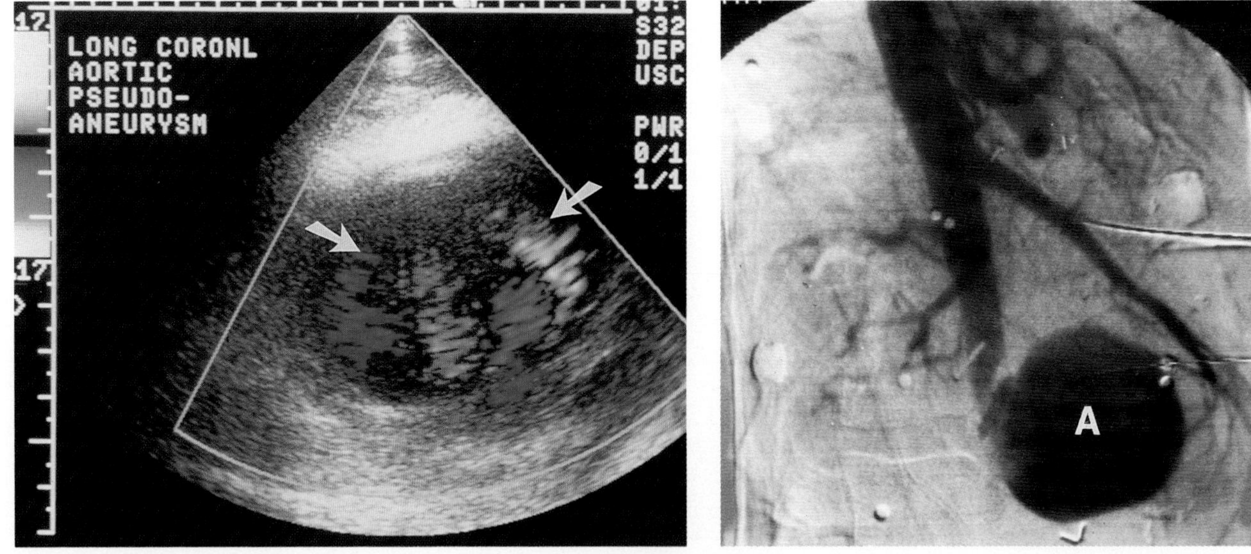

FIG. 7.15. Post-traumatic aortic pseudoaneurysm. **A:** Note large aortic pseudoaneurysm demonstrated with color Doppler sonography (*arrows*). Patient sustained a midabdominal gunshot wound. **B:** Lateral aortogram confirms pseudoaneurysm (A).

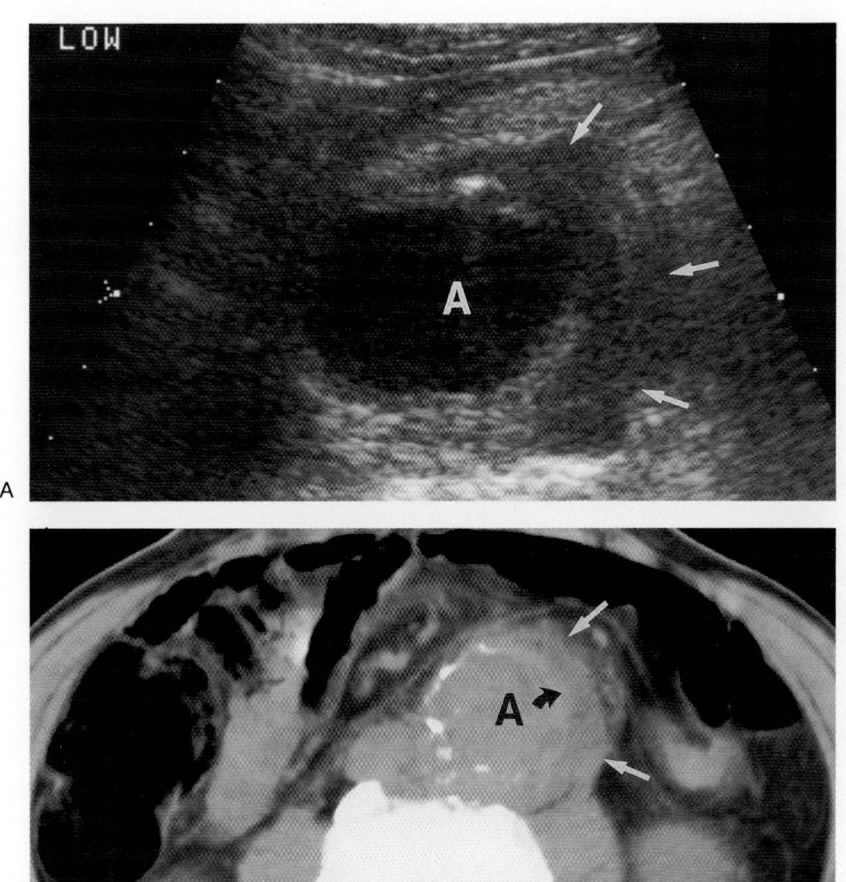

FIG. 7.16. Inflammatory aortic aneurysm. **A:** Transverse sonogram of the aorta demonstrates hypoechoic soft tissue (*arrows*) surrounding a large abdominal aortic aneurysm. **B:** CT scan confirms perianeurysmal inflammatory tissue (*arrows*). A, aneurysm; *curved arrow,* outer wall of aneurysm.

aneurysm. This appearance can be mimicked by either retroperitoneal adenopathy or a periaortic mass. Biopsy may be required for definitive diagnosis. Perianeurysmal fibrosis may cause obstructive uropathy similar to retroperitoneal fibrosis if there is ureteral encasement.

Aortic Grafts and Postoperative Complications of Aortic Surgery

The standard surgical treatment for abdominal aortic aneurysms is replacement of a graft within the native abdominal aorta (15). In general, there is usually an end-to-end or an end-to-side proximal anastomosis (Fig. 7.17). Although sonography is quite reliable for detecting the patency of aortic grafts following surgery, CT, MRI, and indium-labeled white cell scans are the preferred techniques to diagnose surgical complications such as graft infection and aortoenteric fistulas (16–19). Similarly, postoperative pseudoaneurysms at the anastomotic site are best evaluated by CT and MRI.

INFERIOR VENA CAVA

Technique

Sonography is an excellent method to quickly evaluate the suprarenal inferior vena cava. The intrahepatic portion is readily visualized with both grayscale and color Doppler sonography from either a sagittal or coronal plane. In some patients, the infrarenal inferior vena cava may be obscured due to overlying bowel gas. When overlying bowel gas presents a problem, graded-compression scans as well as coronal views through the right flank may aid in visualization of the inferior vena cava.

Abnormalities of the Inferior Vena Cava

Congenital anomalies such as duplications, transposition, and azygous continuation of the inferior vena cava are best evaluated with contrast-enhanced CT or MRI (20). The main indication for sonography is to determine the patency of the inferior vena cava, to exclude tumor invasion, and to diagnose pericaval masses or adenopathy.

Thrombosis of the Inferior Vena Cava

Color Doppler sonography is the technique of choice to evaluate inferior vena cava patency and to exclude thrombosis. The inferior vena cava is very sensitive to respiratory changes as well as right atrial systole. Reversal of flow in the inferior vena cava and hepatic veins may be demonstrated during right atrial systole (Fig. 7.18). The inferior vena cava decreases substantially in size during inspiration and Valsalva's maneuver. The inferior vena cava increases in size with expiration. When the anteroposterior (AP) diameter of the inferior vena cava exceeds 1 cm, congestive heart failure or other causes of raised right atrial pressure should be considered (21).

In obese patients, it is often important to use a lower frequency transducer to obtain adequate color Doppler signal from the inferior vena cava. Color Doppler sensitivity must be maximized by using maximal power gain, low wall-filter, and low pulse repetition frequency. Flash artifacts can be minimized by using breath-held images.

Tumor thrombus from the liver, kidney, and adrenal may extend into the inferior vena cava. Tumor neovascularity within the inferior vena cava may be diagnosed with color Doppler sonography. However, it is often not possible to distinguish bland clot from tumor thrombus (Figs. 7.19 and 7.20).

Leiomyosarcoma

Leiomyosarcoma is a rare primary tumor of the inferior vena cava. This lesion may be difficult at times to differentiate from neoplastic invasion of the inferior vena cava from other primary tumors (22). The inferior vena cava is usually markedly distended by an echogenic mass (Fig. 7.21). The lesion may rarely calcify.

Mechanical Filters and Stents in the Inferior Vena Cava

Inferior vena cava filters are routinely placed for prophylaxis in patients unable to receive anticoagulant therapy for recurrent pulmonary emboli. Complications of filter placement include proximal thrombosis (Fig. 7.19B) and development of paralumbar collaterals. Because of associated artifacts, MRI and CT may have difficulty in imaging metallic stents. Color Doppler sonography is an excellent technique to rapidly diagnose inferior vena caval thrombosis following filter placement. In patients with stenosis of the inferior vena cava, metallic stents may be inserted percutaneously to restore patency. Color Doppler sonography may be useful to evaluate patency following stent placement (Fig. 7.22).

Aortocaval Fistulas

Rarely, an aorta aneurysm may rupture into the inferior vena cava, resulting in a high output aortocaval fistula (23). The inferior vena cava is markedly distended and has a pulsatile venous waveform on spectral Doppler sonogram (Fig. 7.23). Color Doppler sonography may demonstrate the actual site of the fistula in selected patients (Fig. 7.24).

(text continues on page 406)

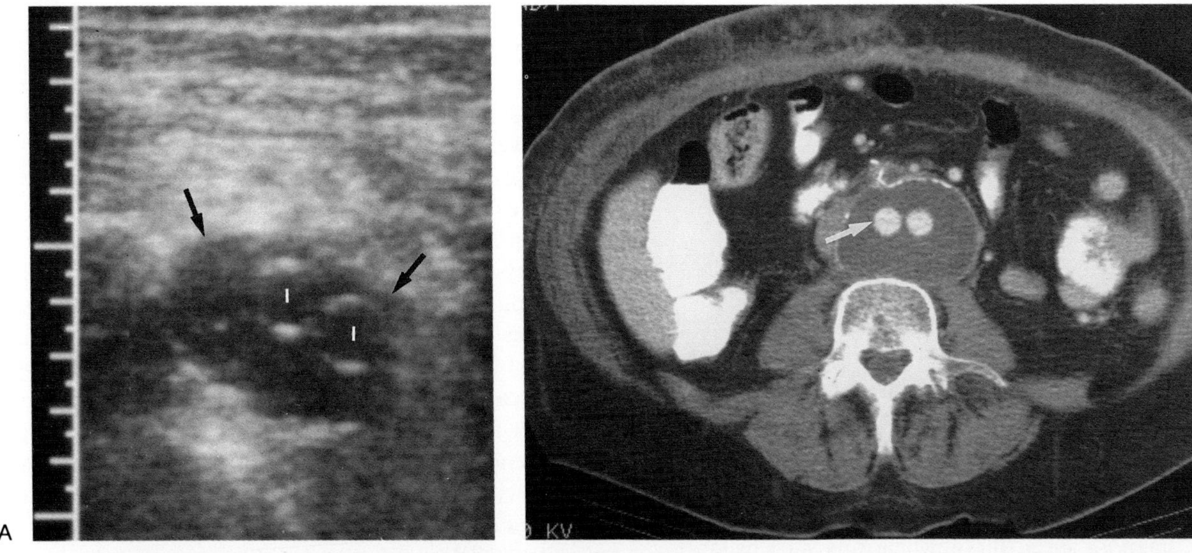

FIG. 7.17. Sonographic appearance of postoperative aortic graft. **A:** Transverse sonogram demonstrates postoperative aortic graft wrapped inside native aorta. I, iliac graft limbs; *arrows,* outer wall of native aorta. **B:** Contrast-enhanced CT scan demonstrates enhancing graft (*arrow*) surrounded by a large amount of thrombus within native aorta. (Case courtesy of Gretchen Gooding, MD, San Francisco, CA.)

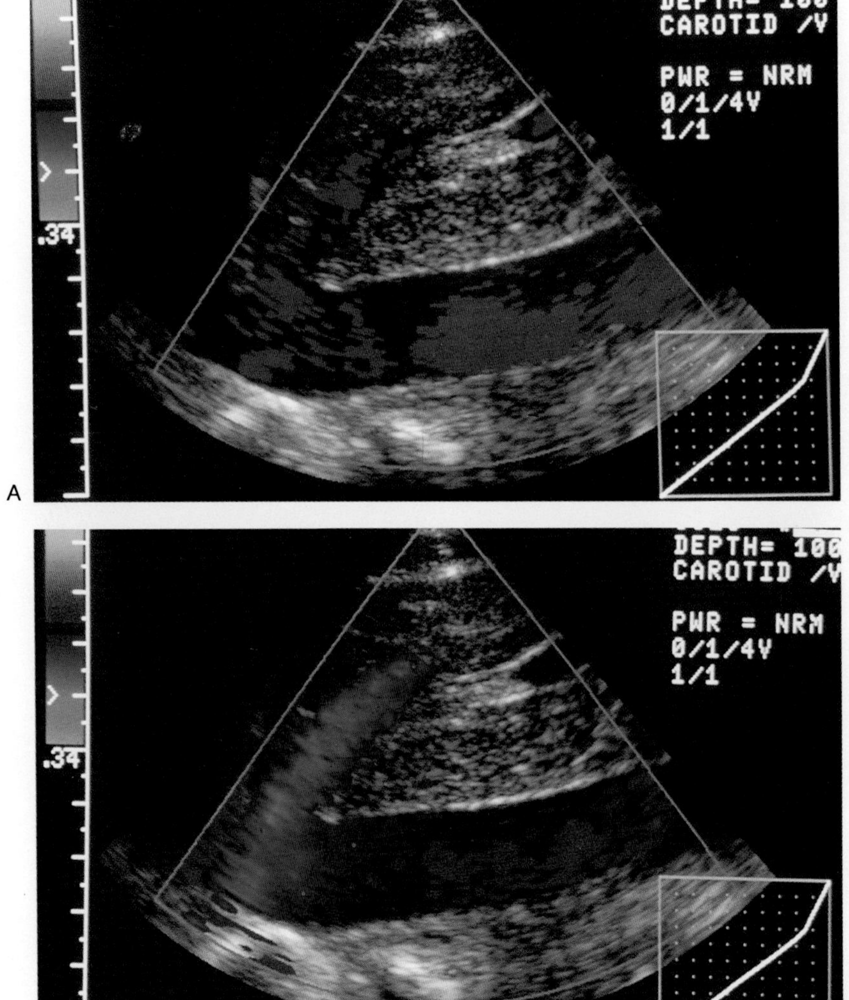

FIG. 7.18. Reversal of flow within the inferior vena cava during right atrial systole. **A:** Color Doppler sonogram demonstrates forward flow during right atrial diastole in the aorta. **B:** Following right atrial systole, there is a reversal of flow into the inferior vena cava and hepatic veins.

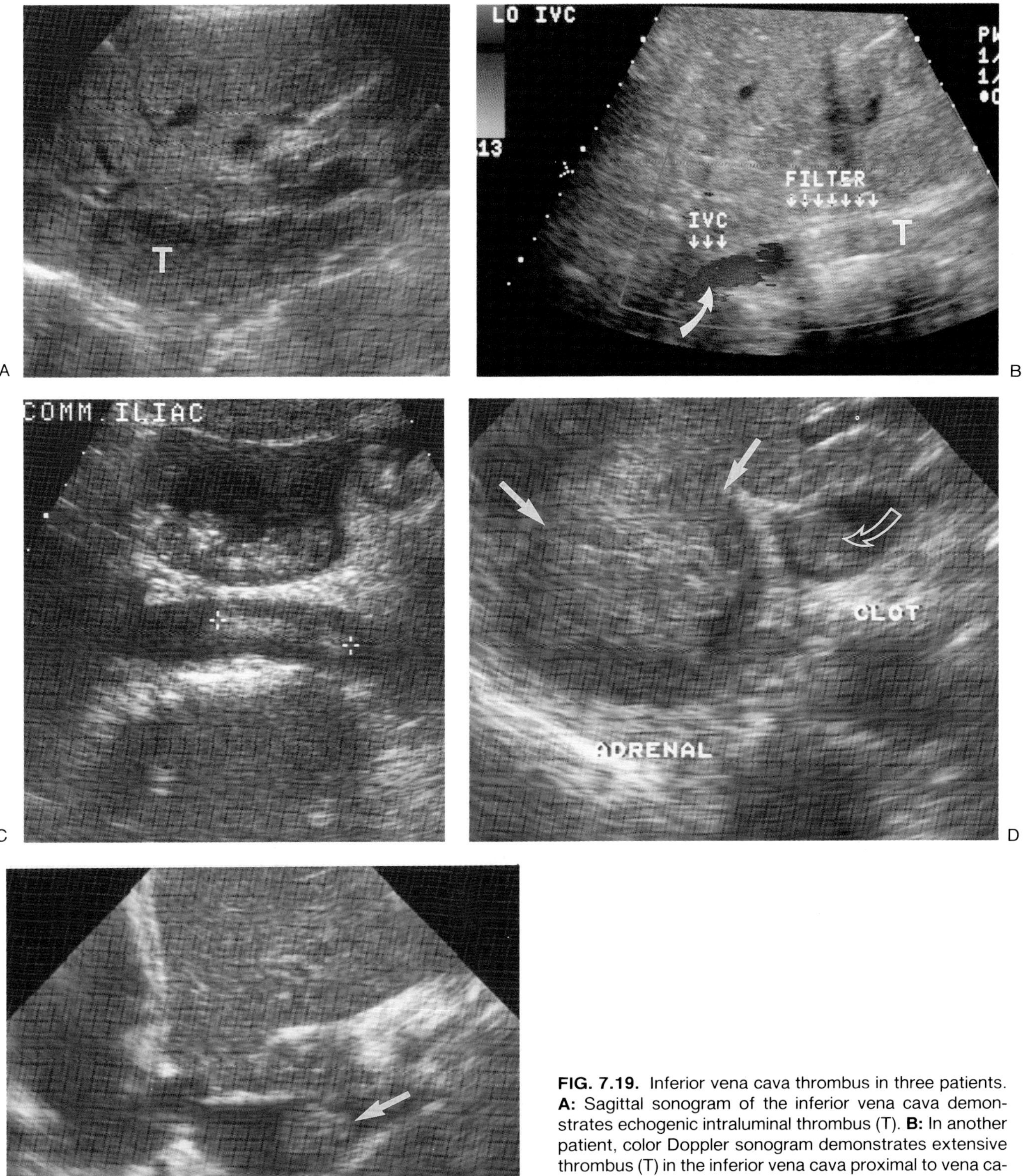

FIG. 7.19. Inferior vena cava thrombus in three patients. **A:** Sagittal sonogram of the inferior vena cava demonstrates echogenic intraluminal thrombus (T). **B:** In another patient, color Doppler sonogram demonstrates extensive thrombus (T) in the inferior vena cava proximal to vena caval filter (*arrows*). Note patency of flow above the filter (*curved arrow*) in the inferior vena cava. **C:** In this same patient thrombus is identified in the left common iliac vein (*cursors*). **D:** In a third patient, a transverse scan of the upper abdomen demonstrates an adrenal carcinoma (*arrows*) with tumor thrombus (*curved arrow*) extending into the inferior vena cava. **E:** Sagittal scan of the same patient demonstrates tumor thrombus (*arrow*) close to the junction of the inferior vena cava with the right atrium.

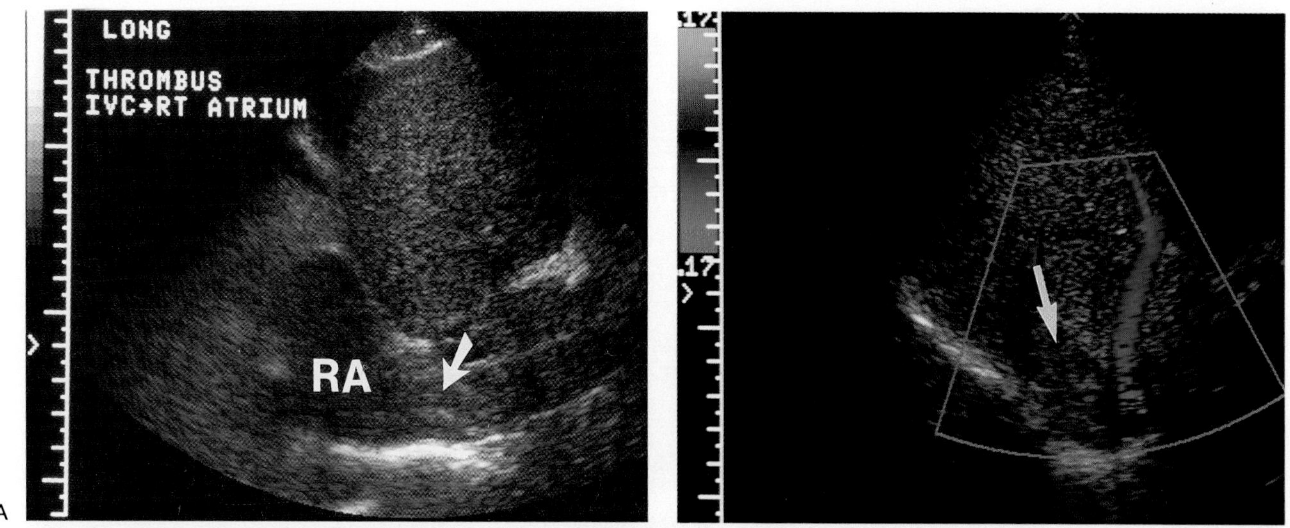

FIG. 7.20. Inferior vena caval thrombus extending into the right atrium. **A:** Sagittal sonogram of the inferior vena cava demonstrates extensive thrombus (T) extending into the right atrium (RA). **B:** Transverse color Doppler sonogram demonstrates patent hepatic vein but large thrombus (*arrows*) in the intrahepatic portion of the inferior vena cava. Patient had metastatic adenocarcinoma.

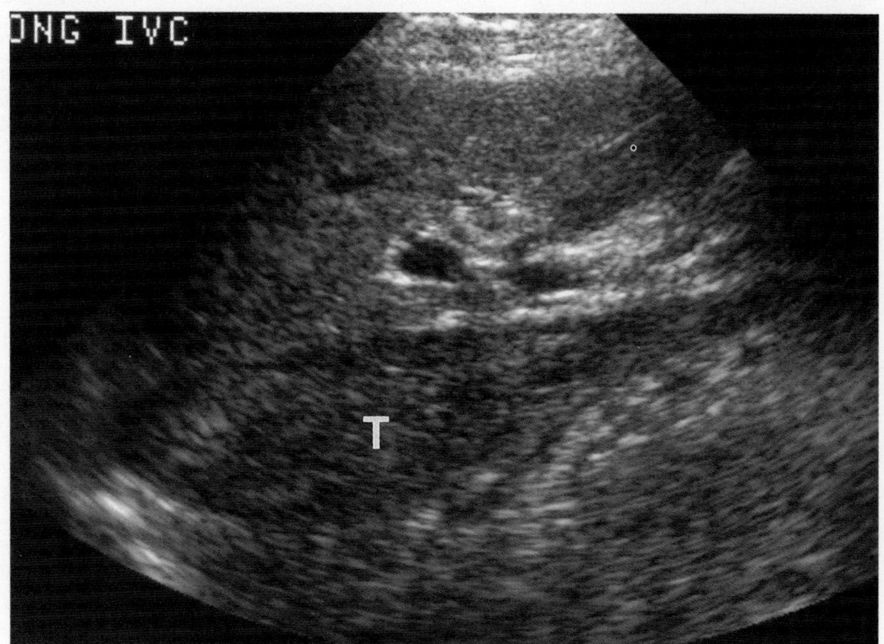

FIG. 7.21. Leiomyosarcoma of the inferior vena cava. Extensive tumor (T) is seen extending throughout the entire inferior vena cava. Surgery revealed primary leiomyosarcoma.

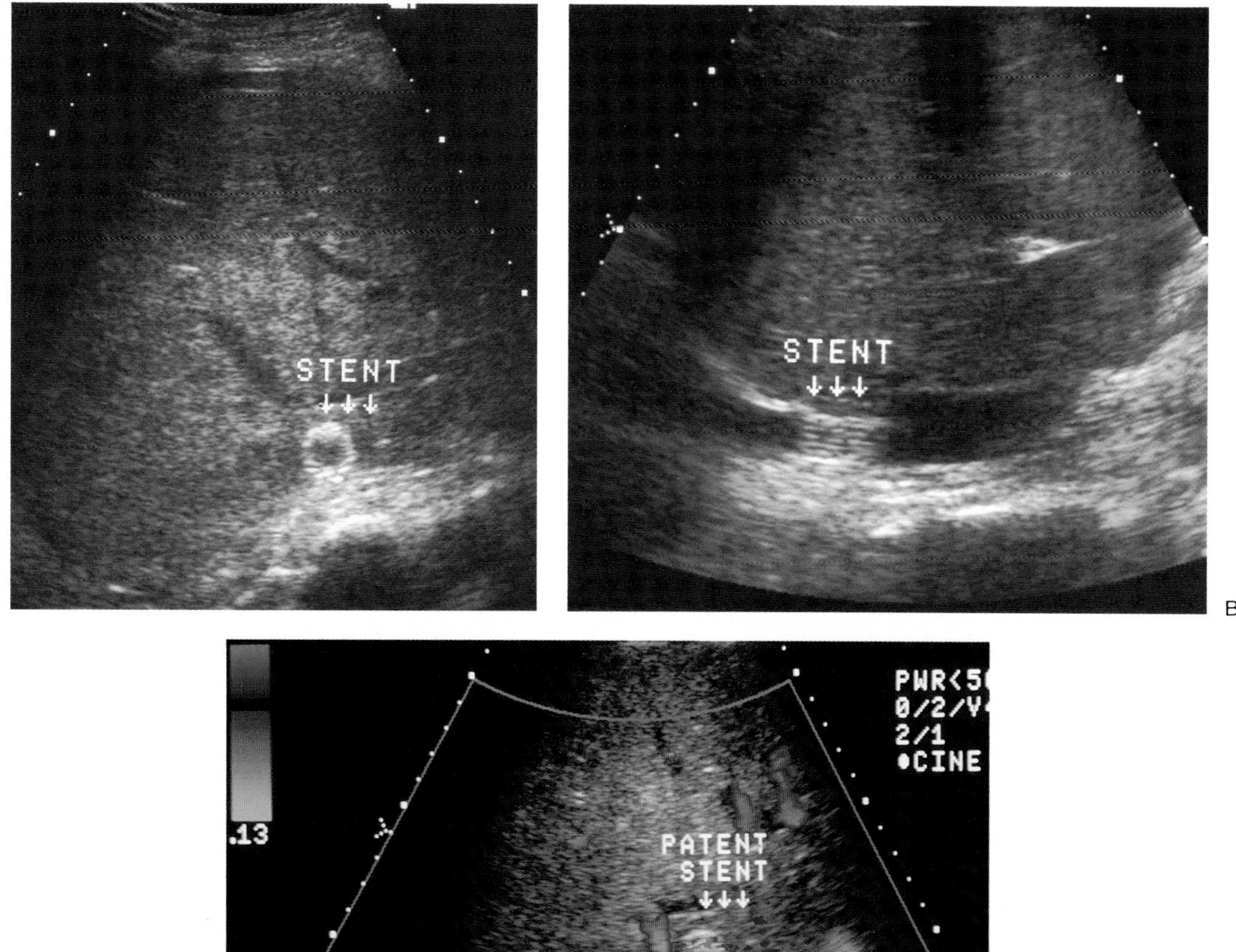

FIG. 7.22. Stenosis of the inferior vena cava treated with a metallic stent. **A:** Transverse scan demonstrates echogenic metallic stent within the intrahepatic portion of the inferior vena cava (*arrows*). **B:** Sagittal scan demonstrates exact position of the stent (*arrows*) within the inferior vena cava. **C:** Color Doppler sonogram demonstrates patency of the cava at the level of the stent (*arrows*).

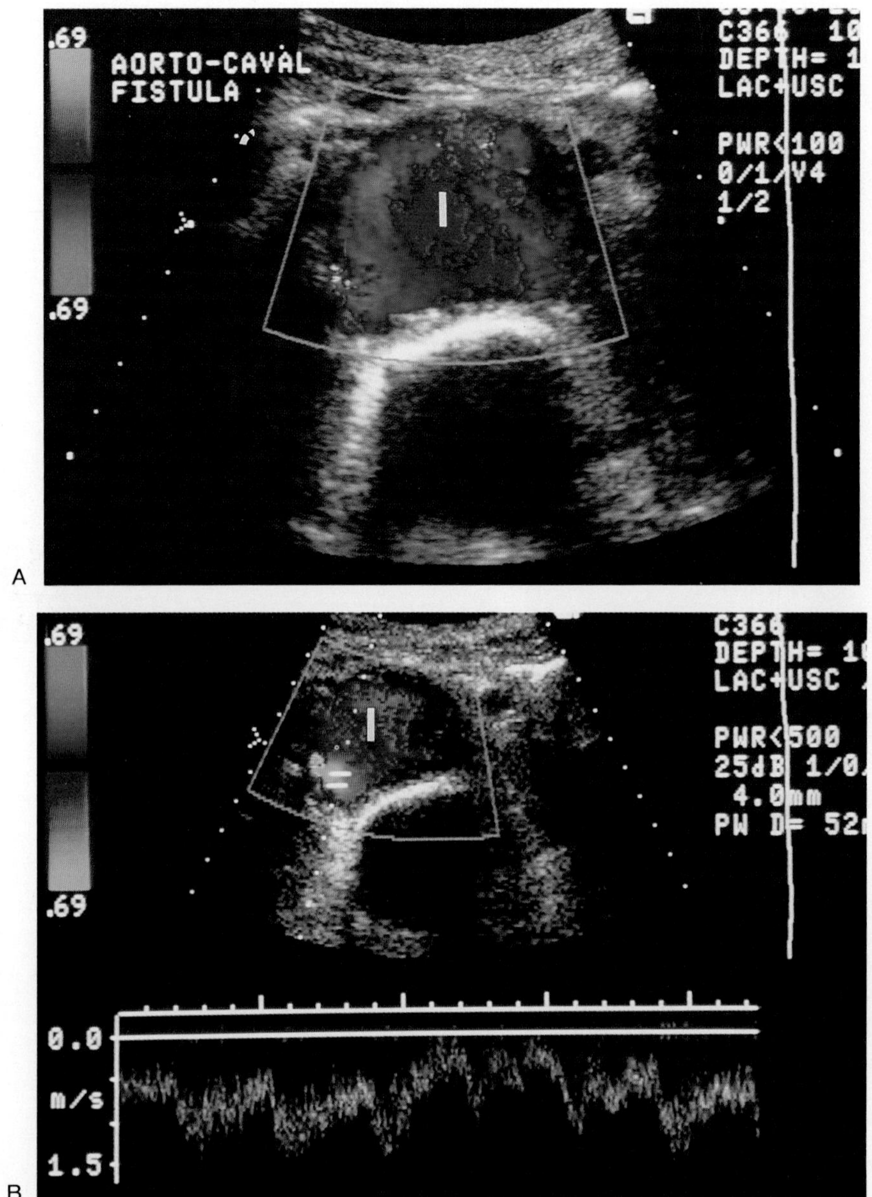

FIG. 7.23. Aortocaval fistula. **A:** Transverse color Doppler sonogram of the inferior vena cava (IVC) demonstrates marked enlargement of the IVC (I) due to aortocaval fistula. **B:** Spectral Doppler sonogram demonstrates characteristic pulsatile venous flow within the IVC (I).

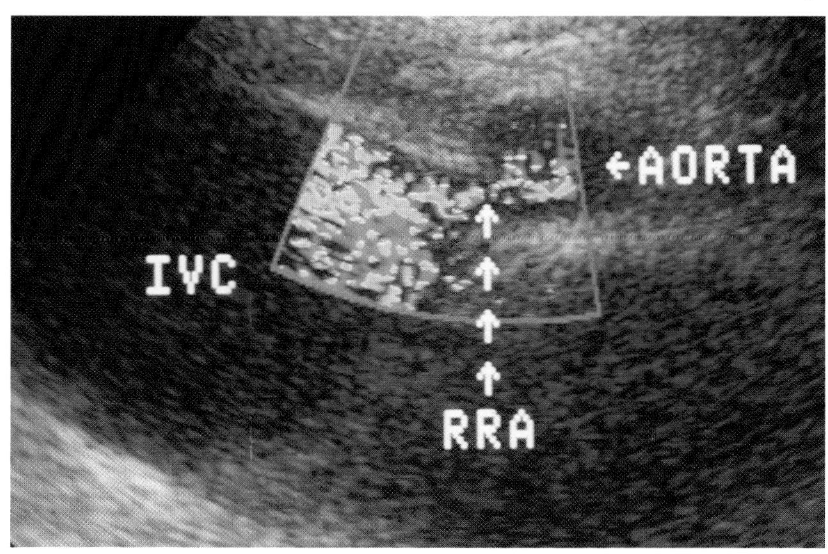

FIG. 7.24. Fistula between renal artery and inferior vena cava (IVC). Transverse color Doppler sonogram demonstrates site of communication (*arrow*) between right renal artery and IVC. Note markedly distended IVC.

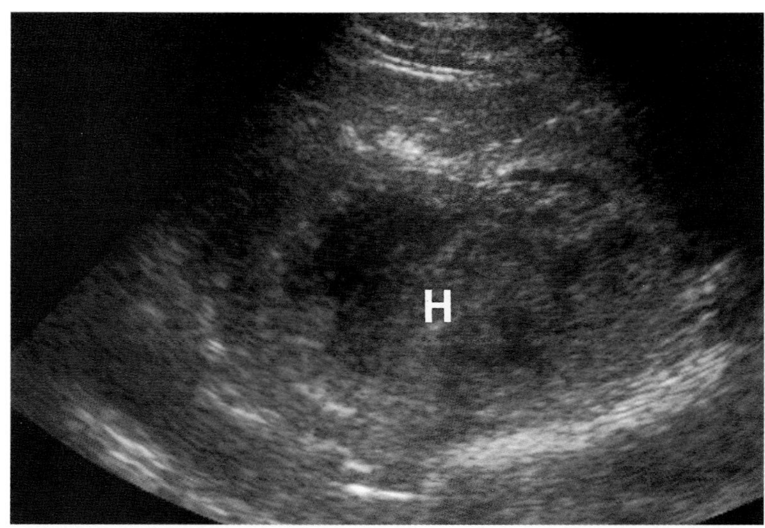

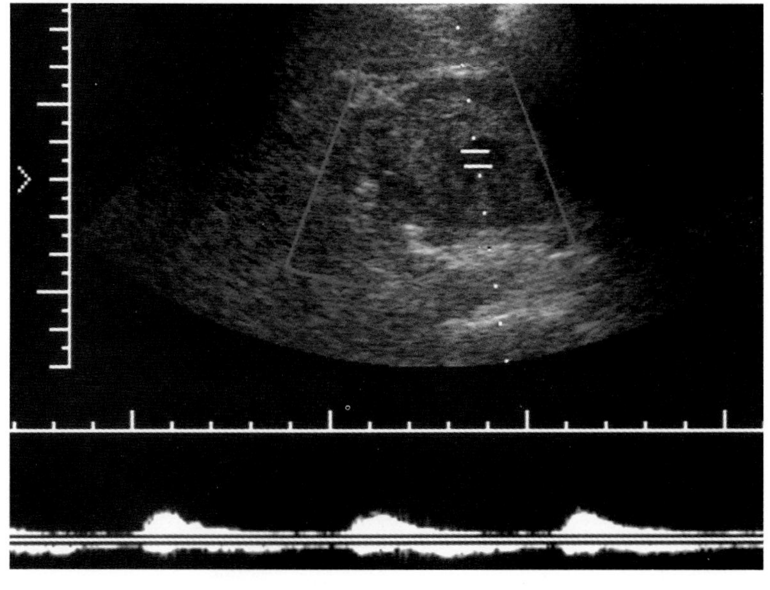

FIG. 7.25. Acute retroperitoneal hemorrhage secondary to ruptured pseudoaneurysm. **A:** Transverse scan demonstrates echogenic hematoma (H) in retroperitoneum. **B:** Spectral Doppler scan demonstrates arterial flow in pseudoaneurysm that had spontaneously bled.

RETROPERITONEUM

In general, most retroperitoneal abnormalities are best assessed by CT or MRI. Even when an abnormality is detected with sonography, CT is often indicated to further define the extent of the lesion or to guide percutaneous biopsy or drainage. Unlike CT, sonography is not able to identify fascial boundaries and extraperitoneal compartments. Similarly, CT excels at demonstrating abnormalities of the retrofascial spaces including the psoas compartment and iliac fossa.

In patients with adequate acoustic access, sonography can detect a variety of retroperitoneal abnormalities including solid and cystic masses and enlarged lymph nodes. Spontaneous retroperitoneal hemorrhage may occur in patients receiving excessive anticoagulation. In the appropriate clinical setting, hypoechoic fluid or echogenic masses (representing clot) suggest the diagnosis of acute hemorrhage (Fig. 7.25).

Retroperitoneal lymph nodes larger than 1.5 cm are generally pathologic. Lymph nodes typically appear sonographically as discrete hypoechoic masses. However, in patients with bulky disease a retroperitoneal "mantle" of adenopathy may appear as a confluent mass, often with a lobulated contour (Fig. 7.26). It is generally not possible to characterize retroperitoneal adenopathy by sonography alone. One advantage of contrast-enhanced CT is the ability to define areas of low-density necrosis within lymph nodes. This suggests either mycobacterial infection or necrotic tumor. Necrosis within lymph nodes is generally not appreciable with sonography (Fig. 7.27). Color Doppler sonography may be of value in demonstrating both para-aortic and paracaval adenopathy (Figs. 7.28 to 7.30).

Sonographically, retroperitoneal cystic masses such as lymphoceles, cystic neoplasms, abscesses, and pancreatic pseudocysts can generally be distinguished from solid retroperitoneal lesions (Figs. 7.31 and 7.32). Not infrequently, however, the sonographic appearance is nonspecific and CT or MRI is required for precise diagnosis. Unlike sonography, CT can specifically diagnose fatty masses (retroperitoneal teratoma and/or liposarcoma) due to their characteristically negative attenuation values. Solid retroperitoneal masses generally require CT-guided biopsy for diagnosis.

Retroperitoneal fibrosis may occur as an idiopathic condition or as a result of methysergide ingestion. This may be mimicked by a mantle of adenopathy from such lesions as metastatic prostate carcinoma, which incite a sclerous and/or desmoplastic reaction in the surrounding tissue. Retroperitoneal fibrosis is also associated with aortic aneurysms (i.e., perianeurysmal fibrosis). Perianeurysmal or retroperitoneal fibrosis may result in ureteral encasement, obstruction, and uremia.

Retroperitoneal and psoas abscesses are generally better demonstrated with CT. Larger abscesses, however, can be identified with sonography in patients with good acoustic access (Fig. 7.33).

REFERENCES

1. Taylor KJW, Burns PN, Woodcock JP, Wells PNT. Blood flow in deep abdominal and pelvic vessels: ultrasonic pulsed-Doppler analysis. *Radiology* 1985;154:487–493.
2. Taylor KJW, Holland S. Doppler ultrasound, I: basic principles, instrumentation and pitfalls. *Radiology* 1990;174:297–307.
3. LaRoy LL, Cormier PJ, Matalon TAS, Patel SK, Turner DA, Silver B. Pictorial essay: imaging of abdominal aortic aneurysms. *AJR* 1989;152:785–792.
4. Russel JGB. Is screening for abdominal aortic aneurysm worthwhile? *Clin Radiol* 1990;41:182–184.
5. Collin J. The epidemiology of abdominal aortic aneurysm. *Br J Hosp Med* 1988;1:64–67.
6. Katz DA, Littenberg B, Cronenwett JL. Management of small abdominal aortic aneurysms: early surgery vs. watchful waiting. *JAMA* 1992;268:2678–2686.
7. Cronenwett JL, Murphy TF, Zelenock GB, et al. Actuarial analysis of variables associated with rupture of small abdominal aorta aneurysms. *Surgery* 1985;98:472–483.
8. Clayton MJ, Walsh JW, Brewer WH. Contained rupture of abdominal aortic aneurysms: sonographic and CT diagnosis. *AJR* 1982;138:154–156.
9. Raptopoulos V, Cummings T, Smith EH. Computed tomography of life-threatening complications of abdominal aortic aneurysm—the disrupted aortic wall. *Invest Radiol* 1987;22:372–376.
10. Shuman WP, Hastrup W Jr, Kohler TR, et al. Suspected leaking abdominal aortic aneurysm: use of sonography in the emergency room. *Radiology* 1988;168:117–119.
11. Kittredge RD, Gordon RB. CT demonstration of dissecting hematoma originating in abdominal aorta. *J Comput Assist Tomogr* 1987;11:279–281.
12. Conrad MR, Davis GM, Green CE, Curry TS III. Real-time ultrasound in the diagnosis of acute dissecting aneurysms of the abdominal aorta. *AJR* 1979;132:115–116.
13. Giyanani VL, Krebs CA, Nall LA, Eisenberg RL, Parvey HR. Diagnosis of abdominal aortic dissection by image-directed Doppler sonography. *JCU* 1989;17:445–448.
14. Sterpetti AV, Hunter WJ, Feldhaus RJ, et al. Inflammatory aneurysm of abdominal aorta: incidence of pathologic and etiologic considerations. *J Vasc Surg* 1989;9:643–650.
15. Gooding GAW. Ruptured abdominal aorta: postoperative ultrasound appearance. *Radiology* 1982;145:781–783.
16. Gooding GAW, Effeney DJ, Goldstone J. The aortofemoral graft: detection and identification of healing complications by ultrasonography. *Surgery* 1981;8:94–101.
17. Elliot JP, Smith RF, Szylagyi DE. Aortoenteric and paraprosthetic–enteric fistulae: problems of diagnosis and management. *Arch Surg* 1974;108:479–490.
18. Low RN, Wall SD, Jeffrey RB Jr, et al. Aortoenteric fistula and perigraft infection: evaluation with CT. *Radiology* 1990;175:157–162.
19. Wilson DG, Seabold JE, Lieberman LM. Detection of aortoarterial graft infections by leukocyte scintigraphy. *Clin Nucl Med* 1983;8:421–423.
20. Mellins HZ. Inferior vena cava obstruction. In: Pollack HM, ed. *Clinical urography*. Philadelphia: Saunders; 1990:2105–2111.
21. Nakao S, Come PC, McKay RG, Ransil BJ. Effects of positional changes on inferior vena cava size and dynamics and correlations with right-sided cardiac pressure. *Am J Cardiol* 1987;59:125–132.
22. Fong KW, Zalev AH. Sonographic diagnosis of leiomyosarcoma of the inferior vena cava: a correlation with computed tomography and angiography. *J Can Assoc Radiol* 1987;38:229–231.
23. Middleton WD, Smith DF, Foley WD. CT detection of aortocaval fistula. *J Comput Assist Tomogr* 1987;11:344–347.

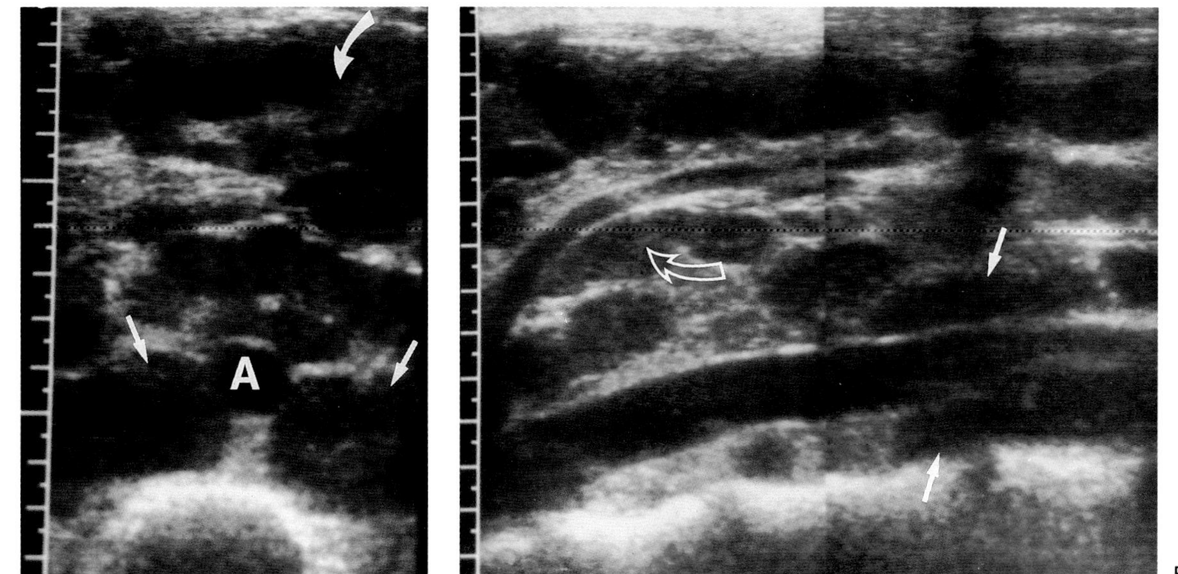

FIG. 7.26. Retroperitoneal and mesenteric adenopathy in AIDS-related lymphoma. **A:** Transverse scan demonstrates enlarged para-aortic nodes (*arrows*) and mesenteric adenopathy (*curved arrows*). A, aorta. **B:** Sagittal scan demonstrates para-aortic (*arrows*) and mesenteric nodes (*curved arrow*).

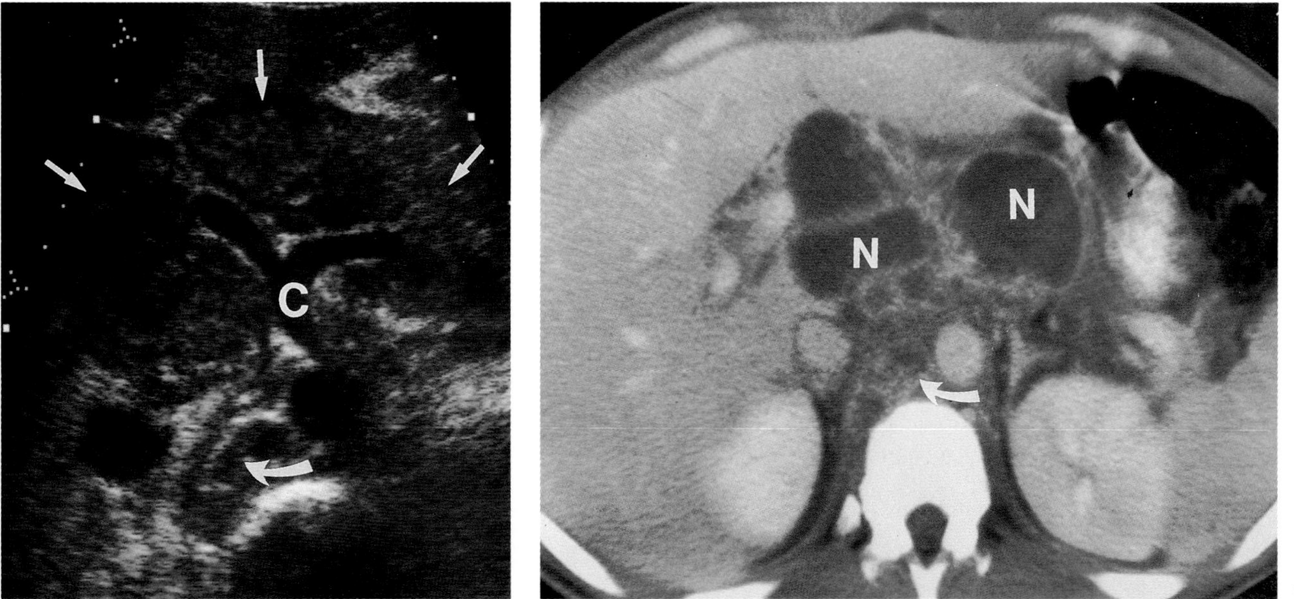

FIG. 7.27. Necrosis within lymph nodes demonstrated by contrast CT. **A:** Transverse scan of celiac axis (C) demonstrates extensive lymphadenopathy (*arrows*). Note retrocrural node (*curved arrow*). **B:** Contrast CT scan reveals extensive necrosis within nodes not evident with sonography (N). Note necrotic retrocrural nodes (*curved arrows*). Patient had AIDS and tuberculous adenitis.

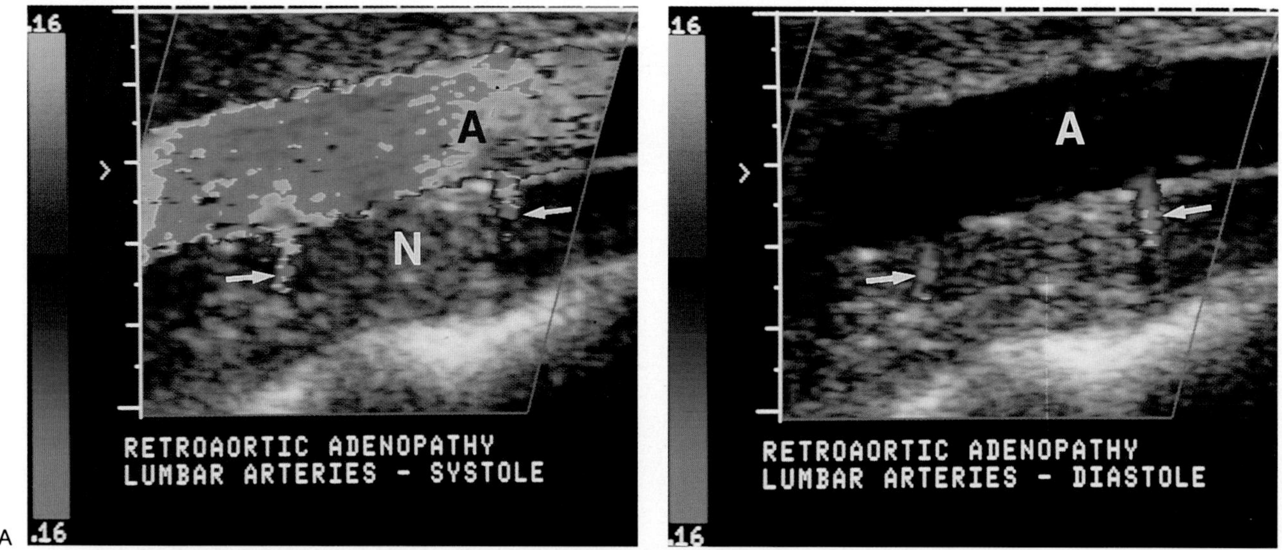

FIG. 7.28. Retroaortic nodal mass from metastatic adenocarcinoma. **A:** Sagittal scan of the aorta (A) during systole demonstrates a hypoechoic nodal mass (N) posterior to the aorta. Note enlarged lumbar arteries (*arrows*) supplying nodes. **B:** Scan taken during diastole. Note lack of flow in aorta (A) but persistent flow within lumbar arteries (*arrows*).

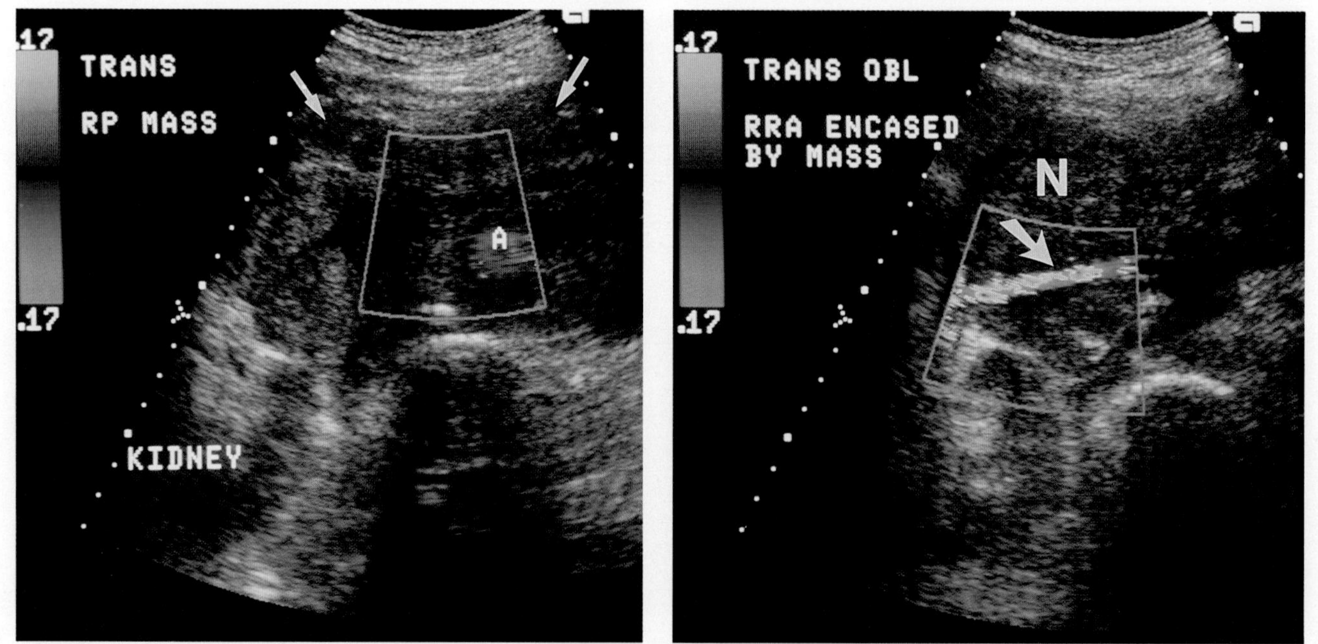

FIG. 7.29. Encasement of right renal artery by nodal mass. **A:** Transverse scan of aorta (A) demonstrates large mantle of para-aortic nodes (*arrows*). **B:** Note encasement of right renal artery (*arrow*) by nodal mass (N). Patient had metastatic germinoma from right testis.

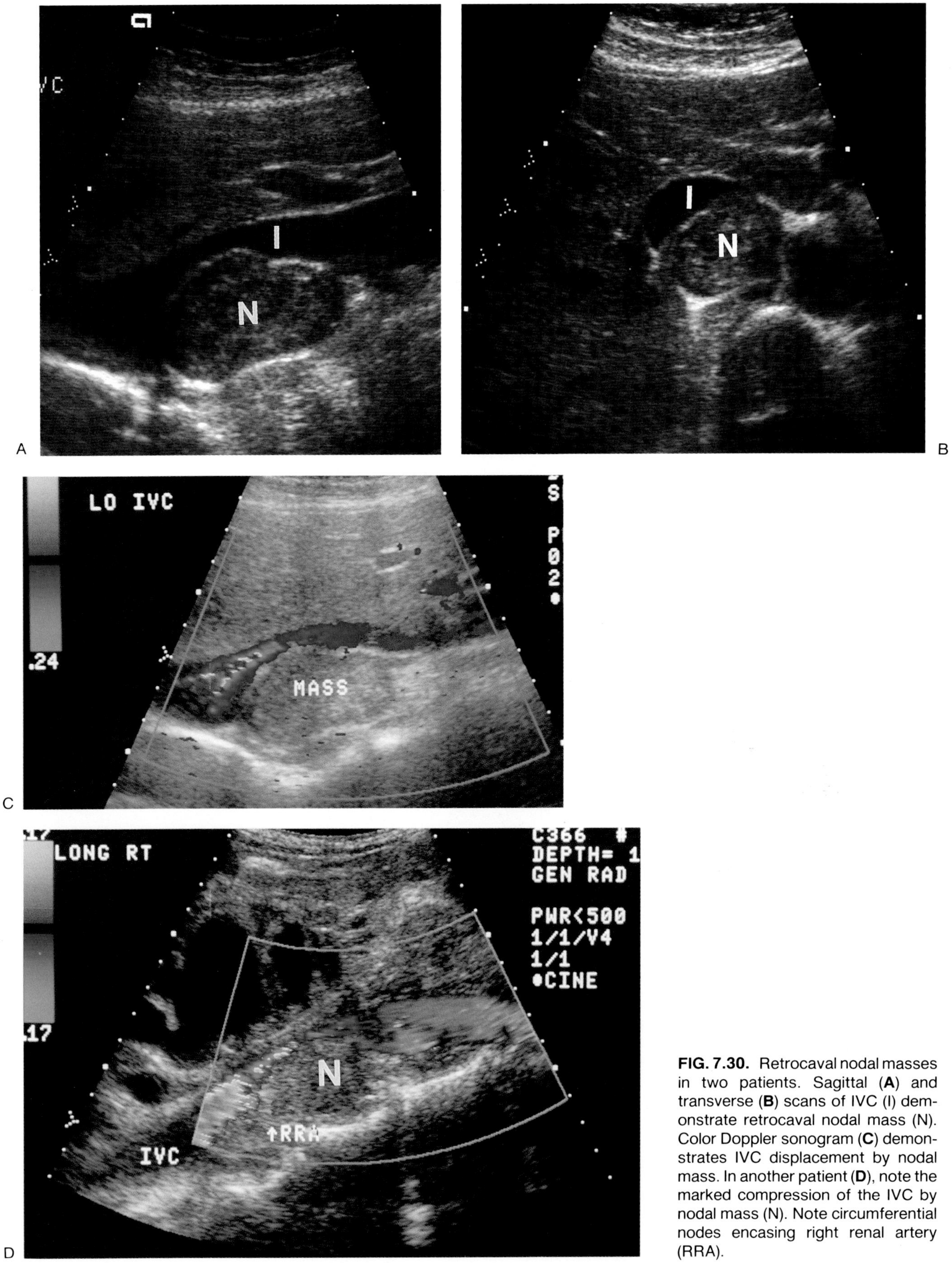

A

B

C

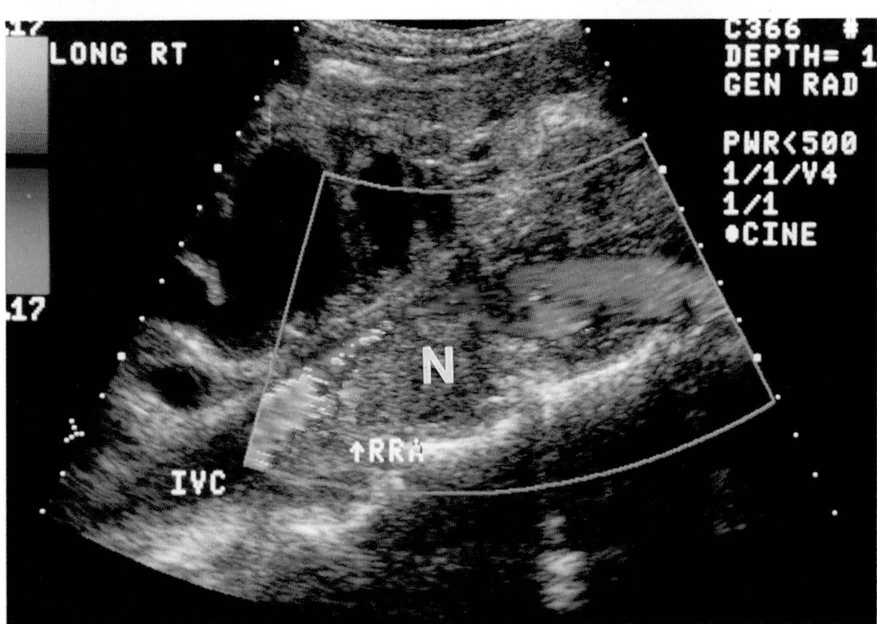

D

FIG. 7.30. Retrocaval nodal masses in two patients. Sagittal (**A**) and transverse (**B**) scans of IVC (I) demonstrate retrocaval nodal mass (N). Color Doppler sonogram (**C**) demonstrates IVC displacement by nodal mass. In another patient (**D**), note the marked compression of the IVC by nodal mass (N). Note circumferential nodes encasing right renal artery (RRA).

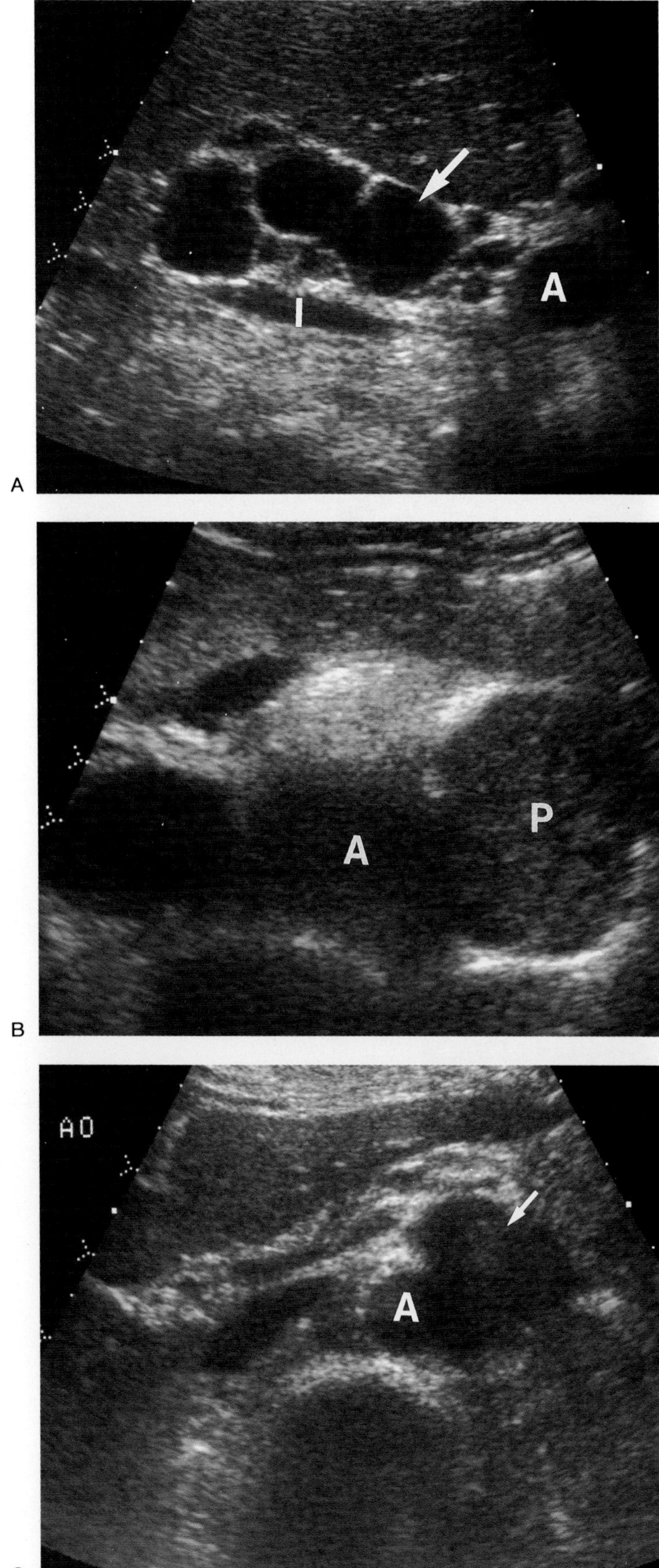

FIG. 7.31. Retroperitoneal masses in three patients. **A:** Complex cystic retroperitoneal mass (*arrow*) represents cystic teratoma. Note multilocular appearance. **B, C:** In another two patients, note the solid para-aortic masses adjacent to the aorta (A). P, pheochromocytoma (in **B**). *Arrow* denotes retroperitoneal fibrosarcoma in (**C**).

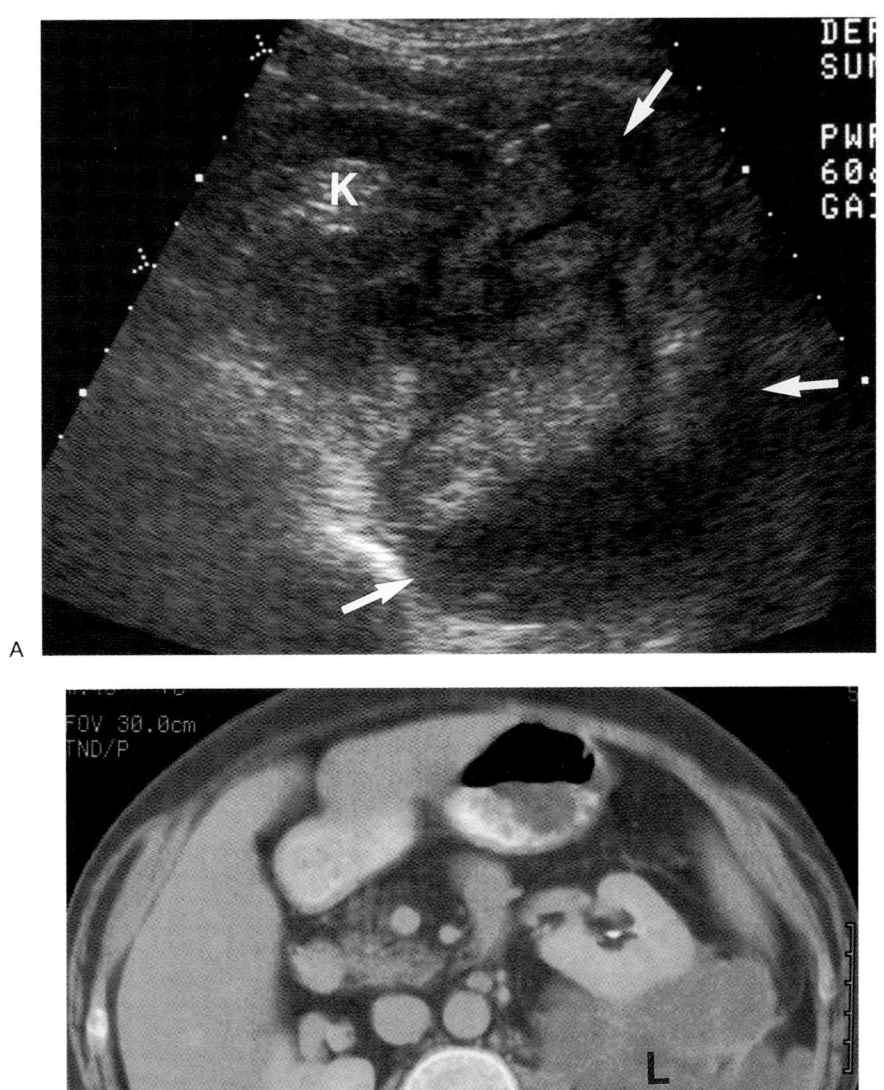

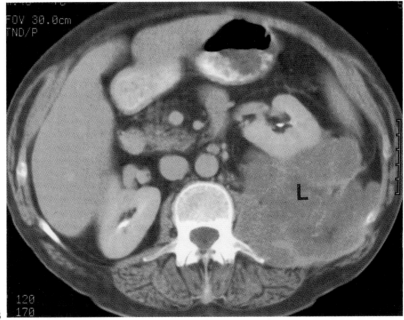

FIG. 7.32. Large retroperitoneal mass. **A:** Solid mass (*arrows*) posterior to left kidney (K) is demonstrated. **B:** CT scan demonstrates lymphomatous mass (L) in posterior pararenal space and perirenal space.

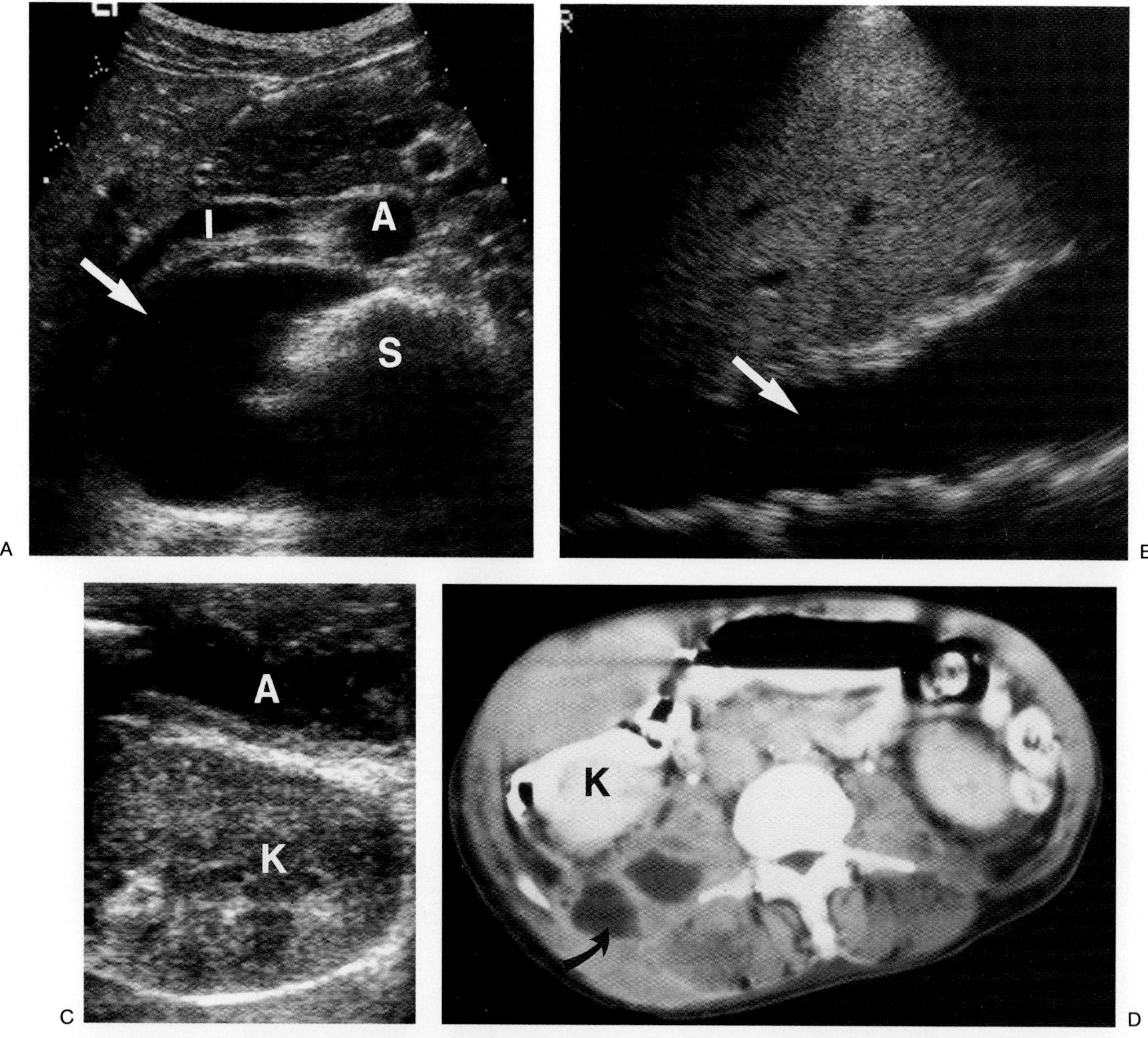

FIG. 7.33. Pyogenic psoas abscesses demonstrated by sonography in two patients. Note large right psoas abscess (*arrows*) on transverse (**A**) and sagittal (**B**) scans. In I, inferior vena cava; A, aorta; S, spine. In another patient (**C, D**), note hypoechoic psoas abscess (A) identified on prone scan (**C**) posterior to the right kidney (K). Contrast CT scan (**D**) demonstrates psoas abscess (*arrow*) posterior to right kidney (K). (Parts C and D courtesy of Eric Olcott, MD.)

Index